Practical
Cytopathology

Practical Cytopathology

Edited by

Robert W. Astarita, M.D.
Associate Clinical Professor
Department of Pathology
University of California, San Diego
School of Medicine
Chief, Division of Anatomic Pathology
Veterans Administration Medical Center
San Diego, California

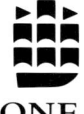

CHURCHILL LIVINGSTONE
New York, Edinburgh, London, Melbourne

Library of Congress Cataloging in Publication Data

Practical cytopathology / edited by Robert W. Astarita.
    p.   cm.
    Includes bibliographical references.
    ISBN 0-443-08469-6
    1. Cytodiagnosis. 2. Biopsy, Needle. I. Astarita, Robert W.
    [DNLM: 1. Biopsy, Needle—methods. 2. Cytodiagnosis—methods.
QY 95 P895]
RB43.P684   1990
616.07′582—dc20
DNLM/DLC
for Library of Congress   89-22257
                                                                                                   CIP

© **Churchill Livingstone Inc. 1990**

All rights reserved. No part of this publication may be reproduced, stored in a retrieval system, or transmitted in any form or by any means, electronic, mechanical, photocopying, recording, or otherwise, without prior permission of the publisher (Churchill Livingstone Inc., 1560 Broadway, New York, NY 10036).

Distributed in the United Kingdom by Churchill Livingstone, Robert Stevenson House, 1–3 Baxter's Place, Leith Walk, Edinburgh EH1 3AF, and by associated companies, branches, and representatives throughout the world.

The Publishers have made every effort to trace the copyright holders for borrowed material. If they have inadvertently overlooked any, they will be pleased to make the necessary arrangements at the first opportunity.

Acquisitions Editor: *Robert A. Hurley*
Assistant Editor: *Nancy Terry*
Copy Editor: *Marian Ryan*
Production Designer: *Jill Little*
Production Supervisor: *Sharon Tuder*

Printed in the United States of America

First published in 1990

Contributors

Robert W. Astarita, M.D.
Associate Clinical Professor, Department of Pathology, University of California, San Diego, School of Medicine; Chief, Division of Anatomic Pathology, Veterans Administration Medical Center, San Diego, California

Carlos W. M. Bedrossian, M.D.
Professor, Department of Pathology, University of Iowa College of Medicine; Director, Division of Cytopathology, University of Iowa Hospitals and Clinics, Iowa City, Iowa

Thomas A. Bonfiglio, M.D.
Professor, Department of Pathology and Laboratory Medicine, University of Rochester School of Medicine; Chief, Department of Anatomic Pathology, University of Rochester Medical Center, Rochester, New York

Kent Bottles, M.D.
Assistant Clinical Professor, Departments of Pathology and Medicine, University of California, San Francisco, School of Medicine; Director, Department of Cytology, San Francisco General Hospital, San Francisco, California

Para Chandrasoma, M.D.
Associate Professor, Department of Pathology, University of Southern California School of Medicine; Chief, Department of Surgical and Anatomic Pathology, LAC-USC Medical Center, Los Angeles, California

Daniel A. Egerter, M.D.
Outpatient Pathology Associate, Fine Needle Aspiration Biopsy Clinic, Sacramento, California

Bernard Gondos, M.D.
Clinical Professor, Department of Pathology, University of California, Los Angeles, UCLA School of Medicine, Los Angeles, California; Director, Department of Pathology, Sansum Medical Clinic, Santa Barbara, California

Prabodh K. Gupta, M.D.
Professor, Department of Pathology and Laboratory Medicine, University of Pennsylvania School of Medicine; Director, Department of Cytopathology, and Director, Cytometry Laboratory, University of Pennsylvania Hospital, Philadelphia, Pennsylvania

Parviz Haghighi, M.D.
Professor, Department of Pathology, University of California, San Diego, School of Medicine; Department of Pathology, Veterans Administration Medical Center, San Diego, California

Darryl G. Heustis, M.D.
Associate Professor, Department of Pathology, Loma Linda University School of Medicine; Medical Director, School of Cytotechnology, Loma Linda University School of Allied Health Professions; Chief of Staff, Jerry L. Pettis Memorial Veterans Hospital, Loma Linda, California

Fritz Lin, M.D.
Professor, Department of Pathology and Oncology, University of Kansas Medical Center School of Medicine; Director, Department of Surgical Pathology and Cytopathology, University of Kansas Medical Center, Kansas City, Kansas

Britt-Marie Ljung, M.D., M.I.A.C.
Associate Professor, Department of Pathology, University of California, San Francisco, School of Medicine; Department of Pathology, University of California Medical Center at San Francisco, San Francisco, California

Theodore R. Miller, M.D.
Clinical Professor and Vice-Chairman, Department of Pathology, University of California, San Francisco, School of Medicine; Director, Department of Cytology, University of California Medical Center at San Francisco, San Francisco, California

Roberta K. Nieberg, M.D.
Professor, Department of Pathology, University of California, Los Angeles, UCLA School of Medicine, Los Angeles, California

Dorothy L. Rosenthal, M.D.
Professor, Department of Pathology, University of California, Los Angeles, UCLA School of Medicine; Head, Cytology Service, UCLA Center for Health Sciences, Los Angeles, California

Preface

Increasingly, clinicians are relying on cytopathologic diagnoses to make immediate treatment and management decisions. Advances in fiberoptic technology, radiographically directed fine needle aspiration, and stereotactic biopsies have enabled physician specialists, pathologists, and interventional radiologists to obtain cytologic specimens rapidly from nearly all body sites with minimal trauma and discomfort. DNA probes, gene rearrangement studies, immunoelectron microscopy, immunocytochemistry, flow cytometry, and image analysis are among the newer modalities that can be applied to cytologic specimens.

Cytopathology now forms the cornerstone for diagnosis in a variety of clinical settings. A successful cytopathology service is predicated upon mastering basic as well as more sophisticated diagnostic skills, both of which are examined in this book.

Practical Cytopathology is intended for community pathologists, service-oriented pathologists at academic institutions, pathology residents, and cytotechnologists. Both nationally and internationally recognized authorities have contributed to this practical text/atlas. Cytopathology is emphasized herein as a clinical pathologic discipline. The book is an eminently readable text, one that may be read at the hospital and brought home in the evening to be read again. Fine needle aspiration of lesions of the breast, thyroid, salivary glands, lymph nodes, pancreas, liver, and biliary tract are thoroughly discussed. Diagnostic criteria for benign and malignant conditions are enumerated for all major organ systems. Finally, color plates complement the black and white microphotographs, which is a major benefit to the text.

Robert W. Astarita, M.D.

Acknowledgments

Had I written the full text of this book myself, it would have come to press sometime in 1992, perhaps in time for the unification of the European Community of nations. More importantly, the reader would have been deprived of the input and expertise of the many excellent contributors, to whom I am deeply grateful. Their insight and dedication truly make the publication of this book an invaluable teaching and learning enterprise.

I am privileged to acknowledge several individuals who have served as mentors and friends, and who have encouraged me to pursue my interests in surgical pathology, hematopathology, and cytopathology. I am indebted to Roger Terry M.D., Emeritus Professor of Pathology, USC School of Medicine; Robert J. Lukes, M.D., Emeritus Professor of Pathology, USC School of Medicine; Clive R. Taylor, M.D. Ph.D., Professor and Chairman, Department of Pathology, USC School of Medicine; Robert M. Nakamura M.D., Chairman, Department of Pathology, Hospital of Scripps Clinic, La Jolla, California; Adelbert D. Cramer, M.D., Codirector, Department of Pathology, Henry Mayo Memorial Hospital, Newhall, California; and Carol Carriere, C.T., A.S.C.P., C.M.I.A.C., Chief Cytotechnologist and Education Coordinator, LAC-USC Medical Center. I also wish to thank Rose Marie Darde, C.T., A.S.C.P., and Alan Olschewski, C.T., A.S.C.P., Anatomic Pathology Supervisor, VA Medical Center, San Diego, for technical assistance and significant contributions to the teaching case files. Finally, excellent clerical support was provided by Susan Harris and Eva Lehman.

Robert W. Astarita, M.D.

Contents

Color plates follow the table of contents.

1. Fundamentals of Cytopathology — 1
   Robert W. Astarita and Daniel A. Egerter

2. Cytology of the Female Genital Tract — 23
   Prabodh K. Gupta, Darryl G. Heustis, Thomas A. Bonfiglio, Roberta K. Nieberg, and Fritz Lin

3. Cytopathology of Irradiation and Chemotherapy — 141
   Parviz Haghighi

4. Fine Needle Aspiration Cytology of the Breast — 163
   Britt-Marie Ljung

5. Cytologic Diagnosis of Respiratory Diseases — 181
   Dorothy L. Rosenthal

6. Fine Needle Aspiration of the Thyroid Gland — 233
   Theodore R. Miller

7. Cytology of the Gastrointestinal Tract — 251
   Kent Bottles and Para Chandrasoma

8. Fine Needle Aspiration of the Pancreas — 279
   Para Chandrasoma

9. Fine Needle Aspiration of the Liver — 291
   Para Chandrasoma

10. Urologic Cytology — 303
    Dorothy L. Rosenthal

11. Cytology of Body Cavity Fluids — 337
    Bernard Gondos

12. Cytology of the Central Nervous System — 357
    Dorothy L. Rosenthal

13. Cytopathology of Lymph Nodes — 379
    Robert W. Astarita

14. Immunocytochemistry — 403
    Carlos W. M. Bedrossian

Index — 459

Practical Cytopathology

Color Plates

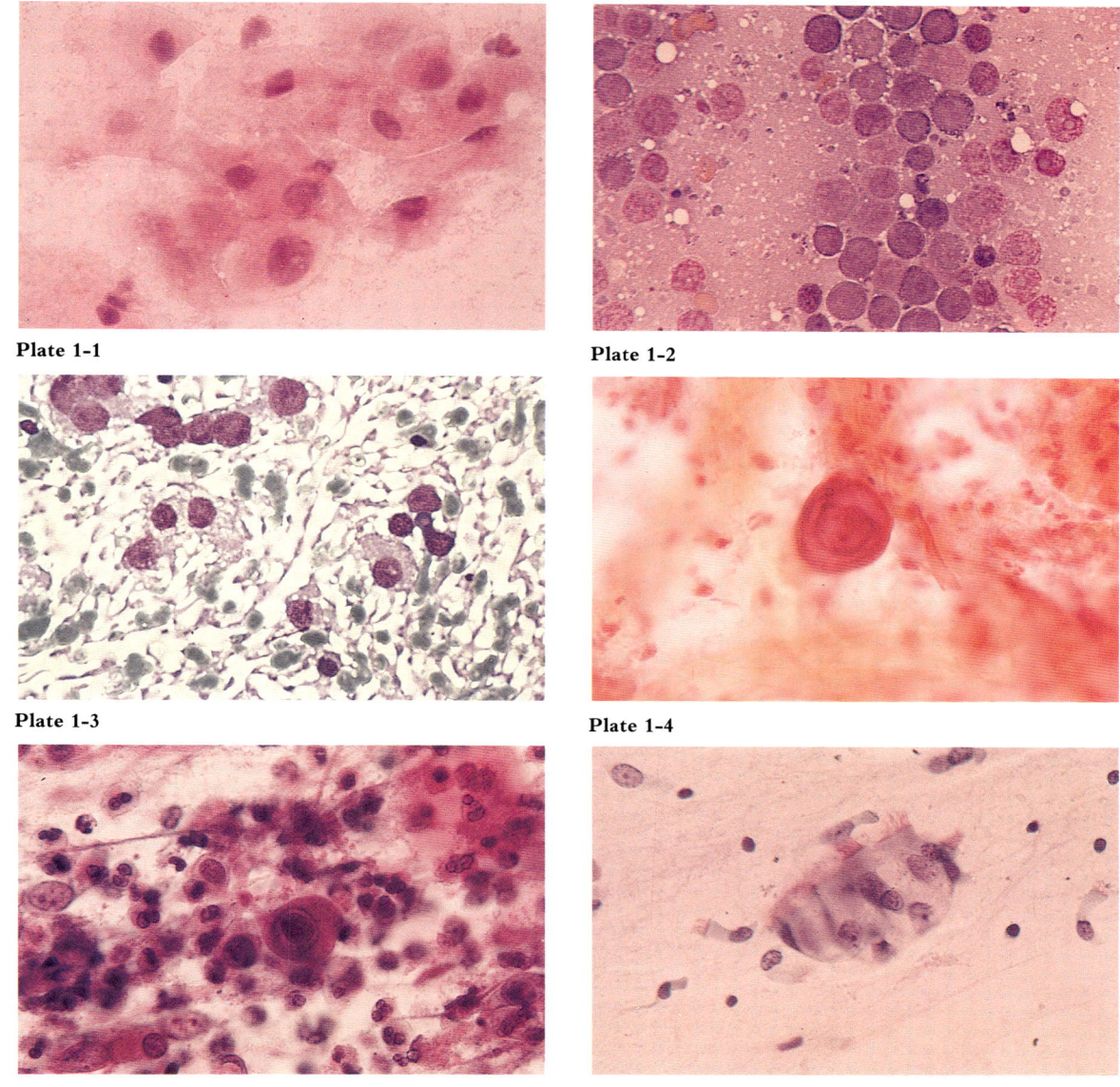

Plate 1-1

Plate 1-2

Plate 1-3

Plate 1-4

Plate 1-5

Plate 1-6

Plate 1-1 (Fig. 1-1) Cervical-vaginal smear showing air-drying artifacts. Note faded homogeneous chromatin pattern and smudged nuclear detail. (Papanicolaou stain, × 250.)

Plate 1-2 (Fig. 1-2) Lymph node FNA showing large neoplastic lymphocytes containing prominent nucleoli. Note background cytoplasmic fragments or "blue blobs." (Wright-Giemsa stain, × 200.)

Plate 1-3 (Fig. 1-3) FNA of palpable testicular mass showing neoplastic cells and tigroid lace-like background, a pattern characteristic of seminoma. (MGG stain, × 250.) (Case courtesy of Torsten Löwhagen, M.D., F.I.A.C., Karolinska Hospital, Stockholm, Sweden.)

Plate 1-4 (Fig. 1-4) Psammoma body showing concentric laminations. (MGG stain, × 200.)

Plate 1-5 (Fig. 1-5) Epithelial cells showing large intranuclear inclusions consistent with cytomegalovirus infection. (Papanicolaou stain, × 250.)

Plate 1-6 (Fig. 1-6) Ribbon of bronchial columnar epithelial cells containing terminal bars and cilia. (Papanicolaou stain, × 250.)

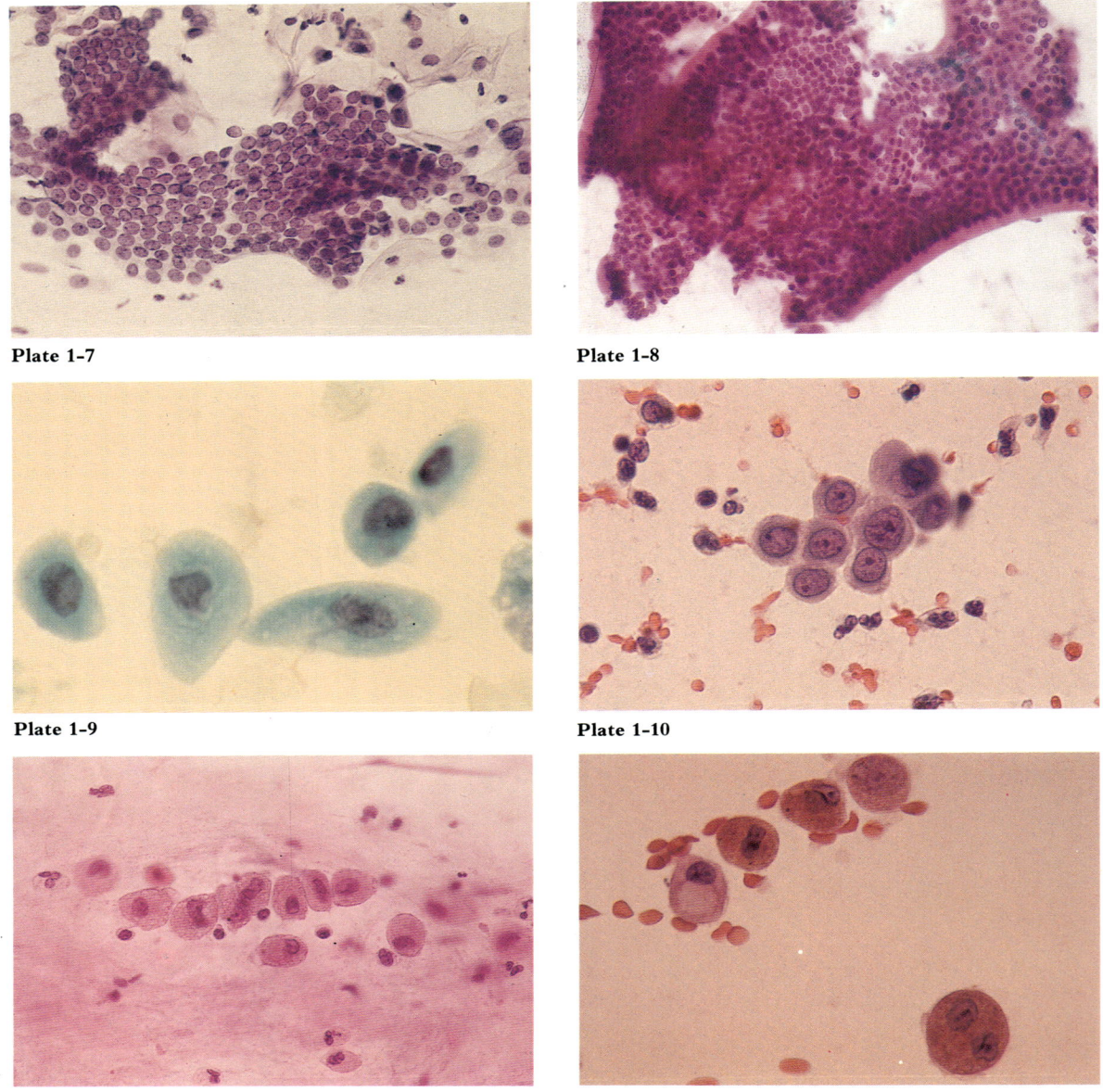

Plate 1-7 (Fig. 1-7) Sheets of benign endocervical cells approaching honeycomb configuration. (Papanicolaou stain, × 125.)
Plate 1-8 (Fig. 1-8) Sheet of benign gastric columnar cells showing honeycomb pattern. (Papanicolaou stain, × 100.)
Plate 1-9 (Fig. 1-9) Transitional cells from voided urine specimen (Papanicolaou stain, × 500.)
Plate 1-10 (Fig. 1-10) Pleural fluid. Haphazardly arranged group of mesothelial cells showing intercellular spaces or "windows." (Papanicolaou stain, × 250.)
Plate 1-11 (Fig. 1-11) Sputum smear showing benign histiocytes with some indented nuclei and bubbly cytoplasm. (Papanicolaou stain, × 160.)
Plate 1-12 (Fig. 1-12) Specimen from lung FNA showing histiocytes containing intracytoplasmic anthracotic pigment and single histiocyte with large cytoplasmic vacuole. (Papanicolaou stain, × 250.)

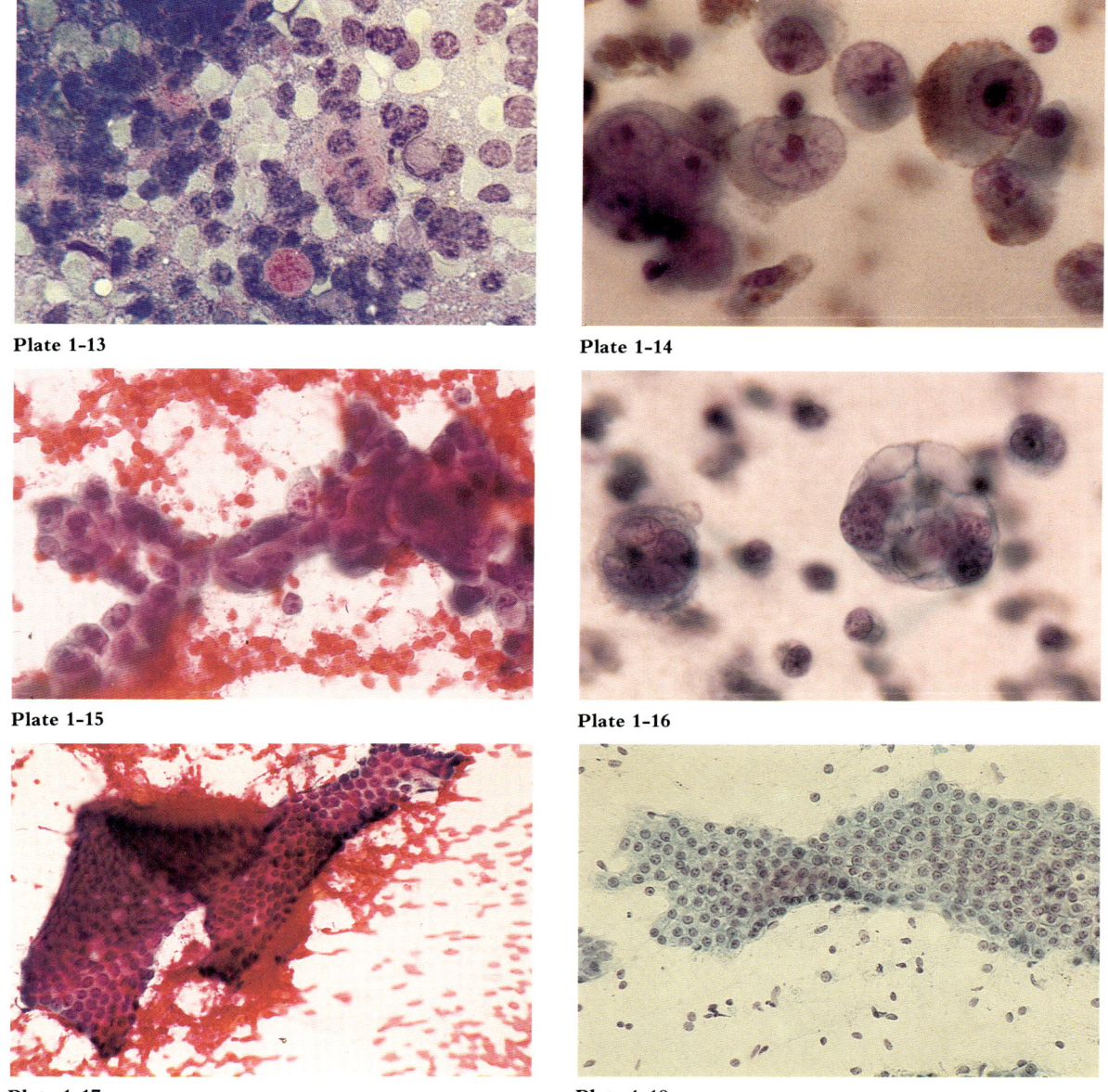

Plate 1-13 (Fig. 1-13) Parotid gland FNA showing small uniform cells surrounding a central metachromatic basement membrane globule characteristic of adenoid cystic carcinoma. (MGG stain, × 250.) (Case courtesy of Torsten Löwhagen, M.D., F.I.A.C., Karolinska Hospital, Stockholm, Sweden.)

Plate 1-14 (Fig. 1-14) Nuclepore filter preparations of pleural fluid showing metastatic malignant melanoma. (Papanicolaou stain, × 450.)

Plate 1-15 (Fig. 1-15) Brushing from mass at ampulla of Vater containing malignant cells from an adenocarcinoma. (Papanicolaou stain, × 200.)

Plate 1-16 (Fig. 1-16) Cell balls representing metastatic adenocarcinoma in pleural effusion. (Papanicolaou stain, × 200.)

Plate 1-17 (Fig. 1-17) Benign cells. Duodenal brushing from ampulla of Vater reveals a monolayered sheet of cells of uniform size and shape. (Papanicolaou stain, × 200.)

Plate 1-18 (Fig. 1-18) FNA of a palpable breast mass showing a sheet of benign ductal cells of uniform size and shape with little overlapping of nuclei. (Papanicolaou stain, × 160.)

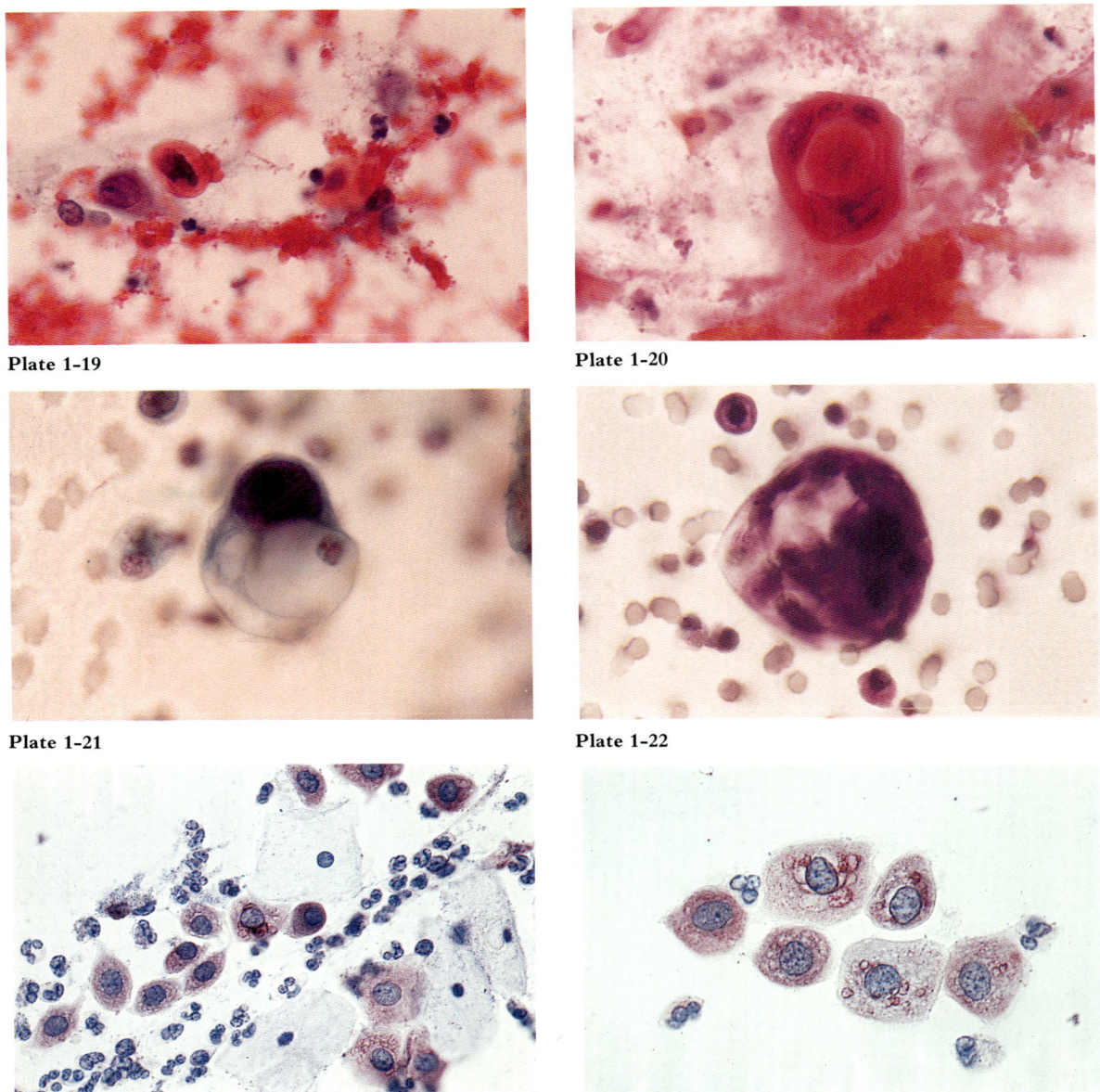

Plate 1-19 (Fig. 1-19) Lung sputum specimen showing malignant squamous cells containing orangeophilic refractile cytoplasm and coal black atypical nuclei. (Papanicolaou stain, × 160.)

Plate 1-20 (Fig. 1-20) Lung sputum from patient with squamous carcinoma illustrating onion skin configuration of keratin pearl and dirty background of tumor diathesis. (Papanicolaou stain, × 250.)

Plate 1-21 (Fig. 1-21) Filter preparation from pleural fluid of metastatic adenocarcinoma showing signet ring configuration, in which the malignant nucleus is displaced by a large intracytoplasmic secretory vacuole. (Papanicolaou stain, × 250.)

Plate 1-22 (Fig. 1-22) Nuclepore filter preparation from pleural fluid containing cell ball configuration characteristic of metastatic breast carcinoma. (Papanicolaou stain, × 250.)

Plate 2-1 (Fig. 2-13B) CVE smear stained with monoclonal antibodies for *Chlamydia trachomatis*. (AEC substrate.)

Plate 2-2 (Fig. 2-14B) Monoclonal staining of Papanicolaou-stained CVE smear for *Chlamydia trachomatis* infection. (AEC substrate.)

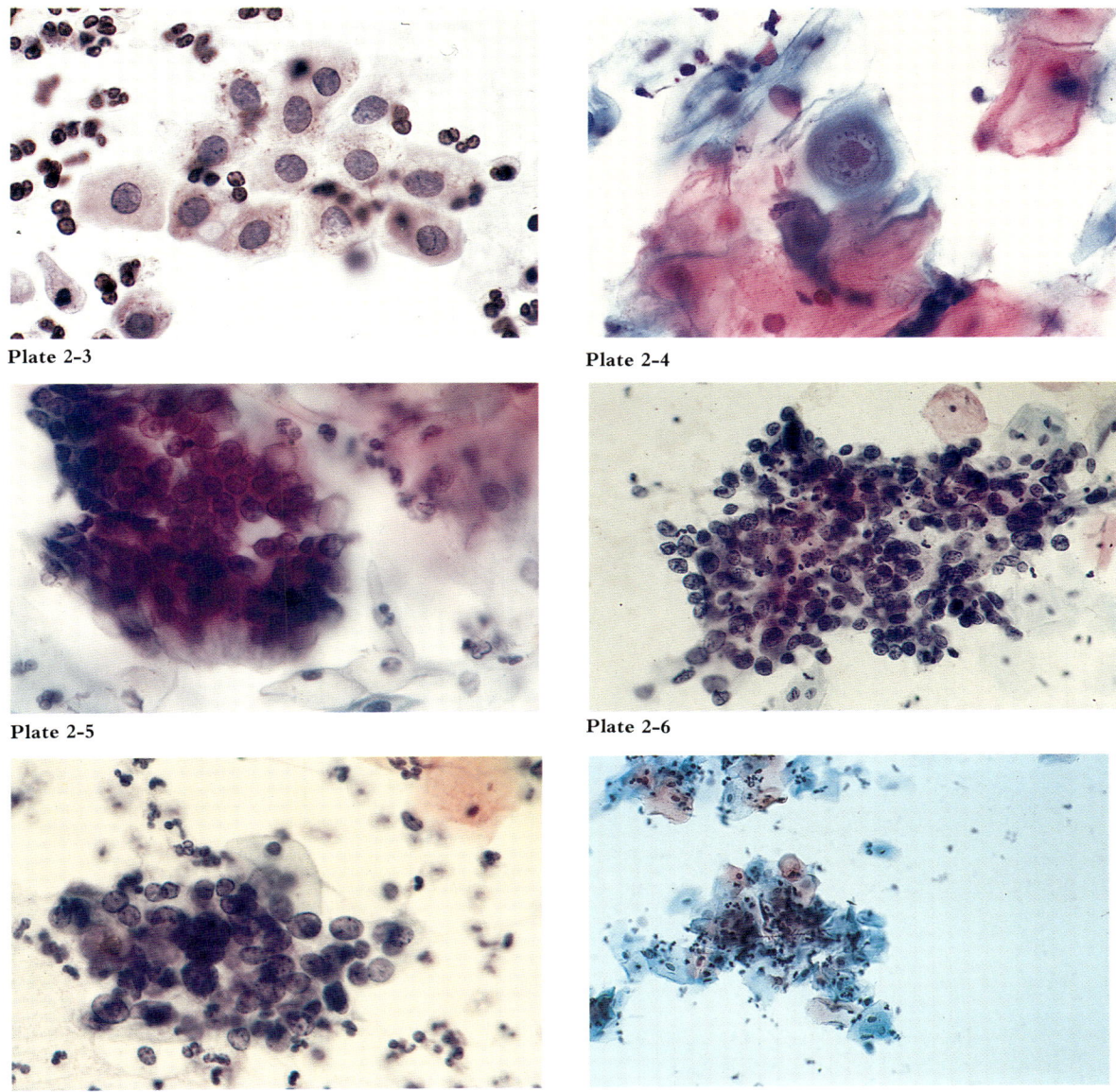

Plate 2-3 (Fig. 2-14C) CVE smear stained with immunoperoxidase technique for *Chlamydia trachomatis* infection using monoclonal antibodies. (DAB substrate.)

Plate 2-4 (Fig. 2-20B) Papanicolaou-stained CVE smear revealing a columnar epithelial cell with distinct, intranuclear, acidophilic, inclusion of CMV infection.

Plate 2-5 (Fig. 2-34) Vaginal smear showing adenosis in a patient exposed to DES in utero. (Papanicolaou stain, × 200.)

Plates 2-6 and 2-7 (Figs. 2-37A,B) CIS of the vulva. A syncytial arrangement of cells, scant to adequate cytoplasm, and a generally clean smear background are seen. (Plate 6, Papanicolaou stain, × 100; Plate 7, Papanicolaou stain, × 200.)

Plate 2-8 (Fig. 2-38) Intertwined squamous cells bound together by the pseudohyphae of Candida species. (Papanicolaou stain, × 100.)

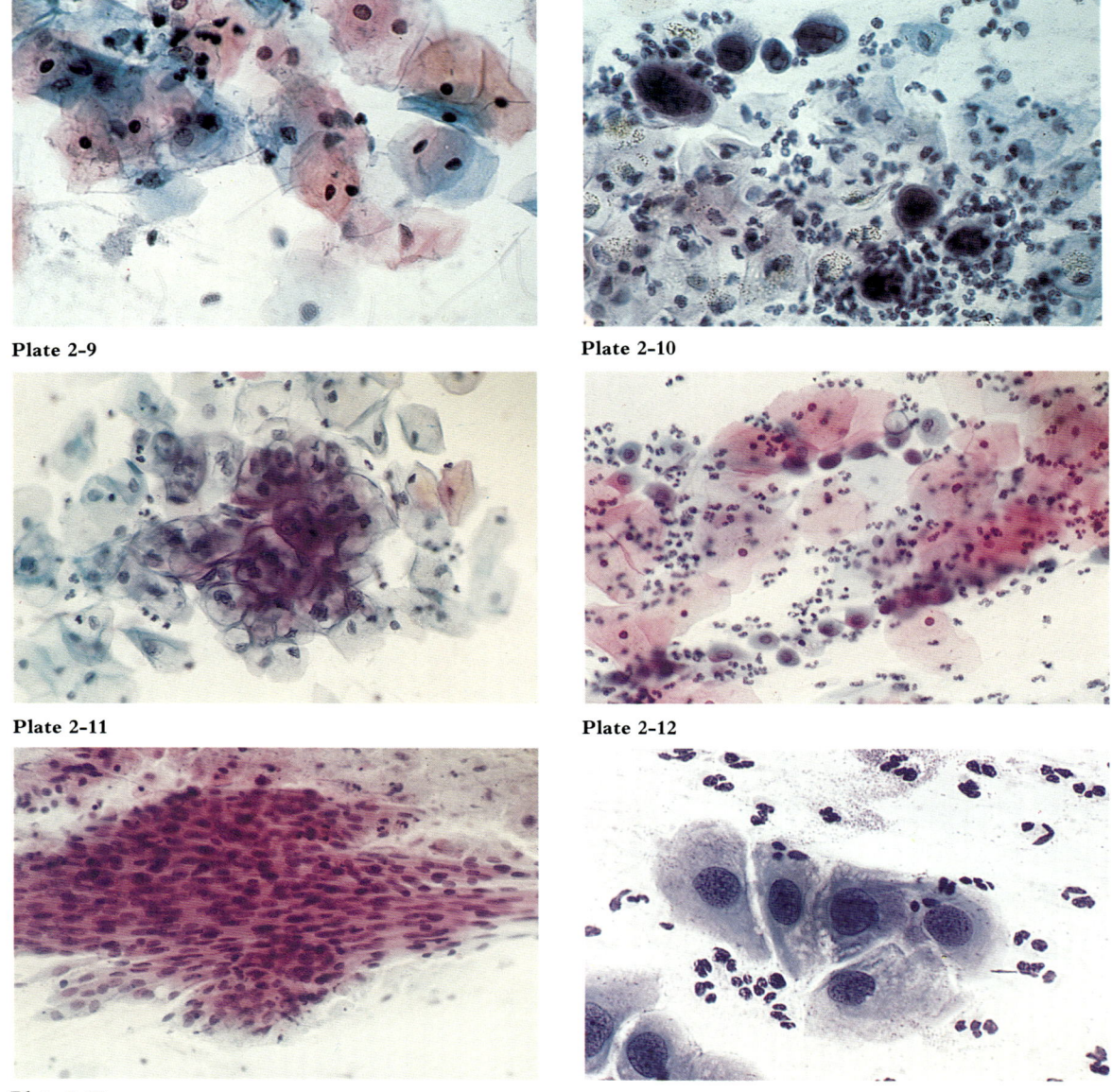

Plate 2-9 (Fig. 2-39) Scattered squamous cells and Leptothrix bacteria. (Papanicolaou stain, × 100.)

Plate 2-10 (Fig. 2-40) Herpes-infected cells showing multinucleation, nuclear molding, and ground-glass nuclei. (Papanicolaou stain, × 100.)

Plate 2-11 (Fig. 2-41) Cluster of condylomatous cells showing enlarged, hyperchromatic, irregular nuclei, perinuclear clearing, and variable condensation of peripheral cytoplasm. (Papanicolaou stain, × 100.)

Plate 2-12 (Fig. 2-43) Small metaplastic squamous cells showing dense cytoplasm and a cookie-cutter configuration. (Papanicolaou stain, × 100.)

Plate 2-13 (Fig. 2-44) An atrophic sheet of squamous cells showing spindle nuclei, bland chromatin, centrally placed nuclei, and adequate cytoplasm. (Papanicolaou stain, × 200.)

Plate 2-14 (Fig. 2-49) Cells derived from a case of slight dysplasia with enlarged hyperchromatic nuclei and mature-appearing cytoplasm. (Papanicolaou stain, × 40.)

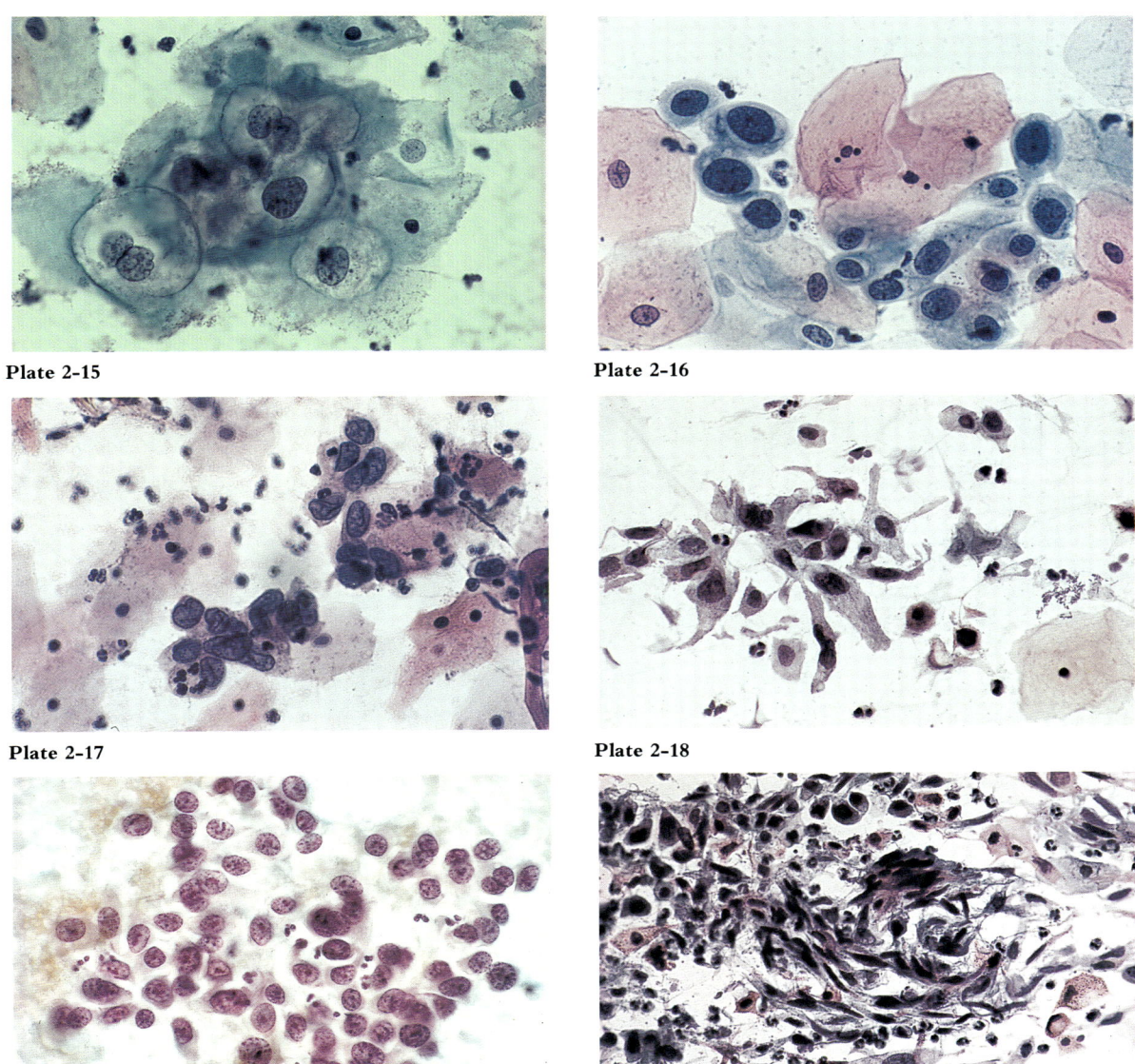

Plate 2-15 (Fig. 2-51) Cells derived from a case of slight dysplasia (CIN I). The degree of nuclear enlargement is evident when the nuclei of the abnormal cells are compared with those of the normal intermediate squamous cells. (Papanicolaou stain, × 200.)

Plate 2-16 (Fig. 2-53) Numerous cells derived from a patient with moderate dysplasia. (Papanicolaou stain, × 200.)

Plate 2-17 (Fig. 2-57) CIS. These cells appear in syncytial aggregates and have nuclei that are arranged irregularly with respect to one another. (Papanicolaou stain, × 200.)

Plate 2-18 (Fig. 2-60) Cells derived from a patient with keratinizing (pleomorphic) dysplasia. (Papanicolaou stain, × 200.)

Plate 2-19 (Fig. 2-64) Cytologic specimen derived from a case of microinvasive carcinoma. (Papanicolaou stain, × 200.)

Plate 2-20 (Fig. 2-68) Cells derived from a patient with keratinizing invasive carcinoma. (Papanicolaou stain, × 100.)

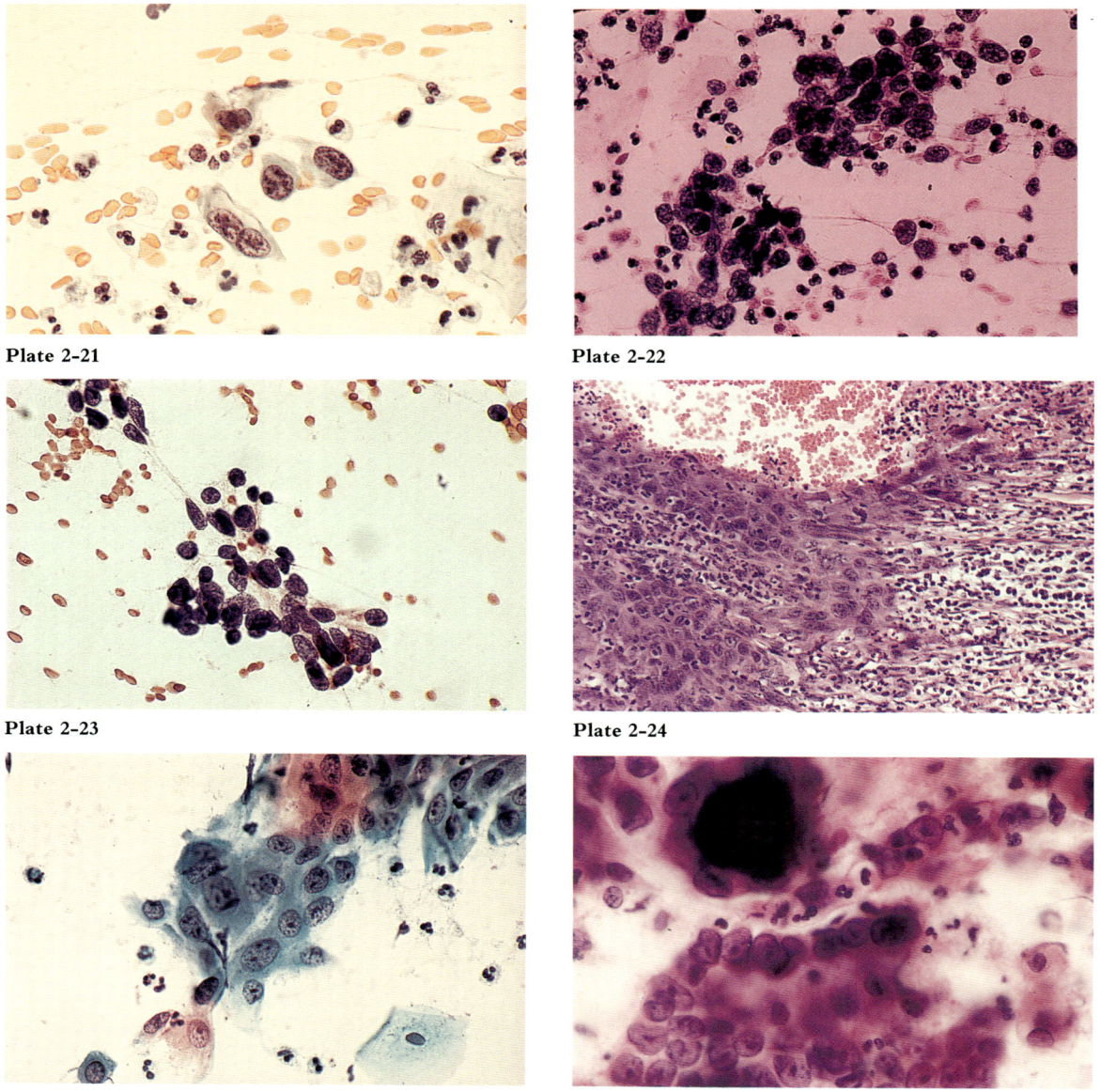

Plate 2-21 (Fig. 2-70) Single tumor cells in a case of nonkeratinizing squamous cell carcinoma of the uterine cervix. (Papanicolaou stain, × 200.)

Plate 2-22 (Fig. 2-72) Small cell carcinoma of the cervix. (Papanicolaou stain, × 200.)

Plate 2-23 (Fig. 2-73) Small cell carcinoma. The presence of nucleoli helps to distinguish this from CIS. (Papanicolaou stain, × 200.)

Plate 2-24 (Fig. 2-74) Tissue section of the cervix showing evidence of inflammation and epithelial repair. (H & E stain × 40.)

Plate 2-25 (Fig. 2-75) Epithelial reparative reaction of the cervix. (Papanicolaou stain, × 200.)

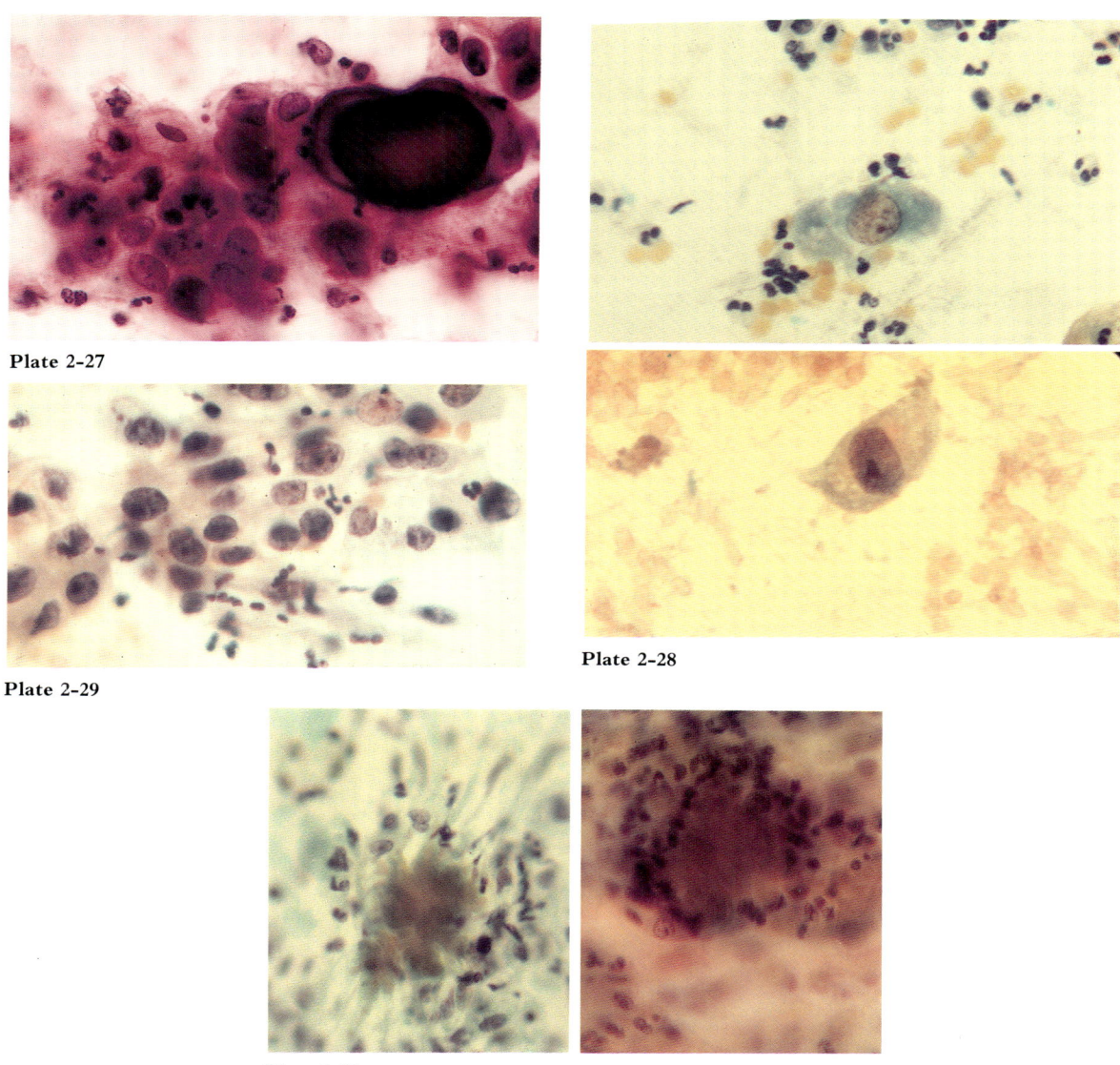

Plate 2-27

Plate 2-28

Plate 2-29

Plate 2-30

Plates 2-26 and 2-27 (Figs. 2-80A,B) Two photographs of endocervical adenocarcinoma displaying prominent psammoma bodies. (Papanicolaou stain, × 200.)
Plate 2-28 (Fig. 2-90A) Single decidual cells in a smear obtained from a pregnant patient.
Plate 2-29 (Fig. 2-90B) Sheets of decidual cells in a pregnant patient with a decidualized polyp protruding through the cervical os. (CVE smear, × 310.)
Plate 2-30 (Fig. 2-94) "Cockelburrs." Hematoidin crystals in a patient who was 7 months pregnant. (CVE smear, × 310.)

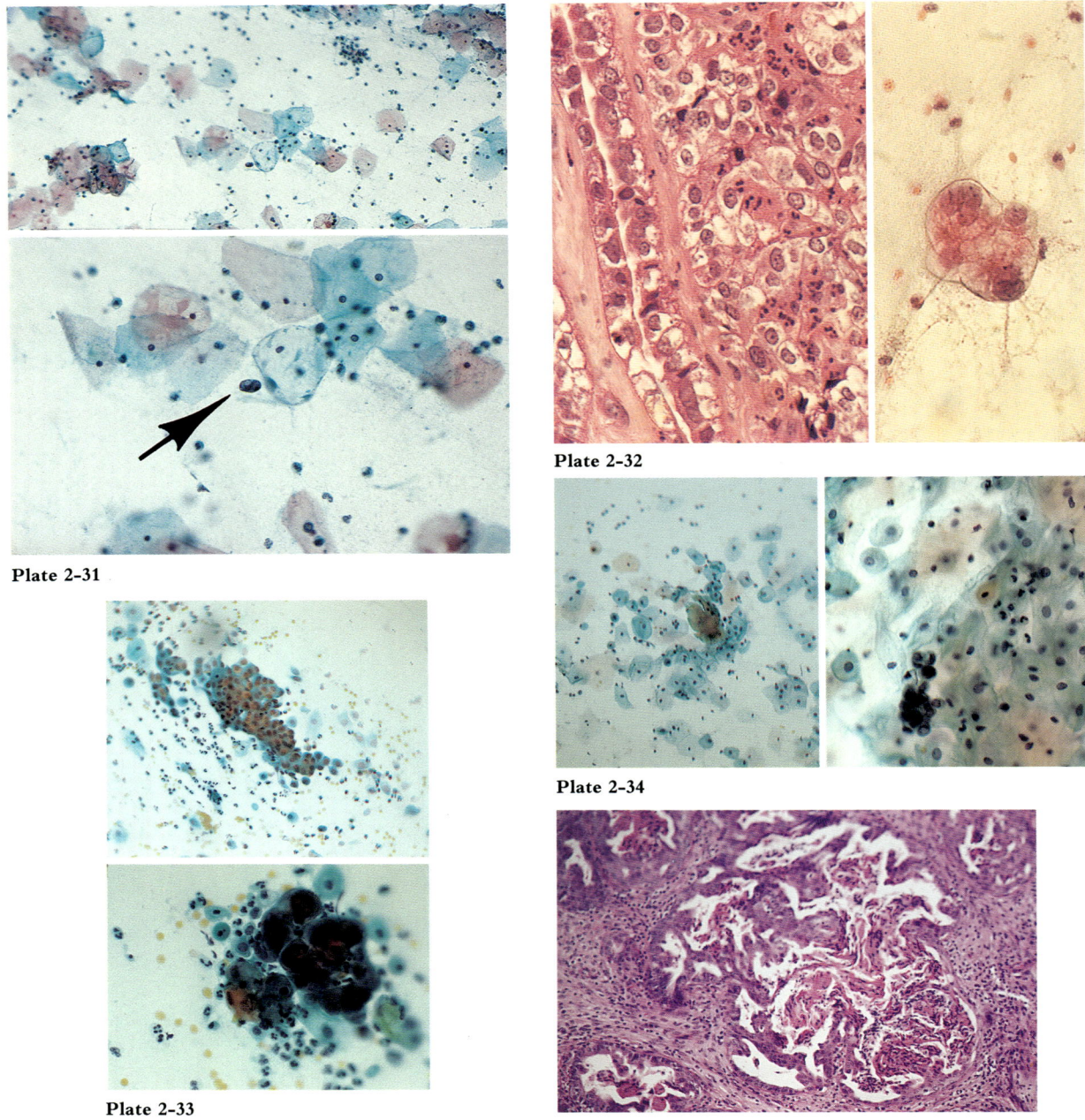

Plate 2-31 (Fig. 2-99) Grade I adenocarcinoma. A single, atypical, endometrial cell (arrow) in a clean smear with elevated estrogenic effect. (Upper: CVE smear, × 120; Lower: CVE smear, × 310.)

Plate 2-32 (Fig. 2-109) (Right) Cell ball from a clear cell adenocarcinoma of the endometrium. (CVE smear, × 400.) (Left) Tissue section of the tumor. (Uterus, hysterectomy, × 400.)

Plate 2-33 (Fig. 2-111) (Bottom) Adenoacanthoma. Irregular cluster of malignant glandular cells with entrapped, atypical, keratinizing squamous cells. (CVE smear, × 500.) (Top) Adenoacanthoma. Benign squamous metaplastic cells with abnormal keratinization. (CVE smear, × 310.)

Plate 2-34 (Fig. 2-112A) (Left) Adenoacanthoma. Keratinaceous material floating in a clean background. (CVE smear, × 120.) (Right) Adenoacanthoma. Tight cluster of low-grade malignant glandular cells. (CVE smear, × 310.)

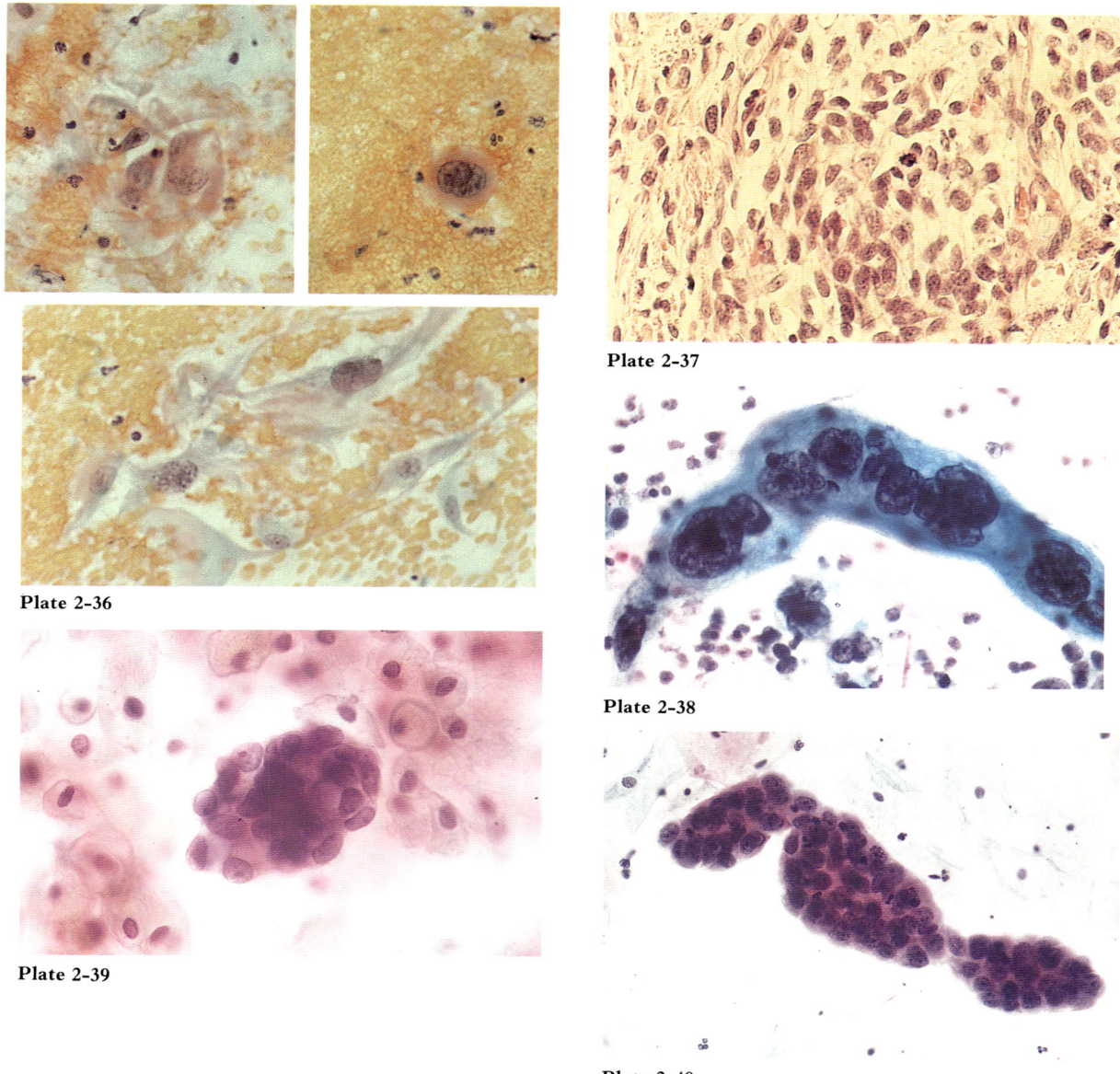

Plate 2-35 (Fig. 2-112B) Adenoacanthoma with keratin production. (Uterine curettage, × 310.)
Plate 2-36 (Fig. 2-115A) Single pleomorphic spindle cells from a stromal sarcoma. (CVE smear, × 400.)
Plate 2-37 (Fig. 2-115B) Stromal sarcoma. (Uterus, hysterectomy, × 400.)
Plate 2-38 (Fig. 2-117) Choriocarcinoma. Malignant syncytiotrophoblasts. (CVE smear, × 450.)
Plate 2-39 (Fig. 2-119) Ovarian carcinoma. The cells are loosely arranged in a cluster, exhibiting a three-dimensional effect. (CVE smear, × 640.)
Plate 2-40 (Fig. 2-120) Ovarian carcinoma. The cells are arranged in a tight cluster without a three-dimensional effect. (CVE smear, × 400.)

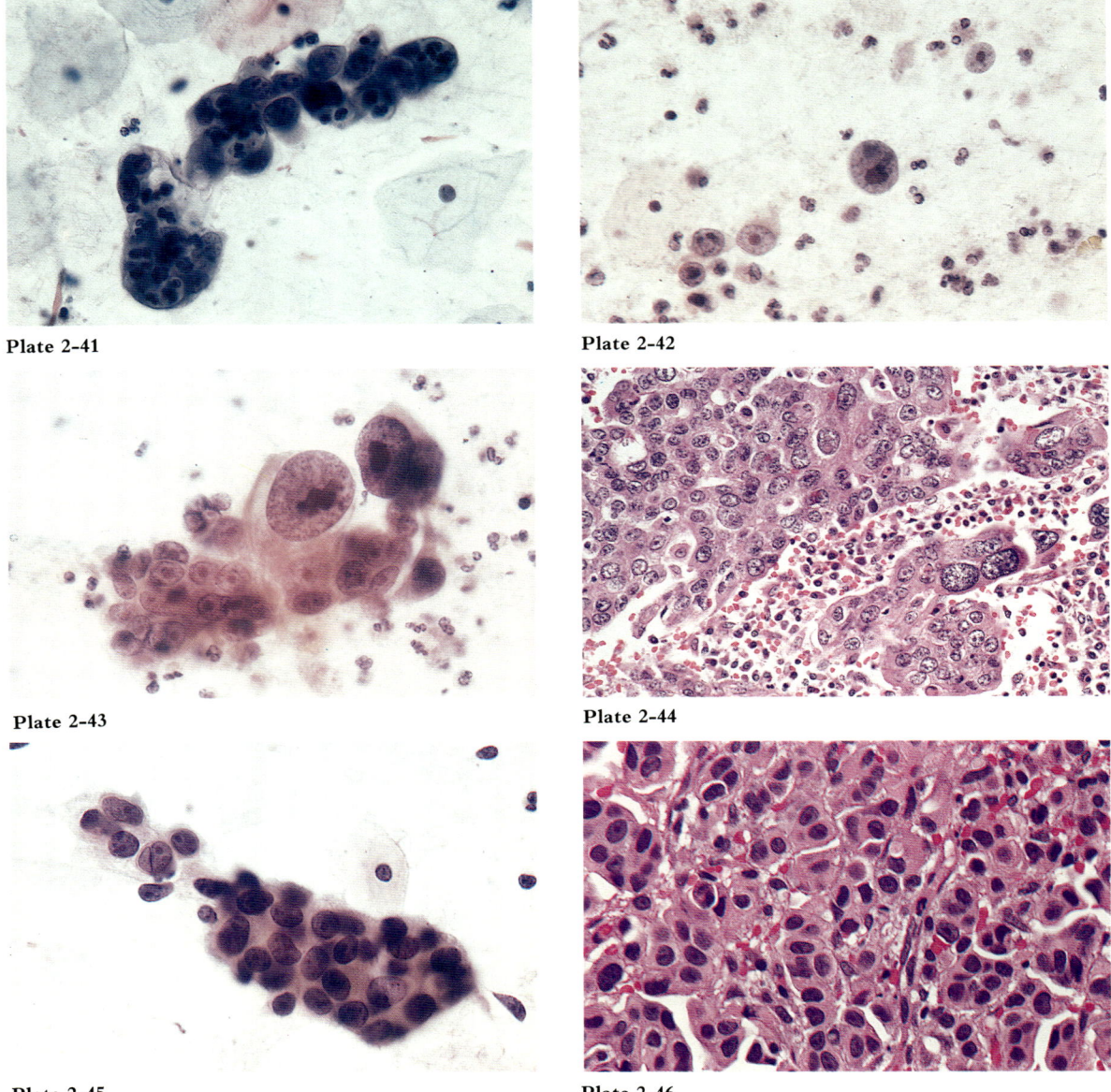

Plate 2-41 (Fig. 2-121) Ovarian carcinoma. Inflammatory cells in the cytoplasm of a loosely arranged cell cluster. (CVE smear, × 640.)

Plate 2-42 (Fig. 2-122A) Ovarian carcinoma. Note the single cells in a poorly differentiated carcinoma (CVE smear, × 640.)

Plate 2-43 (Fig. 2-122B) Ovarian carcinoma. The cells of this poorly differentiated carcinoma exhibit marked variations in size, as well as macronucleoli. (CVE smear, × 640.)

Plate 2-44 (Fig. 2-122C) Ovarian carcinoma. Note the poor differentiation in the same carcinoma as pictured in Plate 43. (× 312.)

Plate 2-45 (Fig. 2-123A) Mammary carcinoma. A cluster of cells that are compactly arranged and exhibit a three-dimensional effect. Note the absence of a tumor diathesis. (CVE smear, × 640.)

Plate 2-46 (Fig. 2-123B) Mammary carcinoma. Histomorphologic confirmation of a metastatic mammary carcinoma involving the uterine cervix. (× 500.)

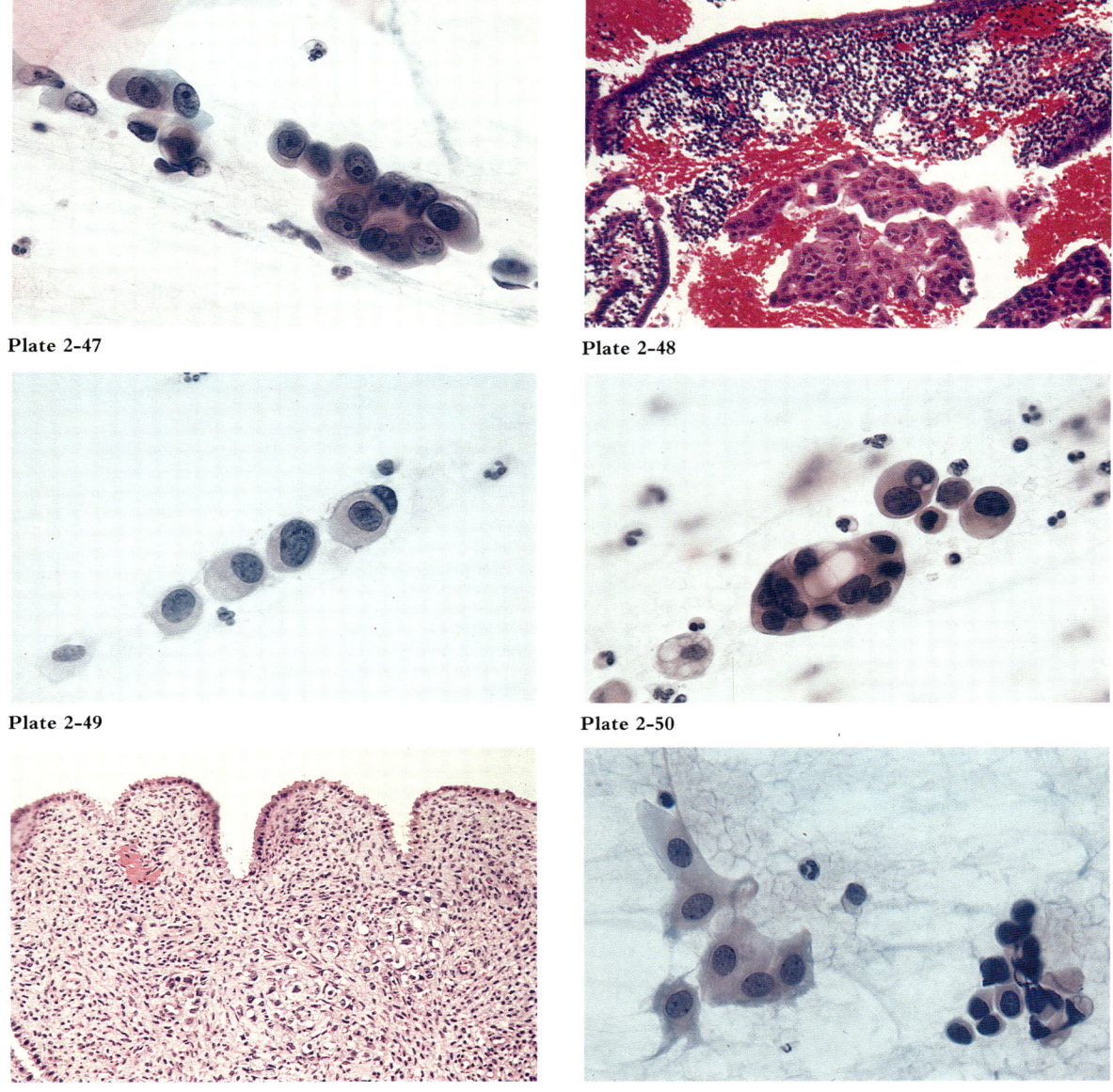

Plate 2-47 (Fig. 2-124A) Mammary carcinoma. Note the compact cellular arrangement, macronucleoli and clean smear background. (CVE smear, × 640.)

Plate 2-48 (Fig. 2-124B) Mammary carcinoma. Histomorphologic confirmation of a metastatic mammary carcinoma involving the endometrium. (× 160.)

Plate 2-49 (Fig. 2-125A) Mammary carcinoma. The small cells in this lobular carcinoma are arranged in a linear fashion. (CVE smear, × 640.)

Plate 2-50 (Fig. 2-125B) Mammary carcinoma. An unusual glandlike feature in a lobular carcinoma. (CVE smear, × 640.)

Plate 2-51 (Fig. 2-125C) Mammary carcinoma. Histomorphologic confirmation of a metastatic lobular carcinoma involving the uterine cervix. (× 160.)

Plate 2-52 (Fig. 2-126A) Mammary carcinoma. Cells derived from a lobular carcinoma are sometimes rather small (right) compared to the parabasal-like cells (left). (CVE smear, × 640.)

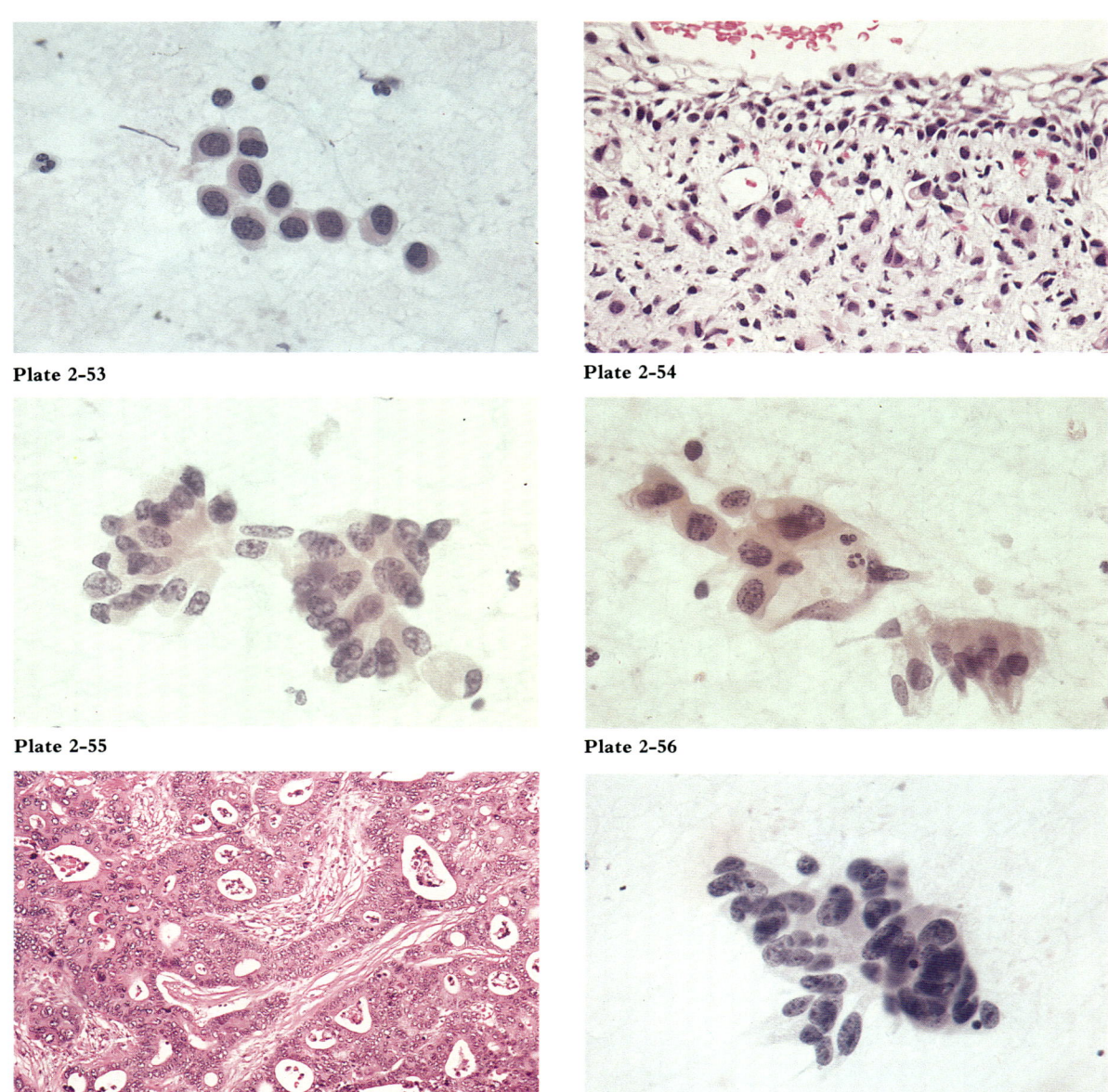

Plate 2-53 (Fig. 2-126B) Mammary carcinoma. These cells from a lobular carcinoma exhibit a lack of cohesiveness. (CVE smear, × 640.)

Plate 2-54 (Fig. 2-126C) Mammary carcinoma. Histomorphologic confirmation of a lobular carcinoma involving the uterine cervix. (× 400.)

Plate 2-55 (Fig. 2-127A) Colonic carcinoma. Low to tall columnar cells, arranged in a palisading fashion, are commonly observed. (CVE smear, × 640.)

Plate 2-56 (Fig. 2-127B) Colonic carcinoma. Note the low columnar cells. (CVE smear, × 640.)

Plate 2-57 (Fig. 2-127C) Colonic carcinoma. Histomorphologic confirmation of colonic carcinoma (× 125.)

Plate 2-58 (Fig. 2-128) Colonic carcinoma. Note the constant feature of columnar cells in a palisading arrangement. (Bronchial brush smear, × 640.)

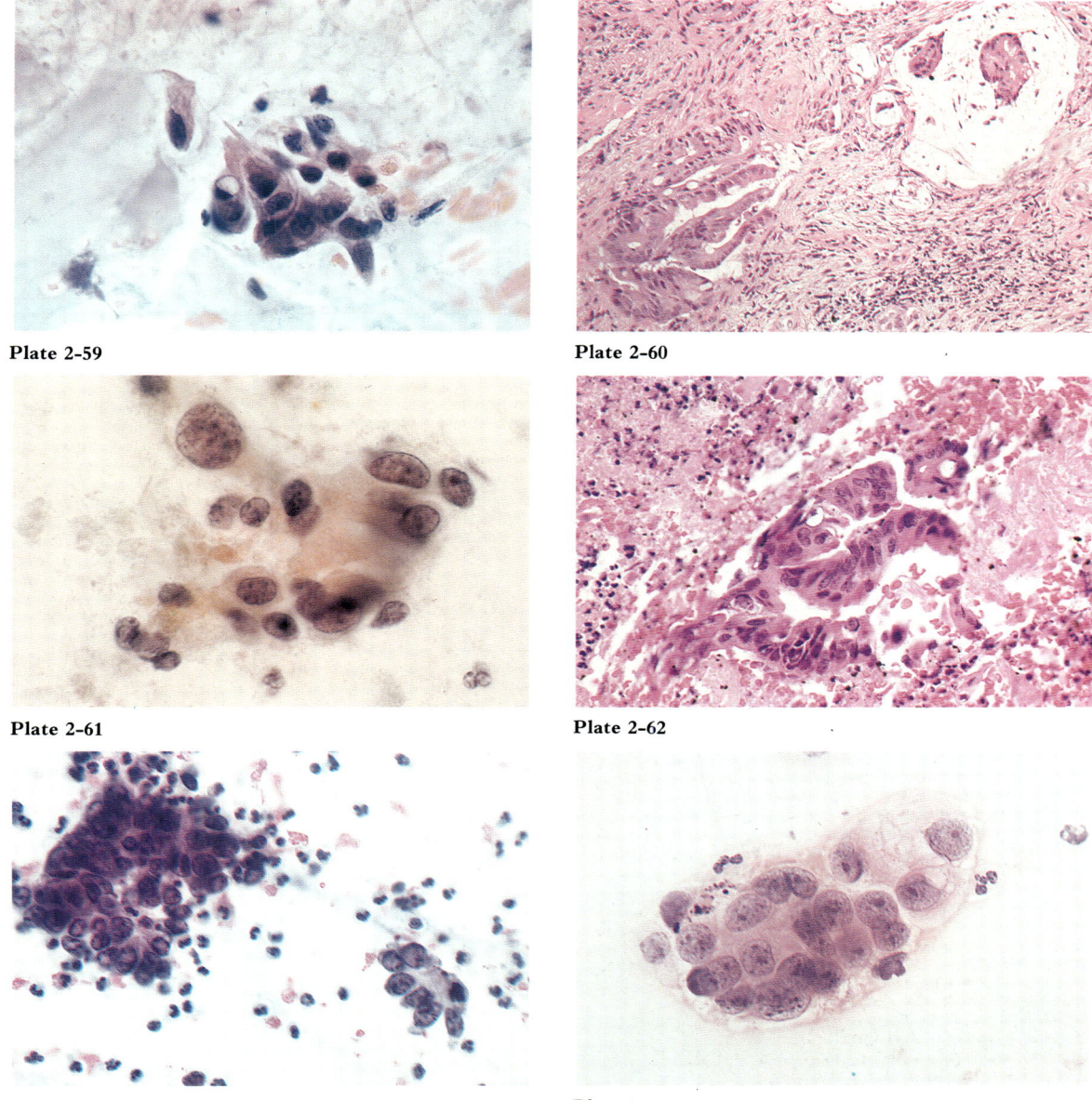

Plate 2-59 (Fig. 2-129A) Colonic carcinoma with mucin. Note the columnar cells and tumor diathesis. (CVE smear, × 640.)

Plate 2-60 (Fig. 2-129B) Colonic carcinoma. Histomorphologic confirmation of a mucin-producing colonic carcinoma. (× 160.)

Plate 2-61 (Fig. 2-130A) Colonic carcinoma. Variations in cellular size are apparent in this poorly differentiated carcinoma. (CVE smear, × 1008.)

Plate 2-62 (Fig. 2-130B) Colonic carcinoma. Histomorphologic confirmation of a carcinoma involving the vagina. (× 312.)

Plate 2-63 (Fig. 2-131) Colonic carcinoma. Small cells derived from a poorly differentiated carcinoma are seen. (CVE smear, × 500.)

Plate 2-64 (Fig. 2-132A) Lung carcinoma. Note the similarity of this carcinoma to an ovarian carcinoma. (CVE smear, × 640.)

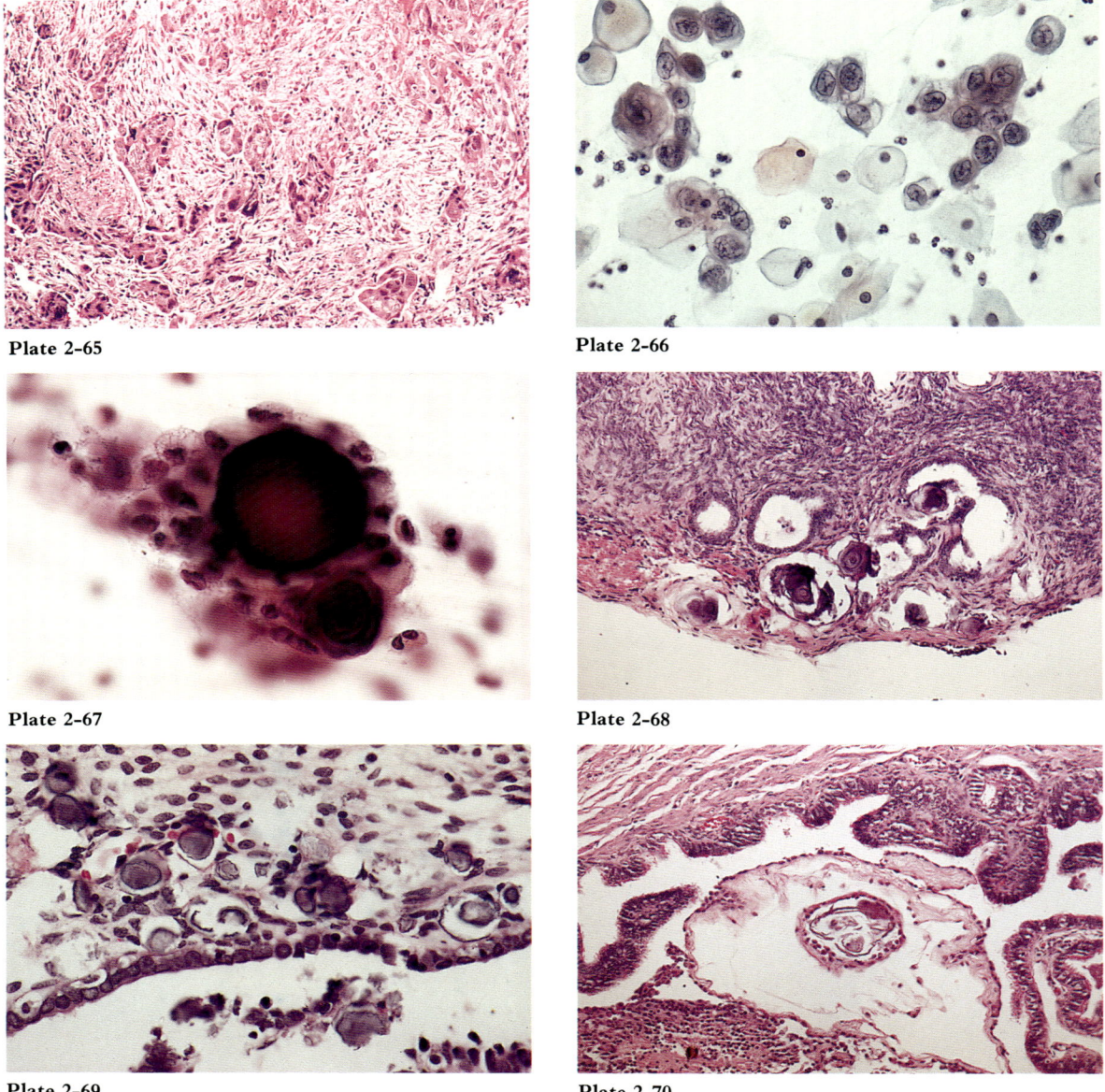

Plate 2-65 (Fig. 2-132B) Lung carcinoma. Histomorphologic confirmation of a lung carcinoma. (× 160.)

Plate 2-66 (Fig. 2-133) Carcinoma of unknown origin. Note that malignant tumor cells are present in an otherwise normal cellular background. (CVE smear, × 400.)

Plate 2-67 (Fig. 2-134A) Psammoma body. Note the absence of malignant tumor cells. (CVE smear, × 800.)

Plate 2-68 (Fig. 2-134B) Histomorphologic confirmation of psammoma bodies in serosal inclusion cysts of the ovary. (× 160.)

Plate 2-69 (Fig. 2-135) Psammoma bodies in the uterine cervix. (× 400.)

Plate 2-70 (Fig. 2-136) Psammoma bodies in the uterine tube. (× 160.)

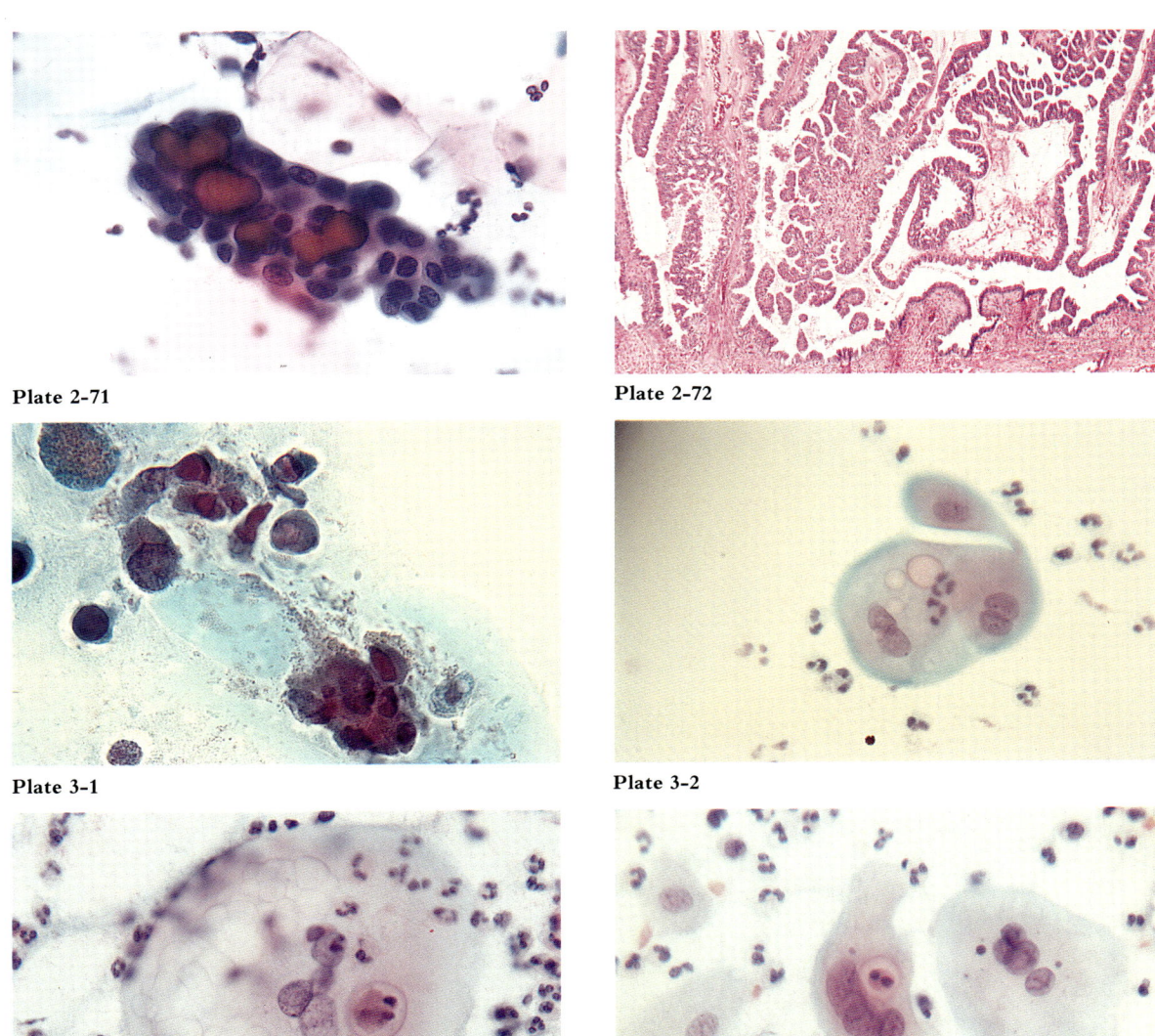

Plate 2-71 (Fig. 2-137A) Note that the epithelial cells do not fulfill the criteria for malignant disease. (CVE smear, × 640.)

Plate 2-72 (Fig. 2-137B) Histomorphologic confirmation of a serous cystadenoma of borderline malignancy (× 64.)

Plate 3-1 (Fig. 3-2) Voided urine specimen showing cyclophosphamide effect. (× 160.)

Plate 3-2 (Fig. 3-4) Radiation effect. Multinucleated intermediate cell with bizarre cell shape. A discrete cytoplasmic vacuole is also seen. (× 160.)

Plate 3-3 (Fig. 3-5) Radiation effect. This intermediate cell shows multinucleation, multiple cytoplasmic vacuoles with one discrete vacuole containing a polymorphonuclear leukocyte nucleus, and polymorphonuclear "superimposition." (× 160.)

Plate 3-4 (Fig. 3-7) Radiation effect, intermediate cells. Note the binucleation and nuclear enlargement, as well as the nucleus of a polymorphonuclear leukocyte within the discrete cytoplasmic vacuole. (× 160.)

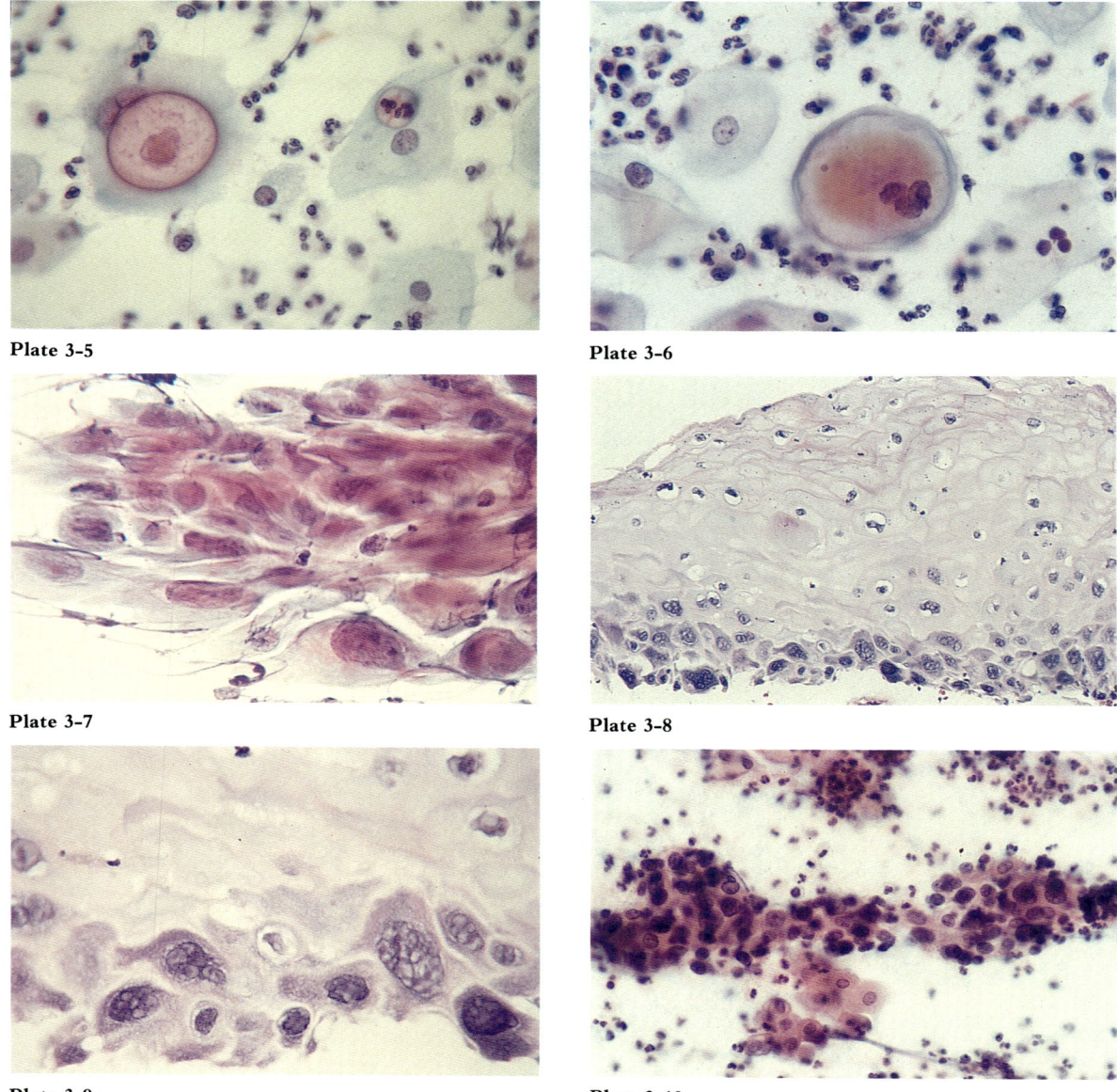

Plate 3-5 (Fig. 3-8) Radiation effect. The intermediate cell on the left shows a single, discrete, cytoplasmic vacuole pushing the double nuclei to one side and containing nuclear material. (× 160.)

Plate 3-6 (Fig. 3-9) Radiation effect. The intermediate cell in the center shows, in addition to trinucleation, a "two-tone" cytoplasm. (× 160.)

Plate 3-7 (Fig. 3-15) Radiation repair. Note the typical repair arrangement of the keratinocytes, as well as the nuclear enlargement that is consistent with radiation effect. (× 160.)

Plate 3-8 (Fig. 3-19) Post-irradiation dysplasia evident on biopsy. (× 50.)

Plate 3-9 Higher magnification of Plate 3-8 shows markedly bizarre cells. (× 160.)

Plate 3-10 Irradiated squamous carcinoma, recurrent. Note the "healthy" appearance of the unaffected cancer cells. (× 100.)

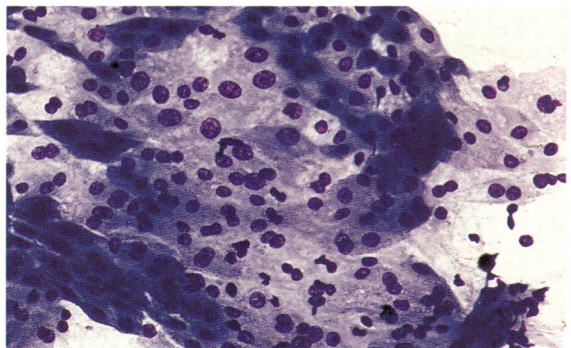

Plate 4-1

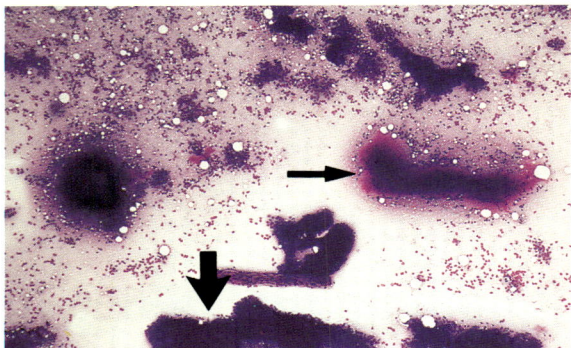

Plate 4-2

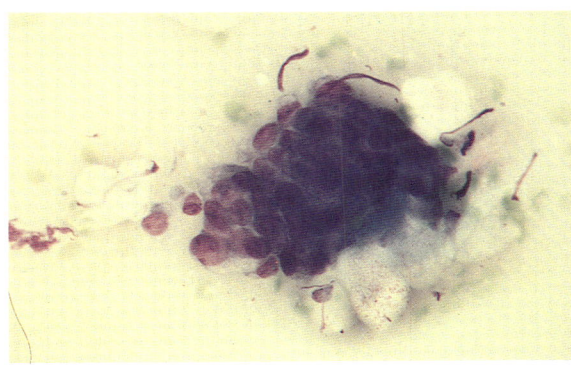

Plate 4-3

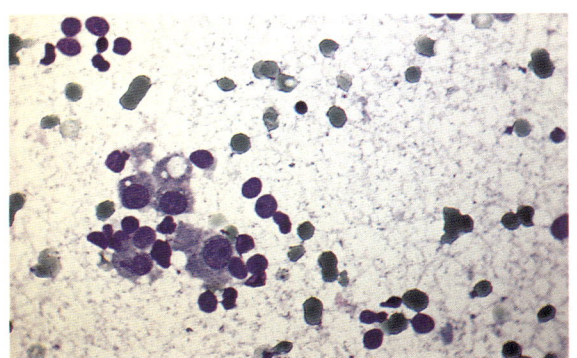

Plate 4-4

Plate 4-5

Plate 4-1 (Fig. 4-5) Benign breast epithelium with apocrine change. (MGG stain, × 100.)

Plate 4-2 (Fig. 4-6) Fibroadenoma, low-power magnification. Marked cellularity, cohesive epithelial clusters, metachromatic stroma (*thin arrow*), and a portion of a small vessel (*thick arrow*) are visible. (MGG stain, × 16.)

Plate 4-3 (Fig. 4-9A) Paget's disease of the nipple. Discohesive, markedly atypical, and large tumor cells are seen.

Plate 4-4 (Fig. 4-9B) Papilloma of the nipple. A cohesive cluster of epithelial cells with mild atypia is evident. (MGG stain, × 160.)

Plate 4-5 (Fig. 4-11) Breast in pregnancy. Small, oval, naked nuclei as well as larger epithelial cells with prominent nucleoli and abundant granular to vacuolated cytoplasm are seen in a proteinaceous background. (MGG stain, × 160.)

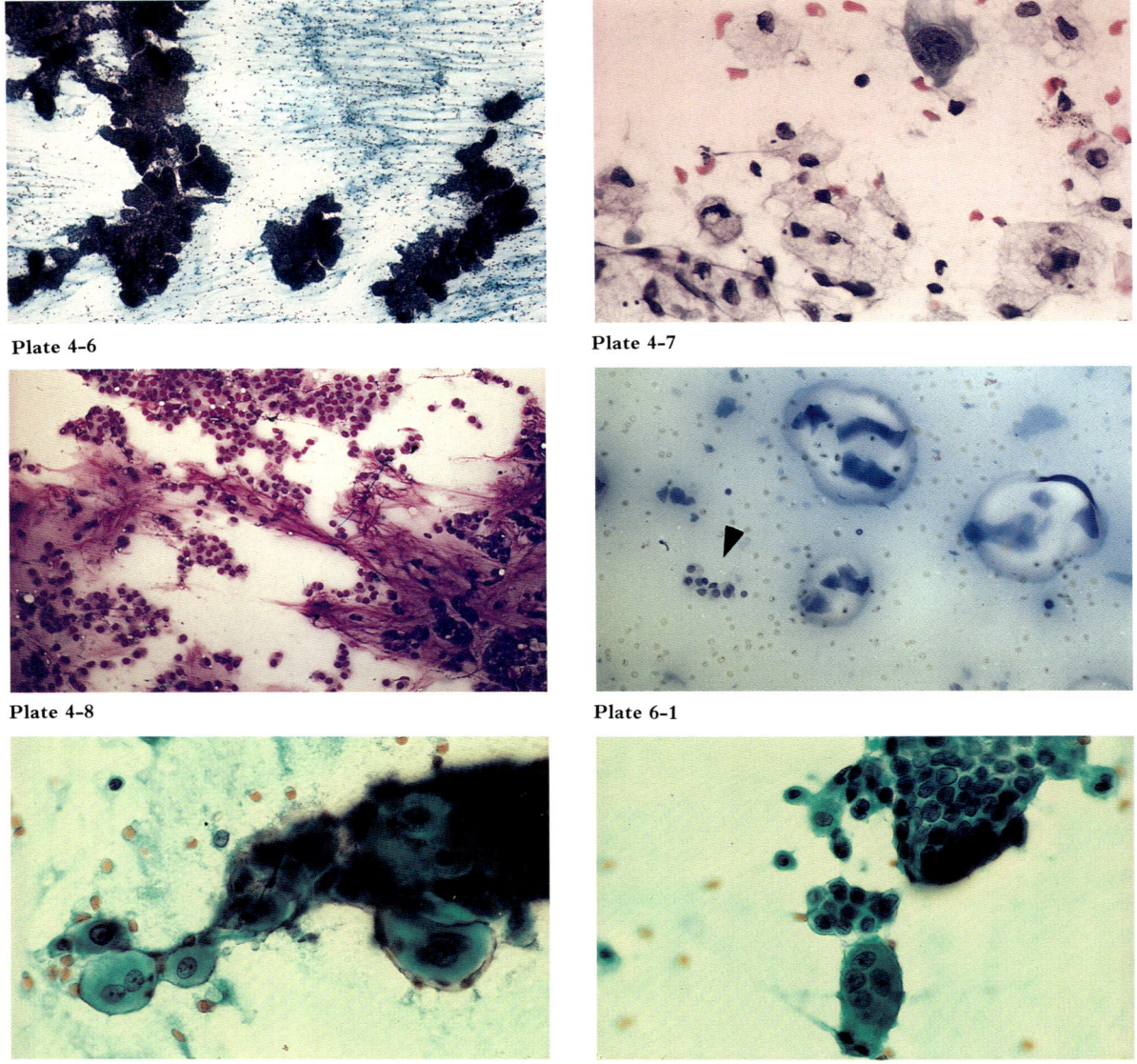

Plate 4-6 (Fig. 4-12) Breast in pregnancy. Smear shows extremely high cellularity and scalloped outline of lobules and distal ducts. (Papanicolaou stain, × 16.)

Plate 4-7 (Fig. 4-13) Fat necrosis. There is one markedly atypical cell with a large nucleus and several prominent nucleoli located next to lipophages with abundant, vacuolated cytoplasm and small nuclei without significant atypia. (Papanicolaou stain, × 160.)

Plate 4-8 (Fig. 4-16) Colloid carcinoma. Abundant metachromatic, stringy, mucinous material is mixed with cancer cells. (MGG stain, × 40.)

Plate 6-1 (Fig. 6-2) A small cluster of benign follicular cells (arrow) are visible in a field of watery blue colloid. (MGG stain, × 10.)

Plate 6-2 (Fig. 6-9) A cluster of cohesive cells from a patient with papillary carcinoma demonstrating metaplastic cytoplasm. (Papanicolaou stain, × 40.)

Plate 6-3 (Fig. 6-12) Three features of papillary carcinoma. The upper portion shows a papillary structure without a demonstrable vessel. In the midportion, there are epithelial cells with well-defined cytoplasms, and in the lower portion of the field is an epithelial giant cell. (Papanicolaou stain, × 40.)

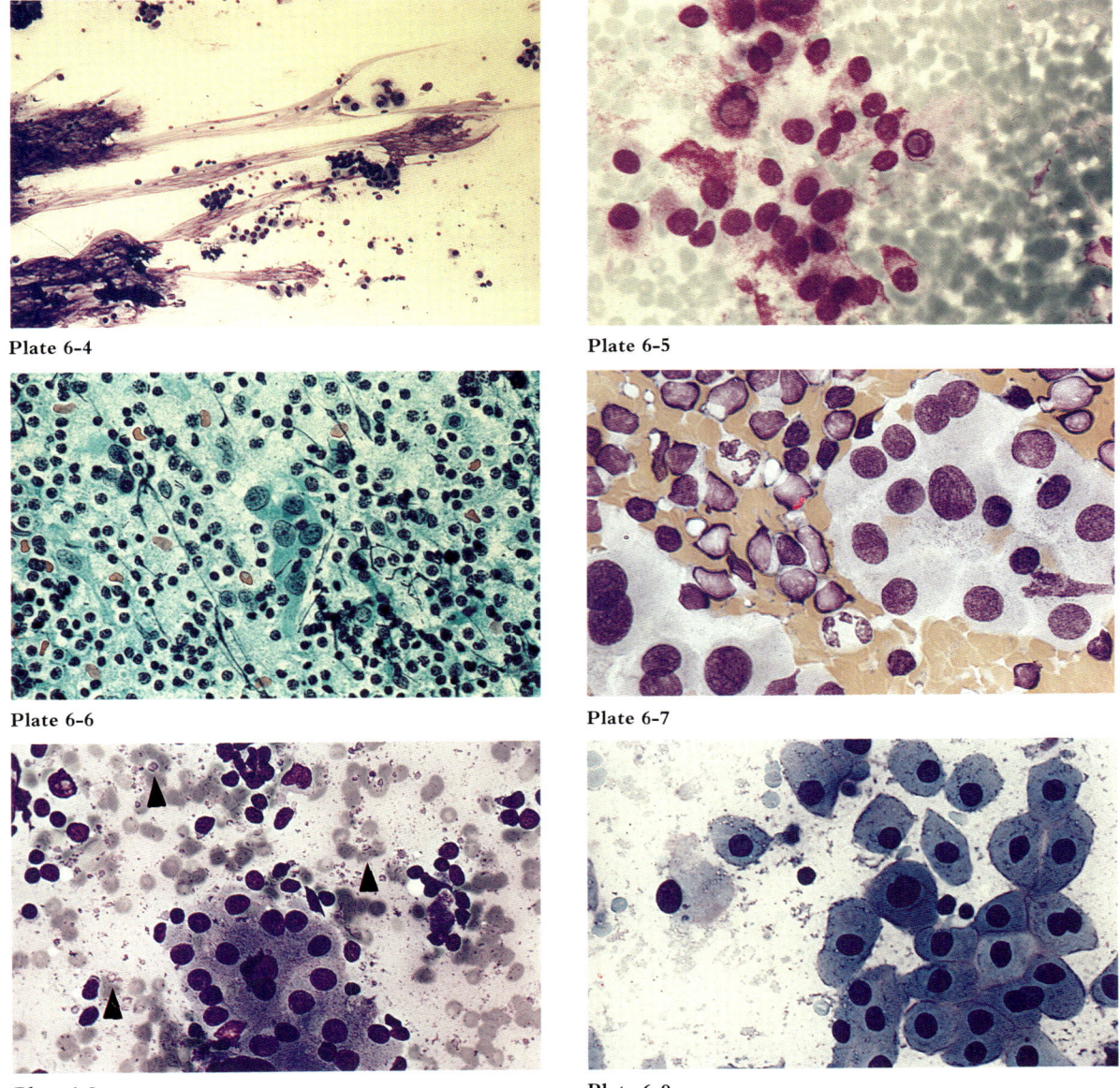

Plate 6-4 (Fig. 6-13) This air-dried smear demonstrates the streaking and smearing effects of "bubble-gum" colloid. (MGG stain, × 10.)

Plate 6-5 (Fig. 6-15) This smear from a medullary carcinoma shows red cytoplasmic granulation as well as nuclear inclusions. (MGG stain, × 40.)

Plate 6-6 (Fig. 6-16) In this example of chronic thyroiditis, a small group of Hürthle cells with abundant granular cytoplasm and lymphocytic background is seen. (Papanicolaou stain, × 20.)

Plate 6-7 (Fig. 6-17) This air-dried smear from a patient with chronic thyroiditis reveals Hürthle cells with abundant, slate-gray cytoplasm. (Wright-Giemsa stain, × 40.)

Plate 6-8 (Fig. 6-18) In this example of chronic thyroiditis, air-dried smears reveal "blue blobs" (arrows), as well as Hürthle cells and lymphoid elements. (MGG stain, × 40.)

Plate 6-9 (Fig. 6-19) Cells with abundant granular cytoplasm in a very discohesive pattern are seen in this example of a Hürthle cell tumor. (MGG stain, × 20.)

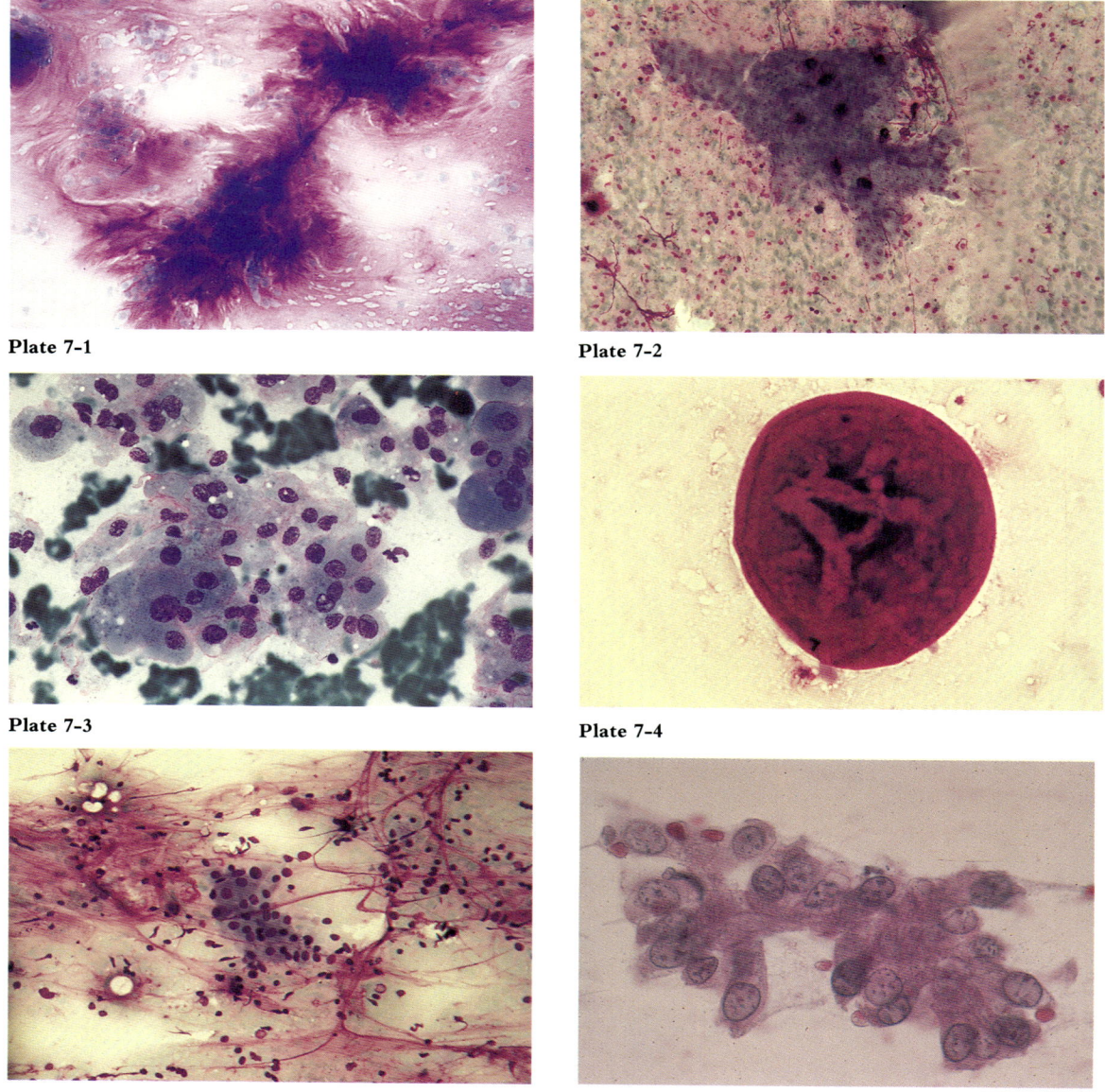

Plate 7-1 (Fig. 7-2) Smear from a pleomorphic adenoma. The stroma of a pleomorphic adenoma stains intensely purple and has a fernlike arrangement. (MGG stain, × 200.)

Plate 7-2 (Fig. 7-5) Smear from a Warthin's tumor showing numerous mast cells with their characteristic red cytoplasmic granules superimposed on a sheet of oncocytes. (MGG stain, × 300.)

Plate 7-3 (Fig. 7-6) Smear from an oncocytoma. The oncocytes show considerable variation in nuclear size, as well as an intensely granular cytoplasm. (MGG stain, × 400.)

Plate 7-4 (Fig. 7-8) Smear of a rigidly spherical stromal ball that is characteristic of adenoid cystic carcinoma. (MGG stain, × 400.)

Plate 7-5 (Fig. 7-11) Smear from a mucoepidermoid carcinoma showing neoplastic cells and extracellular mucin. (MGG stain, × 300.)

Plate 8-1 (Fig. 8-2) ERCP aspirate, smear. Atypical pancreatic ductal epithelial cells are evident in this example of chronic pancreatitis. (H & E stain, × 100.)

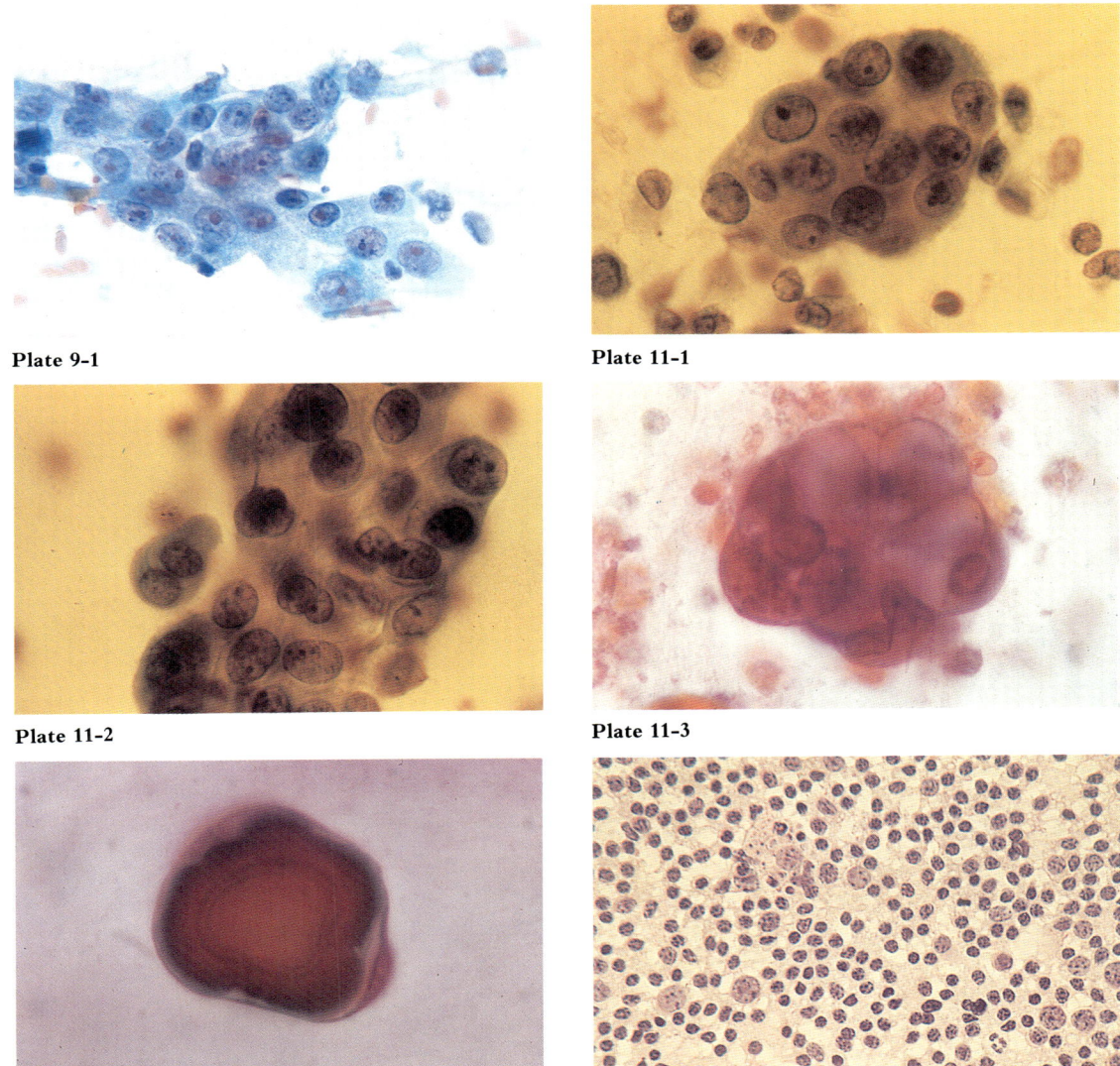

Plate 9-1
Plate 11-1
Plate 11-2
Plate 11-3
Plate 11-4
Plate 13-1

Plate 9-1 (Fig. 9-4) Liver aspiration. A smear reveals well-differentiated hepatocellular carcinoma. (Papanicolaou stain, × 158.)

Plate 11-1 (Fig. 11-7A) Peritoneal mesothelioma in a patient who formerly worked as an asbestos pipe coverer and insulator in a naval shipyard. Note the tight cluster of cells.

Plate 11-2 (Fig. 11-7B) Group of loosely attached cells in ascitic fluid from same patient as Plate 11-1.

Plate 11-3 (Fig. 11-7C) Ascitic fluid from a patient with malignant ovarian tumor exhibits an abundant, clear cytoplasm indicating the presence of mucin.

Plate 11-4 (Fig. 11-7D) Psammoma body, papillary adenocarcinoma of the ovary. The presence of psammoma bodies does not always signify malignant disease, as they may also occur in benign conditions, but there is a high incidence of associated papillary adenocarcinoma.

Plate 13-1 (Fig. 13-1) Smear from lymph node FNA showing a spectrum of small lymphocytes, transformed follicular center cells, and tingible body macrophages indicative of a benign reactive process. (Papanicolaou stain, × 125.)

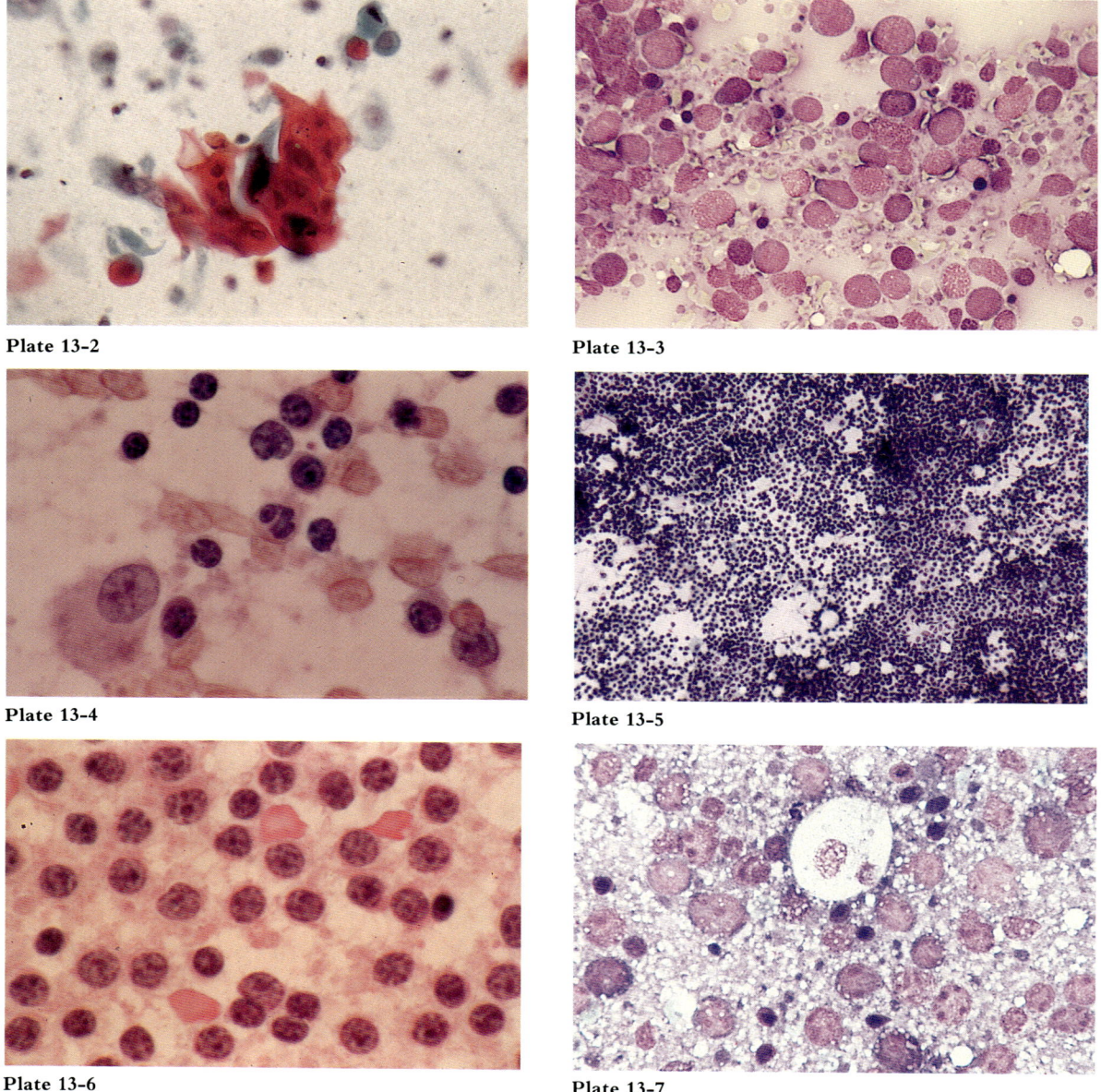

Plate 13-2 (Fig. 13-2) Lymph node FNA specimen containing aggregates of neoplastic squamous cells, in a case of metastatic squamous carcinoma. (Papanicolaou stain, × 200.)
Plate 13-3 (Fig. 13-3) Lymph node FNA smear from patient with malignant lymphoma of the large noncleaved FCC type (centroblastic). (May Grünwald Giemsa stain, × 250.)
Plate 13-4 (Fig. 13-5) Lymph node FNA consistent with reactive lymphoid hyperplasia. (H & E stain, × 320.)
Plate 13-5 (Fig. 13-6A) Lymph node imprint in patient with chronic lymphocytic leukemia. (Wright-Giemsa stain, × 50.)
Plate 13-6 (Fig. 13-6B) Lymph node imprint in case of chronic lymphocytic leukemia. (H & E stain, × 320.)
Plate 13-7 (Fig. 13-8A) Lymph node FNA smear in patient with small noncleaved FCC lymphoma (malignant lymphoma, lymphoblastic, Burkitt type). (May Grünwald Giemsa stain, × 320.) (Case courtesy of Edneia Tani, M.D., Karolinska Hospital, Stockholm, Sweden.)

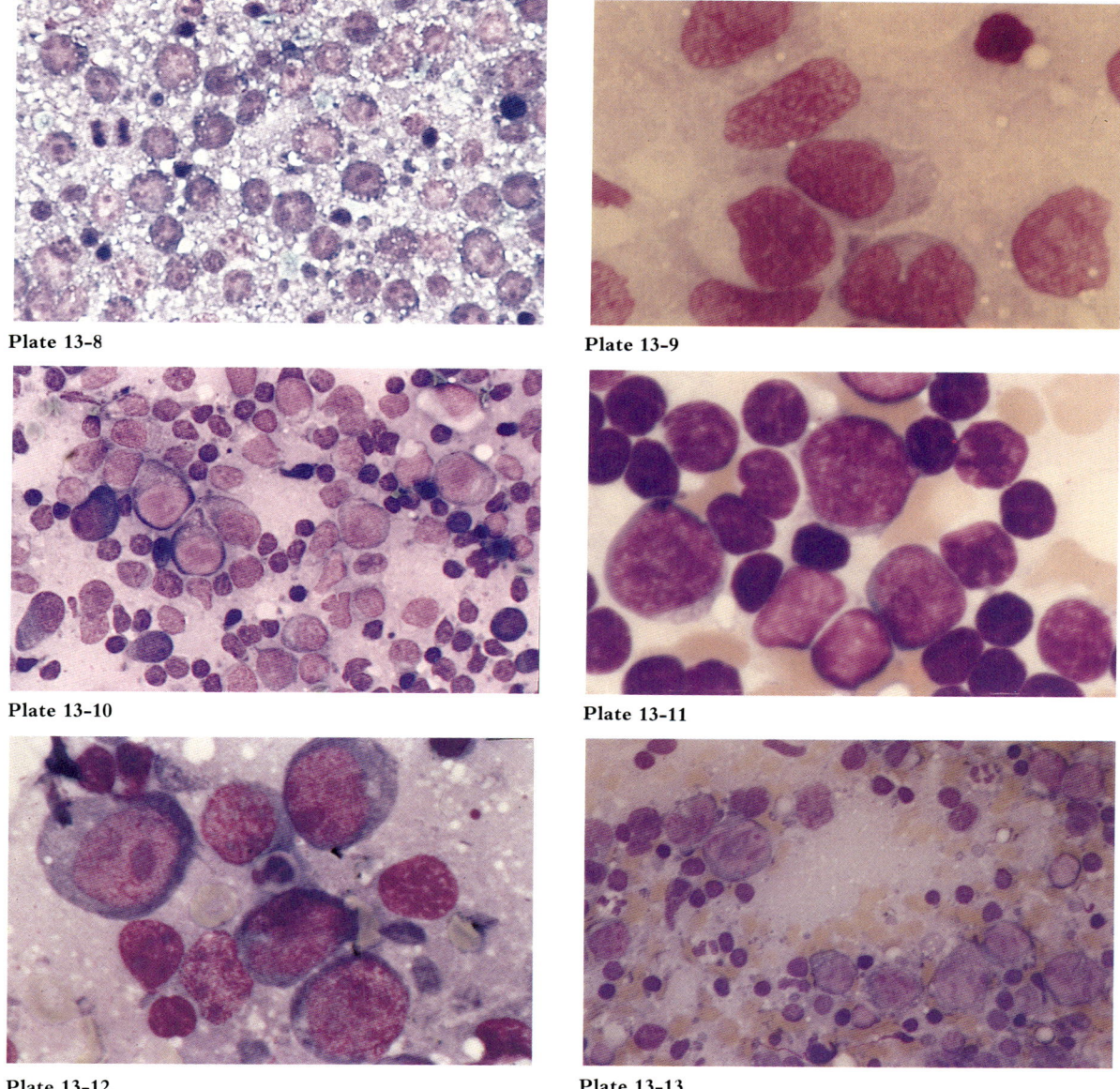

Plate 13-8 (Fig. 13-8B) Lymph node FNA from same patient as Plate 13-7 with relatively monomorphous population of small and intermediate-sized follicular center cells. (May Grünwald Giemsa stain, × 250.)

Plate 13-9 (Fig. 13-9) Lymph node FNA in case of large cleaved follicular center cell lymphoma. (Wright-Giemsa stain, × 630.)

Plate 13-10 (Fig. 13-10A) Reactive lymph node in a patient with proven infectious mononucleosis. Note "spectrum" of lymphocytes and occasional immunoblasts. (May Grünwald Giemsa stain, × 220.) (Case courtesy of Edneia Tani, M.D., Karolinska Hospital, Stockholm, Sweden.)

Plate 13-11 (Fig. 13-10B) Lymph node imprint in a patient with infectious mononucleosis. (Wright-Giemsa stain, × 500.)

Plate 13-12 (Fig. 13-12B) Lymph node imprint from B-cell immunoblastic sarcoma composed of large neoplastic immunoblasts. (Wright-Giemsa stain, × 500.)

Plate 13-13 (Fig. 13-13B) T-cell immunoblastic sarcoma showing immunoblasts with irregular complex nuclear folding. (Wright-Giemsa stain, × 160.)

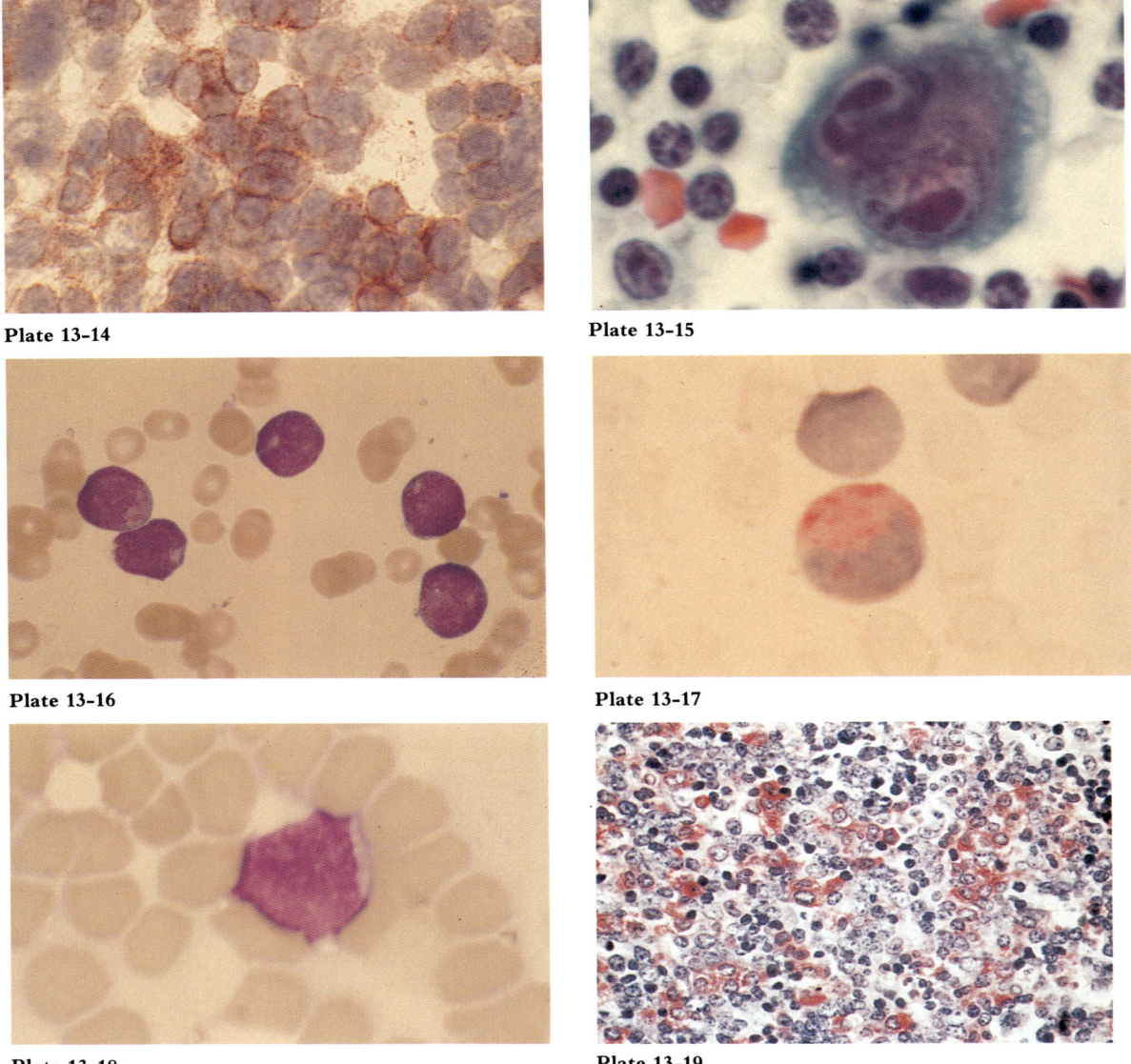

Plate 13-14 (Fig. 13-13C) An example of T-immunoblastic sarcoma in which T-cell origin is confirmed by strong staining of neoplastic cells by a pan-T-cell antibody. (Avidin-biotin-peroxidase complex, × 160.)

Plate 13-15 (Fig. 13-14) Reed-Sternberg cell demonstrating large bilobed nucleus containing huge "owl's eye" nucleoli. (Papanicolaou stain, × 400.)

Plate 13-16 (Fig. 13-16A) Convoluted T-cell lymphoma showing intermediate-sized primitive lymphoid cells (lymphoblasts). (Wright-Giemsa stain, × 320.)

Plate 13-17 (Fig. 13-16B) Convoluted T-cell lymphoma exhibiting positive intracytoplasmic acid phosphatase staining, suggesting T-cell origin. (Acid phosphatase stain, × 500.)

Plate 13-18 (Fig. 13-17A) Primitive blast-like cell in a patient with granulocytic sarcoma or "chloroma." (Wright-Giemsa stain, × 500.)

Plate 13-19 (Fig. 13-17B) Paraffin-embedded, formalin-fixed section from enlarged lymph node in a patient with granulocytic sarcoma. Positive cytoplasmic staining (red) for chloroacetate-esterase (CAE) reveals the primitive myeloid origin of these cells. (Chloroacetate-esterase stain, × 100.)

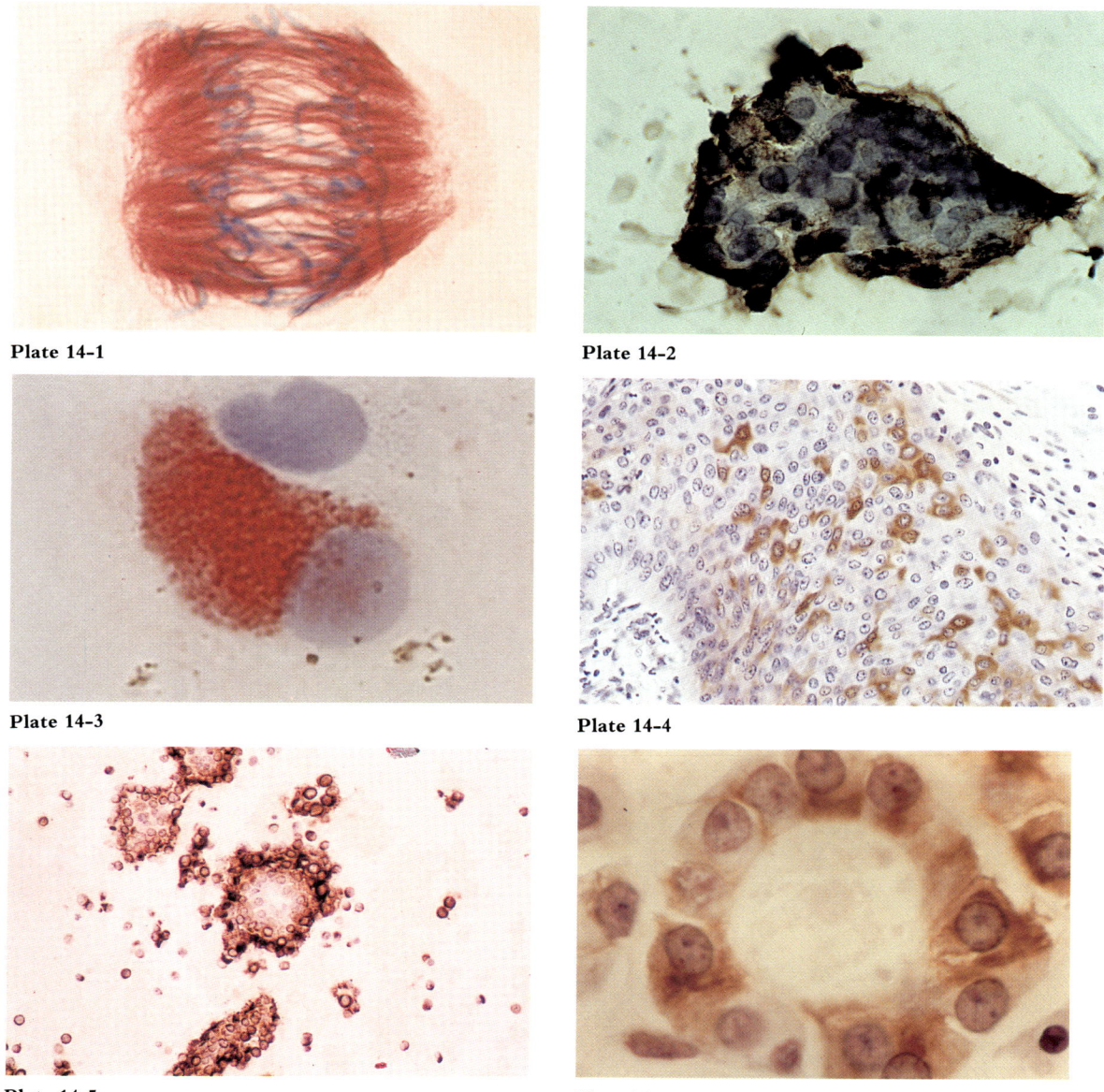

Plate 14-1 (Fig. 14-1) Cell in mitosis. Microtubule spindle is stained red with rabbit antitubulin. Chromosomes are counterstained by toluidine blue. (Courtesy of S. Van Noorden, M.D.)

Plate 14-2 (Fig. 14-2) Giant cell staining positively with HSV antibody.

Plate 14-3 (Fig. 14-3) Papanicolaou smear stained with anti-*Chlamydia* antibody. (Courtesy of T. Kobayashi, M.D.)

Plate 14-4 (Fig. 14-4) Koilocytes stained by synthetic antibody that recognizes HPV-related DNA sequences.

Plate 14-5 (Fig. 14-5) Islet cell tumor of the pancreas stained for keratin with broad spectrum antibody.

Plate 14-6 (Fig. 14-6A) Immunocytochemistry of follicular carcinoma of the thyroid. Neoplastic cells stain for vimentin but colloid does not.

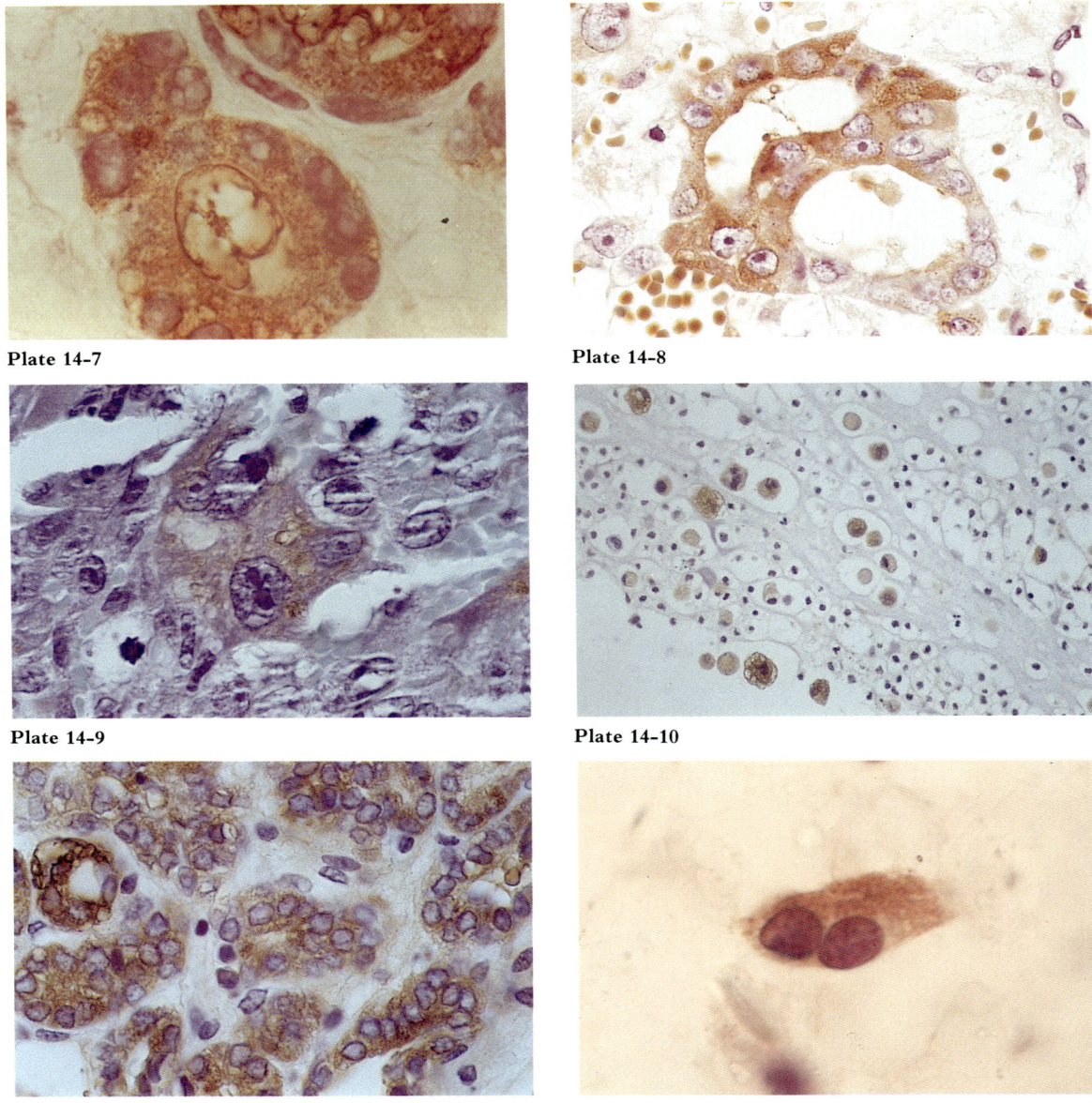

Plate 14-7 (Fig. 14-6B) Immunocytochemistry of follicular carcinoma of the thyroid. Both follicular cells and colloid stain for thyroglobulin.
Plate 14-8 (Fig. 14-7) Embryonal carcinoma staining positively for alphafetoprotein.
Plate 14-9 (Fig. 14-8) Choriocarcinoma. Syncytiotrophoblastic giant cell staining positively for BHCG.
Plate 14-10 (Fig. 14-9) Malignant epithelial cells in pleural effusion stain positively for EMA, while background mesothelial cells do not.
Plate 14-11 (Fig. 14-10) Follicular variant of papillary carcinoma staining positively for thyroglobulin.
Plate 14-12 (Fig. 14-11) Neoplastic C-cells staining positively for calcitonin.
Plate 14-13 (Fig. 14-12) Adenocarcinoma by routine cytologic stains. (Left) With MGG, intracellular mucin appears blue and floculent. (Right) With Papanicolaou the secretory product is retracted from the cell membrane and surrounded by a halo.

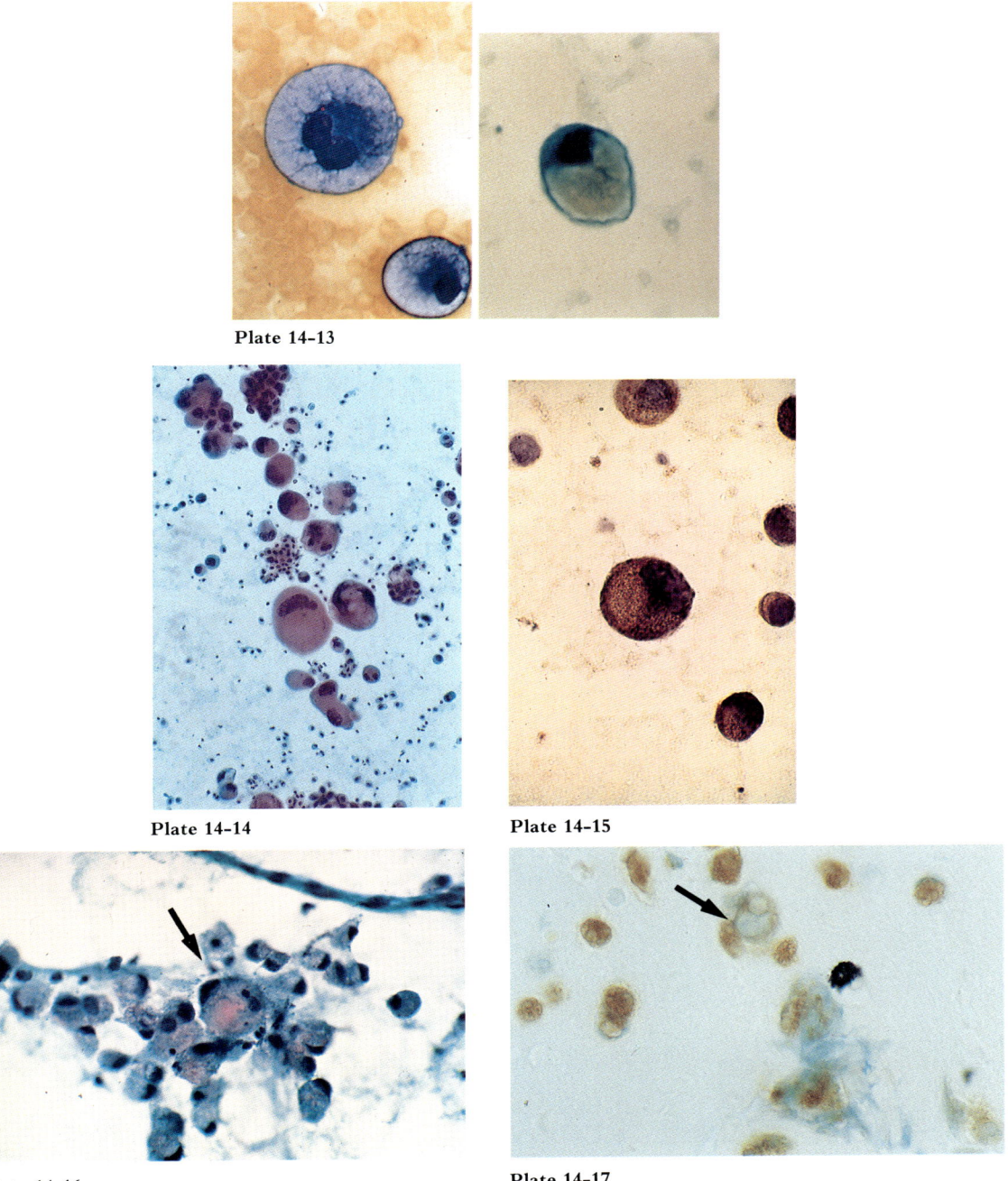

Plate 14-14 (Fig. 14-13A) Metastatic adenocarcinoma. The large tumor cells show partial vacuolization of the cytoplasm with the Papanicolaou stain.
Plate 14-15 (Fig. 14-13B) Metastatic adenocarcinoma. Positivity of the CEA immunostain is evenly distributed throughout the cytoplasm.
Plate 14-16 (Fig. 14-14) Mucicarmine stain of adenocarcinoma cells. Note faint positivity within the cytoplasm of the tumor cells (*arrow*).
Plate 14-17 (Fig. 14-15) Two markers of glandular differentiation combined in the same stain. The CEA appears brown while alcian blue delineates mucin droplets in the cytoplasm (*arrow*).

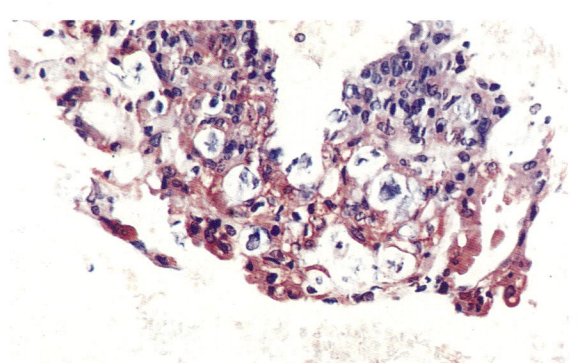

Plate 14-18

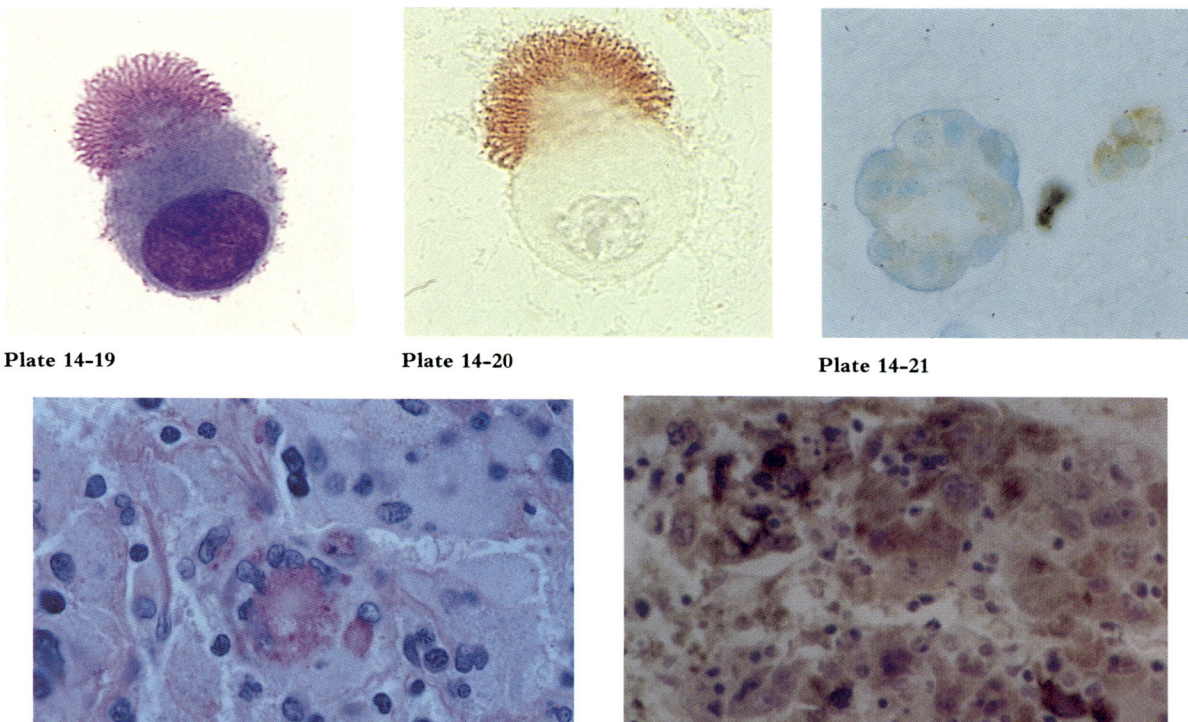

Plate 14-19 **Plate 14-20** **Plate 14-21**

Plate 14-22 **Plate 14-23**

Plate 14-18 (Fig. 14-16) Bone FNA stained with PSA. Strong immunopositivity in small gland neoplasm indicates prostatic origin of metastasis.
Plate 14-19 (Fig. 14-17A) Serous cystadenocarcinoma of the ovary. With the Giemsa stain, a tuft of cilia is noted in the apex of the cell. (Courtesy of T. Kobayashi, M.D.)
Plate 14-20 (Fig. 14-17B) Serous cystadenocarcinoma of the ovary. Immunostain with anti-CA-125 antibody clearly delineates a ciliary tuft. (Courtesy of T. Kobayshi, M.D.)
Plate 14-21 (Fig. 14-18) Lung adenocarcinoma stained by alcian blue/CEA.
Plate 14-22 (Fig. 14-19A) Cell block from hepatocellular carcinoma showing PAS-positive cytoplasmic inclusions.
Plate 14-23 (Fig. 14-19B) Cell block from hepatocellular carcinoma. Many of the bizarre tumor cells are positive for AFP.

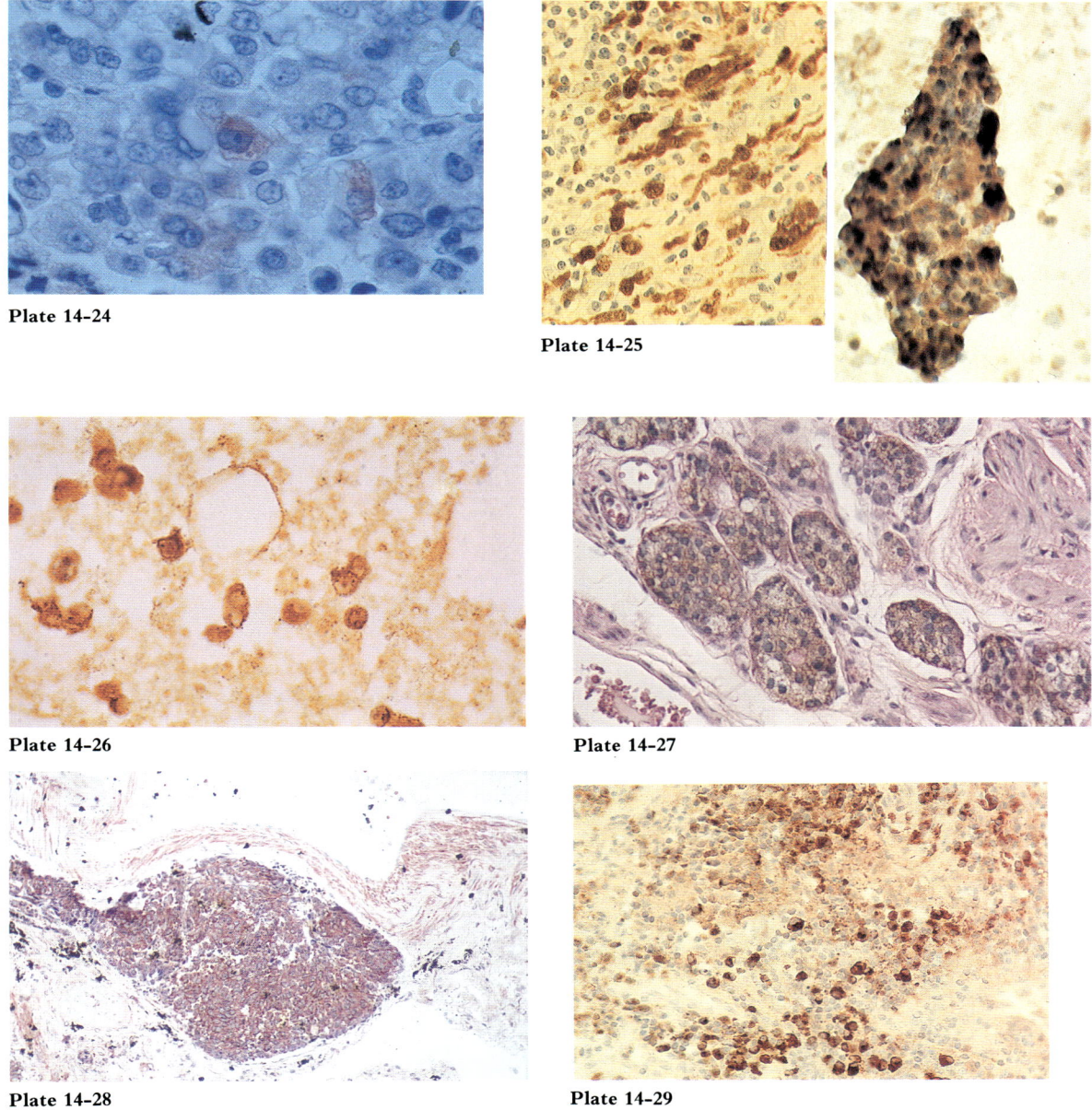

Plate 14-24 (Fig. 14-20) Hepatocellular carcinoma stained for A_1AT. Note variable positivity of individual tumor cells typical of this marker.

Plate 14-25 (Fig. 14-21) S100 positivity in melanoma. (Left) Positive tumor cells are noted within a necrotic portion of the tumor. (Right) A cluster of tumor cells from the FNA shows strong cytoplasmic immunostaining.

Plate 14-26 (Fig. 14-22) Islet cell tumor staining positively for gastrin.

Plate 14-27 (Fig. 14-23) Adenocarcinoid demonstrated by a combined stain. Immunopositivity for chromogranin appears brownish and reticular, while glandular mucin appears rose-colored.

Plate 14-28 (Fig. 14-24) Lymph node biopsy specimen stained for NSE. The positivity of the oat cell carcinoma in the center contrasts with the anthracotic pigment on the left and the negative lymph node on the right.

Plate 14-29 (Fig. 14-25) Large cell lymphoma stained for LCA. Note bright red diffuse positivity accomplished with the use of AEC as the chromogen.

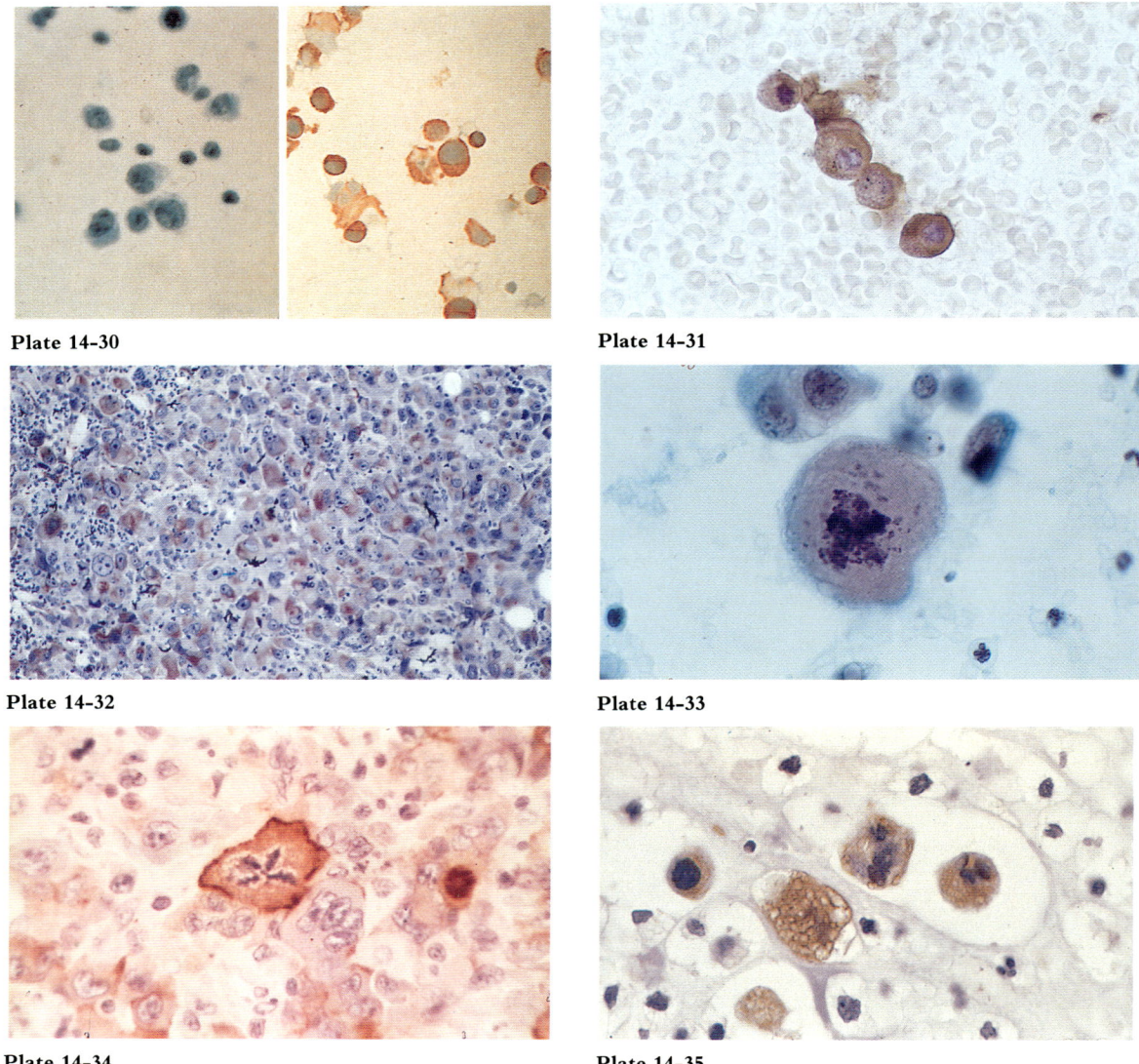

Plate 14-30 (Fig. 14-26) Plasmacytoma in pleural effusion. (Left) Malignant cells with eccentric nuclei are delineated with Papanicolaou stain. (Right) Strong immunopositivity for κ chain only confirms the monoclonal nature of the proliferation.

Plate 14-31 (Fig. 14-27) Thymoma. Larger epithelioid cells stain positively for cytokeratin.

Plate 14-32 (Fig. 14-28) Leiomyosarcoma in B5 fixed material stained for desmin. Note the faint, salmon-colored positivity of the large tumor cells. (Courtesy of B. Atkinson, M.D.)

Plate 14-33 (Fig. 14-29A) Malignant cells with abnormal mitoses. With Papanicolaou stain the giant cell is bizarre and undifferentiated. (Courtesy of B. Atkinson, M.D.)

Plate 14-34 (Fig. 14-29B) Malignant cells with abnormal mitoses. The strong A_1ACT positivity is typical of malignant fibrous histiocytoma. (Courtesy of B. Atkinson, M.D.)

Plate 14-35 (Fig. 14-30) Metastatic carcinoma staining positively for CEA.

1
Fundamentals of Cytopathology

Robert W. Astarita
Daniel A. Egerter

Cytopathology is defined as the study of cells that have exfoliated freely from tissue surfaces or that have been collected by brushing, scraping, washing, or by needle aspiration.[1-5] The diagnostic cytopathologist must be able to diagnose a variety of benign and malignant conditions by examining cells microscopically from almost anywhere in the body. Cytologic specimens are collected from mucosal surfaces, including oral cavity, bronchus, esophagus, stomach, vagina, cervix, endometrium, and bladder, to name a few. Skin, soft tissue, breast, thyroid, lymph node, and bone may be sampled by fine needle aspiration (FNA). Masses presenting in intra-abdominal sites, pelvic organs, and retroperitoneum frequently are investigated by ultrasound or by computed tomography (CT)-directed aspiration needle biopsy, precluding the necessity for invasive surgical exploration. Sputum, effusions, urine, and cerebrospinal fluid (CSF) are collected and processed for cytologic examination as well. Table 1-1 lists the common body sites from which cytologic samples are prepared. These specimens are diagnostic in most cases, influencing the patient's clinical management and treatment.

Despite the excellent credibility that experienced cytopathologists have earned, the limitations of this discipline must be acknowledged. It is axiomatic that a poorly obtained specimen or poorly fixed sample precludes interpretation in most cases. Bloody smears, smears that are too thick, smears that have air-dried before ethanol fixation (Fig. 1-1, Plate 1-1), and samples that have undergone degeneration because of excessive delay in processing usually render the specimen technically unfit for interpretation.

Poor sampling represents another diagnostic pitfall. Cervical-vaginal-endocervical (CVE) specimens that do not contain endocervical cells and sputum samples that do not contain "dust cells" are also indicative of an inadequate sample. This is the kind of problem that can lead to a false-negative interpretation. These facts must be brought to the attention of the patient's physician so that the procedure is repeated and a representative specimen obtained. Another limitation is an incomplete history. For example, omission of a history of chemotherapy, of radiation therapy, or of known renal calculi increases the possibility of a false-positive diagnosis of malignancy.

Table 1-1 Origins of Cytology Specimens

Body Site	Specimen
Female genital tract	Vaginal smear
	Cervical smear
	Cervical scrape
	Endocervical aspiration
	Endometrial aspiration
	FNA of palpable mass
	Radiologically guided FNA
Respiratory tract	Sputum
	Bronchial aspirates and washings
	Bronchial brushing
	Radiologically guided FNA
Oral cavity	Scrape
	FNA of palpable mass
Urinary tract	Urine
	Urinary tract washings and brushings
	Radiologically guided FNA
GI tract	Brushings
	Washings
	Radiologically guided FNA
Body fluids	Pleural, pericaridal, ascitic fluids
	Cerebrospinal fluid
Salivary glands	FNA
Lymph nodes	FNA
Breast	FNA
	Nipple secretions
Prostate	FNA
Pancreas	FNA
Thyroid	FNA

Examination of a slide requires a systematic approach to ensure that the entire sample is examined. The number of cases and number of slides screened per day should be limited to avoid compromising the thoroughness of the examination. Screening guidelines have been proposed and will be incorporated into federal and state regulations for most laboratories. The person responsible for screening the slide must exercise diligence in identifying the critical cells and noncellular structures in the smear.

During the screening procedure, the slide is placed on the stage with the label consistently located to the left or right of the observer. (By convention, the slide label is located to the left of the observer, in most laboratories.) The slide is first screened at low-power magnification. Significant cells and structures that are identified are then examined under high dry magnification. The critical cells are then circled or dotted. The oil immersion lens is seldom employed in cytology, although it can be useful in assessing bacterial and other infectious agents or for detailed study of nuclear or cytoplasmic structures.

An overview of the material submitted is best appreciated at low power. At this time, the cellularity, cell organization, background and staining quality can be assessed. The background of the smear provides valuable clues for the cytopathologist who is disciplined enough to analyze it in every case. For example, the presence of a tumor diathesis (necrotic tumor cytoplasm) in a cervical specimen is one of the many criteria that support the diagnosis of invasive squamous cell carcinoma.[6] In FNA May-Grünwald-Giemsa (MGG)-stained air-dried smears, the presence of extracellular "blue blobs" (Fig. 1-2, Plate 1-2) or lymphoglandular bodies (fragments of lymphocytic cytoplasm of varying size) indicates that the material was obtained from organized lymphoid tissue.[7] Lymphoglandular bodies are present in both benign and malignant lymphoid proliferations and are useful in distinguishing some non-Hodgkin's lymphomas from undifferentiated carcinomas. The background tigroid (Fig. 1-3, Plate 1-3) lacy appearance seen in testicular seminomas[7] in MGG-stained smears constitutes another useful diagnostic clue.

Recognition of noncellular structures also contributes to diagnostic accuracy. The presence of psammoma bodies (Fig. 1-4, Plate 1-4), while present in both benign and malignant conditions, may help establish the diagnosis of papillary thyroid cancer,[8] salivary gland acinic cell tumors,[9] and ovarian serous tumors.[4] Infectious agents can be overlooked quite easily, unless the observer is alert to them. Viral inclusions of cytomegalic inclusion disease (Fig. 1-5, Plate 1-5), cysts of toxoplasmosis, intracytoplasmic histoplasmosis, cysts of *Pneumocystis carinii,* and a variety of other infectious agents are identifiable in cytologic smears. The finding of hooklets of *Echinococcus* in a liver FNA with only necrotic debris and a few benign liver cells transforms an apparently nondiagnositic specimen into an interpretive coup.[10]

Examination of single cells and clusters at high-power magnification should follow scanning at low

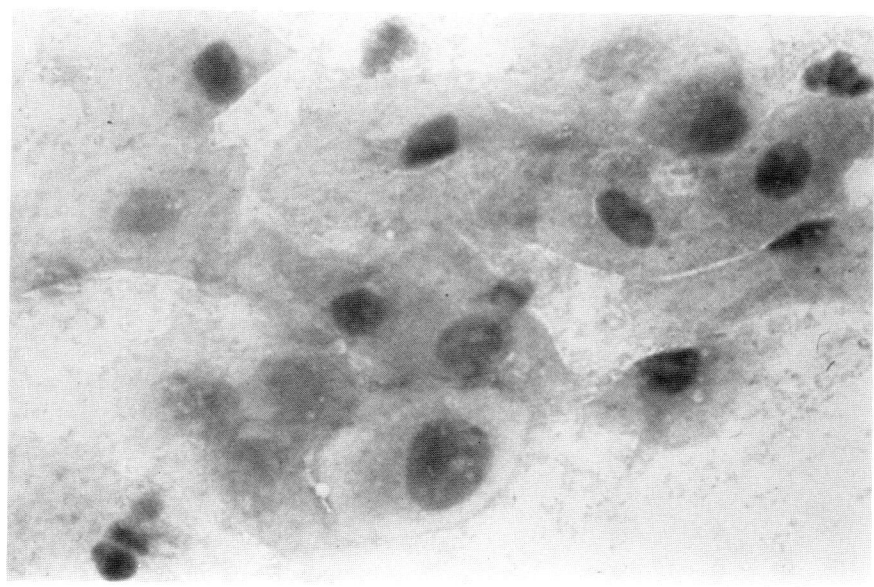

Fig. 1-1 Cervical-vaginal smear showing air-drying artifacts. Note faded homogeneous chromatin pattern and smudged nuclear detail. (Papanicolaou stain, × 250.) (See Plate 1-1.)

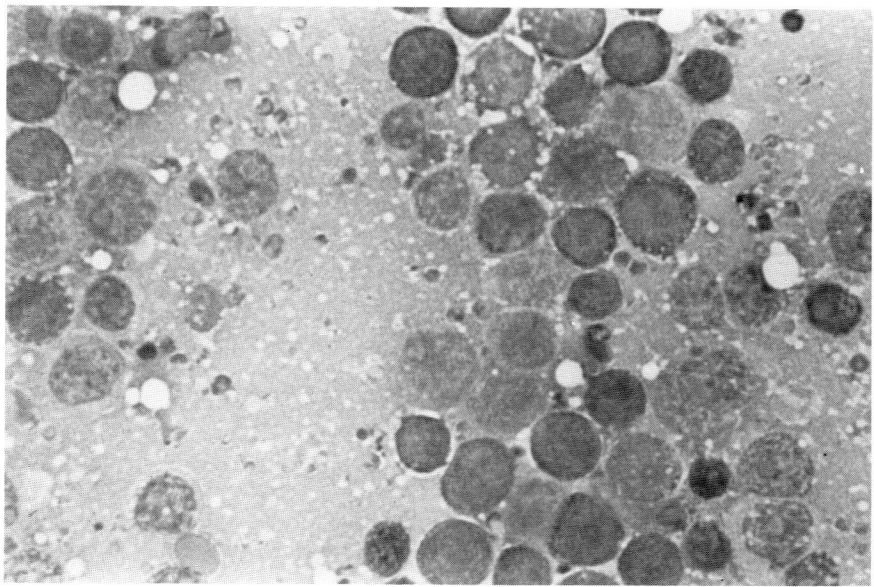

Fig. 1-2 Lymph node FNA showing large neoplastic lymphocytes containing prominent nucleoli. Note background cytoplasmic fragments or "blue blobs." (Wright-Giemsa stain, × 200.) (See Plate 1-2.)

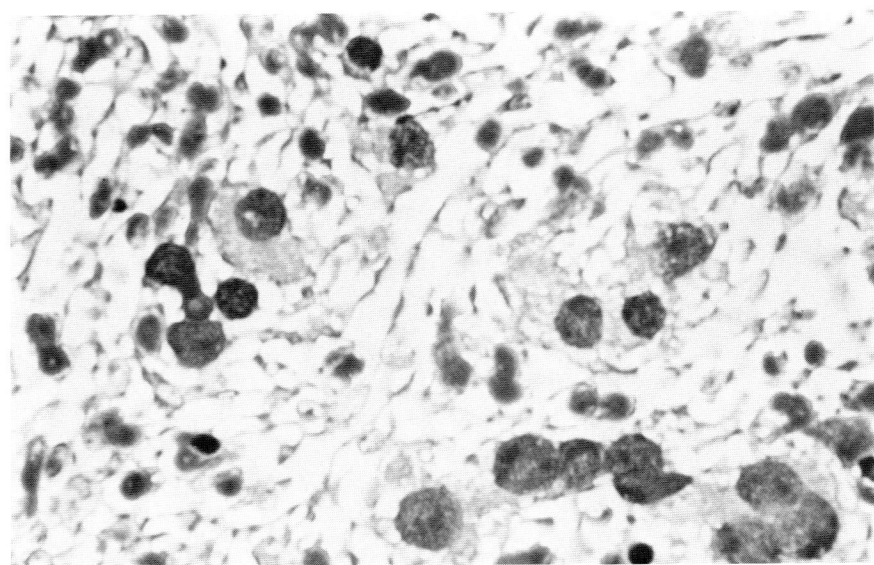

Fig. 1-3 FNA of palpable testicular mass showing cells and tigroid lace-like background, a pattern characteristic of seminoma. (MGG stain, × 250.) (See Plate 1-3.) (Case kindly contributed by Torsten Löwhagen, M.D., F.I.A.C., Karolinska Hospital, Stockholm, Sweden.)

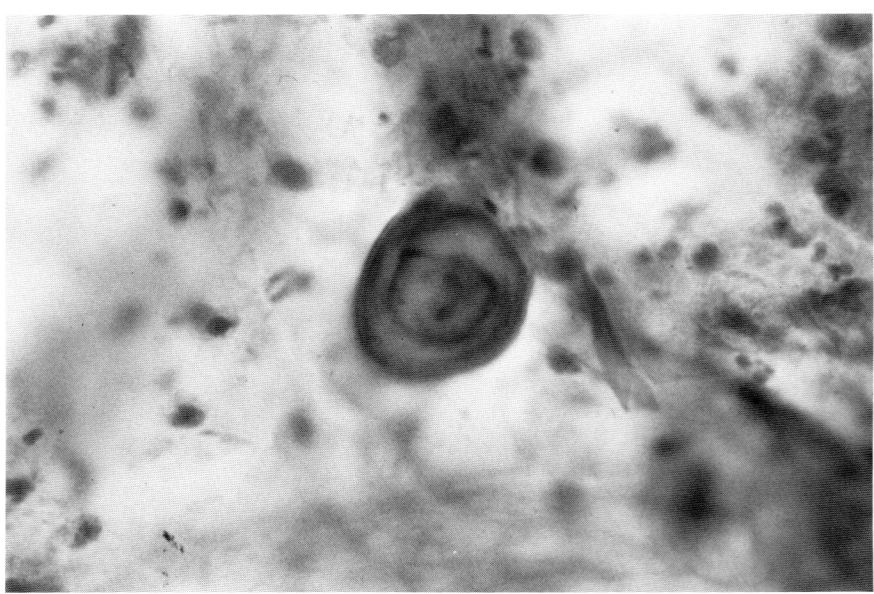

Fig. 1-4 Psammoma body showing concentric laminations. Psammoma bodies are associated with a variety of benign and malignant papillary neoplasms. (MGG stain, × 200.) (See Plate 1-4.)

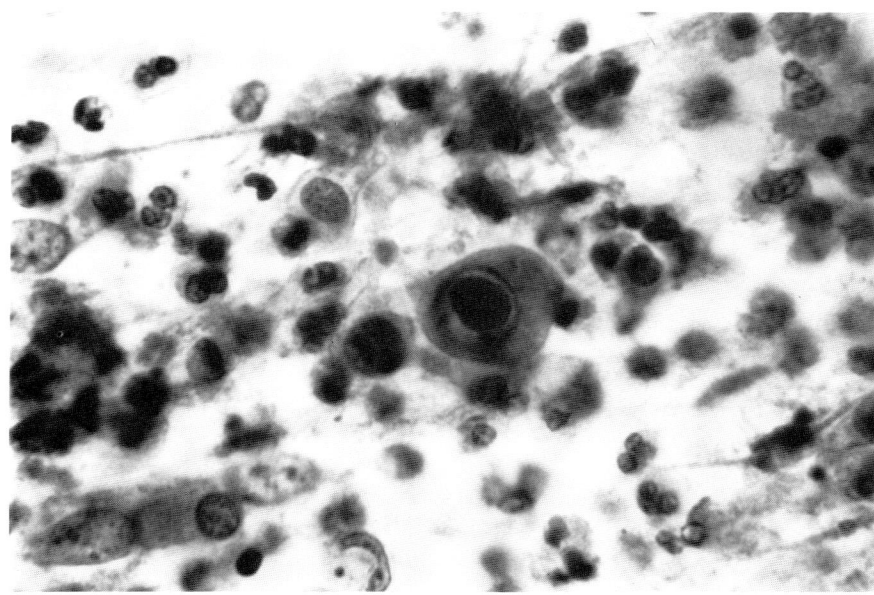

Fig. 1-5 Epithelial cells showing large intranuclear inclusions consistent with cytomegalovirus infection. (Papanicolaou stain, × 250.) (See Plate 1-5.)

power. Estimating nuclear and cell size is important in evaluating aberrations from normal. The presence of red blood cells (7.5 μm) and small lymphocytes (8 μm) in most samples provides an excellent built-in standard (check cells) against which other cells may be measured.

CYTOLOGY OF NORMAL CELLS

In order to recognize and diagnose the spectrum of benign and malignant disorders, the clinician must first come to terms with normal cell morphology. A basic histology text and atlas should be consulted. Subsequently, a variety of cytology specimens should be screened and reviewed under appropriate supervision so that the clinician can become familiarized with normal cell parameters.

Benign ciliated columnar epithelial cells are recognized easily when oriented about their long axes (Fig. 1-6, Plate 1-6); however, these cells may be present in sheets and look entirely different when viewed en-face or on-end. Endocervical columnar cells (Fig. 1-7, Plate 1-7) and gastric mucosal columnar cells (Fig. 1-8, Plate 1-8) often exhibit sheetlike and honeycomb configurations. Examining the peripheral borders of such arrangements of cells usually enables the observer to identify longitudinally oriented columnar cells. Without this clue, the novice might otherwise interpret these cells as squamous epithelial cells.

Identification of superficial cells, intermediate cells, and parabasal cells and recognition of their relative proportions in a CVE smear are important in assessing a woman's hormonal status in the reproductive years, both during pregnancy and during the peri- and postmenopausal years.

Normal transitional cells usually exfoliate as single caudate cells, rounded cells, and flat squamous-like cells. Transitional cells may also exfoliate as small aggregates (Fig. 1-9, Plate 1-9). Nuclear/cytoplasmic ratios are somewhat greater than those of benign squamous cells. In reactive conditions, transitional cells may show chromatin clumping, hyperchromatism, and multinucleation. Instrumentation or the presence of renal calculi may produce tissue fragments or large clumps of transitional cells simulating papillary carcinoma.

Normal mesothelial cells present on inner body surfaces, such as pleura and peritoneum, exfoliate singly or in small haphazardly arranged clusters

6 PRACTICAL CYTOPATHOLOGY

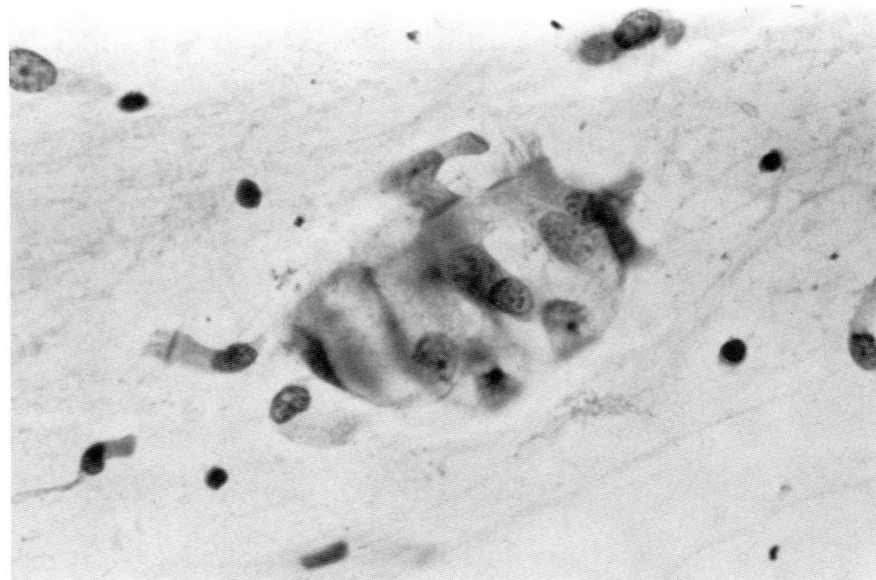

Fig. 1-6 Ribbon of bronchial columnar epithelial cells containing terminal bars and cilia. (Papanicolaou stain, × 250.) (See Plate 1-6.)

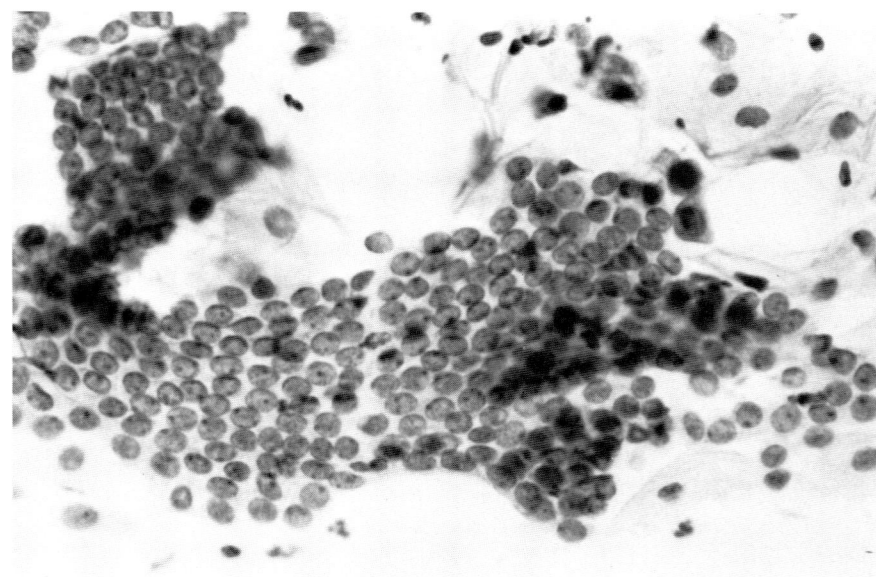

Fig. 1-7 Sheets of benign endocervical cells approaching honeycomb configuration. Columnar origin is more difficult to ascertain when cells are oriented en face. (Papanicolaou stain, × 125.) (See Plate 1-7.)

FUNDAMENTALS OF CYTOPATHOLOGY 7

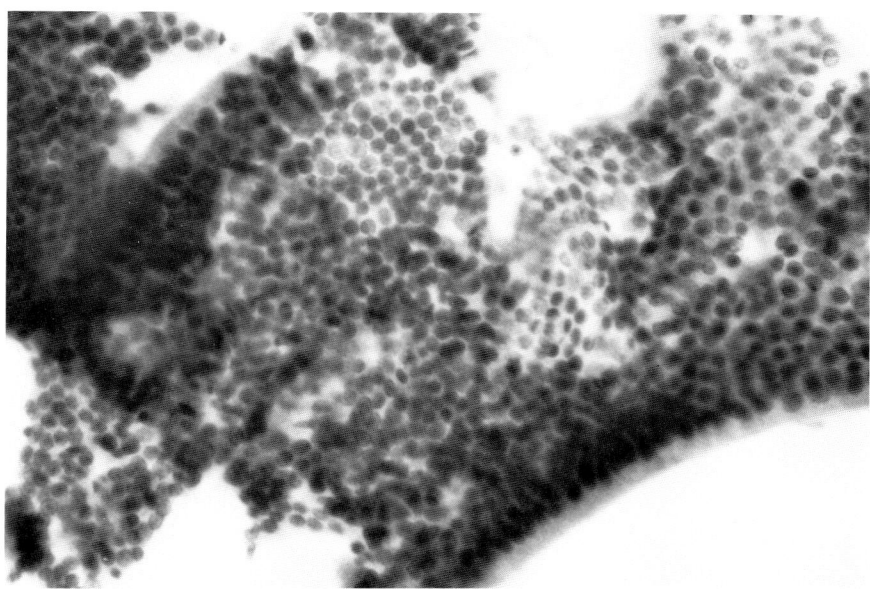

Fig. 1-8 Sheet of benign gastric columnar cells showing honeycomb pattern. Columnar origin is detectable at periphery of this tissue fragment. (Papanicolaou stain, × 100.) (See Plate 1-8.)

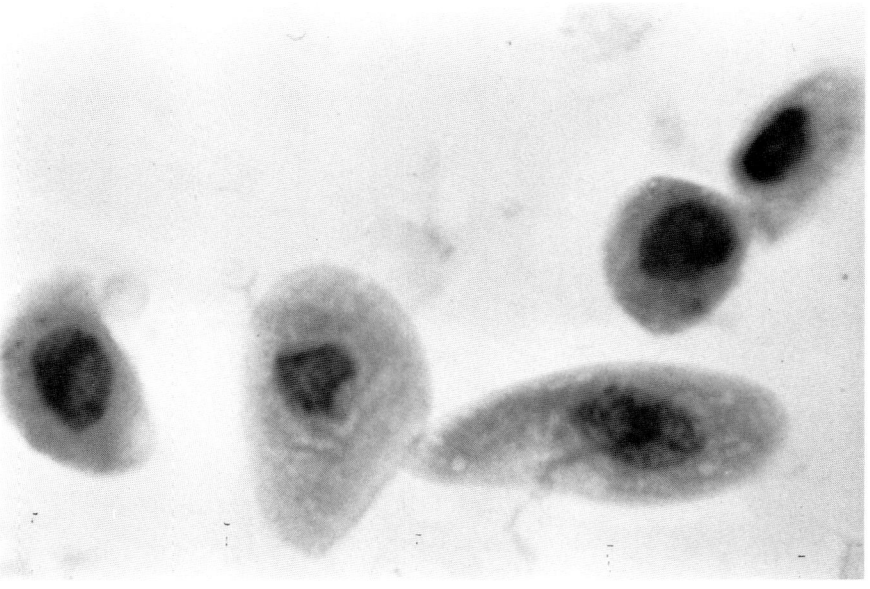

Fig. 1-9 Transitional cells from voided urine specimen (Papanicolaou stain, × 500.) (See Plate 1-9.)

8 PRACTICAL CYTOPATHOLOGY

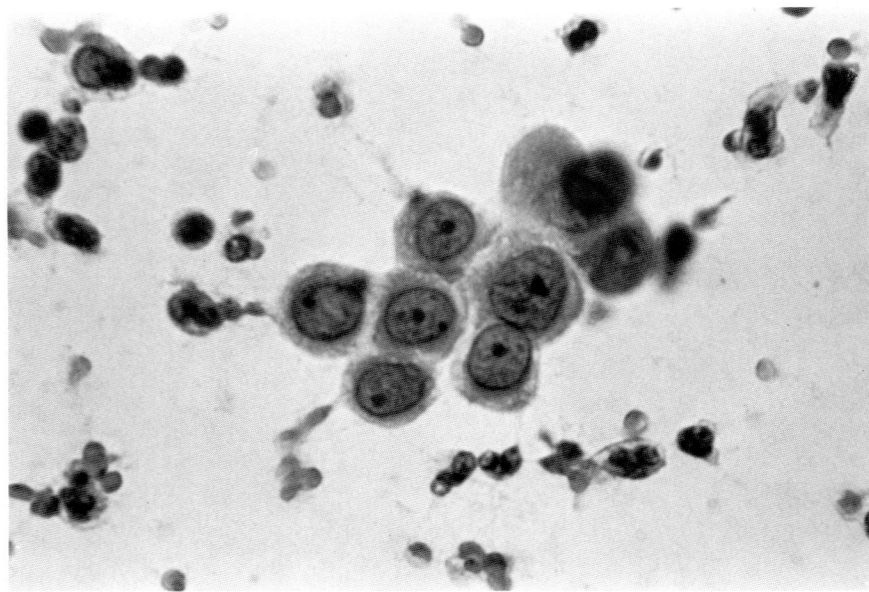

Fig. 1-10 Pleural fluid. Haphazardly arranged group of mesothelial cells showing intercellular spaces or "windows." (Papanicolaou stain, × 250.) (See Plate 1-10.)

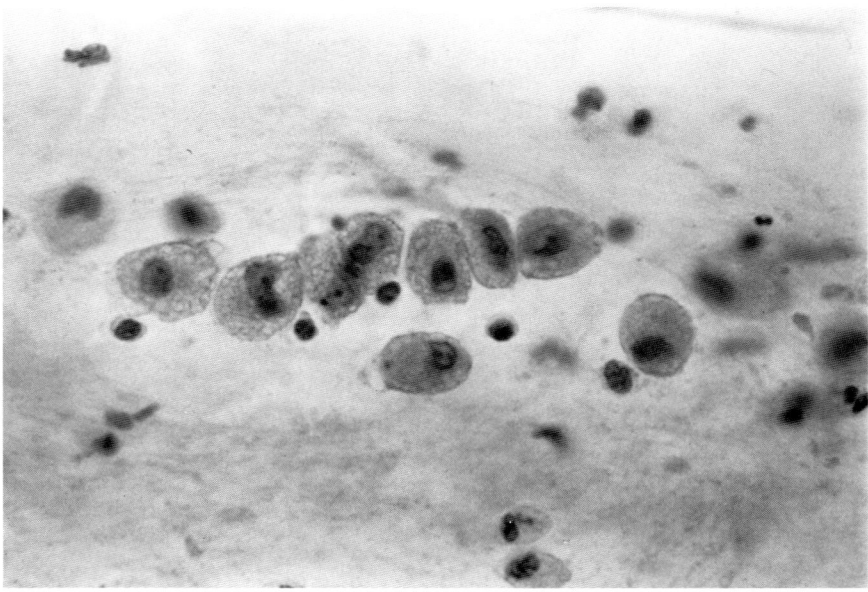

Fig. 1-11 Sputum smear showing benign histiocytes with some indented nuclei and bubbly cytoplasm. (Papanicolaou stain, × 160.) (See Plate 1-11.)

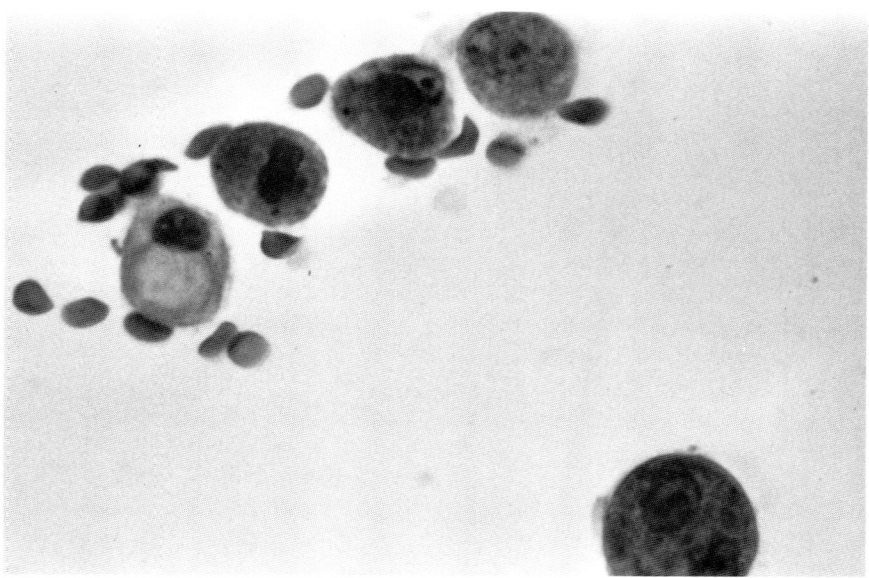

Fig. 1-12 Specimen from lung FNA showing histocytes contaiining intracytoplasmic anthracotic pigment and single histiocyte with large cytoplasmic vacuole. (Papanicolaou stain, × 250). (See Plate 1-12.)

showing intercellular spaces or "windows" (Fig. 1-10, Plate 1-10). Reactive mesothelial cells may demonstrate multicellular aggregates, coarsely granular chromatin, and prominent nucleoli, simulating malignancy in some conditions (e.g., pulmonary infarct). Benign mesothelial cells may contain large intracytolasmic vacuoles mimicking malignant signet-ring type cells in an adenocarcinoma. In these cases, the observer must be confident that the nuclear criteria for malignancy are met before making a diagnosis of malignancy. Other criteria for the diagnosis of a malignant effusion are enumerated in Chapter 11.

Benign histiocytes (Fig. 1-11, Plate 1-11), are most often identified as single cells; however, they may present as cell aggregates showing a haphazard arrangement. Histiocyte nuclei are usually vesicular and eccentrically oriented. Reactive histiocytes may show indented kidney bean-like nuclei or multiple nuclei. Coarse chromatin aggregates, irregular nuclear membranes, prominent nucleoli, and increased mitoses may all be seen in activated histiocytes. The cytoplasm usually is bubbly or vacuolated and sometimes contains anthracotic pigment such as seen in the "dust cells" (Fig. 1-12, Plate 1-12) from a good sputum sample.

CYTOLOGIC CRITERIA OF MALIGNANCY

There is no single cytologic feature that establishes a malignant diagnosis. Once made, the diagnosis of malignancy determines therapeutic action. Surgery, chemotherapy, and/or radiation therapy may follow the diagnosis of malignancy, with all the potential benefits and consequences for the patient. This diagnosis must be made objectively, with complete confidence and thorough knowledge of the patient's clinical history and laboratory studies.

There are cytologic criteria that, taken together, argue strongly in favor of a diagnosis of malignancy.[11] These criteria are not cast in stone, however. In fact, there are rare benign lesions that fulfill malignant criteria and, conversely, there are malignant neoplasms that appear deceptively bland. For example, the spindle cells seen in an FNA from an early nodular fasciitis (a benign reactive proliferation), may exhibit nuclear pleomorphism, hyperchromatism, increased mitoses, and prominent macronucleoli.[4] By contrast, cells from an adenoid cystic carcinoma of the parotid gland may appear deceptively benign.[7] In this case, the cytologic diagnosis of adenoid cystic carcinoma is established by the identification of characteristic rigidly spherical stromal balls or metachromatic basement membrane globules as seen in MGG-stained specimens (Fig. 1-13, Plate 1-13).

Recognizing these limitations, it is important to become familiar with the general cytologic criteria of malignancy, the nucleus of the cell representing the focal point of our examination (Table 1-2). Nuclei are viewed at high-power magnification. Variation in nuclear shape, size, and staining quality (Fig. 1-14, Plate 1-14), as well as increased nuclear size in proportion to cytoplasmic content, nuclear hyperchromatism, irregular nuclear contours, abnormal chromatin distribution, enlarged irregular nucleoli (Fig. 1-14, Plate 1-14), abnormal mitoses, and loss of cell cohesion argue in favor of a diagnosis of malignancy.[12]

Malignant nuclei are usually larger than their benign counterparts and demonstrate a high nuclear/cytoplasmic ratio. The increased nuclear size of malignant cells generally correlates with increased amounts of DNA and DNA-associated proteins. Malignant nuclei often exhibit marked variation (Figs. 1-15 and 1-16, Plates 1-15 and 1-16) in size and shape,[11-13] in contrast to benign cells, which contain more uniform nuclei (Fig. 1-17, and 1-18, Plates 1-17 and 1-18).

Malignant nuclei usually demonstrate irregular nuclear contours and projections, indentations, sharp angulated borders, and irregular nuclear membrane thickening. When malignant cell groups are present, nuclear molding is observed in which nuclear borders follow the contour of cytoplasmic vacuoles or cell membranes. For example, nuclear molding is a distinctive feature in cases of small cell undifferentiated carcinoma (oat cell carcinoma).

Examination of the nuclear chromatin pattern is an essential step in distinguishing malignant nuclei from benign nuclei. Benign chromatin patterns are characterized by an even, uniformly granular distribution. Malignant nuclei show an uneven distribution of coarse clumped chromatin, irregular angulated "cookie cutter sharp" chromatin, increased basophilic staining (hyperchromasia), irregular condensation of chromatin along the nuclear membrane, parachromatin clearing, and large irregular angulated nucleoli.

While malignant cells may contain multiple nuclei and increased mitoses, these features do not represent

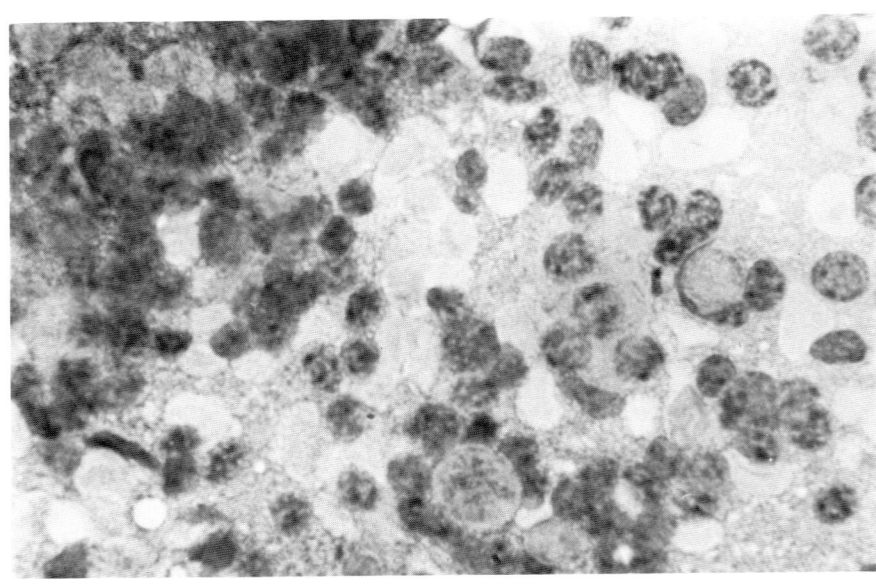

Fig. 1-13 Parotid gland FNA showing small uniform cells surrounding a central metachromatic basement membrane globule characteristic of adenoid cystic carcinoma. (MGG stain, × 250.) (See Plate 1-13.) (Case courtesy of Torsten Löwhagen, M.D., F.I.A.C., Karolinska Hospital, Stockholm, Sweden.)

Table 1-2 Nuclear Criteria of Malignancy

Nuclear size	Usually larger than benign counterparts; malignant nuclei variable in size
Nuclear-cytoplasmic ratio	Increased
Nuclear shape	Moderate to marked variation in nuclear shape
Nuclear molding	Secondary criterion suggestive of malignancy, especially in small cell undifferentiated carcinomas
Nuclear membrane	Irregular thickening, angulation; indentations and projections
Chromatin	Uneven chromatin distribution, variation in chromatin size and shape; coarse, clumped, irregular, and sharply angulated chromatin ("cookie-cutter sharp"); parachromatin clearing
Number of nuclei	Multinuclearity unreliable malignant criterion; malignant cells may contain multiple nuclei but variation among nuclei and malignant nuclear features more important
Mitoses	Increased mitoses unreliable malignant criterion; look for abnormal mitoses and aneuploidy

dependable criteria for malignancy. Since benign reactive or reparative cells may exhibit similar features, the cytologist must concentrate on the more compelling nuclear characteristics of malignancy already described.

Cytoplasmic features contribute relatively little to the diagnosis of malignancy. For some observers, a high nuclear/cytoplasmic ratio raises the question of malignancy. While this statement may be valid for large cells, it does not hold up for small cells, such as reserve cells or lymphocytes, which normally contain scant cytoplasm. Another pitfall that must be avoided is interpreting a truly bare nucleus (from a degenerated cell that has lost part or all of its cytoplasm) as indicative of malignancy because of an apparently increased nuclear/cytoplasmic ratio. Ciliated bronchial columnar cells may fragment in some inflammatory conditions, leaving behind a nucleated cytoplasmic portion and an anucleate ciliated cytoplasmic tuft (ciliocytophthoria). The degenerated nucleated portion of the cell may mimic dysplasia or malignancy. Intact cells should be evaluated, while degenerated cells should be avoided at all costs.

Cytoplasmic features can be helpful in the classification of malignant tumors. For example, most squamous carcinomas (Fig. 1-19, Plate 1-19) contain sharp cell borders, an outer hyaline-like ectoplasm, and an inner amorphous endoplasm in which the nucleus is found. Concentric cytoplasmic refractile rings, marked orangeophilia, and keratin pearl formation (Fig. 1-20, Plate 1-20) may be seen in cases of squamous carcinoma as well. Squamous carcinoma is often characterized by the presence of malignant spindle cells and by "tadpole" cells that contain abnormal coal black nuclei at the head of the cell, and an endoplasmic spiral core (Herxheimer's spiral) extends to the tail. The interface between the endoplasmic spiral core and the surrounding ectoplasm appears as a refractile structure in these cells. Cells exhibiting a tadpole configuration and malignant nuclear features are essentially diagnostic of squamous carcinoma.

Cytoplasmic characteristics may also prove useful in cases of adenocarcinoma, in which single secretory type vacuoles are present in some cases, displacing the nucleus to the periphery in a signet ring configuration (Fig. 1-21, Plate 1-21). Frequently there is a loss of cytoplasm at the nuclear/vacuolar cytoplasmic angle. This phenomenon, in combination with malignant nuclear abnormalities, is diagnostic of adenocarcinomas.

Cell relationships and the architecture of tissue fragments that may be present in cytologic specimens also prove revealing. For example, most adenocarcinomas exfoliate as cell groups and aggregates, sometimes exhibiting a common cytoplasmic border, or community border. Squamous carcinomas more often exfoliate as single cells. Malignant effusions arising from adenocarcinomas of the breast usually present as cell balls (Figs. 1-19 and 1-22, Plates 1-19 and 1-22). Effusions arising from adenocarcinomas

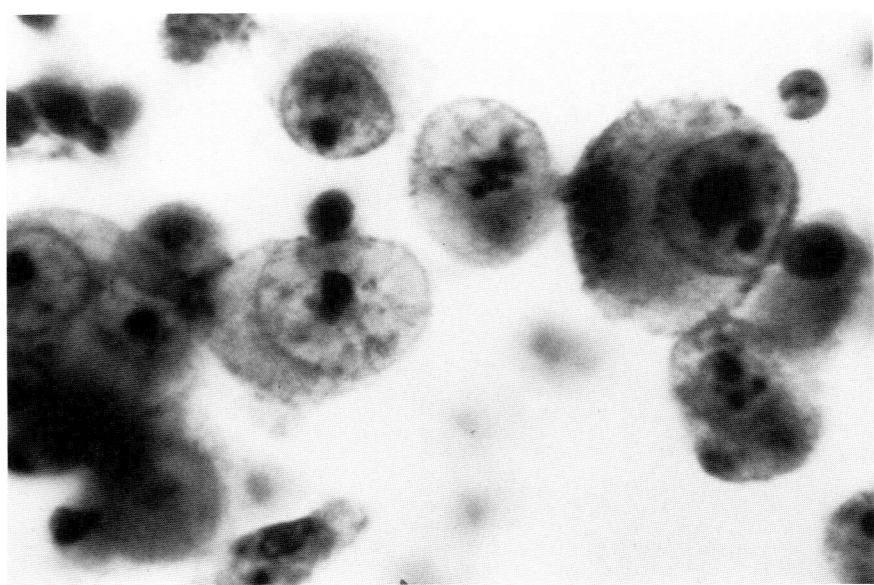

Fig. 1-14 Nuclepore filter preparations of pleural fluid showing metastatic malignant melanoma. Cells exhibit anisonucleosis, anisochromatosis, increased nuclear cytoplasmic ratios, prominent irregular nucleoli, and intracytoplasmic melanin pigment. (Papanicolaou stain, × 450.) (See Plate 1-14.)

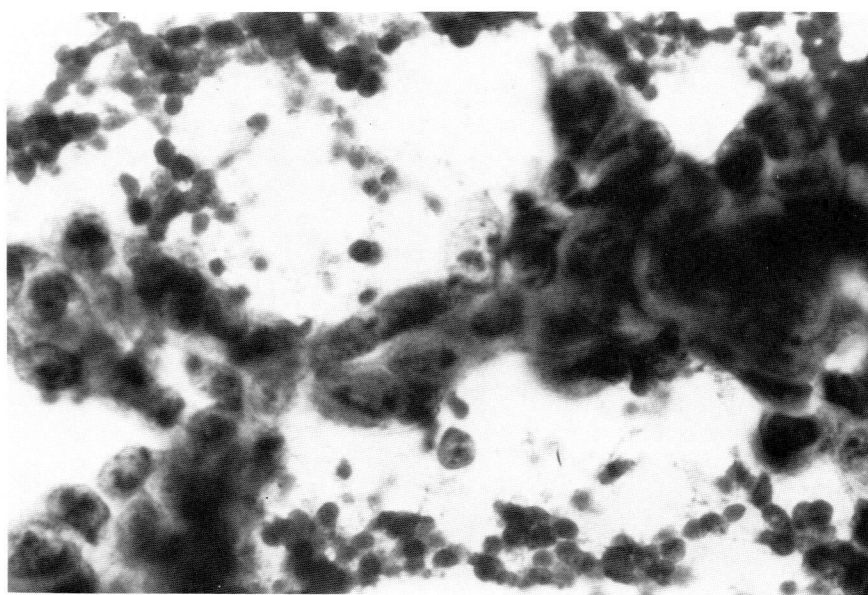

Fig. 1-15 Brushing from mass at ampulla of Vater containing malignant cells from an adenocarcinoma. The cells are pleomorphic and show irregular distribution of chromatin, high nuclear/cytoplasmic ratios, and prominent nucleoli. (Papanicolaou stain; × 200.) (See Plate 1-15.)

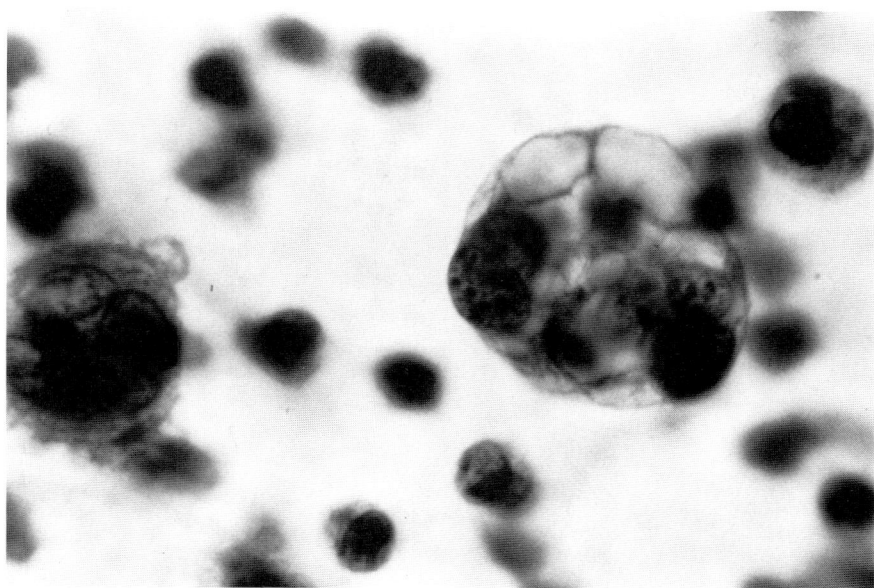

Fig. 1-16 Cell balls representing metastatic adenocarcinoma in pleural effusion. Malignant cells show overlapping nuclei, irregular distribution of chromatin, nuclear variation in size and shape, irregular nuclear outlines, and large intracytoplasmic vacuoles. (Papanicolaou stain, × 200.) (See Plate 1-16.)

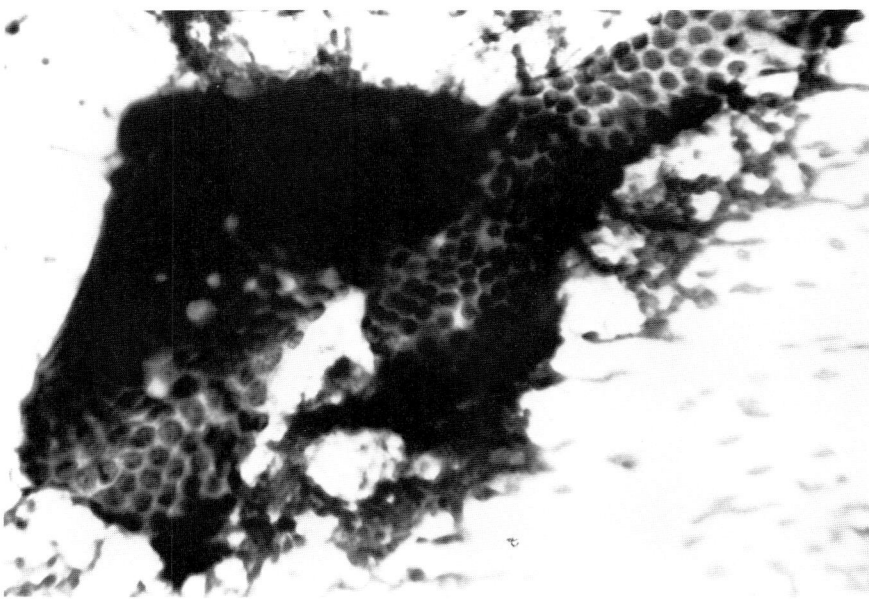

Fig. 1-17 Benign cells. Duodenal brushing from ampulla of Vater reveals a monolayered sheet of cells of uniform size and shape. Chromatin is evenly distributed, and nucleoli are inconspicuous. (Papanicolaou stain, × 200.) (See Plate 1-17.)

14 PRACTICAL CYTOPATHOLOGY

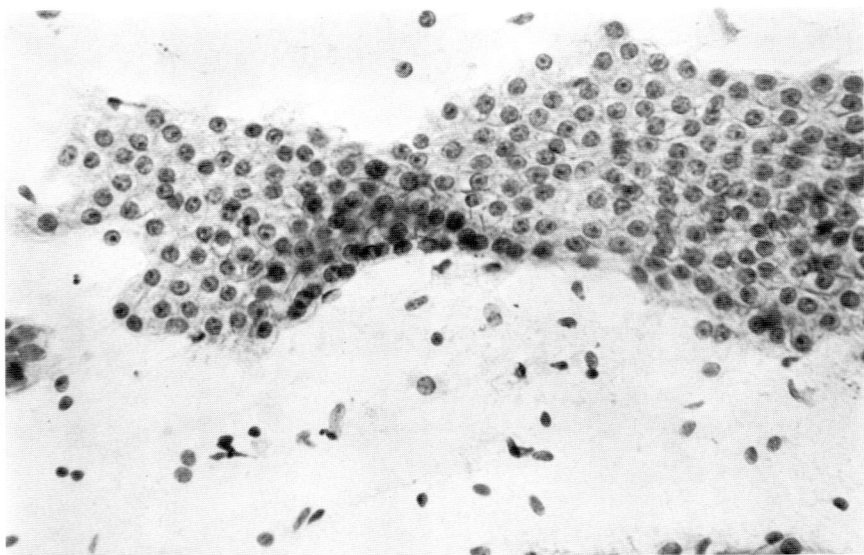

Fig. 1-18 FNA of a palpable breast mass showing a sheet of benign ductal cells of uniform size and shape with little overlapping of nuclei. Note scattered single naked nuclei in background, characteristic of benign breast specimens. (Papanicolaou stain, × 160.) (See Plate 1-18.)

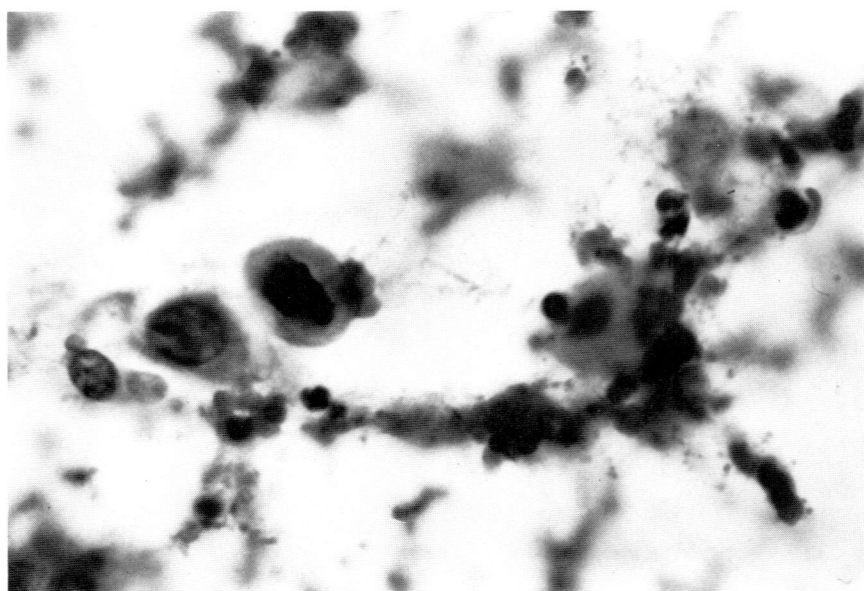

Fig. 1-19 Lung sputum specimen showing malignant squamous cells containing orangeophilic refractile cytoplasm and coal black atypical nuclei. (Papanicolaou stain, × 160.) (See Plate 1-19.)

FUNDAMENTALS OF CYTOPATHOLOGY 15

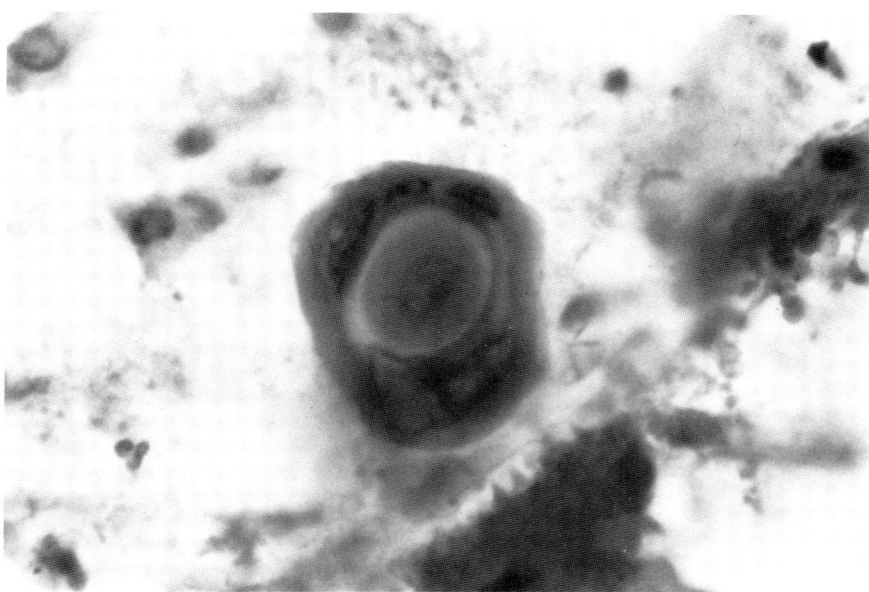

Fig. 1-20 Lung sputum from patient with squamous carcinoma illustrating onion skin configuration of keratin pearl and dirty background of tumor diathesis. (Papanicolaou stain, × 250.) (See Plate 1-20.)

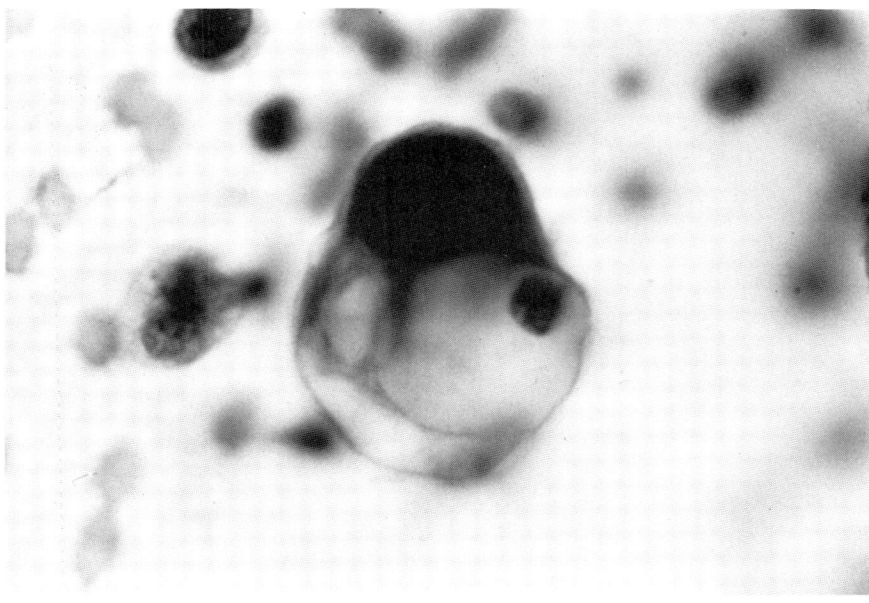

Fig. 1-21 Filter preparation from pleural fluid of metastatic adenocarcinoma showing signet ring configuration, in which the malignant nucleus is displaced by a large intracytoplasmic secretory vacuole. (Papanicolaou stain, × 250.) (See Plate 1-21.)

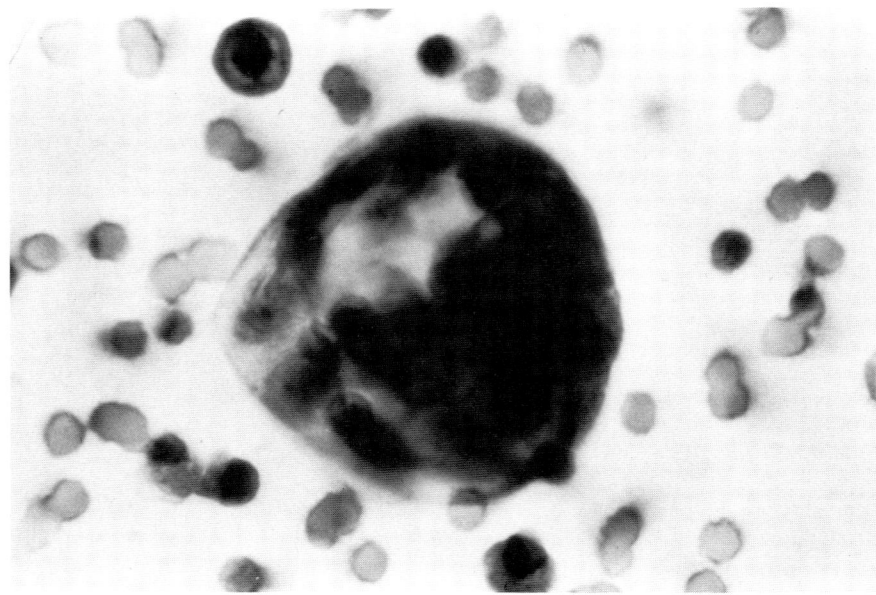

Fig. 1-22 Nuclepore filter preparation from pleural fluid containing cell ball configuration characteristic of metastatic breast carcinoma. (Papanicolaou stain, × 250.) (See Plate 1-22.)

of the ovary may present as cell balls or papillary aggregates of cells. Papillary configurations of cytologically malignant cells are also seen in FNA specimens from thyroid, lung, and other midline organs.

CYTOLOGIC METHODS AND TECHNIQUES

The accuracy of cytologic diagnosis is predicated on a representative specimen, optimal fixation, and adequate preparation and staining of the samples obtained. A detailed account of cytologic techniques is beyond the scope of this book, and the reader is encouraged to consult any of the following references for a more comprehensive treatment of the subject.[1-3] A brief discussion of cytologic techniques follows here.

After preparing smears rapid fixation is required to preserve cytologic detail. Delay in fixation results in air-drying artifacts. The fixation of choice for most aspiration biopsy smears is 95 percent ethanol; it can also be used as a final fixative for smears made from fresh fluids or from fluids prefixed in 50 percent ethanol.

CVE and other smears are sometimes sprayed with a coating fixative. Commercial coating fixatives and some hairsprays with a high alcohol content may be used with good results, especially when specimens are mailed to an outside reference center for staining and interpretation. When an aerosol-type fixative is used, the smears should be sprayed immediately from a distance of approximately 10 to 12 inches. The appropriate distance for optimal fixation should be determined on site by testing the spray fixative at varying distances from the slide. Water-soluble coating fixatives should be removed before staining by immersing the slides in two solutions of 95 percent ethanol for 5 to 10 minutes each.

When bloody smears are encountered, RBC may be hemolyzed using Carnoy's fixative. However, smears should not be allowed to stand in this fixative for more than 5 minutes, or nuclear detail will suffer. It is important that Carnoys' fixative be prepared fresh, since it deteriorates with time, forming hydrochloric acid. Carnoy's fixative should not be used with Nuclepore or Gelman filters, since it will damage them.

Fluid specimens are preserved in a variety of ways, depending on the source. Those cells bathed in high protein-containing fluids, such as pleural and peritoneal body fluids, remain well preserved for 1 to 2 days. Bronchial aspirates and sputums that contain considerable mucus may be refrigerated for up to 24 hours with reasonable cell preservation.[1] Specimens from CSF and urine with a low mucus and protein content must be processed immediately, however, or prefixed, since rapid enzymatic deterioration of cells occurs. Prefixation is defined as a fluid specimen collected in a medium that preserves morphology up to the time the slide is prepared.[1] Cells requiring prefixation are usually added in equal volume to a 50 percent ethanol solution, although other fixatives may be employed as well (e.g., Soccomanno's fixative). Cytologic specimens from stomach contain hydrochloric acid, which is destructive to cells. Such specimens should be collected on ice and processed immediately to avoid cell damage.

Most cytologic specimens, including those obtained by FNA, are sufficiently concentrated to allow for preparation of thin-layered direct smears on glass slides. By contrast, direct smears from 10 ml CSF or 100 ml of pleural fluid are impractical because of cell dilution in the fluid. Techniques that have been developed to solve this problem are enumerated here. While applauding the advantages of these methods, cytopathologists must also recognize the unique artifacts that may result from their use.

In many cases, simple centrifugation at 600 gravities for 10 minutes concentrates cells in a button. After most of the supernatant is discarded, the button in resuspended and smeared directly onto glass slides. Membrane filters are another way to concentrate suspended cells. The three commercially available brands, Gelman (Scientific Products, McGraw Park, IL 60085), Millipore (Millipore Filter Corp., Bedford, MA 01730), and Nuclepore (Wallabs, P.O. Box 455, Fairfax, CA 94930), are thin membranes through which fluid is drawn by a vacuum while cells of a minimum diameter are retained. The filter is then mounted on a slide, fixed, and stained. Urine and body fluids should be collected fresh because prefixation coagulates proteins that can clog filters. Prefixation also renders cells rigidly spherical interferring with the quality of the filter preparation. Some investigators suggest washing urine and body fluid specimens through successive centrifugation steps to remove salts, proteins, and debris, which can clog filters.[1] Final filter preparations are fixed in 95 percent ethanol and Papanicolaou stained in most laboratories.

For fluid specimens with few cells, cytocentrifugation concentrates cells onto a 6-mm circle on a glass slide, while the supernatant is absorbed by filter paper. Elegantly uniform smears of suspended tumor cell suitable for immunoperoxidase staining may be achieved with this method.[14] When an especially cell poor specimen is encountered (e.g., CSF), precentrifugation of the fluid may be necessary. Air-dried Romanowsky-stained (i.e., Wright's, MGG, Diff-Quik) cytocentrifuge preparations are particularly useful for examining inflammatory cells and hematologic malignancies. Artifacts of cytocentrifugation include flattening and enlargement of all cells, cell lysis, and air-drying of ethanol-fixed, Papanicolaou-stained specimens. Exaggeration of irregularities of nuclear contour also occurs, a fact that may prove spuriously alarming when evaluating cytocentrifuged lymphocytes.

Sputum specimens frequently contain large amounts of ropy viscous mucus, which makes it difficult to transfer the sample to slides in a uniform manner. The addition of an ethanol-based Carbowax fixative such as Saccamano's fixative and blending at high speed in a Waring Blendor will break up the mucus.[15] Alternatively, a mucolytic agent such as Mucolexx (Lerner Laboratories, Stamford, CT 06920) can be used.[1] After concentration by centrifugation the cells are spread evenly on a slide.

One of the oldest methods of processing fluids (usually effusions) is the preparation of cell blocks for histologic examination. First fluids may be centrifuged fresh to concentrate cells for preparation of smears, after which fixative is added and the specimen is centrifuged again to concentrate cells as a button. The supernatant is decanted and the tissue pellet is removed, wrapped in lens paper, or embedded in melted agar and processed routinely for paraffin section.[1] Plastic-embedded sections also can be prepared for application of immunohistochemistry and enzyme histochemistry techniques.[16] The advantages of cell blocks include the potential to make many sections for special stains and other ancillary studies. Tissue architecture may also be revealed when tissue fragments are included in the sections. It has also been reported that the use of the cell blocks may contribute to additional diagnoses.[17] The disadvantages of this method include increased time and expense and the loss of important nuclear and cytoplasmic detail due to the increased number of processing steps. While well-prepared cytologic smears yield results equal or superior to that of cell blocks, preparation of cell blocks is worthwhile, since opportunities to perform special studies and assess tissue architecture are enhanced.

Special stains are indicated in cytologic specimens just as they are in surgical pathology. For example, mucicarmine, and Alcian blue are helpful in detecting mucin production, and methyl green pyronin (MGP) is useful in the differential staining of DNA and RNA and in assessing cytoplasmic RNA content in high-turnover lymphomas and other malignant neoplasms. Infectious agents are detected with standard bacterial, fungal, and mycobacterial stains.[10] Previously stained slides can be decolorized and restained with virtually any stain.

Cytologic material is also suitable for ancillary studies such as immunocytochemistry[18–21] and enzyme cytochemistry,[22,23] nucleic acid hybridization,[24] transmission electron microscopy (TEM)[25,26] and scanning electron microscopy (SEM),[27] flow cytometric quantitation of DNA,[28–32] computer-based image analysis of cells,[33] and measurements of DNA synthesis.[4] Just as in histology, immunocytochemistry can help in the differential diagnosis of poorly differentiated neoplasms seen in cytologic preparations.[34–36] Important treatment decisions may be influenced by immunocytochemical characterization of lymphoid tumors[14,21] and by evaluation of estrogen receptors in breast cancer diagnosed from FNA.[37] Important prognostic information can be derived from typing of human papillomavirus in cervical intraepithelial neoplasia (CIN) using nucleic acid probes.[24] DNA analysis of tumors can be performed on aspirated and exfoliated tissue.[38,39] It appears that the assessment of nuclear aneuploidy and other characteristics will prove important in determining prognosis and treatment.[40] In the future, these techniques may allow us to classify tumors more accurately and to predict their biologic behavior more precisely.

FINE NEEDLE ASPIRATION

At many centers, the cytopathologist performs as well as interprets FNA. FNA diagnosis is most accurate when the same qualified person performs the aspiration, prepares the smears and interprets the biopsy.[41–43] For palpable masses, a 22-gauge or 25-gauge needle (attached to a syringe mounted onto a syringe holder) is introduced into the mass through alcohol-wiped skin. The dominant hand manipulates the syringe holder, and the other hand fixes the mass between two fingers. The biopsy is performed by moving the needle back and forth within the mass while varying the angle of the needle and exerting suction on the syringe. The procedure is terminated by releasing the negative pressure before removing the needle. Pressure is applied to the biopsy site by an assistant or by the patient while the aspirator prepares alcohol-fixed slides for Papanicolaou[44] and hematoxylin and eosin (H & E) staining, and air-dried slides for MGG staining. Unless one is dealing with a cyst, all of the diagnostic material should be contained in the needle, not in the syringe itself. After the cyst fluid is drained completely, a repeat FNA of any residual mass is indicated.[5]

Preparation of the aspirate smear is a critical step. A good smear results in an evenly distributed monolayer of cells. The smear must be fixed immediately in 95 percent ethanol for Papanicolaou or hematoxylin and eosin (H & E) staining or air-dried for Romanovsky-type staining (MGG stain, Wright's, Diff-Quik). Other fixatives such as absolute alcohol, formal-acetone, cold-buffered acetone may be used to improve antigen preservation for immunocytochemistry studies. We routinely use both air-dried and alcohol-fixed smears. Generally, Romanovsky type stains yield more information about the cytoplasm, while the Papanicolaou stain provides excellent nuclear detail (Table 1-3).

Drying artifacts may occur in Papanicolaou-stained slides when smears dry before fixation. The hallmarks of air-drying include a faded homogeneous chromatin pattern and blurring of nuclear detail (Fig. 1-1). Because these artifacts seriously hinder accurate interpretation, ethanol fixation must occur immediately after the smear is made. In unskilled hands, an artifactually distorted, crushed, thick, or dried smear is encountered, which defies interpretation by the most experienced cytopathologist.[7]

Anyone performing FNA must be adept at the four basic smearing methods that have been developed to address varying consistencies of the aspirated sample. Learning these methods is best accomplished by practicing the maneuvers under the close supervi-

Table 1-3 Comparison of Air-Dried and Wet-Fixed Smears: General Properties

	Air-dried MGC	Wet-fixed Papanicolaou
Cell and nuclear size	Exaggerated, differences enhanced	Comparable to tissue sections
Nuclear detail	Fair	Excellent
Cytoplasmic detail	Well demonstrated	Poorly demonstrated
Nucleoli	Not always discernable	Well demonstrated
Stromal components	Well shown and often differentially stained	Poorly demonstrated
Partially necrotic tissue	Poor definition of cell details	Good definition of single intact cells
Tissue fragments	Cells poorly seen due to heavily stained ground substance	Individual cells usually seen clearly

(Modified from Orell et al.,[5] with permission.)

sion of an expert. Although perfecting these techniques requires actual hands-on experience, an excellent article by Abele et al.[45] on this subject provides a good starting point for the novice.

Material obtained from FNA is also suitable for viral, fungal, mycobacterial, and bacterial culture. In cases in which infection is suspected, an additional aspirate is performed; the material is rinsed in fetal calf serum (FCS) and distributed for various microbiological studies. At San Francisco General Hospital, where infectious diseases are prevalent in the large refugee and acquired immune deficiency syndrome (AIDS) populations, aspirates routinely are submitted for culture.[46] Success of culture depends upon the amount of material submitted with greater yields correlating with increased volumes of aspirate.[5]

LABORATORY ORGANIZATION

The operation of a quality cytology laboratory requires a nucleus of competent well-trained cytotechnologists, a viable documented quality control program, and appropriate supervision and leadership provided by the chief cytotechnologist and the attending pathologist. Accurate interpretation of cytologic abnormalities is dependent, to a large degree, on the technical quality of an adequate and representative specimen. Optimal specimen collection requires instruction of clinicians who obtain their own specimens in their offices or at satellite facilities. When specimens are collected in-house, active participation on the part of the cytotechnologist and pathologist improves specimen yield and overall technical quality. Communication lines between the clinician and the cytologist must be kept open at all times and a team approach to diagnostic cytopathology fostered.

Proposed federal and state legislation mandates workload guidelines for cytotechnologists, proficiency testing, and inspection and certification of laboratories engaged in on-premises screening. Rescreening of negative cases, reporting of unsatisfactory specimens, and adherence to strict quality-assurance guidelines also are required. These standards are met in most laboratories; however, oversights by a small minority of laboratories have led to sensational press accounts of errors in diagnosis and of widespread recognition of the shortcomings of the "Pap mill" mentality.

Accurate patient and specimen identification, documentation of the time a specimen is collected or received, prompt reporting of results, and long-term retention of reports and slides constitute sound elements of laboratory practice. A record of all previous surgical pathology and cytology diagnoses on a patient should be available at the time the case is screened and relevant slides from previous material reviewed if indicated. After initial screening, a hierarchical system of review is indicated (by the senior cytotechnologist and/or the pathologist) in any specimen that is positive or suspicious of malignancy or in cases that constitute a diagnostic problem. There should be no hesitation in seeking the opinion of an outside consultant when faced with a difficult and perplexing case. Additional specimens should be requested when the diagnosis remains in doubt.

Cases in which there is a major discrepancy between the clinical diagnosis and the cytologic diagnosis should be rescreened. Rarely are slides mislabeled or specimens transposed. Every effort should be made to avoid such potential catastrophic errors by prelabeling slides and filters with both patient name and accession number and by avoiding interruptions during case preparation. Contamination of slides prepared from one patient with malignant cells from another patient constitutes an additional source of error. For this reason, solutions and stains should be filtered and replaced daily and known contaminated reagents immediately discarded. Specimens that are known to shed cells are best stained in separate dishes and the staining solutions filtered after each case. Mounting media are another source of contamination and should periodically be examined under the microscope.

Printed guidelines for handling potentially hazardous chemicals and infections specimens should be provided in every laboratory. At the most basic level, protective clothing (including laboratory coat and gloves) is recommended, and specimen preparation under a hood is advised. Mouth pipetting of specimens is prohibited, as is eating, smoking, or drinking in the laboratory. Potentially infectious specimens and materials should be discarded in appropriately labeled leak-proof containers for autoclaving prior to disposal.[1] Handwashing constitutes a simple but most effective practice in reducing the risk of infection.

Participation in continuing education programs and workshops by the pathologist and the cytotechnologist allows for exchange of ideas, advancement of the field, and improved patient care. Such opportunities should be vigorously supported by the laboratory director and by the hospital administration.

REFERENCES

1. Koss IG; Diagnostic Cytology and Its Histolopathologic Bases. 3rd Ed. Philadelphia, JB Lippincott, 1979
2. Keebler CM, Reagan JW (eds): A Manual of Cytotechnology. 6th Ed. American Society of Clinical Pathology, 1983
3. Naib AM (ed): Exfoliative Cytopathology. 3rd Ed. Little, Brown, Boston, 1985
4. Koss LG, Woyke S, Olszewski W: Aspiration Biopsy: Cytologic Interpretation and Histologic Bases. Igaku-Shoin, New York, 1984
5. Orell SR, Sterrett GF, Walters MN-I, Whitaker D: Manual and Atlas of Fine Needle Aspiration Cytology. Churchill Livingstone, Edinburgh, 1986
6. Wied GL, Keebler CM, Koss LG, Reagan JW: Compendium on Diagnostic Cytology. 6th Ed. Tutorials of Cytology, International Academy of Cytology, Chicago, 1988
7. Linsk JA, Franzen S: Clinical Aspiration Cytology. JB Lippincott, Philadelphia, 1983
8. Miller TR, Bottles K, Holly EA, et al: A step-wise logistic regression analysis of papillary carcinoma of the thyroid. Acta Cytol (Praha) 30:285, 1986
9. Bottles K, Löwhagen T: Psammoma bodies in the aspiration cytology diagnosis of acinic cell tumors. Acta Cytol (Praha) 29:191, 1985
10. Bottles K, Miller TR, Jeffrey RB Jr, et al: Aspiration cytology characterization of inflammatory masses. West J Med 144:695, 1986
11. Nieburgs HE: Malignancy associated cellular (MAC) markers. p 23. In Wied GL, Keebler CM, Koss LG, Reagan JW: Compendium on Diagnostic Cytology. 6th Ed. Tutorials of Cytology, International Academy of Cytology, Chicago, 1988
12. Frost JK: The Cell in Health and Disease. An Evaluation of Cellular Morphologic Expression of Biologic Behavior. S. Karger, Basel, 1986
13. Koss LG: Diagnostic Cytology and Its Histopathologic Basis. JB Lippincott, Philadelphia, 1979
14. Tani EM, Christensson B, Porwit A, Skoog L: Immunocytochemical analysis and cytomorphologic diagnosis on fine needle aspirates of lymphoproliferative disease. Acta Cytol (Praha) 32:209, 1988
15. Saccomano G, Saunders RP, Archer VE, Wood BG: Concentrations of carcinoma or atypical cells in sputum. Acta Cytol (Praha) 7:305, 1963
16. Cohen MB, Miller TR, Beckstead JH: Fine needle aspiration biopsy and plastic embedding: A combination of two techniques. Lab Invest 56:14A, 1987
17. Richardson HL, Koss LG, Simon TR: Evaluation of concomitant use of cytological and histocytological techniques in recognition of cancer in exfoliated material from various sources. Cancer 8:948, 1955
18. DeLellis RA, Sterngerger LA, Mann RB, et al: Immunoperoxidase techniques in diagnostic pathology. Am J Clin Pathol 71:483, 1979
19. Falini B, Taylor CR: New developments in immunoperoxidase techniques and their applications. Arch Pathol Lab Med 107:105, 1983
20. Kennett RH, McKearn TJ, Bechtol KB (eds): Monoclonal Antibodies and Hybridomas: A New Dimension in Biological Analyses. Plenum, New York, 1980
21. Martin SE, Zhang HZ, Magyarosy E, et al: Immunologic methods in cytology: Definitive diagnosis of non-Hodgkin's lymphomas using immunologic markers for T- and B-cells. Am J Clin Pathol 82:666, 1984
22. Miller TR, Bottles K, Abele JS, et al: Neuroblastoma diagnosed by find needle aspiration biopsy. Acta Cytol (Praha) 29:461, 1985

23. Wasastjerna C, Ekelund P: The amino acid naphthylamidase reaction of the bile canaliculi in liver smears. Acta Cytol (Praha) 18:23, 1974
24. Lorincz AT, Lancaster WD, Kurman RJ, et al: Characterization of human papilloma viruses in cervical neoplasias and their detection in routine clinical screening. p. 225. In Peto R, zur Hausen H (eds): Banbury Report. Vol. 21: Viral Etiology of Cervical Cancer. Cold Spring Harbor Laboratory, Cold Spring Harbor, NY, 1986
25. Akhtar M, Ali MA, Owen EW: Application of electron microscopy in the interpretation of fine needle aspiration biopsies. Cancer 48:2458, 1981
26. Stark P, Hildebrandt-Stark HE: Electron microscopy of cells obtained by fine needle aspiration biopsy of lung lesions. Radiology 22:327, 1982
27. Domagala W, Kahan AV, Koss LG: A simple method of preparation and identification of cells for scanning electron microscopy. Acta Cytol (Praha) 23:140, 1979
28. Atkin NB, Kay R: Prognostic significance of madal DNA value and other factors in malignant tumors based on 1465 cases. Br J Cancer 40:210, 1979
29. Gaub J, Auer G, Zetterberg A: Quantitative cytochemical aspects of a combined Feulgen naphthol yellow S staining procedure for the simultaneous determination of nuclear and cytoplasmic proteins and DNA in mammalian cells. Exp Cell Res 92:323, 1975
30. Auer G, Caspersson T, Wallgren A: DNA content and survival in mammary carcinoma. Anal Quantum Cytol 2:161, 1980
31. Zetterberg A, Esposti P-L: Prognostic significance of nuclear DNA levels in prostatic carcinoma. Scand J Urol Nephrol 55(suppl):53, 1980
32. Koss LG, Wolley RC, Schreiber K, et al: Flow microfluorometric analysis of nuclei isolated from various normal and malignant human epithelial tissues. J Histochem Cytochem 25:565, 1977
33. Boon ME, Lowhagen T, Willems JS: Planimetric studies on fine needle aspirations from follicular adenoma and follicular carcinoma of the thyroid. Acta Cytol (Praha) 24:145, 1980
34. Koprowski H, Steplewski Z, Herlyn D, et al: Study of antibodies against human melanomas produced by somatic cell hybrids. Proc Natl Acad Sci USA 75:3405, 1978
35. Kennett RH, Gilbert F: Hybrid myelomas producing antibodies against a human neuroblastoma antigen present in fetal brain. Science 203:1120, 1979
36. Herlyn M, Steplewski Z, Herlyn D, et al: Colorectal carcinoma specific antigen: Detection by means of monoclonal antibodies. Proc Natl Acad Sci USA 76:1438, 1979
37. Azavedo E, Baral E, Skoog L: Immunohistochemical analysis of estrogen receptors in cells obtained by fine needle aspiration from human mammary carcinomas. Anticancer Res 6:263, 1986
38. Tribukait B, Esposti PL, Ronstrom L: Tumour ploidy for characterization of prostatic carcinoma: Flow-cytofluorometric DNA studies using aspiration biopsy material. Scand J Urol Nephrol 55 (suppl):59, 1980
39. Tsou KC, Hong DH, Varello M et al: Flow cytometric DNA analysis as a diagnostic aid for cervical condyloma and cancer. Cancer 54:1778, 1984
40. Barlogie B, Drewinko B, Schumann J, et al: Cellular DNA content as a marker of neoplasia in man. Am J Med 69:195, 1980
41. Fox CH: Innovation in medical diagnosis: The Scandinavian curiosity. Lancet 1:1387, 1979
42. Koss LG: Thin needle aspiration biopsy. (Editorial). Acta Cytol (Praha) 24:13, 1980
43. Christopherson WM: Cytologic detection and diagnosis of cancer: Its contributions and limitations. Cancer 51:1201, 1983
44. Bottles K, Miller TR, Cohen MB, Ljung BM: Fine needle aspiration biopsy: Has its time come? Am J Med 81:525, 1986
45. Abele JS, Miller TR, King EB, et al: Smearing techniques for the concentration of particles from fine needle aspiration biopsies. Diagn Cytopathol 1:59, 1985
46. Bottles K, McPhaul LW, Volberding P: Fine-needle aspiration biopsy of patients with the acquired immunodeficiency syndrome (AIDS): Experience in an outpatient clinic. Ann Intern Med 108:42, 1988

2
Cytology of the Female Genital Tract

Prabodh K. Gupta
Darryl G. Heustis
Thomas A. Bonfiglio
Roberta K. Nieberg
Fritz Lin

Basic Principles
Prabodh K. Gupta

Cytopathology of the lower female genital tract has been most effective in proper identification of the preneoplastic and neoplastic lesions of the cervix and the vagina, as well as the various infections involving this region. The technique of sample collection is associated with a high level of patient acceptability, as it causes little discomfort to the patient and has no serious complications. Sampling of large mucosal areas is easily obtained and epithelial lesions can be detected and diagnosed accurately. The natural history of the lesion and the effects of various treatment modalities can be investigated using noninvasive procedures.

A number of techniques and smears are available and recommended for sampling of genital tract lesions. Specimens generally include exfoliated cells, forcibly removed or abraded cells, and aspirated cellular samples. For suspected disease of the lower genital tract, the most commonly used smears involve samples of vaginal pool material and scrapings or aspiration of the endocervical contents, representing the cells of the transformation zone. An adequate sampling of this area and its contents on the smear are more important than the occurrence of endocervical columnar cells, squamous metaplastic cells, or mucus. The quantity and quality of os mucus is variable and is dependent upon a number of factors, including the day of the menstrual cycle, hormonal status, contraceptive practice, and concomitant infection.

Proper and rapid fixation of cellular samples is essential. The recommended fixative is 95 percent ethyl alcohol, although spray fixative, when applied according to the manufacturer's instructions, is adequate and convenient. The patient should be advised against douching during the 24 hours preceding the vaginal specimen collection. Menstrual contents generally render the specimen unsatisfactory, as do excessive cytolysis secondary to progesterone effect and heavy inflammation and degeneration. Lower genital tract smears tend to be less than optimal during the first four days of menses and among women taking oral contraceptives.[1]

SAMPLING TECHNIQUES

A number of techniques are available for sampling the lower genital tract. The most commonly employed include the following.

1. *Vaginal pool smear.* The specimen for a vaginal pool smear is obtained from the accumulated contents of the posterior fornix of the vagina by a spatula or aspirator. These samples represent material from the cervix, vagina, uterine cavity, and even the fallopian tubes. In vaginal pool material, cells are often poorly preserved, and early cervical dysplastic lesions are inadequately represented. This specimen, however, is useful in the detection of endometrial or ovarian lesions and hormonal changes.
2. *Pancervical specimen.* A pancervical specimen is obtained by either a spatula aspiration, or an endocervical swab, and represent samples of the transformation zone and any developing cervical cancer.[2] In my experience, cotton swab specimens are somewhat inferior to those obtained either by the pancervical scraping or endocervical aspiration techniques. Recently, various endocervical brushes have been introduced for specimen collection. These provide good sampling of the endocervical canal, but some experience in the proper interpretation of the cellular changes is necessary.
3. *Vaginopancervical (Fast) smear.* The vaginopancervical (Fast) smear, which is recommended by Frost, is a good technique for routine population screening.[3] Briefly, it involves use of vaginal pool material from the posterior fornix and a pancervical scraping specimen, both of which are spread on a single glass slide.
4. *Triple smear method (cervical-vaginal-endocervical, or CVE smear).* The triple smear method is advocated by Wied and Bahr.[4] It contains three distinct samples representing the vaginal wall, ectocervix, and endocervix. This technique is particularly useful in localization of a lesion and for cytohormonal evaluation.
5. *Irrigation smears.* Irrigation smears of various types have been advocated from time to time.[5,6] However, they are inferior to any direct sampling technique, as they do not adequately detect early neoplastic lesions.
6. *Endometrial cytologic samplings.* The endometrial cytologic techniques that are most commonly employed include aspiration (Isaac and Mi-mark), washings (Gravlee jet wash), endometrial brushings (Ayre, Johnston and Stromby), and endometrial microbiopsies. These procedures can be reliable and accurate.[7,8] They are highly specialized and expensive, and require special cytomorphologic interpretation.

CYTOPATHOLOGIC REPORTING

Use of the Papanicolaou classification is not recommended; however, if it is used, it must be accompanied by a descriptive report and set of recommendations. The morphologic findings and report should be presented in a manner similar to that used by anatomic pathology laboratories, and these documents should serve as effective means of accurate and precise communication, not only with the other pathologists, but most importantly, with the attending clinicians, in order to facilitate appropriate clinical management. Unsatisfactory smears, resulting from such factors as inadequate sampling, air-drying, bleeding, cytolysis, or obscuring inflammation and necrosis, should be identified properly and cited in the body of the report. Various cytohormonal patterns and infective organisms should be identified and reported. Infections are accurately detectable in vaginal smears, occur far more frequently than do preneoplastic and neoplastic changes, and are most often treatable.

CYTOHORMONAL EVALUATION

An appropriately collected and stained lower genital tract smear can be used to assess the hormonal status of a patient. A lateral vaginal wall smear, obtained by scraping the upper one third of the canal, is the recommended sample. The vaginal pool smear is generally satisfactory for this purpose, but the ectocervical scrape smear is not.

Among the cells normally found in smears of the lower genital tract, squamous cells—especially those obtained from the upper third of the lateral vaginal wall—most faithfully reflect the hormonal changes occurring in the body.[9] The squamous cells seen in vaginal smears are of three basic types: superficial, intermediate, and parabasal (Figs. 2-1 to 2-3). The predominant cell type varies according to hormonal balance. Squamous superficial cells are identified by their polygonal shape, thin cytoplasm, and central pyknotic nucleus. Intermediate cells are also polygonal and thin, but they contain a vesicular nucleus that may reveal chromatinic threads and a heterochromatic Barr body at the periphery of the nuclear envelope. Parabasal cells are generally oval or round and have a thick, homogeneous cytoplasm and a nucleus that is variable in its texture. They may be either vesicular or pyknotic.

In response to the influence of estrogen hormones, squamous cells become thin, flat, and orangophilic in their tinctorial staining character. However, this staining reaction is variable, and should not be used as an absolute indicator of estrogenic activity. The cytoplasm may contain varying numbers of brownish-black, keratohyalin granules. The nuclei of these cells are pyknotic and are less than 6 μm in diameter.

Intermediate cells, which are thin and flat and have vesicular nuclei, respond to the progestogen hormone. Steroids also cause a proliferative arrest of the epithelium, with predominance of intermediate cells. Large quantities of progestogen, as may occur in the late luteal phase of the menstrual cycle, in pregnancy, and in some oral contraceptive users, cause cytolysis, with disintegration of the cytoplasm of these cells. Clumping of the intermediate cells with folding of the free margins (navicular cells) is also commonly seen. During pregnancy, intracytoplasmic glycogen

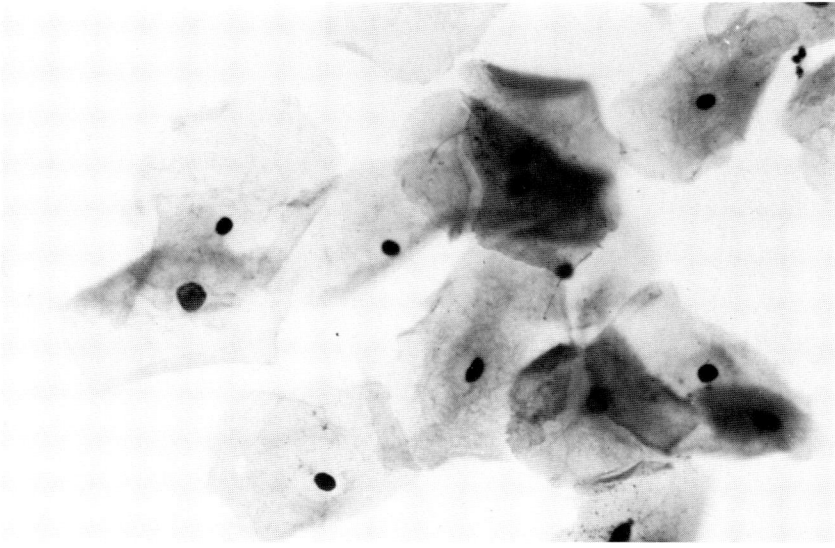

Fig. 2-1 CVE Smear. Note the numerous polygonal superficial cells. These cells are very pale, transparent, and contain small pyknotic nuclei. An occasional intermediate cell is also seen. (Papanicolaou stain.)

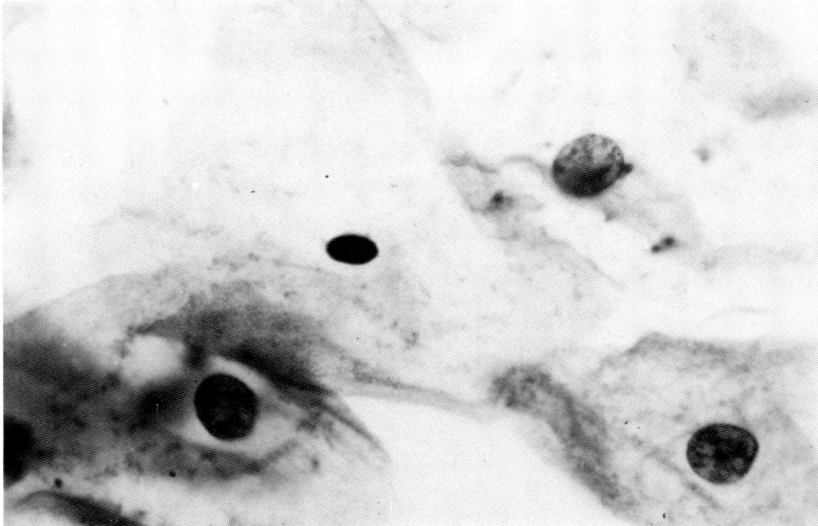

Fig. 2-2 CVE smear containing three intermediate cells and one superficial cell. In this higher magnification, the nuclear details of the intermediate cells are clearly visible. Intermediate cells and superficial cells can have similar tinctorial features; however, their nuclear configurations are entirely different. The vesicular nuclei of intermediate cells reveal chromatinic details. (Papanicolaou stain.)

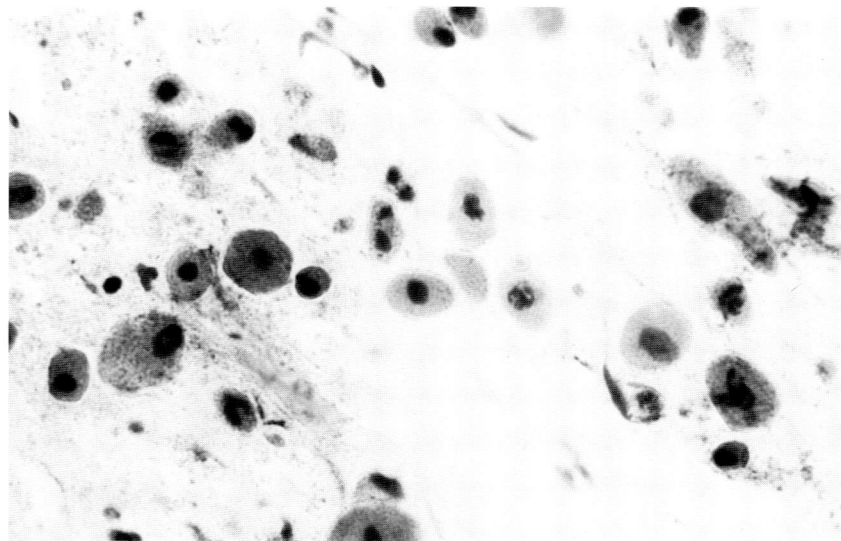

Fig. 2-3 Parabasal cells. The cells in this preparation of CVE material are seen as small, round or oval cells with relatively thick cytoplasm. These cells most often occur singly. They can lose their delicate cytoplasm and appear as bare nuclei. The nuclei of such cells can either be vesicular or pyknotic. (Papanicolaou stain.)

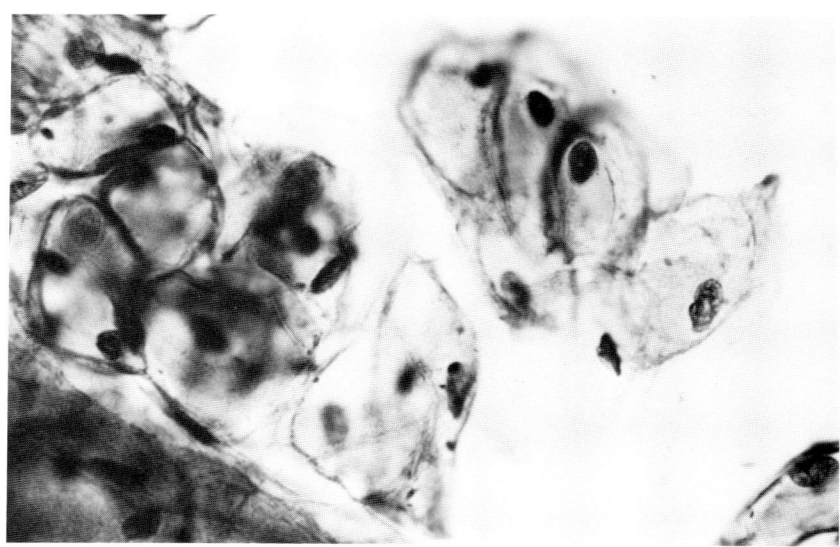

Fig. 2-4 CVE smear obtained during pregnancy. Note the groups of intermediate cells with vesicular nuclei. These cells have folded (navicular) shapes and tend to stick together, forming small clumps of cells. Occasionally, prominent cytolysis causes a disintegration of the cell cytoplasm. Such preparations contain numerous bare nuclei only. Occasionally, numerous bacillary organisms (lactobacilli) can be observed in cervical-vaginal smears obtained during pregnancy. (Papanicolaou stain.)

accumulates in these cells, and may be observed as areas of golden-brown pigment upon staining with the Bismarck brown stain, one of the components of the original Papanicolaou recipe (Fig. 2-4).

Hormonal agents, including thyroxin, testosterone and related androgens, vitamins, tetracycline, and digoxin are some of the common substances that affect squamous epithelial maturation.

Maturation Index

The maturation index (MI) is the most widely used method for hormonal evaluation reporting. One hundred well-spread squamous cells are counted and grouped according to type (parabasal, intermediate, or superficial). There proportions are expressed in terms of an MI. Some investigators do not believe in the actual counting of the proportions of squamous cells, and instead express cytohormonal changes in terms of a predominant pattern that is compatible with the day of the menstrual cycle or the hormonal makeup of the individual.

Normal MIs, as observed during active reproductive life, are presented in Table 2-1.

Table 2-1 Normal Hormonal Values

Stage of Hormonal Development	Maturation Index (%) (Parabasal/Intermediate/Superficial)
Neonatal	0/90/10
Infancy	80/20/0
Preovulatory	0/40/60
Postovulatory	0/70/30
Pregnant	0/95/5
Menopausal	0/80/10
Postmenopausal	70/30/0, 100/0/0, or 0/100/0

Abnormal Hormonal Patterns

Abnormal hormonal values may be observed in women with either primary amenorrhea caused by ovarian, pituitary, or adrenal dysfunction and testicular feminizing syndromes, or secondary amenorrhea caused by endocrine lesions, including Chiari-Frommel syndrome, Simmonds' disease, and pituitary and ovarian tumors with hormonal activity, such as granulosa cell tumor or luteal cysts, arrhenoblastomas, and hilar cell tumors. More commonly, however, endometrial lesions, solid and cystic tumors of the ovary, including cystadenoma and carcinoma of the fallopian tubes, and metastatic tumors, including those of the breast and lung, are all associated with abnormal hormonal findings and may be manifested by a pronounced estrogen effect. In fact, any woman who is 10 years or more postmenopausal and whose vaginal smear demonstrates more than 10 percent superficial cells, in the absence of a known cause for such change, should be investigated for ovarian or endometrial lesions.

The vaginal component of the Fast smear or a specific lateral vaginal wall scraping or vaginal component or the CVE smear are recommended for cytohormonal evaluation. Ectocervical smears and endocervical samples are not recommended for hormonal evaluation.

Table 2-2 Common Infectious Conditions Detectable in CVE Smears

Bacterial agents
Neisseria gonorrhoeae
Gardnerella vaginalis
Granuloma inguinale
Actinomyces species
Chlamydia trachomatis
Viral agents
Herpes simplex virus (HSV)
Cytomegalovirus (CMV)
Human papillomavirus (HPV)
Molluscum contagiosum
Fungal agents
Candida albicans
Trichophyton species
Parasitic agents
Trichomonas vaginalis
Entamoeba histolytica

INFLAMMATION, INFECTION, AND SEXUALLY TRANSMITTED DISEASES

Although originally intended to test for the early detection of cervical cancer, a cervical-vaginal smear is more often used for the detection and diagnosis of non-neoplastic conditions of the lower genital tract, including those of the vagina, cervix, endocervix, and endometrium. Infectious processes occur more commonly than neoplastic changes and are often easily treatable. The proper diagnosis of these specific infections, based upon the specific morphologic features, can be most valuable in determining proper clinical management. It must be constantly borne in mind that, in cytopathologic diagnosis of infections, a high degree of specificity and accuracy is more important than sensitivity and false diagnosis rates. Whenever possible, all cytodiagnoses of infectious diseases should be corroborated by clinical examination or other appropriate methods, including serologic or immunologic testing and cultures.

The most common infectious conditions detectable in cervical-vaginal smears with a high degree of accuracy are listed in Table 2-2. It must be appreciated that almost all of these conditions occur in a polymicrobial environment. The host reacts to these conditions, and the accompanying cellular changes, inflammation, and degeneration must be considered to be part of the so-called vaginal infectious complex. All of these features not only obscure the infective organisms, but also alter them morphologically, making correct identification and diagnosis difficult.

Bacterial Infections

NEISSERIA GONORRHOEAE

Neisseria gonorrhoeae are gram-negative diplococci that may be observed within the polymorphonuclear leukocytes in vaginal smears. These organisms are best detected toward the edges of the smears, which generally are poorly preserved and air-dried. Cytodiagnosis of gonococcal infection should not be made, and it is strongly recommended that the presence of these organisms, as detected on Papanicolaou-stained vaginal smears, should not be reported.[10] Rather, bacterial culture should be performed for a definitive diagnosis.

GARDNERELLA VAGINALIS

First identified by Dr. Herman Gardner, *Gardnerella vaginalis* is a frequent cause of nonspecific vaginitis or bacterial vaginitis.[11] Organisms are diagnosed by recognizing so-called clue cells which, although originally described in wet-mounted unstained preparations, can be diagnosed accurately

CYTOLOGY OF THE FEMALE GENITAL TRACT **29**

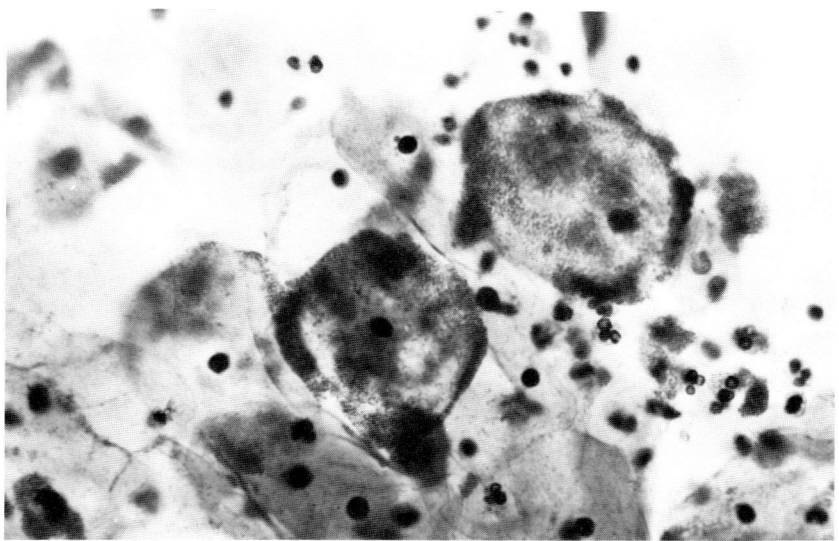

Fig. 2-5 CVE smear revealing *Gardnerella vaginalis*. Note the two squamous cells that are covered over by the organisms. This smear contains some inflammatory exudate; patients in whom this is evident may be symptomatic. (Papanicolaou stain.)

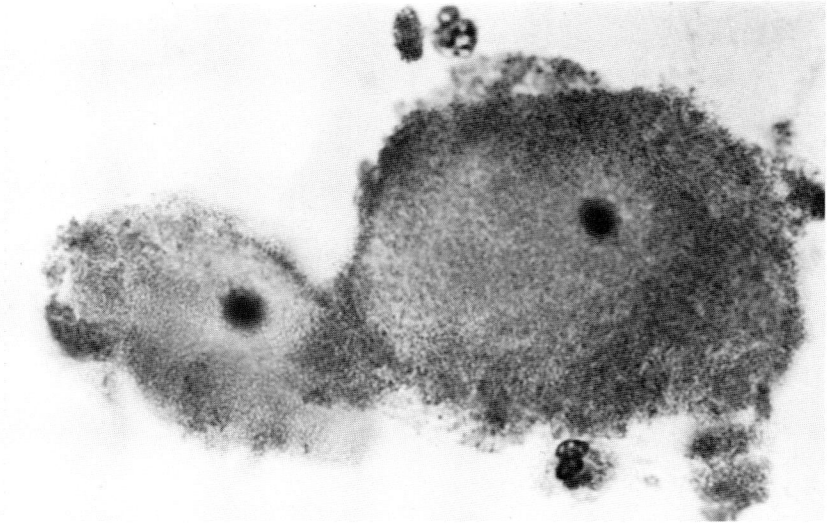

Fig. 2-6 A higher magnification of *Gardnerella vaginalis* infection. Note the coccobacillary organisms that are covering the surfaces of two infected cells, as well as the spread of the infected organisms beyond the outline of the cells. The extension of the organisms beyond the outline of the squamous cell is an important diagnostic feature. (Papanicolaou stain.)

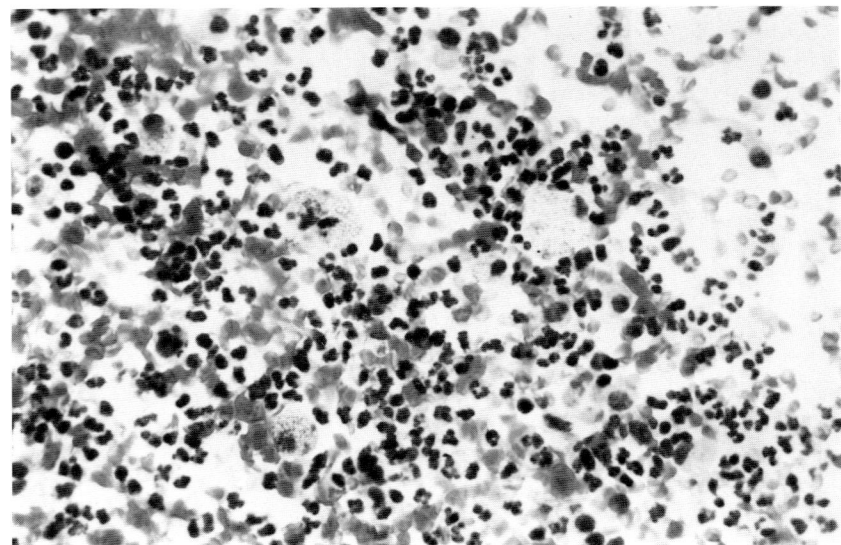

Fig. 2-7 CVE scrape smear in a patient with Granuloma inguinale. Note the acute inflammatory exudate that is intermixed with macrophages and red blood cells.

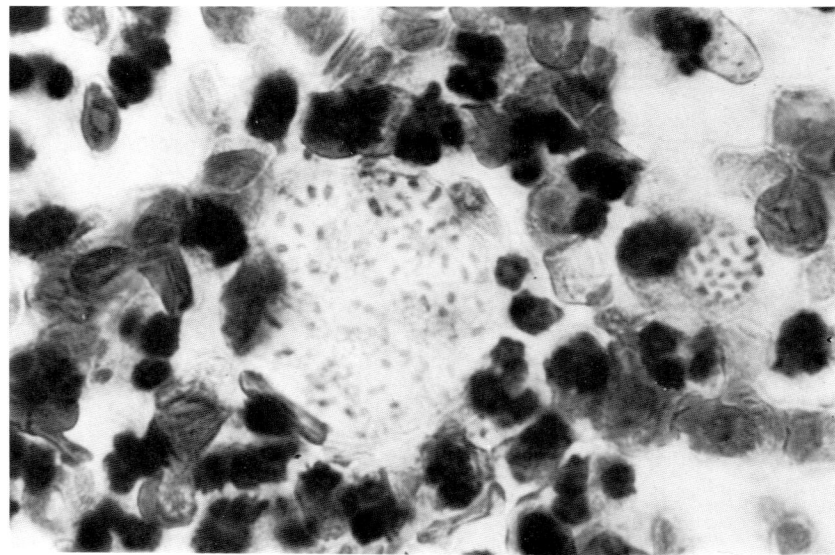

Fig. 2-8 A higher magnification of the case seen in Figure 2-7. Note the two macrophages that contain intracytoplasmic Donovan bodies, which are seen as elongated, safety-pin–shaped structures. These organisms tend to occur in small groups and in lobulated forms. (Papanicolaou stain.)

with Papanicolaou-stained smears. The affected cell is a squame that is covered over with numerous coccobacillary organisms. These organisms, to be diagnostic, spread beyond the cell margin of the squamous cells and appear as molten wax drippings. Variable or no inflammation may be present in the smears. Nearly 40 percent of women with Gardnerella infection are asymptomatic (Figs. 2-5 and 2-6).

GRANULOMA INGUINALE

Granuloma inguinale is not very common in the Northeast United States, but it is widespread in distribution. Clinically, this ulcerogranulomatous lesion may resemble a neoplastic growth. It is caused by gram-negative, encapsulated coccobacillary organisms. Diagnostic organisms (Donovan bodies) occur as intracytoplasmic, safety-pin-shaped structures within lobulated masses inside the foamy macrophages. The background is necrotic and contains numerous, acutely inflammatory cells. Careful evaluation of the foamy macrophages and identification of Donovan bodies are necessary to confirm the diagnosis (Figs. 2-7 and 2-8).

ACTINOMYCES

Although genital Actinomyces infections have become uncommon in most major medical centers, some cases may still be observed among women using intrauterine devices (IUDs) for contraception and among those with other foreign bodies in place, such as pessaries or surgically implanted metal clips.[12] These infections present as large, irregular masses of hematoxylin-stained aggregates (variously called Gupta bodies or Gupta lesions) that contain numerous, parallel, filamentous branching structures.[13,14] The infectious organisms are gram-positive and can be stained with silver stain and immunostaining techniques. Most cases involve *Actinomyces israelii*. In women who have used an IUD for a prolonged period, these filaments may become calcified. Infection may cause a tissue reaction of the Splendore-Hoeppli phenomenon type (Figs. 2-9 to 2-11).

Actual "sulphur granules," which are typically seen in classic, suppurative actinomycotic lesions, are only rarely observed in vaginal-cervical smears (Fig. 2-12). When these granules are present, affected women are symptomatic, complaining of a foul-smelling, chronic vaginal discharge. A fair number of women harboring Actinomyces in the lower genital tract may be asymptomatic, but they are at increased risk of pelvic inflammatory disease, including tubo-ovarian abscesses and the secondary complications of infertility and dissemination of actinomycotic infection.[15–17]

Infection with Chlamydia trachomatis

Chlamydial infection is the most common sexually transmitted infection that localizes to the columnar epithelium of the endocervix. The disease may disseminate to involve the endometrium, the fallopian tubes, or other organs. It has been documented to affect the atrophic parabasal-type epithelium of the cervix and vagina.

Nearly 40 percent of the women harboring *Chlamydia* are asymptomatic. Infection, especially among symptomatic young women, can be fairly accurately diagnosed by tissue culture or by recently introduced monoclonal antibody staining techniques. A high degree of correlation has been documented between monoclonal antibody staining for Chlamydia in cervical-vaginal specimens and McCoy culture studies.

Routinely stained cervical smears often contain evidence of chlamydial infection. A presumptive diagnosis, to be confirmed by appropriate cultures or monoclonal staining, can be made in the presence of an acute inflammatory background in the smear and the identification of small and transformed lymphocytes, histiocytes and metaplastic cells. These changes, although nonspecific, are most commonly observed in women with active chlamydial infection.[18]

In some symptomatic patients and other healthy women harboring a Chlamydial infection, specific cytomorphologic changes can be seen in well-prepared and stained cervical-vaginal smears.[19] Intracytoplasmic aggregates of small coccoid elementary bodies can be seen among the columnar metaplastic cells. (Fig. 2-13, Plate 2-1). These aggregates generally have poorly defined outlines, but some may be compact and dense. These intermediate and reticular forms are often associated with rarefaction, a moth-eaten appearance, and some large inclusions within the cytoplasm of the infected cells (Figs. 2-14A & B,

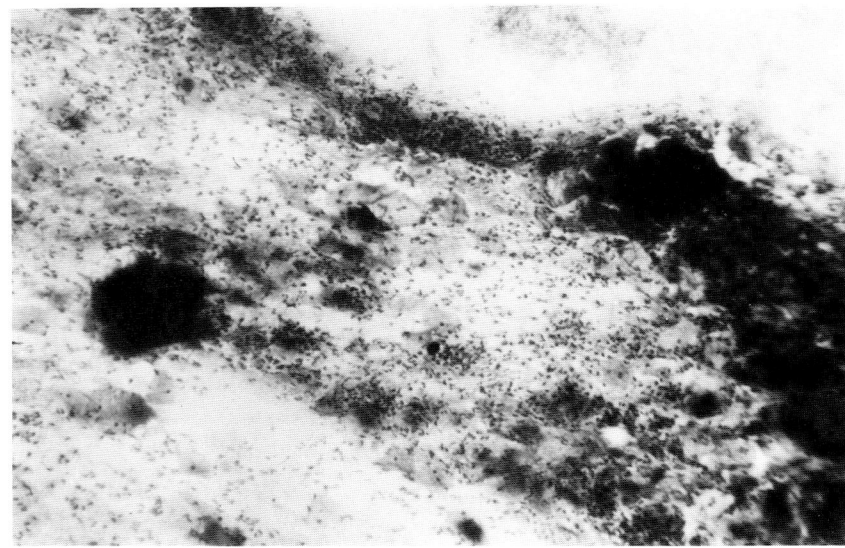

Fig. 2-9 CVE smear containing groups of Actinomyces organisms, which appear as dark clumps. (Papanicolaou stain.)

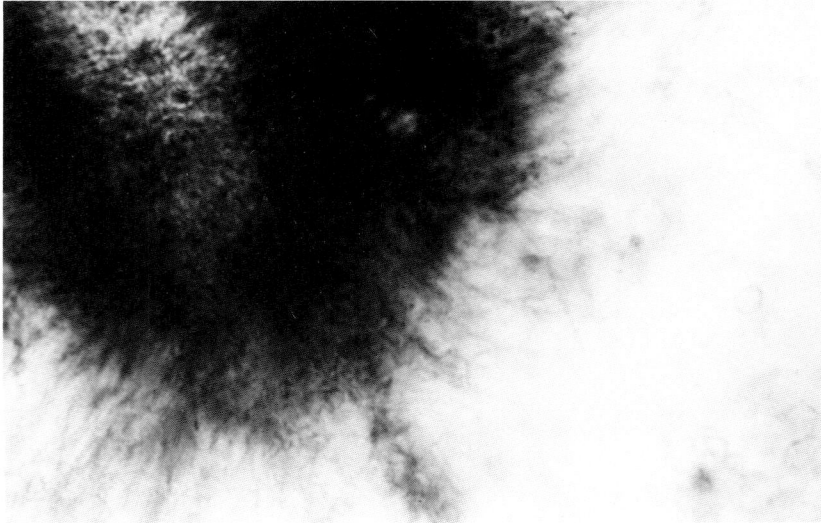

Fig. 2-10 A higher magnification of one of the clumps shown in Fig. 2-9 that reveal Actinomyces. Note the numerous, radiating, parallel, filamentous structures. These organisms show acute angle branching, which is better appreciated on Gram or silver stains. (Papanicolaou stain.)

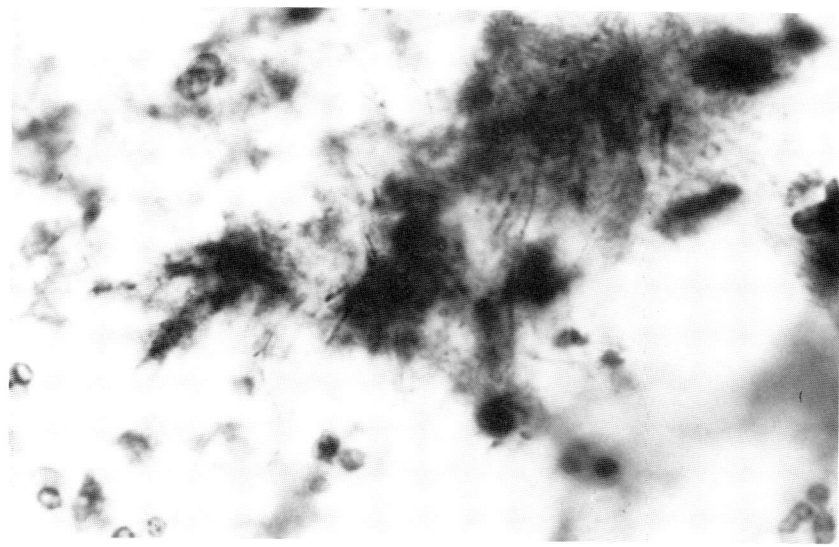

Fig. 2-11 CVE smear showing Actinomyces organisms. Note that the filamentous organisms are thick and appear to be beaded. Such an appearance is common after prolonged use of an IUD. This patient had an IUD in place for more than 3 years. (Papanicolaou stain.)

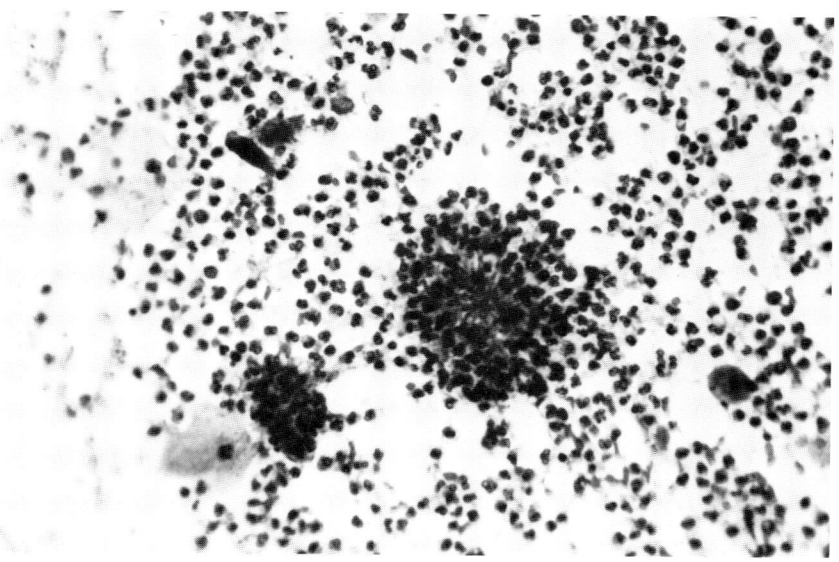

Fig. 2-12 CVE smear of a sulfur granule. Such configurations of Actinomyces infection, although common in tissue preparations, are only occasionally seen in cervical smears. When present, however, the patients invariably are symptomatic, complaining of a profuse, foul-smelling, brownish vaginal discharge. (Papanicolaou stain.)

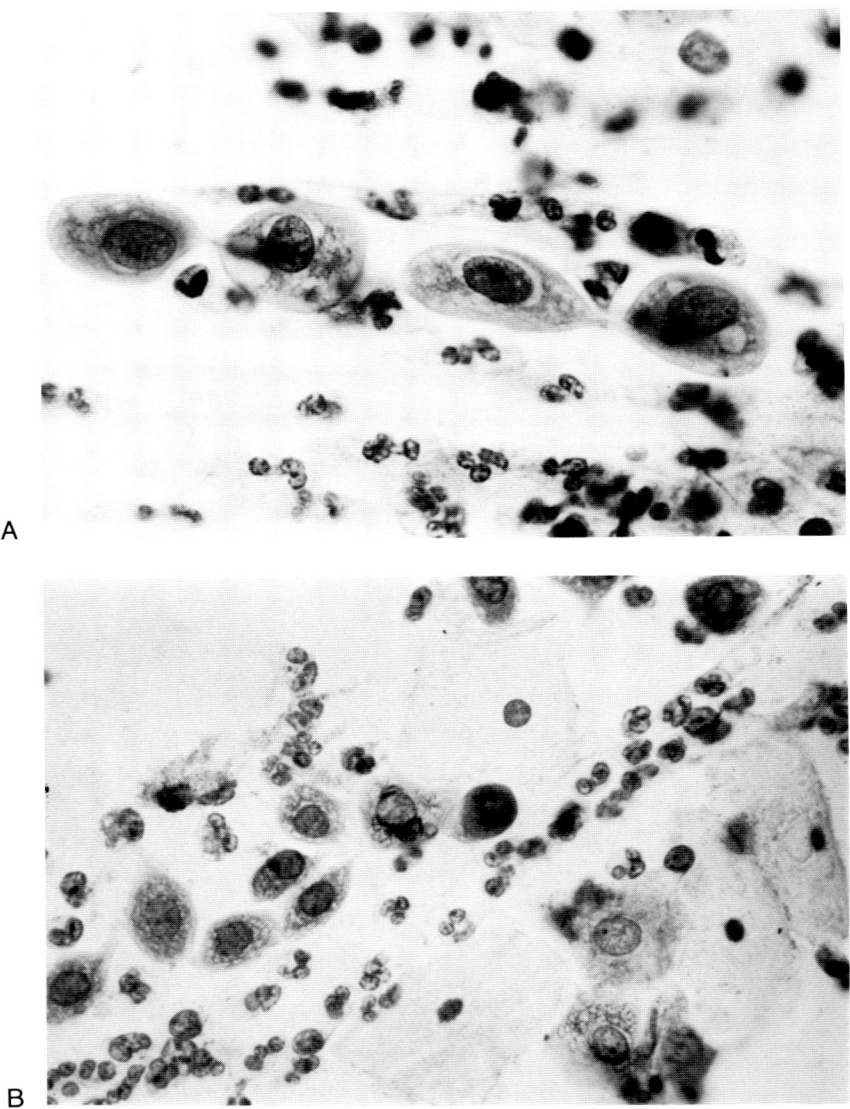

Fig. 2-13 (A) CVE smear revealing *Chlamydia trachomatis* infection. Note the acute inflammatory background of the smear which contains a number of metaplastic columnar cells. These cells have a rarefied appearance, and contain numerous, small, coccoid, intracytoplasmic, elementary bodies. The large vacuoles present in some of these cells represent degenerative changes. (Papanicolaou stain.) **(B)** CVE smear stained with monoclonal antibodies for *Chlamydia trachomatis*. Immunostaining was performed following a routine Papanicolaou stain. The smear was not destained. Note the presence of intracytoplasmic Chlamydia infection within the columnar epithelial cells. (AEC substrate.) (See Plate 2-1.)

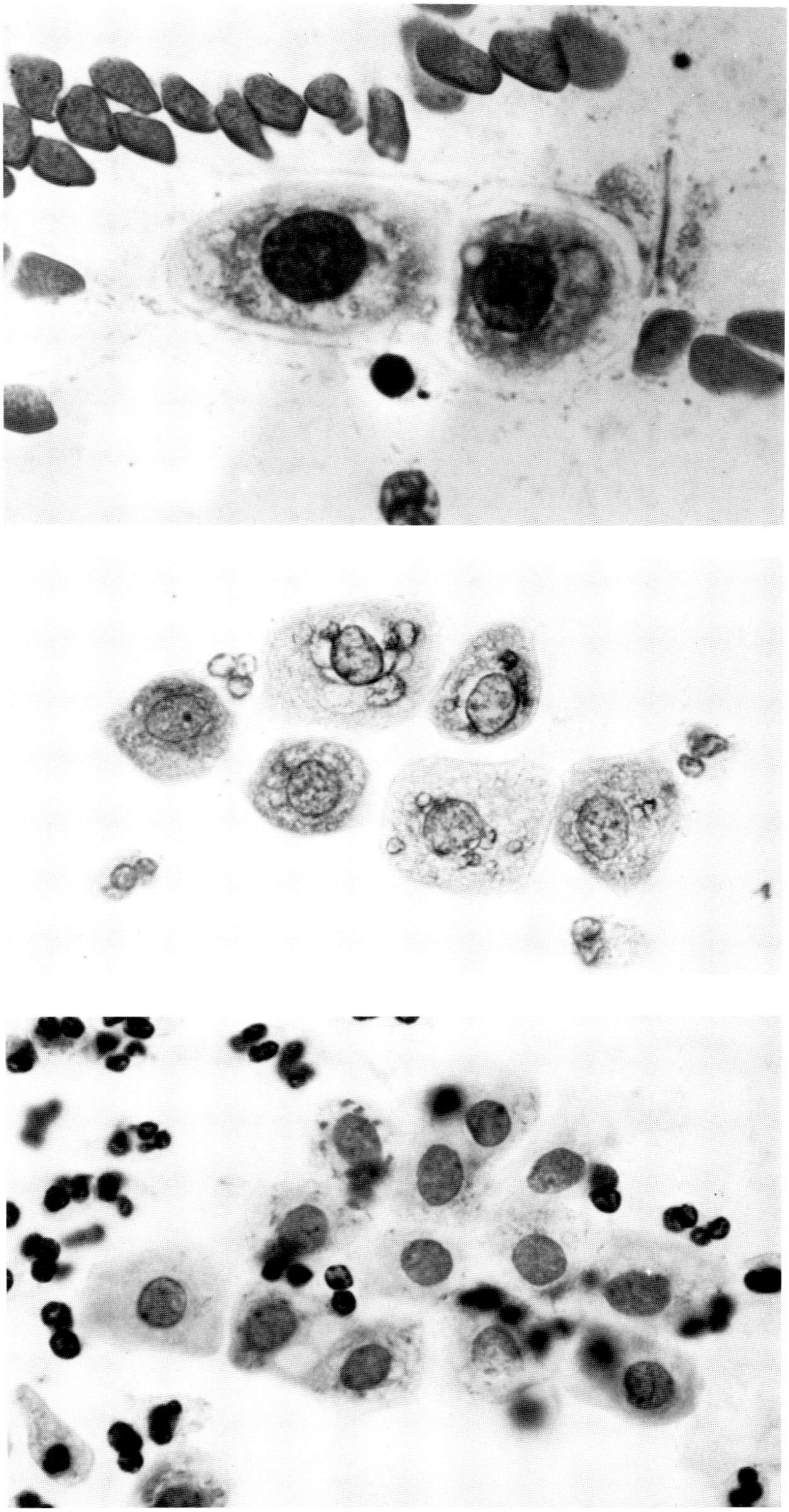

Fig. 2-14 **(A)** CVE smear revealing columnar metaplastic epithelial cells. These cells contain larger intracytoplasmic inclusions that represent the reticular and intermediate forms of the life cycle of *Chlamydia trachomatis* infection. (Papanicolaou stain.) **(B)** Monoclonal staining of Papanicolaou-stained CVE smear for *Chlamydia trachomatis* infection. Note the intracytoplasmic, large structures that are similar to those seen in Fig. A. These structures are considered to represent the reticular and intermediate forms of *Chlamydia trachomatis* infection. (AEC substrate.) (See Plate 2-2.) **(C)** CVE smear stained with immunoperoxidase technique for *Chlamydia trachomatis* infection using monoclonal antibodies. Intracytoplasmic elementary bodies and intermediate forms are clearly visible in this preparation. Note the large vacuoles in the cytoplasm which do not stain for *Chlamydia trachomatis*. The presence of such vacuoles should not be considered to be pathognomonic for *Chlamydia trachomatis* infection. (DAB substrate.) (See Plate 2-3.)

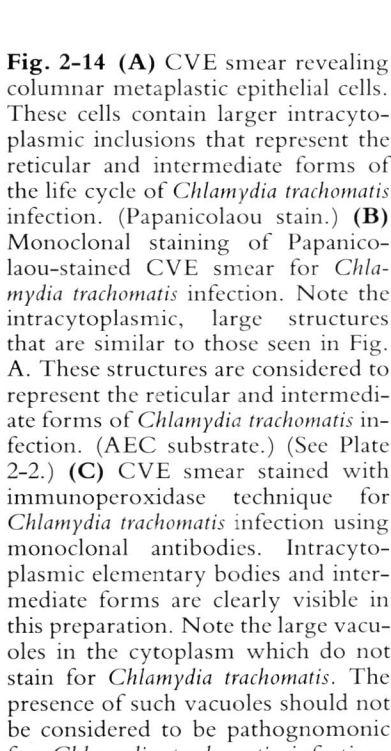
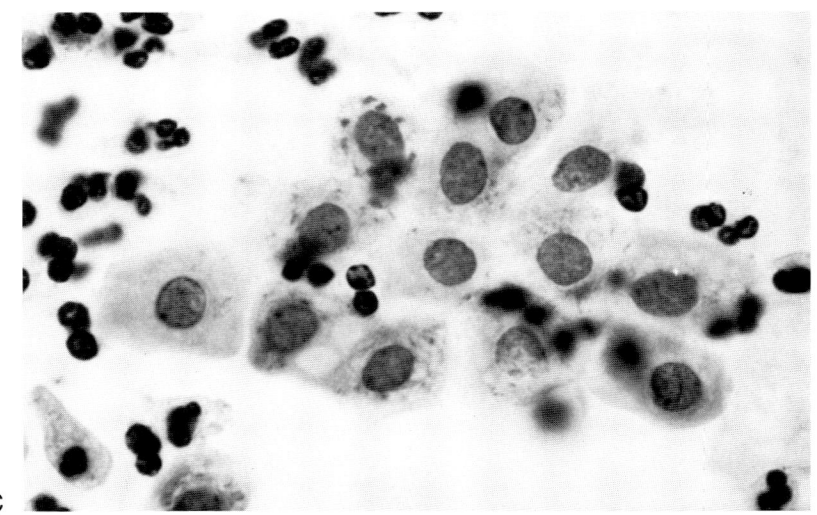

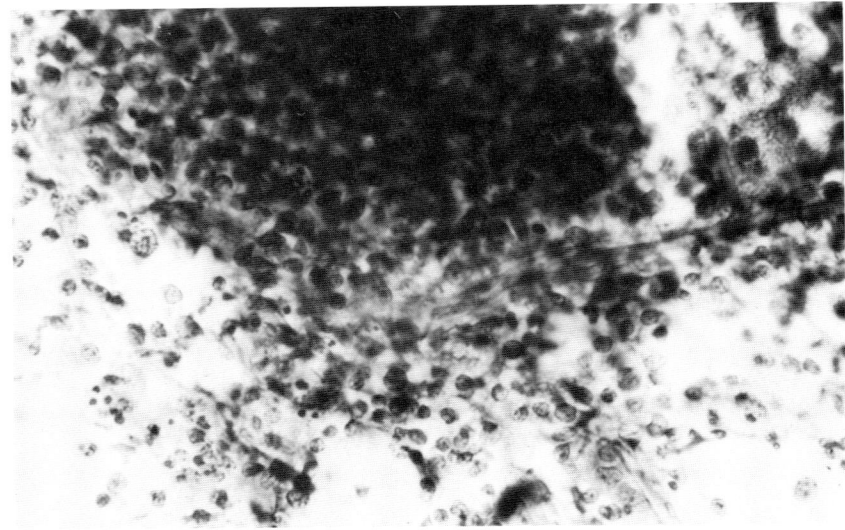

Fig. 2-15 CVE smear revealing cytomorphologic features of follicular cervicitis. Such preparations contain a variable number of mature lymphocytes. Occasionally, a germinal center capillary, as seen in this smear, is also present. A few tingible body macrophages are recognizable. (Papanicolaou stain.)

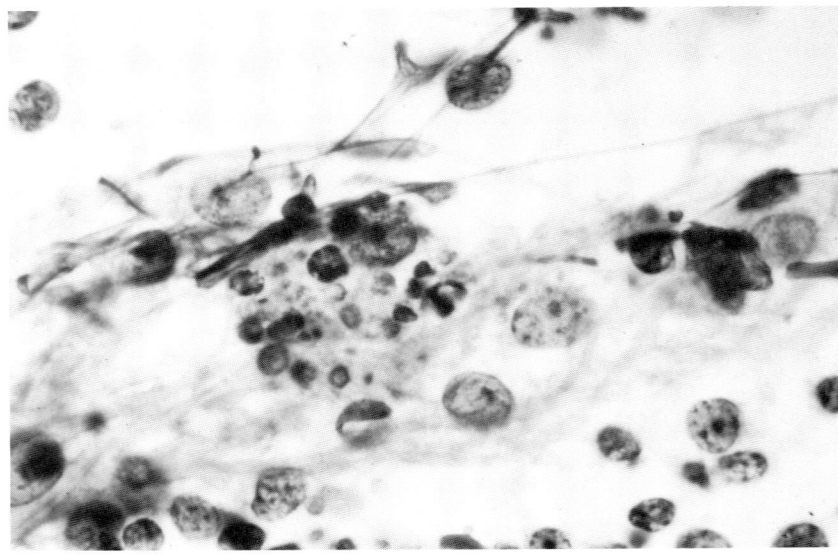

Fig. 2-16 A higher magnification of the smear seen in Fig. 2-16. Note the large tingible body macrophage containing numerous ingested leukocytic fragments. The presence of such macrophages must be established before rendering a diagnosis of follicular cervicitis. (Papanicolaou stain.)

Plates 2-2, 2-3). Varying degrees of cellular degeneration are common. Degenerative changes, which are generally conspicuous with distinct vacuolar margins, should not be confused with the chlamydial infection. Intracytoplasmic mucus, radiation-induced changes, and precipitated proteins can all mimic chlamydial inclusions. In suspicious cases, infection can be confirmed by monoclonal antibody staining of Papanicolaou-stained smears. A high degree of correlation is found between the cytodiagnosis of chlamydial infection and the results of monoclonal and tissue culture techniques.

Monoclonal antibodies can be used to localize the intracellular infection within the tissues of the endocervix, the endometrium, and the fallopian tubes (unpublished observation) (Fig. 2-14C).

Follicular cervicitis is a specific entity that, in nearly 50 percent of affected patients, has been found to be associated with chlamydial infection. Numerous lymphoid cells, as well as germinal center macrophages (tingible bodies), are diagnostic. A few plasma cells, an occasional true lymphoid follicle, and a follicular capillary may be seen. Tingible body macrophages are large (15 to 25 μm), have irregular outlines, and contain phagocytosed nuclear remnants and debris (Figs. 2-15 and 2-16).

Viral Infections

The most commonly diagnosed viral infections of the female genital tract include herpes simplex virus (HSV), also known as herpes genitalis, cytomegalovirus (CMV), and human papillomavirus (HPV) infections.

HERPES SIMPLEX

Herpes simplex is a fairly common genital infection that affects the squamous epithelium of the vulva, vagina, and cervix. Infection may ascend to involve the endocervical or endometrial epithelium.

The cellular changes that are characteristic of herpes simplex infection include multinucleation of the infected squamous or metaplastic-type cells. The nuclei of these cells exhibit peculiar internuclear molding and characteristic chromatinic liquefaction (Fig. 2-17). The nuclear chromatin in the infected cells takes on a watery, ground-glass or gelatinous appearance. Some cells contain the typical acidophylic intranuclear inclusion. It must be realized that multinucleation per se is not a feature of herpes infection; the accompanying chromatinic changes and the presence of intranuclear inclusions are more helpful diagnostically (Fig. 2-18). In the absence of typical inclusions, only a presumptive diagnosis of herpes should be rendered.

Primary and secondary herpetic infections cannot be differentiated by cytologic methods because, quite commonly, cells with and without intranuclear inclusions may be seen in the same smear, sometimes within the same large, multinucleated form. Type I and type II herpes can be distinguished from each other by the appropriate antibody staining reaction.

CYTOMEGALOVIRUS INFECTION

CMV infection is only infrequently diagnosed by cytology specimens obtained from the female genital tract. This infection involves endocervical and endometrial cells. Infected cells, unlike those in herpes viruses, are generally not enlarged. Multinucleation may be observed, with a gelatinous chromatin pattern within the giant cell configuration. The inclusions, although commonly acidophilic, may be amphophilic and disproportionately large. A number of women may have concomitant herpes and CMV infections. Most infected women are asymptomatic. Viral cultures are helpful in establishing a definitive diagnosis (Figs. 2-19, 2-20, Plate 2-4).

HUMAN PAPILLOMAVIRUS INFECTION

HPV is one of the most common sexually transmitted infections. Besides causing warty condyloma acuminatum lesions, HPV is also often associated with flat, condyloma planus lesions that, in most cases, represent dysplasia or cervical intraepithelial neoplasia (CIN). These lesions occur on the cervix starting at the transformation zone, as well as on the vagina and vulva, and in the perianal and anal regions. Presently, there are at least 50 types of HPV known to infect humans. Types 6 and 11 are often found in association with warty lesions, whereas types 16, 18, and 33, among others, often accompany severe cervical dysplastic lesions (CIN II–III) and squamous carcinoma. On morphologic examination, the cellular changes associated with both high- and

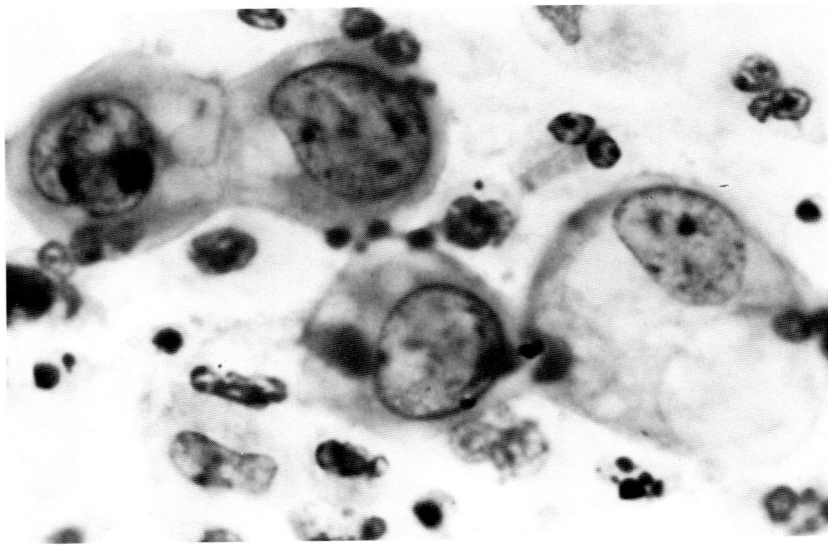

Fig. 2-17 CVE smear revealing evidence of early herpes infection. Note the metaplastic-type cells with relatively uniformly dispersed chromatin patterns. The watery chromatin in such nuclei tends to migrate to the edge of the nucleus, leaving a rather pale, uniformly stained nucleus. Such changes should be considered suggestive of viral infection and should be reported cautiously. (Papanicolaou stain.)

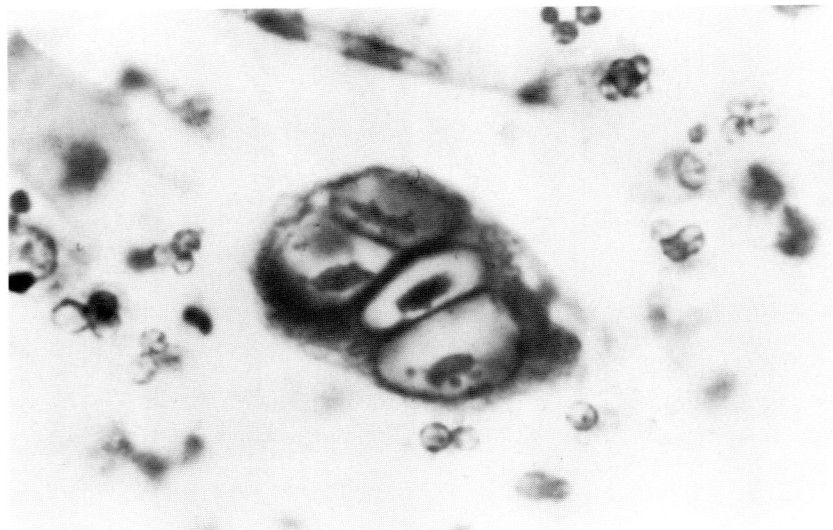

Fig. 2-18 CVE smear showing herpes infection. Note the multinucleated giant cell that contains nuclei revealing internuclear molding. The chromatin margination to the nuclear envelopes is clearly seen, leaving a rather clear nucleus. These nuclei contain large intranuclear inclusions that generally are acidophilic. (Papanicolaou stain.)

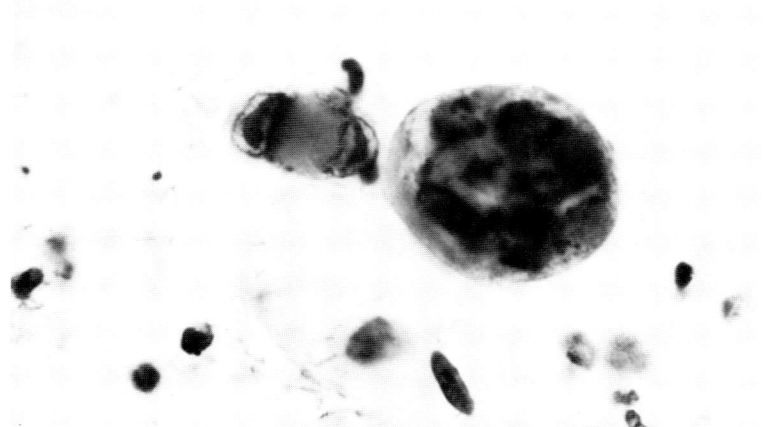

Fig. 2-19 CVE smear showing CMV infection. Note the multinucleated cell with an extremely poorly preserved chromatin pattern. CMV infection generally involves the endocervical-type cells, which do not necessarily enlarge. Two such cells seen in this picture reveal distinct, large, intranuclear inclusions. (Papanicolaou stain.)

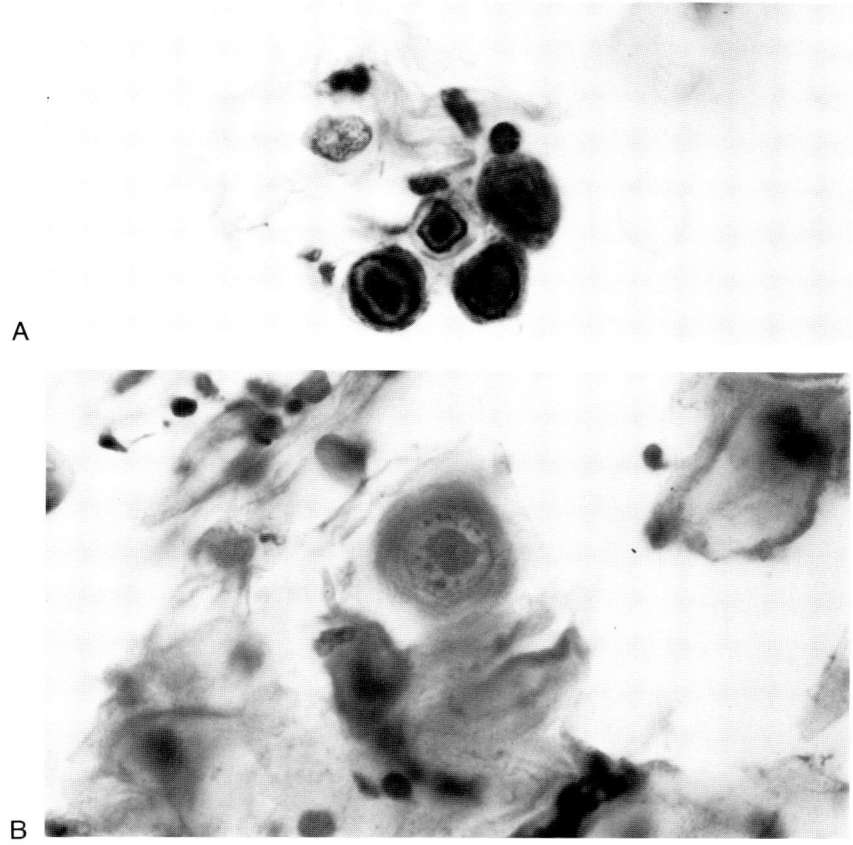

Fig. 2-20 (A) Papanicolaou-stained smear showing CMV infection. Note that a number of columnar, metaplastic-type cells appear individually. These cells contain large, basophilic, intranuclear inclusions that are surrounded by nuclear chromatin clearing. The margination of the intranuclear chromatin to the cell margin produces a distinct nuclear ring, as seen in these cells. An intermediate cell is also present in the field. **(B)** Papanicolaou-stained CVE smear revealing a columnar epithelial cell with distinct, intranuclear, acidophilic inclusion of CMV infection. (See Plate 2-4.)

low-virulence HPV appear to be similar, although evidence suggests that koilocytic changes probably occur most commonly in with HPV of low virulence (Types 6 and 11).

On cytologic examination, HPV infection is recognized by the occurrence of large aggregates or clumps of squamous epithelial cells (Fig. 2-21). The individual squamous cell is dense, with peripheral cytoplasmic condensation. The cellular margins are blunted and the cell acquires a more oval or rounded form in contrast to the typical polygonal appearance (Fig. 2-22). Cytoplasmic transparency is often lost. Generally, a perinuclear halo or a cavity appears, which has a crisp, distinct margin. The nucleus may be euplastic or dysplastic, or degenerated in appearance. It is frequently located to one side of the perinuclear halo (Fig. 2-23). This typical koilocytic change may not be obvious in each smear. Varying degrees of binucleate and multinucleate parakeratotic changes may be present (Fig. 2-24).[20,21]

Sometimes, HPV infection may involve immature metaplastic-type cells. These cells are somewhat larger and more pleomorphic than those in typical metaplasia, and generally are not accompanied by inflammation. These infected cyanophilic cells may be hyperchromatic and may exhibit peripheral cytoplasmic condensation and poorly defined koilocytic changes (Fig. 2-25).

The presence of HPV infection can be confirmed in nearly 65 percent of cases by appropriate antigen antibody staining (Fig. 2-26). These antigens are found most commonly in warty and low-grade dysplastic (CIN I) lesions.[22] The occurrence of integrated viral DNA can be demonstrated by DNA detection techniques, including Southern blot and in situ hybridization studies which are HPV DNA-specific and which can be performed using cervical-vaginal smears and paraffin-processed tissues (Fig. 2-27).[23]

MOLLUSCUM CONTAGIOSUM

Molluscum contagiosum, an RNA virus infection, can be diagnosed by identifying the large, acidophilic, intracytoplasmic inclusions that appear within the infected squamous epithelial cells. The nuclei of these cells are generally compressed, indistinct, and matted along one side of the cell border. The nucleus should be identified definitively before designating the acidophilic cellular structures as inclusions.

Fungal Infections

CANDIDA

Candida albicans is the most commonly observed fungal infection of the lower genital tract. Other species of the organism may cause infection, but they cannot be distinguished morphologically from each other. Nearly one third of the women with vaginal candidiasis are asymptomatic.

Both filamentous and yeast forms of Candida organisms are seen. These are delicate, elongated structures with a pseudoseptate pattern, acute angle branching, and multiple budding yeast forms (Fig. 2-28). Although pure yeast forms may represent an overgrowth of opportunistic infection, the presence of filamentous forms in a smear is believed to be evidence of tissue invasion (Fig. 2-29).

TRICHOPHYTON

Trichophyton and other cutaneous filamentous fungal forms can sometimes be observed as contaminants from the vulvar region in the cervical-vaginal smear. On morphologic examination, they do not exhibit yeast forms or a pseudoseptate pattern, and should be able to be distinguished from Candida organisms. Traditionally, they are not reported as vaginal infections.

Parasitic Infestations

TRICHOMONAS VAGINALIS

Trichomoniasis, a protozoal infection, is the most common parasitic infection observed in the female genital tract. Although most patients are symptomatic, some women, especially after hysterectomy, may be asymptomatic carriers. The infection can be transmitted to men, causing prostatic disease.

A presumptive diagnosis of trichomoniasis can be rendered by observing Leptothrix, which are long, filamentous, bacterial structures that commonly occur in conjunction with trichomonads and that exhibit a "BB shot" or "cannonball" configuration (Figs. 2-30 and 2-31).[24] These latter structures may represent squamous epithelial cells that are covered over by protozoal organisms and phagocytosed, in turn, by polymorphonuclear leukocytes and macro-

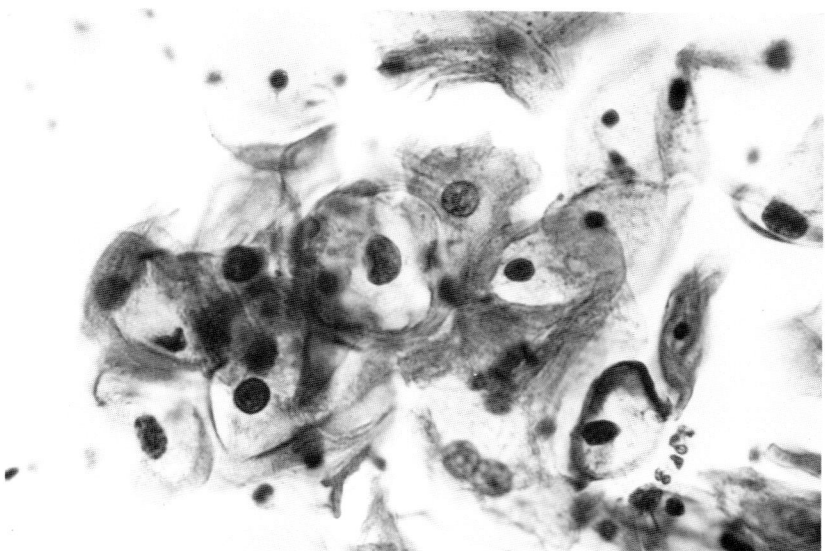

Fig. 2-21 CVE smear revealing cytomorphologic changes secondary to HPV infection. Note that the infected cells have lost their normal polygonal shapes, the margins have become rounded, the cells are aggregated in close proximity, and there is peripheral cytoplasmic condensation. Perinuclear clearing of varying degrees is also present. A few cells appear as typical koilocytes. (Papanicolaou stain.)

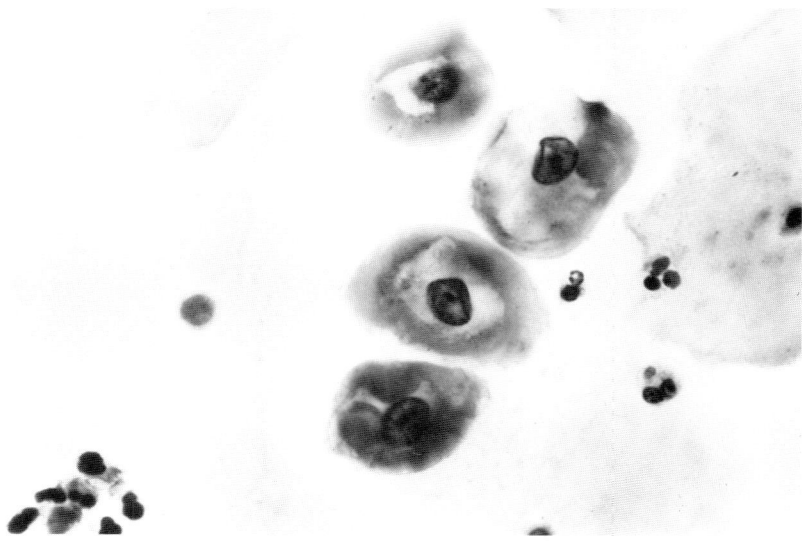

Fig. 2-22 CVE smear revealing morphologic changes secondary to HPV infection. Note the four central cells with the adjoining cells. These cells, although squamous in origin, are somewhat immature in appearance, with marginal blunting, rounding of the edges, and peripheral cytoplasmic condensation. (Papanicolaou stain.)

42 PRACTICAL CYTOPATHOLOGY

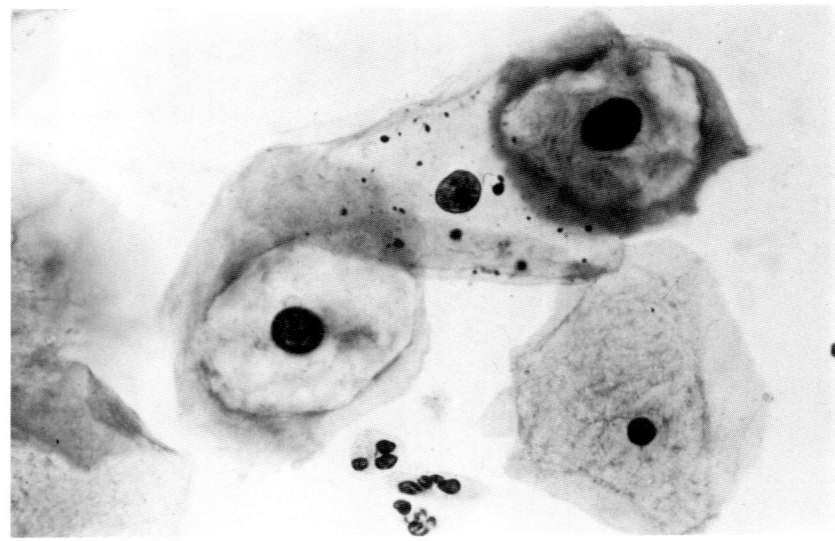

Fig. 2-23 CVE smear showing cytomorphologic changes secondary to HPV infection. Compare the two typical koilocytes seen in this smear with the normal squamous cells that are present. The former are not transparent, and they show distinct perinuclear clearing. The margin of such clearing is very distinct and crisp. (Papanicolaou stain.)

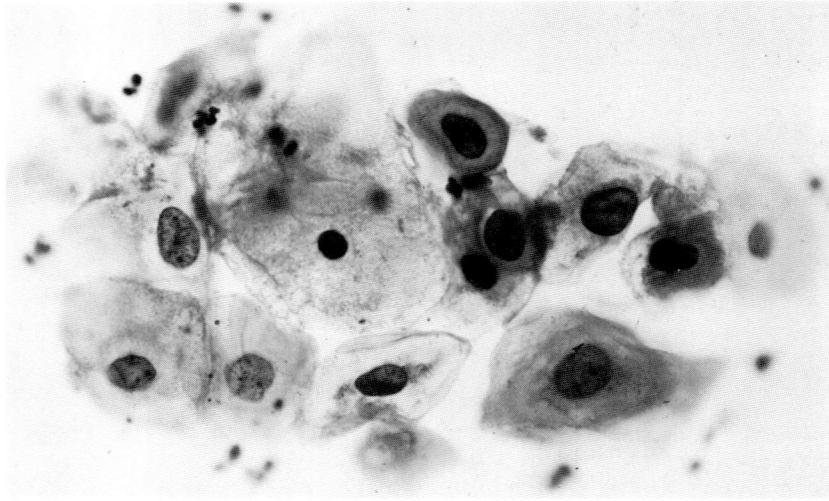

Fig. 2-24 CVE smear showing evidence of HPV infection. The cells are parakeratotic. (Papanicolaou stain.)

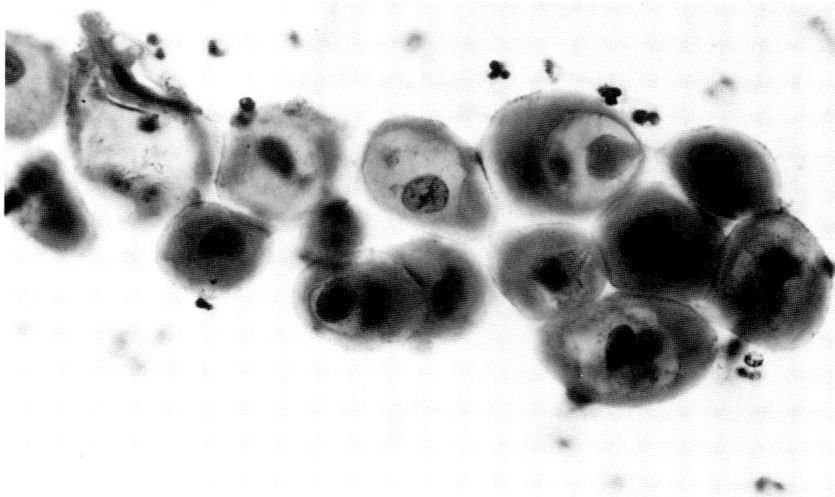

Fig. 2-25 CVE smear showing evidence of HPV infection. The infected cells stain cyanophilic by conventional Papanicolaou staining technique. These cells are metaplastic in nature; however, they have the typical cytomorphologic features of HPV infection. (Papanicolaou stain.)

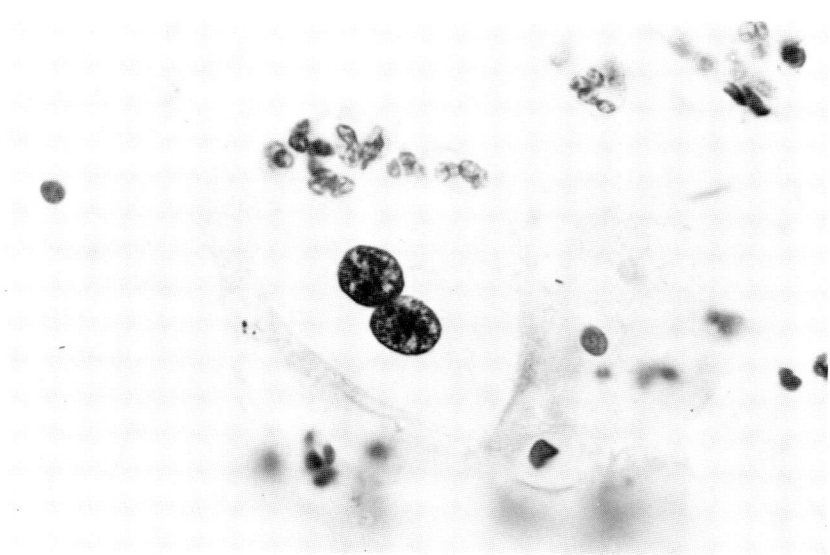

Fig. 2-26 CVE smear revealing a binucleate cell that stains positive for HPV capsid antigen. Such staining can be performed on smears previously stained with Papanicolaou stain without necessarily destaining them. The destaining procedure may actually produce nonspecific staining reactions and inconsistent results. (Peroxidase antiperoxidase staining with DAB staining; no counterstain.)

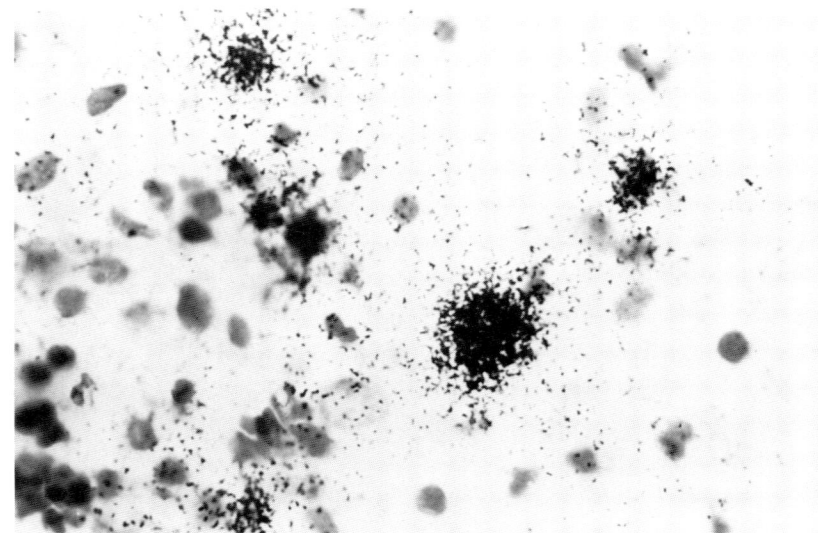

Fig. 2-27 In situ hybridization performed on a CVE smear using an S-35-labeled HPV-16 DNA probe. The infected cells show heavy nuclear radiolabeling. (Autoradiograph; no counterstain.)

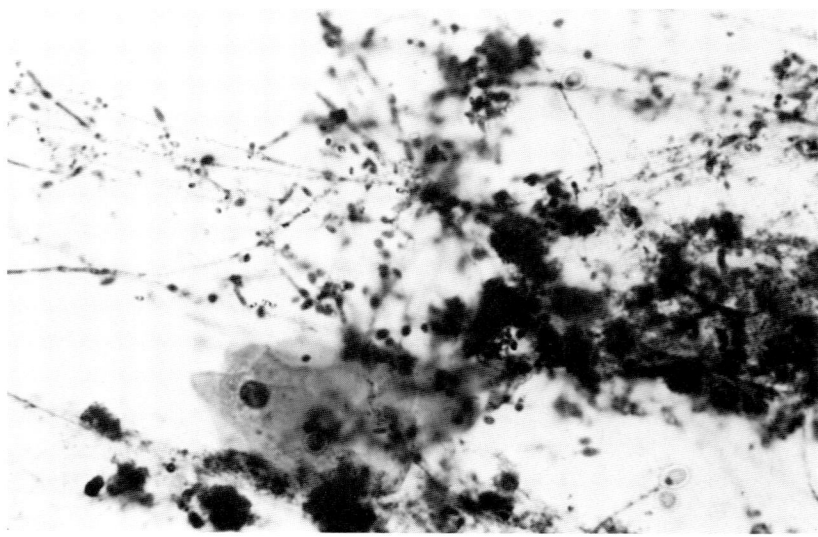

Fig. 2-28 CVE smear showing numerous filamentous forms in a pseudoseptate arrangement and some budding yeast forms of Candida organisms. These organisms cannot easily be differentiated from *Torulopsis* infection. (Papanicolaou stain.)

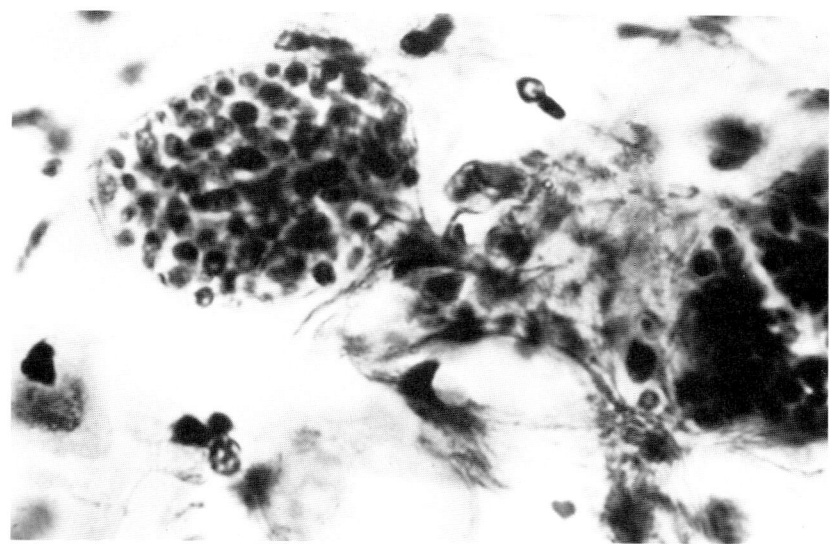

Fig. 2-29 CVE smear revealing intracystic yeast forms in a patient with candidiasis. These forms may represent an asymptomatic infection. (Papanicolaou stain.)

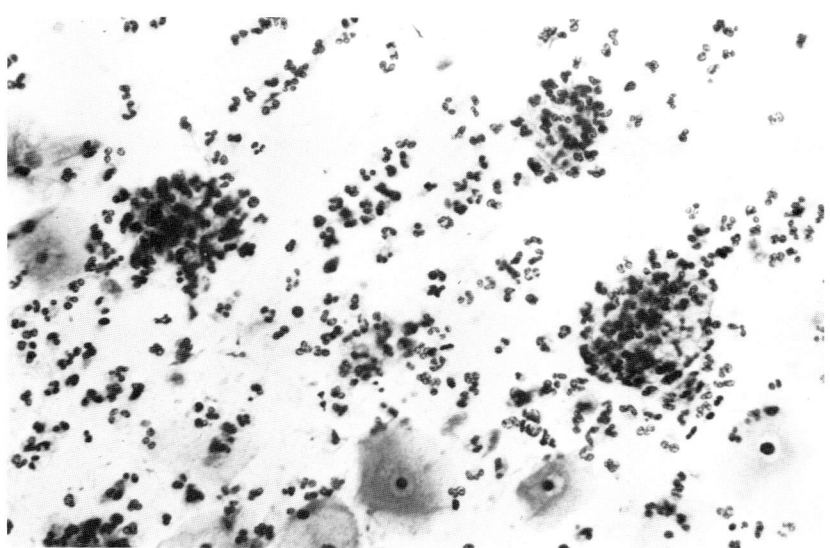

Fig. 2-30 CVE smear revealing aggregates of polymorphonuclear leukocytes occupying the surface of squamous epithelial cells. These aggregates, also called "cannonballs" or "BB shots" are often associated with *Trichomonas vaginalis* infection. The organisms per se must be identified before making a diagnosis of Trichomonas infection. (Papanicolaou stain.)

46 PRACTICAL CYTOPATHOLOGY

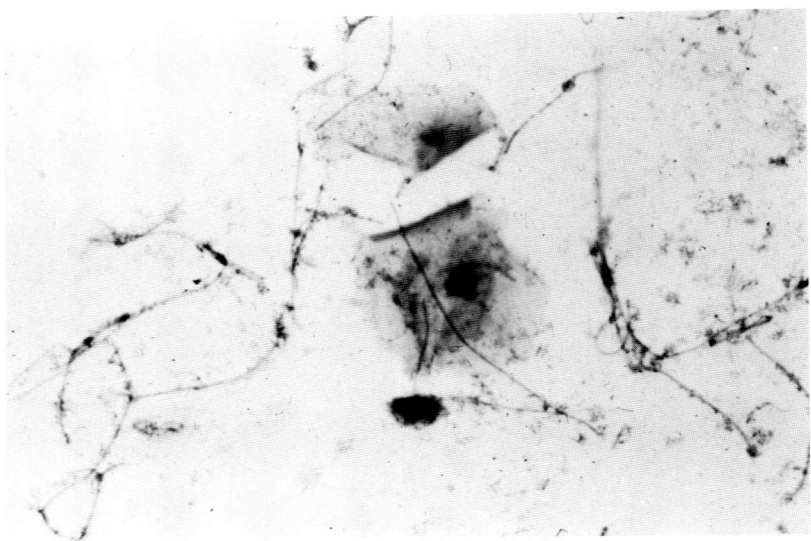

Fig. 2-31 CVE smear revealing numerous filamentous Leptothrix organisms. These bacterial forms frequently accompany Trichomonas infection. (Papanicolaou stain.)

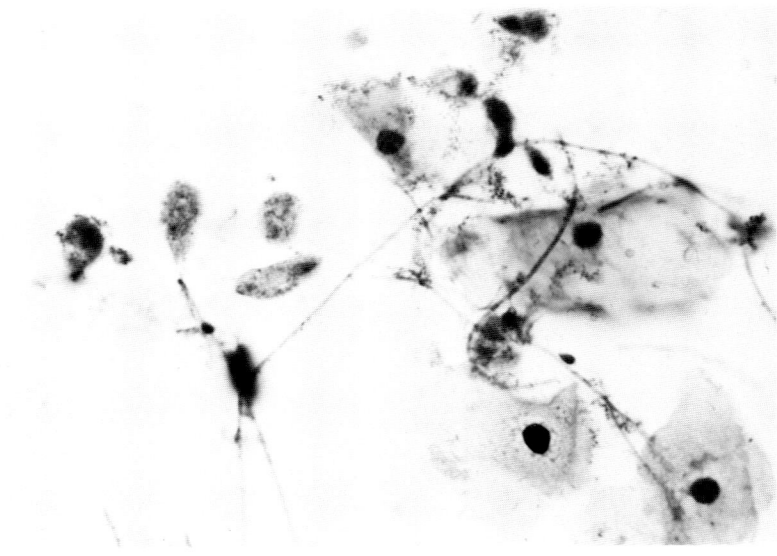

Fig. 2-32 CVE smear showing *Trichomonas vaginalis*. These organisms vary in shape and size. However, they all contain a pale, faint but distinct, vesicular nucleus. Some contain intracytoplasmic granules as well. (Papanicolaou stain.)

phages. Similar structures can occur in the absence of Trichomonas, also.

Trichomonas organisms occur as round to oval to irregularly shaped pale structures that vary in size from the diameter of the nucleus of a neutrophil to that of a parabasal cell, or even larger. Flagella, which are so typical of motile organisms, are not seen in Papanicolaou-stained preparations. The color of the organisms is variable, and generally follows the staining pattern of most of the cells in a smear. To be diagnostic, a distinct, pale, vesicular nucleus must always be identified within the cytoplasm of these structures (Fig. 2-32). Bare nuclei resulting from cytolysis, degenerating leukocytes, as occur in heavy inflammation, and atrophic epithelial cells that frequently occur in postmenopausal states must all be distinguished from true trichomonads. When carefully diagnosed, the cytodiagnosis of Trichomonas infection is quite accurate, and results are comparable to those obtained from hanging drop and culture detection systems.[25]

ENTAMOEBA HISTOLYTICA

Entamoeba histolytica infection is uncommon in this country. The organisms occur as histiocyte-like structures that contain ingested red blood cells within the cytoplasm.

Vaginal and Vulvar Cytology
Darryl G. Heustis

CYTOLOGY OF THE VAGINA

Vaginal cytology may be studied either by examination of the contents of the posterior fornix, or by direct smears of a lesion.

Inflammatory Lesions of the Vagina

Infectious leukorrhea of the vagina is caused by the same spectrum of inflammatory organisms and viruses that affects the cervix, including herpes, Candida, Leptothrix, trichomonads, and Gardnerella. These diseases present with the same cytologic changes that they do elsewhere in the female genital tract. The vaginal epithelium is most susceptible when there is absence of full maturation.[26]

Vaginal parasitosis is not usually found. Parasitic ova are usually due to contamination.[27] Some vaginal parasites, such as *Enterobius vermicularis, Ascaris lumbricoides,* and Microfilariae, have been associated with the use of IUDs.[28]

Benign Tumors of the Vagina

Vaginal adenosis is a condition involving mucus-secreting columnar epithelium in women who were exposed to diethylstilbestrol (DES) in utero. This drug was commonly used between the mid-1940s and the mid-1960s to prevent and treat complications of pregnancy. DES exposure interferes with the transformation of fetal vaginal columnar epithelium to squamous epithelium, with consequent retention of columnar epithelium. Thus, areas of adenosis are characterized by sheets of mucus-producing columnar cells that are identical to normal endocervical cells, and that commonly display honeycomb and picket-fence arrangements (Figs. 2-33 and 2-34, Plate 2-5). As it is impossible to distinguish cells of vaginal adenosis from normal and reactive endocervical cells, separate vaginal smears must be obtained to establish the diagnosis. Women with vaginal adenosis also commonly exhibit areas of squamous metaplasia.[29]

48 PRACTICAL CYTOPATHOLOGY

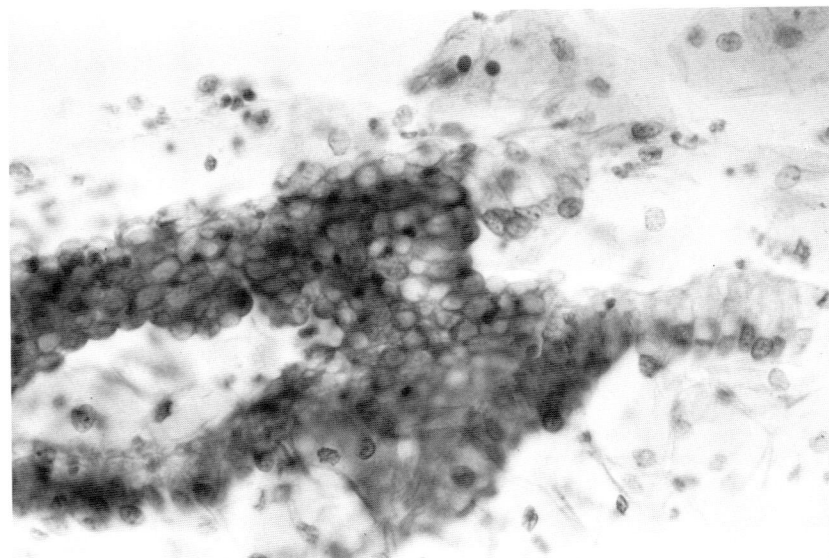

Fig. 2-33 Large cluster of tall columnar epithelium from a vaginal smear showing uniform size and shape. The patient had been exposed to DES in utero. (Papanicolaou stain, × 100.)

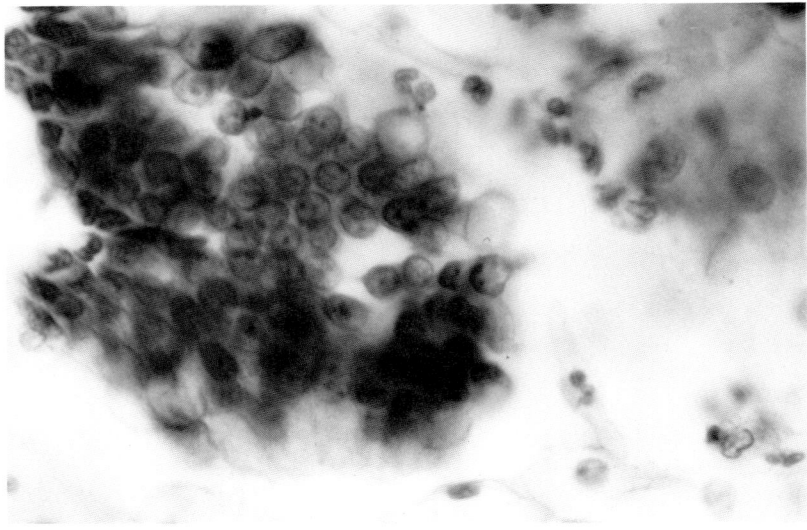

Fig. 2-34 Vaginal smear showing adenosis in a patient exposed to DES in utero. Note the picket-fence arrangement of the cells and their similarity to endocervical cells. (See Plate 2-5.) (Papanicolaou stain, × 200.)

Other benign tumors of the vagina include Gartner's cysts, fibromas, leiomyomas, hemangiomas, and condyloma. All of these occur only rarely.

Malignant Tumors of the Vagina

METASTATIC CARCINOMA

The most common malignant tumor of the vagina is metastatic carcinoma. Common sites of origin include the uterine cervix, endometrium, ovary, intestine, and urinary bladder. Obese or diabetic women who present with cytolytic or markedly karyopyknotic vaginal smears exhibit high intrinsic estrogen activity, and may be at risk for endometrial carcinoma.[30] Ovarian carcinoma cells can be differentiated from endometrial carcinoma, as the cells of the former are usually larger, often overlap, and have prominent nucleoli.

PRIMARY MALIGNANT TUMORS

Primary malignant tumors of the vagina occur only rarely, and *squamous cell carcinoma* is the most common of these. Nearly 50 percent of the cases of invasive squamous cell carcinoma of the vagina are associated with in situ or invasive squamous cell carcinoma of the cervix.[31,32] The cells exhibit cytologic features similar to those of squamous cell carcinoma of the cervix, including bizarre cells, orangeophilia, tadpole cells, and pearl formations. Primary *clear cell adenocarcinoma* of the vagina accounts for 1 percent of all invasive carcinomas of the female genital tract.[33] An increased incidence in recent years has been associated with diethylstilbestrol use. Two main cell types—clear cells and hobnail cells—have been reported.[34] The clear cells are large cells that have delicate, transparent cytoplasm and, in most cases, single, round nuclei (Fig. 2-35). These cells may occur singly or in clusters. The hobnail cells are small and generally round, with minimal cytoplasm, although clear cell differentiation can occur. They have an increased nuclear/cytoplasmic ratio, and the chromatin often appears somewhat dense. Although both cell types may have nucleoli, these are not usually prominent. The smear background may vary from being clean to exhibiting neutrophils, blood, and debris. This tumor is similar to adenocarcinoma of the endocervix, although the cells commonly show less nuclear clearing and the nucleoli are less prominent.

Other malignant tumors of the vagina are very rare. They include sarcoma and melanoma.

CYTOLOGY OF THE VULVA

Although most vulvar lesions are apparent, accessible, and easily biopsied, cytology may provide not only a more rapid means of obtaining diagnostic information, but also an alternative approach in those patients who refuse consent for biopsy.

The normal vulvar surface exfoliates not only superficial squamous cells, but also anucleated squames, from the labia majora. Inflammatory cells are rare or absent. Cells are best obtained by vigorous scraping with a spatula after application of physiologic saline to prevent drying and to decrease cellular distortion.

Inflammatory Lesions

Molluscum contagiosum is a viral disease characterized by intracytoplasmic, oval, orangeophilic inclusions in epithelial cells. These inclusions may be free in the smears upon degeneration of the host cell.

Gonorrheal vulvitis is a bacterial disease presenting with gram-negative diplococci within neutrophils or on the surface of squamous cells. Degeneration and necrosis may be present. A culture is required to establish a definitive diagnosis.

Granuloma inguinale is a disease caused by gram-negative nonmotile bacteria that are commonly found in the cytoplasm of neutrophils, histiocytes, and plasma cells (Donovan bodies). The bacterium often assumes the shape of a closed safety pin. An association between granuloma inguinale and squamous cell carcinoma has been reported.[29]

Herpes genitalis is a viral disease that produces small vesicles or ulcerations on the vulva. Cytologic specimens demonstrate the characteristic ground-glass appearance of the nuclei, as well as intranuclear eosinophilic inclusions.

Lymphogranuloma venereum is caused by a Bedsonian agent, and presents as small, intracytoplasmic inclusions within histiocytes. These are commonly surrounded by a halo.

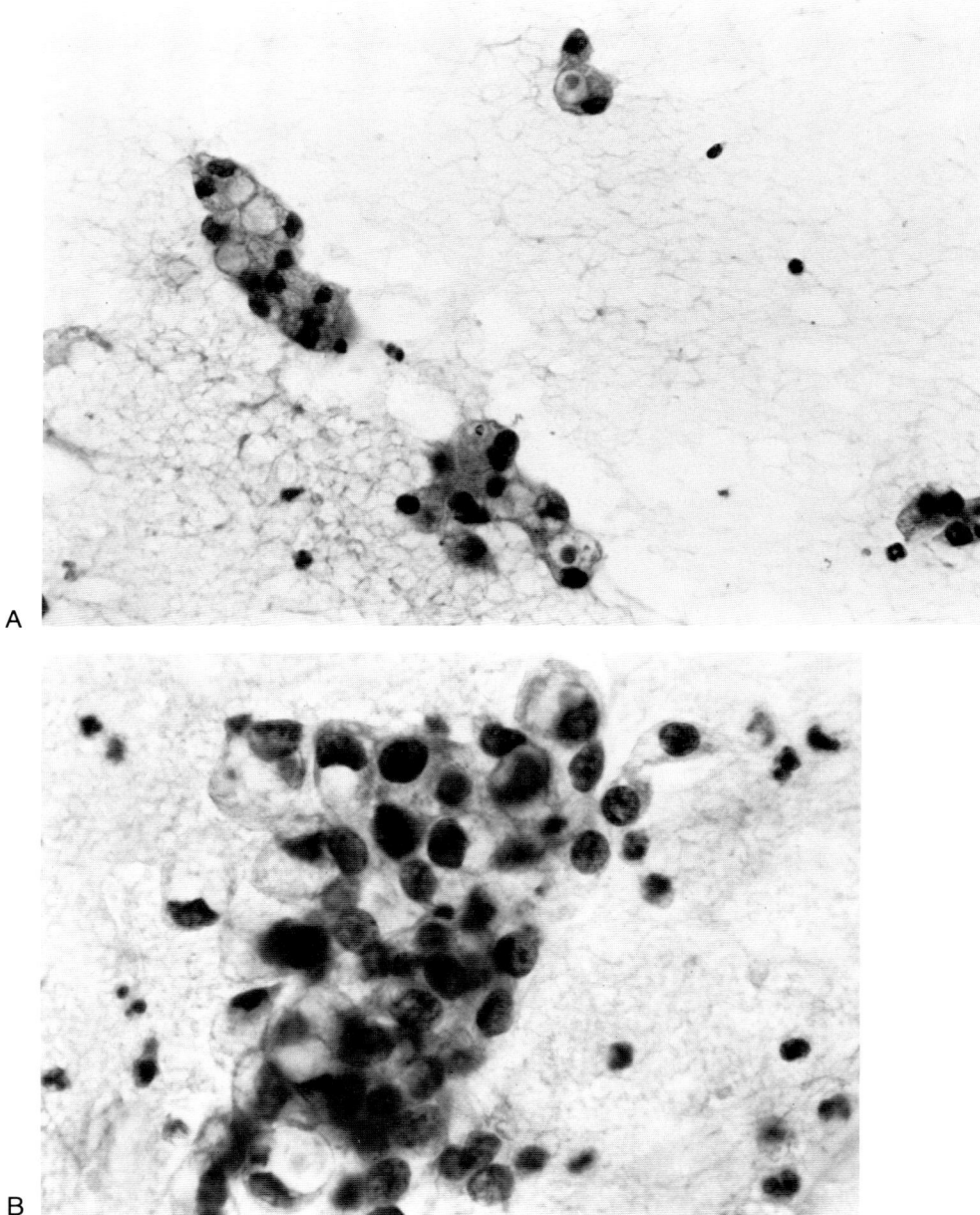

Fig. 2-35 (A,B) Clear cell carcinoma of the vagina. Note the partially vacuolated cytoplasm, the irregularly dispersed, finely granular chromatin, and the suggestion of a glandular (endocervical) origin. (Fig. A, Papanicolaou stain, × 100; Fig. B, Papanicolaou stain, × 200.)

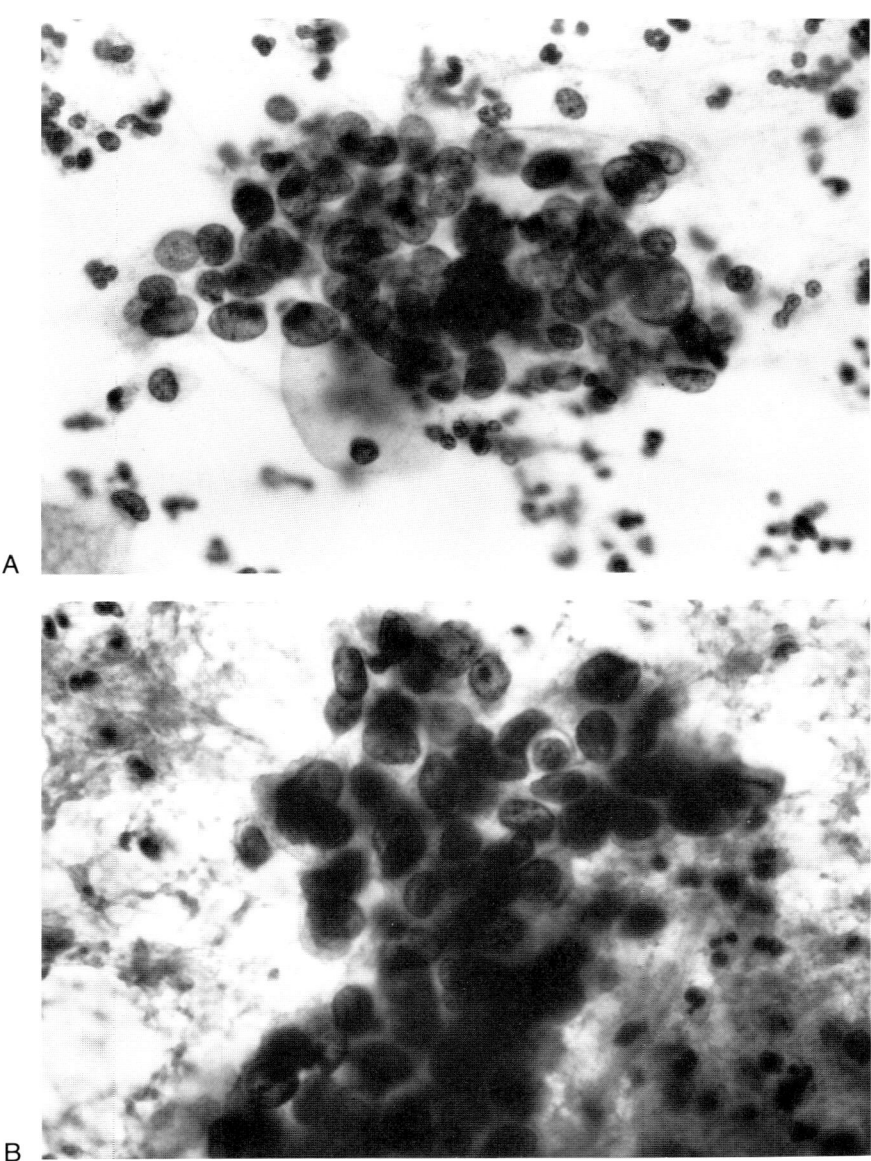

Fig. 2-36 (A,B) Carcinoma in situ of the vulva. Note the syncytial arrangement of the cells with variation in nuclear size and a general absence of nucleoli. Prominent, coarse chromatin granules are easily seen. (Papanicolaou stain, × 200.)

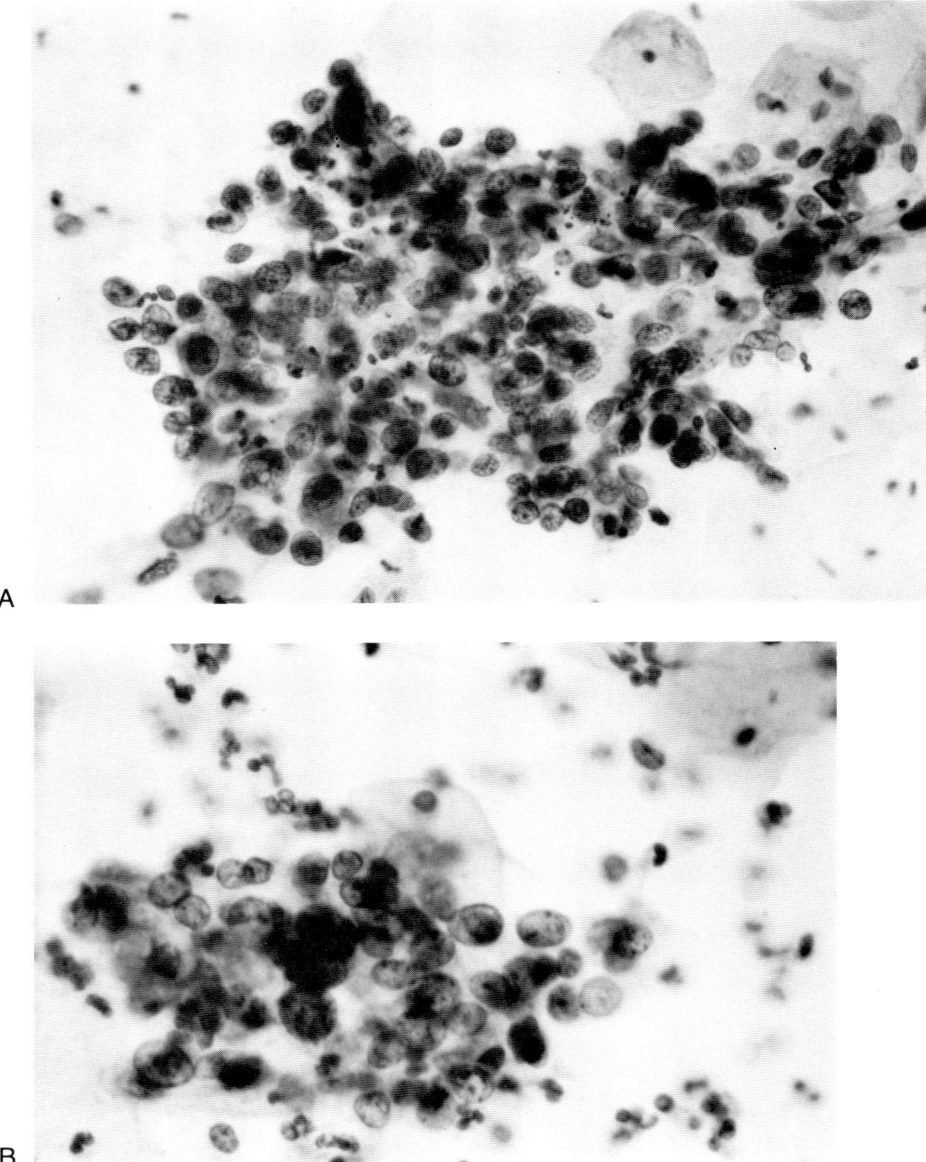

Fig. 2-37 (A,B) CIS of the vulva. A syncytial arrangement of cells, a scant to adequate cytoplasm, and a generally clean smear background are evident. (Fig. A, Papanicolaou stain, × 100; Fig. B, Papanicolaou stain, × 200.) (See Plates 2-6, 2-7.)

BENIGN TUMORS OF THE VULVA

Condyloma acuminatum is the most common benign tumor of the vulva.[26] Although most lesions respond to podophyllin, a few continue to grow and must be removed by other measures, such as electrocautery. Cytologic evaluation reveals squamous cells that display perinuclear cavitation and prominent, hyperchromatic nuclei.

Other benign tumors of the vulva can be cystic or solid. The cystic lesions include Bartholin gland cysts, sebaceous cysts, epidermal inclusion cysts, and wolffian cysts. Among the solid tumors are fibromas, leiomyomas, hemangiomas, lipomas, hidradenomas, and granular cell myoblastomas.

MALIGNANT TUMORS OF THE VULVA

Squamous Cell Carcinoma

Vulvar malignancies constitute about 5 percent of all gynecologic cancers, the most common of which is squamous cell carcinoma.[35] Atrophy of the vulvar skin in older women is associated with excessive keratinization (leukoplakia), which is a precursor of squamous cell carcinoma.[26]

CIS of the vulva (Bowen's disease) resembles carcinoma in situ of the cervix (Figs. 2-36 and 2-37, Plates 2-6 and 2-7). The cells show hyperchromatic or pyknotic nuclei with scant to adequate cytoplasm. Nucleoli are usually absent. The cells may exhibit irregular shapes and sizes, with some very large cells present. The smear background usually shows no significant necrosis. Surface keratin may be seen in the smears.

Invasive squamous cell carcinoma of the vulva yields large numbers of orangeophilic, pleomorphic tumor cells. The cells are commonly found in groups and often display multinucleation. The nuclei are hyperchromatic and vary greatly in size and shape. Cytoplasm is thick and often generous. The smear background commonly displays necrotic debris and inflammatory cells.

Malignant Melanoma

Most malignant melanomas of the female genital tract occur in the vulva.[26] Cytologically, the single, large malignant cells with prominent nucleoli resemble melanoma cells seen from other locations. Multinucleation is common, but the cells may or may not display melanin pigment granules. Holmquist and Torres[36] recently reported a primary malignant melanoma in the female genital tract that presented in an unusual cytologic pattern. In this case, the cytologic findings of spindle-shaped cells and nuclei, coupled with a lack of pigment, suggested a possible leiomyosarcoma.

Benign Disorders of the Cervix
Darryl G. Heustis

INFECTIOUS DISORDERS

Inflammation of the cervix may be caused by a multitude of benign conditions, but the principle initiators are bacteria, fungi, protozoans, and viruses.

Any of these agents can evoke an inflammatory cellular response that affects squamous epithelial cells and that is characterized by any or all of the following features:

1. Prominent nuclei with perinuclear halos

2. Pleomorphic cytoplasmic contours, often with poorly defined borders
3. Amphophilic cytoplasmic staining
4. An empty or salt-and-pepper chromatin pattern
5. Cytolysis
6. Vacuolization
7. Karyorrhexis and pyknosis
8. Widespread MI

These cellular changes are often accompanied by an increased number of neutrophils, an increased amount of blood, and histiocytes that show active phagocytosis.

Döderlein Bacilli

Döderlein bacilli, which are gram-positive rods, are normal inhabitants of the lower female genital tract that stain basophilic with Papanicolaou stains. Enzymatic cytolysis of intermediate squamous cells commonly occurs. Seen in 40 percent of normal smears and in patients with dysplasia and carcinoma in situ (CIS), the bacillus is only seen in 10 percent of patients with early invasive squamous carcinoma and less than 1 percent of those with advanced cancers.[37]

Gardnerella (hemophilus) vaginalis

Gardnerella (hemophilus) vaginalis is a gram-negative short rod that stains dark blue with Papanicolaou. The organism preferentially accumulates on the surfaces of mature squamous cells, giving their cytoplasm a characteristic grainy appearance (clue cells). Only a mild inflammatory reaction is usually seen.

Chlamydia

Chlamydia organisms are coccobacilli that have an affinity for the cytoplasm of squamous metaplastic and endocervical cells in which the eosinophilic and cyanophilic coccoid structures appear to be surrounded by clear zones. Chlamydial vaginal infections can be transmitted to newborn infants during delivery, causing resultant ophthalmic infections.

Candida Species

Candidiasis is the most common fungal infection of the female genital tract. It is frequently associated with diabetes, pregnancy, oral contraceptives, and antibacterial and immunosuppressant medications.

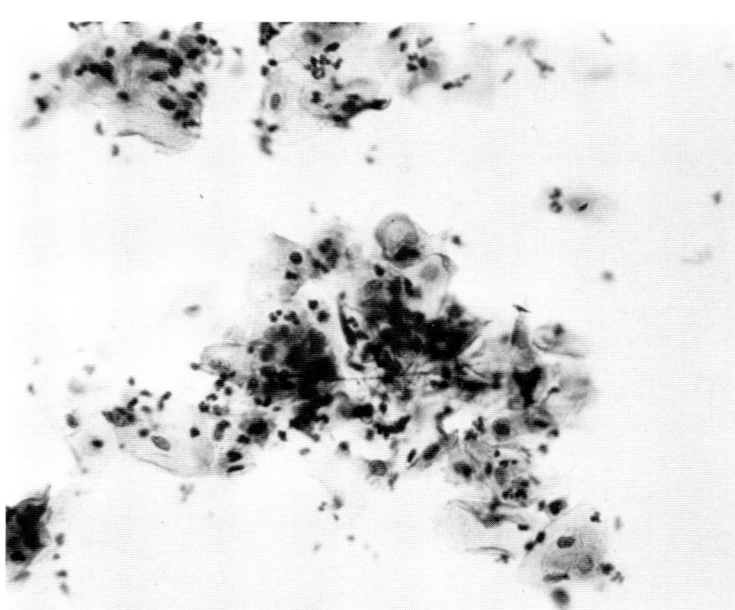

Fig. 2-38 Intertwined squamous cells bound together by the pseudohyphae of Candida species. (Papanicolaou stain, × 100.) (See Plate 2-8.)

The segmented pseudohyphae and tiny spores stain faint blue or pink, and commonly intertwine groups of squamous epithelial cells (yielding the so-called flowers-on-a-lei arrangement) (Fig. 2-38, Plate 2-8). A mild acute inflammatory reaction is often present. Although culture is the best way to diagnose candidiasis, cervical smears have detected up to 80 percent of the infections that were confirmed by culture.[38]

Trichomonads

The small, pear-shaped, flagellated trichomonad prefers an elevated vaginal pH. This organism appears greenish-blue on Papanicolaou stain and exhibits a faint, elongated nucleus and occasional red cytoplasmic granules (Fig. 2-39, Plate 2-9). Associated findings include Leptothrix, coccoid bacteria, squamous metaplasia, acute inflammation, and a shift to the right in MI for an increased estrogen effect. Squamous cells commonly show perinuclear halos, and neutrophils often surround the protozoans. Cytoplasmic fragments and stripped nuclei are commonly misinterpreted as trichomonads.

Herpes Simplex Virus

HSV penetrates the nucleus of squamous or endocervical cells. These nuclei become glassy, acquiring a ground-glass appearance. Multinucleation is common, but the nuclei tend to crowd together (or mold) rather than to overlap (Fig. 2-40, Plate 2-10). Irregular intranuclear inclusions are often present, and may be surrounded by a halo or clear zone. Ng and associates have postulated that the inclusions are a strong indication of a recurrent rather than a primary herpetic infection,[39] but Vesterinen's group has found no such differences.[40] The differential diagnosis includes degenerating endocervicals, multinucleated giant cells, atypical squamous metaplastic cells, and adenocarcinoma.

Condyloma

A product of HPV, condyloma produces two distinctive cell types—koilocytes and dyskeratocytes—which are important in establishing the diagnosis.[41] Koilocytes are usually intermediate squamous cells that display perinuclear cavitation and thickened cytoplasmic borders. Binucleation is common. The nuclear chromatin is either finely granular, smudged, or pyknotic. Dyskeratocytes are small, mature squamous cells that often stain bright orange. These cells exhibit nuclear findings that are similar to those of koilocytes, but that lack the perinuclear cavitation.

Atypical Condyloma

A variant of condyloma, first described in 1981,[42] displays enlarged, hyperchromatic nuclei that appear

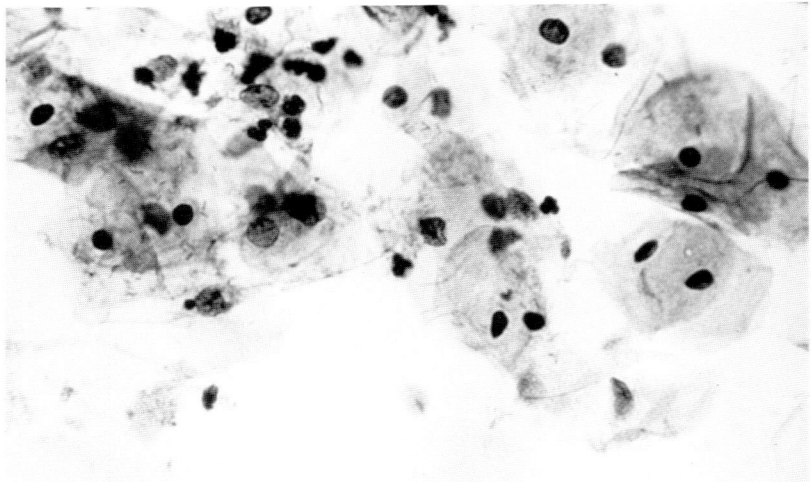

Fig. 2-39 Scattered squamous cells and Leptothrix bacteria. Note the trichomonad in the lower center of the field. (Papanicolaou stain, × 100.) (See Plate 2-9.)

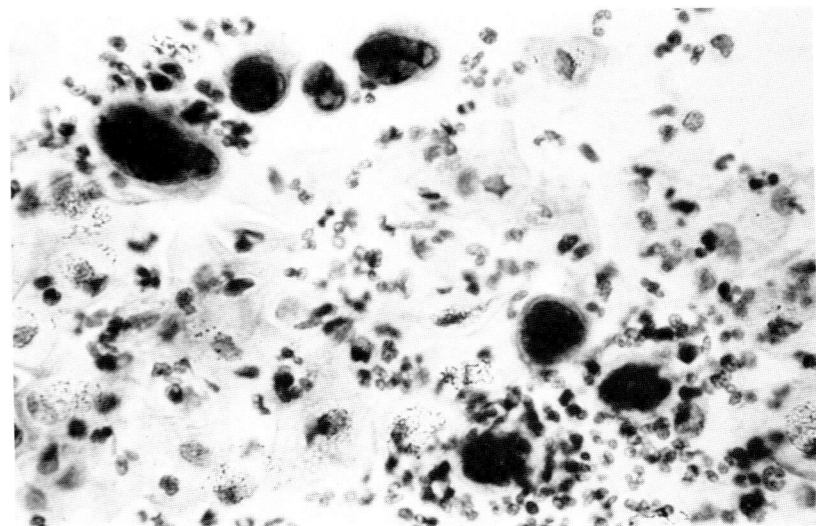

Fig. 2-40 Herpes-infected cells showing multinucleation, ground-glass nuclei and nuclear molding. (Papanicolaou stain, × 100.) (See Plate 2-10.)

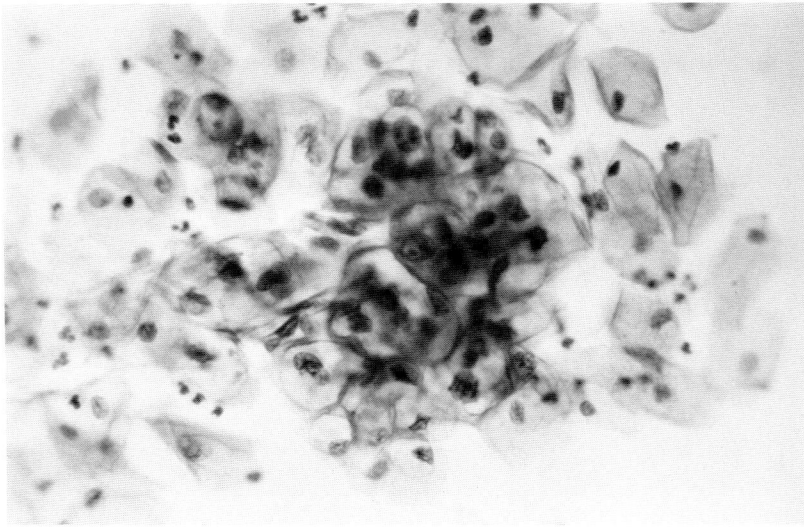

Fig. 2-41 Cluster of condylomatous cells showing enlarged, hyperchromatic, irregular nuclei, perinuclear clearing, and variable condensation of peripheral cytoplasm. (Papanicolaou stain, × 100.) (See Plate 2-11.)

to be dysplastic. Indeed, condyloma may be associated with the spectrum of intraepithelial neoplasia and squamous carcinoma. The cytoplasm is often keratinized, and koilocytes are not always present. When they are, this condition is often diagnosed as dysplasia with koilocytosis. Some forms of atypical condyloma may be confused with CIS or squamous carcinoma (Figs. 2-41, 2-42, Plate 2-11).

DISORDERS UNRELATED TO INFECTION

The cervical epithelium may show growth alterations designed for protection from various internal and external stimuli.

Hyperkeratosis

Hyperkeratosis is a benign protective reaction in which stratified squamous epithelium forms a granular layer and surface keratin. Clinically, this keratinized surface is often referred to as leukoplakia. On cytologic examination, hyperkeratosis appears as anucleated squamous cells, which are often yellow and which may occur singly or in clusters.

Parakeratosis

Parakeratosis is another protective change that is characterized by layers of small, compact squamous cells with pyknotic nuclei. Cytologically these cells may appear singly or as sheets of miniature squamous cells with orangeophilic cytoplasm, strap or spindle forms, and pyknotic nuclei.

Squamous Metaplasia

The most common protective reaction of the cervix is squamous metaplasia. Fragile columnar cells at the squamocolumnar junction of the endocervical canal are replaced by more durable squamous cells. The metaplastic squamous cells are smaller than normal squames, are pleomorphic, and are often arranged in small clusters (in a so-called cookie-cutter arrangement) (Fig. 2-43, Plate 2-12).

Atypical Squamous Metaplasia

In atypical squamous metaplasia, various abnormalities of metaplastic cells are evident. These may include nuclear enlargement, binucleation, irregular nuclear contours, and slight hyperchromatism.

Irradiation

Radiation therapy usually causes degeneration because of its direct toxic effect. Vacuolization of both the nucleus and cytoplasm, increased cell size, pleomorphism with bizarre shapes, multinucleation, and a two-tone cytoplasm may result from radiation exposure.

Folic Acid Deficiency

Folic acid deficiency may also cause enlargement of squamous cells. In such cases, the nucleocytoplasmic ratio remains constant, and the cell changes resemble those seen with radiation effect except that pleomorphism and bizarre cellular configurations are uncommon.

Atrophy

Atrophy is associated with an estrogen deficiency, and the smears are composed primarily of parabasal cells that are shed singly or in sheets. Individual cells commonly exhibit a central, round nucleus that is surrounded by dense, often scant cytoplasm. The atrophic sheets may show either round or elongated nuclei that are often pyknotic (Fig. 2-44, Plate 2-13). The following atrophic changes can mimic squamous cell carcinoma.

1. Parabasal cells in patients with folic acid deficiencies can show marked variations in size and shape, with generous amounts of cytoplasm.[43]
2. Nuclear pyknosis can simulate the hyperchromatism of malignant squamous cells. Diagnosis can be particularly difficult if the nuclei are spindle-shaped.
3. The smear background commonly consists of old and fresh blood, neutrophils, macrophages, and cellular debris, all of which may be associated with squamous cell carcinoma.
4. Large numbers of parabasal cells can imitate CIS, and atrophic sheets may appear as syncytial groups.
5. Cells from a dry vaginal mucosa may produce false eosinophilia (air-drying).[37]

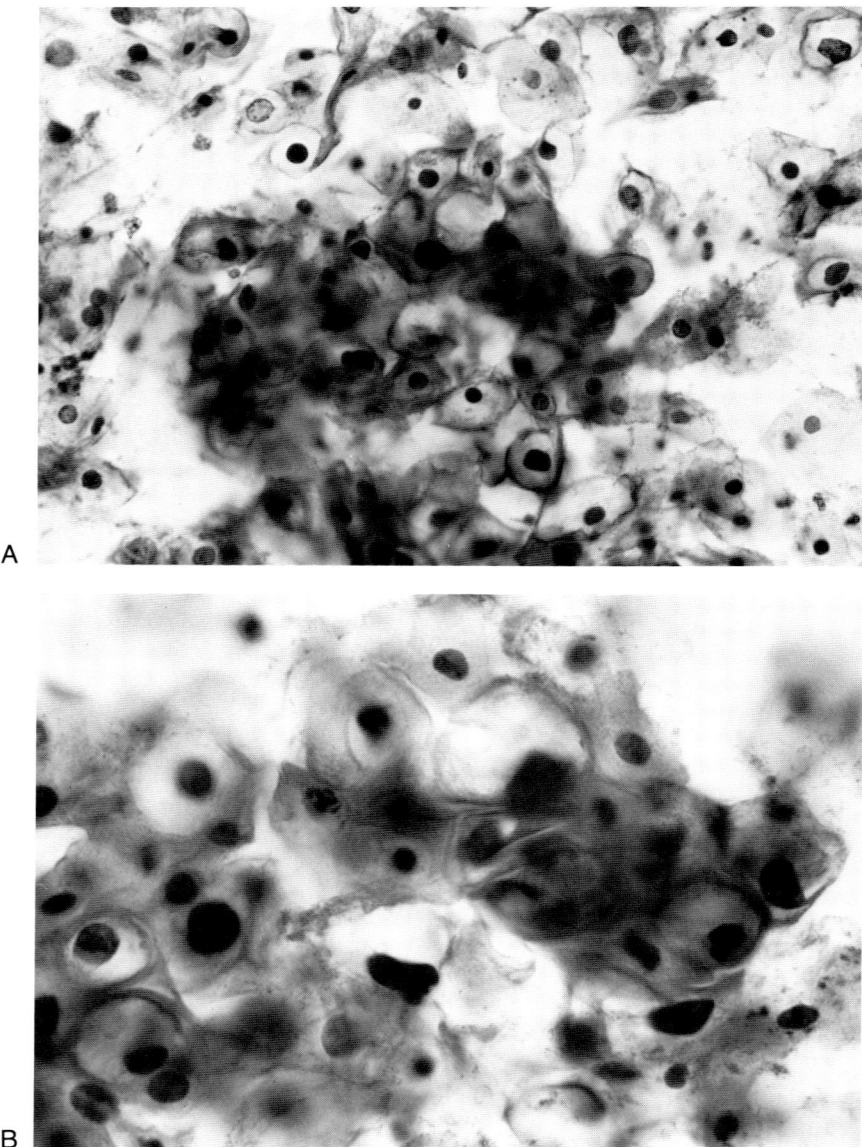

Fig. 2-42A & B Two photographs of atypical condyloma showing pronounced perinuclear cavitation and thickened cytoplasmic borders. The high power view shows atypical hyperchromatic nuclei of variable size and shape. (Fig. A, Papanicolaou stain, × 100; Fig. B, Papanicolaou stain, × 200.)

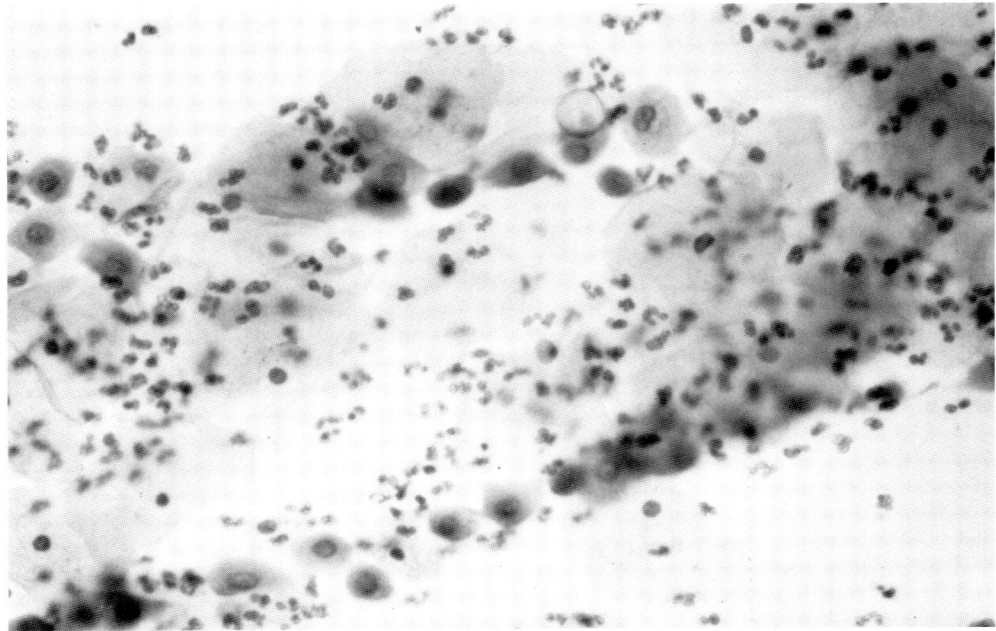

Fig. 2-43 Small metaplastic squamous cells showing dense cytoplasm and a cookie-cutter configuration. (Papanicolaou stain, × 100.) (See Plate 2-12.)

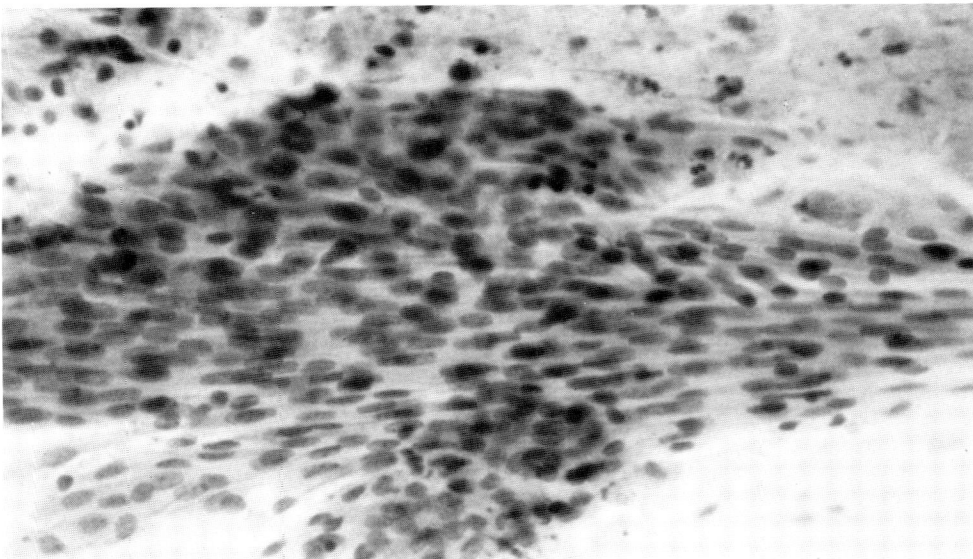

Fig. 2-44 An atrophic sheet of squamous cells showing spindle nuclei, bland chromatin, centrally placed nuclei, and adequate cytoplasm. (Papanicolaou stain, × 200.) (See Plate 2-13).

Reparative Changes

Reparative changes can be found in both glandular and squamous epithelial cells. The cell changes usually represent a response to an injurious stimulus, such as inflammation, irradiation, or chemical or physical trauma. The most common findings include

1. Distinct cell borders
2. Sheets of cells, with single cells rarely being seen
3. Ribbon-like cytoplasmic extensions
4. Eosinophilic nucleoli, either single or multiple
5. Finely granular chromatin
6. Maintenance of nuclear polarity
7. Inflammatory exudate

The differential diagnosis includes endocervical adenocarcinoma and large cell CIS. In endocervical adenocarcinoma, the smear background is usually clean, isolated cells or syncytial groups are present, and cells may overlap. In large cell CIS, the smear usually reveals coarse chromatin, single cells, and a clean background. Macronucleoli are often rare, and cell borders are indistinct.

Cytopathology of Dysplasia, Carcinoma In Situ, and Invasive Carcinoma of the Uterine Cervix

Thomas A. Bonfiglio

DYSPLASIA AND CARCINOMA IN SITU

The development of invasive squamous cell carcinoma of the uterine cervix is antedated by a preinvasive intraepithelial process that may be recognized both on histologic and cytologic examination. The histologic patterns included under the broadly descriptive phrase of "preinvasive cervical neoplasia" are diverse and heterogeneous. This spectrum of neoplastic changes is associated with a variety of abnormal cell types. A careful consideration of the morphologic aspects of these cells permits the cytopathologist not only to detect the presence of the disease process, but also to determine with a high degree of accuracy the histologic appearance of the tissue of origin.

Morphologic Features and Subclassification of Dysplasia and Carcinoma In Situ

A number of subclassification systems have been advocated for the precursor lesions of squamous cell carcinoma; these have previously been reviewed in the literature.[44-46] Currently, two classifications are most commonly utilized. The classification system that is older and more widely accepted by pathologists uses the terms slight (mild), moderate, and marked (severe) dysplasia, as well as CIS, whereas the more recently advocated terminology uses the term *cervical intraepithelial neoplasia* (CIN) for the whole spectrum of neoplastic reactions. This term is further modified by categorizing the lesions according to grades, with grade I corresponding to slight dysplasia, grade II referring to moderate dysplasia, and grade III encompassing both marked dysplasia and CIS.[47]

The intraepithelial phase of the neoplastic process (dysplasia) is characterized by disordered development of the squamous epithelium. This is manifested histologically by a proliferation of primitive cells beginning in the lower portions of the epithelium; by nuclear abnormalities, including hyperchromasia and increased nuclear size; and by mitotic abnormalities, including increased numbers of mitoses and, in many cases, the presence of abnormal mitotic figures. In general, the more the appearance of the epithelium deviates from the normal patterns of cervical epithelium, the more severe the process is judged to be. In practice, the term slight dysplasia is applied when the proliferation of primitive cells is confined to the lower one third of the epithelium (Fig. 2-45). Moderate dysplasia refers to those lesions in which primitive cells involve the middle one third of the epithelium. As the upper one third of the epithelium becomes involved by primitive cells, the dysplasia is considered to be marked (Fig. 2-46). If the entire thickness of the epithelium is replaced by the proliferation, the lesion is termed CIS (Fig. 2-47). As the process increases in severity, mitoses are found at higher and higher levels in the epithelium. Abnormal mitoses also may be identified—rarely in slight dysplasias, but commonly in the most severe reactions. Fu and colleagues have demonstrated that the presence of abnormal mitoses correlates well with the presence of an aneuploid cell population and is predictive of those lesions that are most likely to progress.[48]

Two morphologic tissue patterns can be used in addition to CIN grade in categorizing dysplasia. The first and most common pattern is characteristic of the usual type of lesion that arises in the transformation zone. This is referred to as the nonkeratinizing type and, as used in this chapter, also includes those lesions that are designated by Patten as metaplastic dysplasia.[44] The tissue manifestations of this type of lesion are depicted in Figures 2-45 to 2-47. The second type of lesion is much less common. It usually occurs on the portio of the cervix, and is termed keratinizing because of the marked keratinization of many of the component cells. Marked cellular pleomorphism also characterizes this lesion, and this has led some to refer to the process as "pleomorphic dysplasia." With keratinizing dysplasia (Fig. 2-48), no distinction is made between marked dysplasia and CIS as the process, by its nature, always demonstrates evidence of cell differentiation and therefore does not fit into the accepted definition of classical CIS.

The cytologic manifestations of dysplasia and CIS reflect the morphologic manifestations of these processes, as seen in tissue samples. The pattern of the cellular sample derived from the various epithelial processes under consideration can be predicted from a study of the appearance of the cells in tissue biopsy specimens taken from involved areas (Table 2-3). The cells sampled by the cervical scrape technique are, of course, derived from the superficial cell layers of the epithelium, and represent the cells seen in the more superficial portions of the epithelium of the proliferations.

It is important to emphasize that dysplasia is a full-thickness abnormality, even in slight cases. Although the proliferation of primitive cells does not involve the full thickness of the epithelium, in lesions of less severity than CIS, all cases of dysplasia demonstrate nuclear abnormalities, including increased size and hyperchromasia, even in the superficial portions of the reaction. It is also important to appreciate that dysplastic reactions often demonstrate cellular features indicative of HPV infection, and that this finding does not alter the diagnosis if the other features of dysplasia are present. Indeed, it is the combination of the cellular hyperplasia in the proliferating zone of the epithelium and the HPV-induced nuclear and cytoplasmic changes that is believed to constitute the dysplastic lesion.[49]

Biology of Cervical Neoplasia

Although the etiology of squamous cervical carcinoma and its precursor lesions has not been definitively established, evidence gathered over the past 10 years strongly implicates HPVs as having a major role in the process. Classic genital warts have been recognized for decades, and koilocytosis was first de-

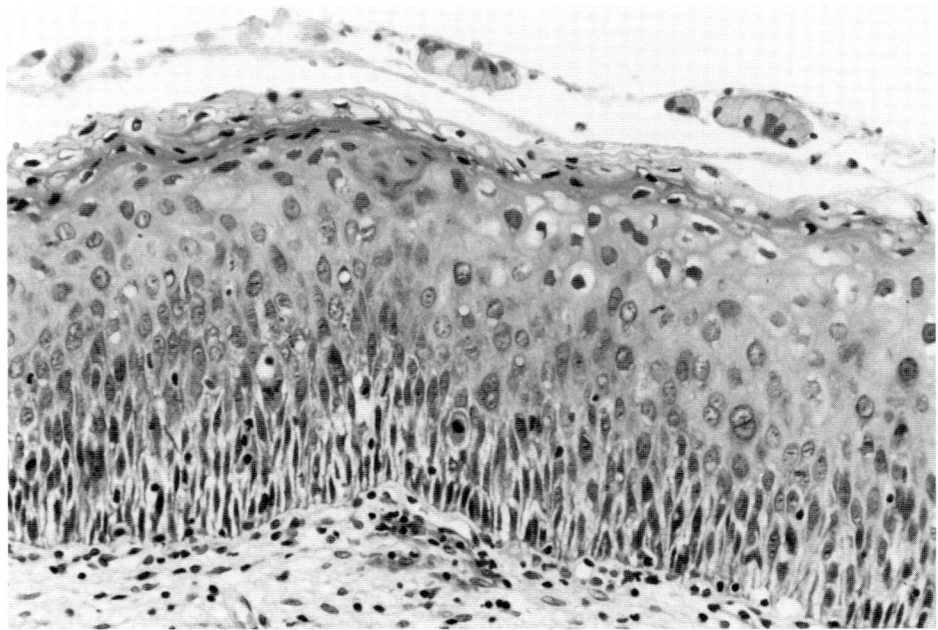

Fig. 2-45 Slight dysplasia (CIN I). Undifferentiated cells are confined to the lower one third of the epithelium. Note the koilocytotic features exhibited by the cells in the more superficial portions of the reaction. (H & E stain, × 40.)

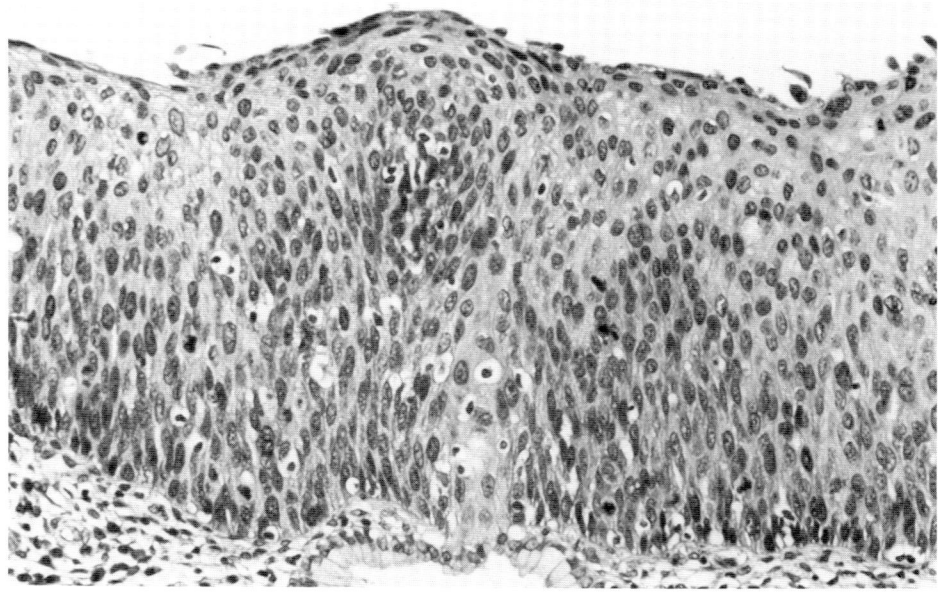

Fig. 2-46 Marked dysplasia (CIN III). Undifferentiated cells extend into the upper one third of the epithelium. Mitoses are present high in the proliferation. Koilocytosis is not evident. (H & E stain, × 40.)

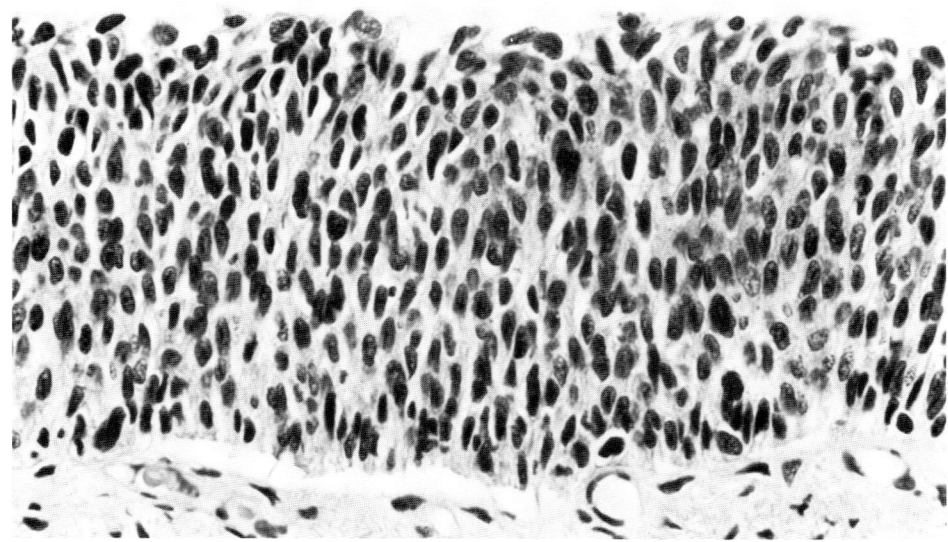

Fig. 2-47 CIS (CIN III). The entire thickness of the epithelium consists of cells that appear to be undifferentiated. Mitoses (which are not evident in the illustration) are present in the upper portion of the epithelium. (H & E stain, × 40.)

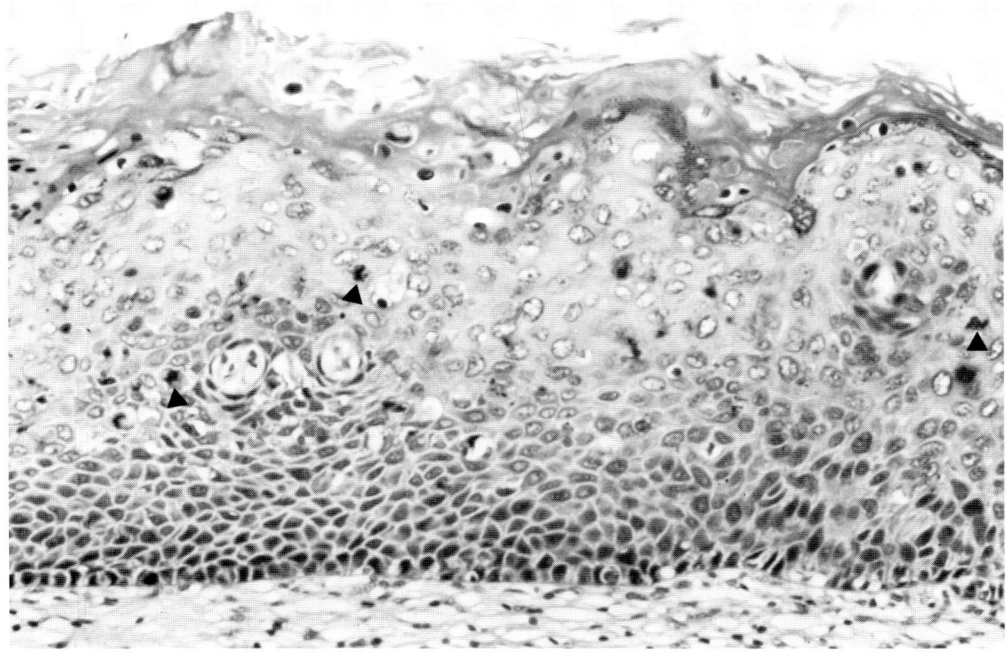

Fig. 2-48 Keratinizing dysplasia. Note the surface keratotic layer, numerous mitoses (*arrows*), and koilocytotic features that are consistent with viral effect. (H & E stain, × 40.)

Table 2-3 Morphologic Features of Dysplasia, CIS and Invasive Carcinoma

	Dysplasia	CIS	Invasive Carcinoma
Slide background	Clean	Clean	Dirty (diathesis)
Number of abnormal cells	Usually >500	Usually >500	Usually >500
Arrangement of abnormal cells	Isolated or in sheets	Isolated or syncytial	Isolated or syncytial
Relative nuclear area	50%	50%	50%
Chromatin pattern	Hyperchromatic; finely granular	Hyperchromatic; finely or coarsely granular	Hyperchromatic; coarsely granular, with clearing
Macronucleoli	Absent	Absent	Present
Micronucleoli	Not usually identifiable	Not usually identifiable	Present
Coexisting abnormality	Atypia	Dysplasia	Dysplasia and CIS

scribed as a distinctive cytologic feature by Koss and Durfee in 1956.[50] It was not until 1976, however, that Meisels and Fortin[51] and Purola and Savia[52] elucidated the facts that flat lesions of the uterine cervix exist and are caused by HPV, and that these lesions are part of the spectrum of squamous neoplasia.

Epidemiologic data add evidence to the association of this virus with carcinogenesis. Sexual promiscuity, an early age at first intercourse, poor hygiene, and low socioeconomic class are factors that are associated with both squamous cell carcinoma and HPV infection. CIN associated with HPV infection seems to have the same progression, persistence, and regression rates as those described before the association between neoplasia and HPV was recognized.[53] In addition, animal models demonstrating the progression from condyloma to carcinoma exist, and cases in which this transformation has occurred in humans have now been well documented.[54,55]

Immunocytochemical studies demonstrate viral antigen in 50 to 60 percent of condylomas and cases of dysplasia. Viral particles can be detected by electron microscopy in a similar percentage of cases. Southern blot analysis and recently described in situ hybridization techniques have demonstrated HPV DNA in 90 to 95 percent of dysplasias and 90 percent of carcinomas of the uterine cervix.[53,55] Most recently, Stoler and Broker have also demonstrated viral messenger RNA within the cytoplasm of cells of invasive squamous cell carcinoma.[56]

As we consider the changes within the spectrum of preinvasive cervical neoplasia, certain important considerations must be kept in mind with regard to the biologic potential of the various lesions. The intraepithelial neoplastic process at any given point is not necessarily progressive. Slight to moderate dysplasia, for example, may not necessarily progress, but may either persist at that stage or regress. Likewise, not every case of carcinoma in situ, if left untreated, progresses to invasive carcinoma. This points to the likelihood that not all cases currently designated carcinoma in situ are true intraepithelial cancers. It also suggests that, at least in some patients, immunologic or other factors may cause a reversal in the neoplastic process. It should also be pointed out that, although the morphologic criteria for classifying these lesions at each step in this spectrum are rather well defined, the biologic behavior or potential of the stages is not. Indeed, certain cases of moderate dysplasia have the same biologic potential as cases of marked dysplasia; likewise, many cases of marked dysplasia have the same biologic potential as those classified as CIS.

As stated earlier, the changes associated with dysplasia and CIS often coexist with features associated with papillomavirus. There is evidence that the type of papillomavirus associated with the dysplastic process may have a bearing on prognosis. For example, HPV types 16, 18, and 31 are most often associated with high-grade intraepithelial neoplasia and invasive carcinoma, whereas types 6 and 11 are associated with more benign lesions.[55-58] It is possible that, with the accumulation of information about the role of the various types of HPVs in carcinogenesis, a new categorization of dysplastic lesions with improved correlation with prognosis may be possible. Until further data are available, the consensus of most experts in the field is that intraepithelial neoplastic changes of the cervix should be classified according to the well-established, traditional criteria, regardless of any cytologic evidence of HPV.[59]

Cytologic Features of Dysplasia and Carcinoma In Situ

The cytologic features of dysplasia and CIS, which have been well established by numerous studies,[60–63] have also been summarized in detail by Patten.[44] This discussion focuses on the features that are of the greatest importance in the evaluation of cervical smears, as well as the application of these features to the assessment of the degree of severity of a lesion. A summary of the cytologic characteristics of the individual types of dysplasia is also provided.

ARRANGEMENT OF CELLS

Abnormal cells in cases of dysplasia usually appear singly in cytologic samples. Small microbiopsies are occasionally seen. The cells in such aggregates are arranged in sheets (Fig. 2-49, Plate 2-14). The cells derived from CIS may also be isolated, but frequently appear as aggregates in a syncytial arrangement (Fig. 2-46). The identification of true syncytial aggregates is the single most important consideration in the differential diagnosis of dysplasia and CIS. The presence of true syncytial aggregates of abnormal cells implies the presence of at least CIS in the sampled cervix.

CYTOPLASMIC CHARACTERISTICS

The nature of the cytoplasm provides information regarding the maturity of the cell. Cells derived from dysplastic processes generally have a polygonal or round to oval configuration. An exception to this may be found in cases of keratinizing dysplasia in which the cells may be quite pleomorphic, with numerous, elongated, spindled, and caudate forms. The cytoplasm is relatively abundant in the better-differentiated cells associated with the less severe dysplasias, but is scant in those cells derived from more advanced lesions.

NUCLEAR AREAS

Cells derived from cases of dysplasia have nuclei in the range of 150 to 200 μm^2 in diameter. The size varies somewhat with the differentiation of the dys-

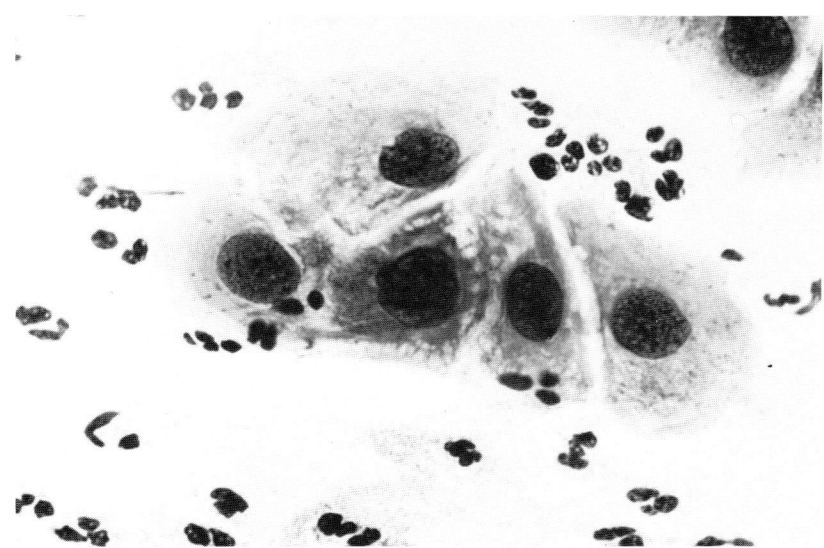

Fig. 2-49 Cells derived from a case of slight dysplasia with enlarged hyperchromatic nuclei and mature-appearing cytoplasm. They are arranged in a loose sheet and have well-defined borders. (Papanicolaou stain, × 40.) (See Plate 2-14.)

plastic process. Nuclei in cases of CIS may range in diameter from 75 to 200 μm^2; in practice, this has led to three categories of CIS that are based on nuclear size—small, intermediate, and large cell types.[39] In evaluating nuclear size on a smear, the nuclei of normal cells may be used as reference points. The nucleus of a normal intermediate squamous cell measures approximately 35 μm^2, whereas that of a cell derived from immature squamous metaplasia measures approximately 50 μm^2.

CHROMATIN PATTERNS

In general, three chromatin patterns are associated with dysplasia. The nuclei of cells derived from dysplastic reactions may have either a finely granular, evenly distributed chromatin; a finely granular, evenly distributed chromatin with some chromatin clumping; or a dense, deeply staining, opaque chromatin. The last pattern is common only in the keratinizing type of lesion. A finely granular, evenly distributed chromatin pattern may also be seen in cells derived from CIS. In some cases of CIS, however, evenly distributed, coarsely granular chromatin is seen. Irregular chromatin distribution, or the phenomenon referred to as nuclear clearing, is not seen in intraepithelial reactions (Fig. 2-50).

Cytologic Evaluation of Severity

The degree of severity of an intraepithelial process is evaluated cytologically by a consideration of individual cells. The features of individual cells that relate to severity include the morphologic characteristics of the nucleus and the cytoplasm, as well as the nuclear/cytoplasmic ratio. With increasing severity of the intraepithelial process, there is decreasing cytoplasmic maturity. A mature, well-defined cytoplasm in a well-differentiated cell is seen in reactions of slight severity. With more advanced lesions, the amount of cytoplasm decreases and appears progressively more immature (resembling that of metaplastic cells) until the extreme of cellular immaturity is reached in cells derived from cases of CIS (Figs. 2-51 to 2-56, Plates 2-15, 2-16). Concomitantly, there is an increase in

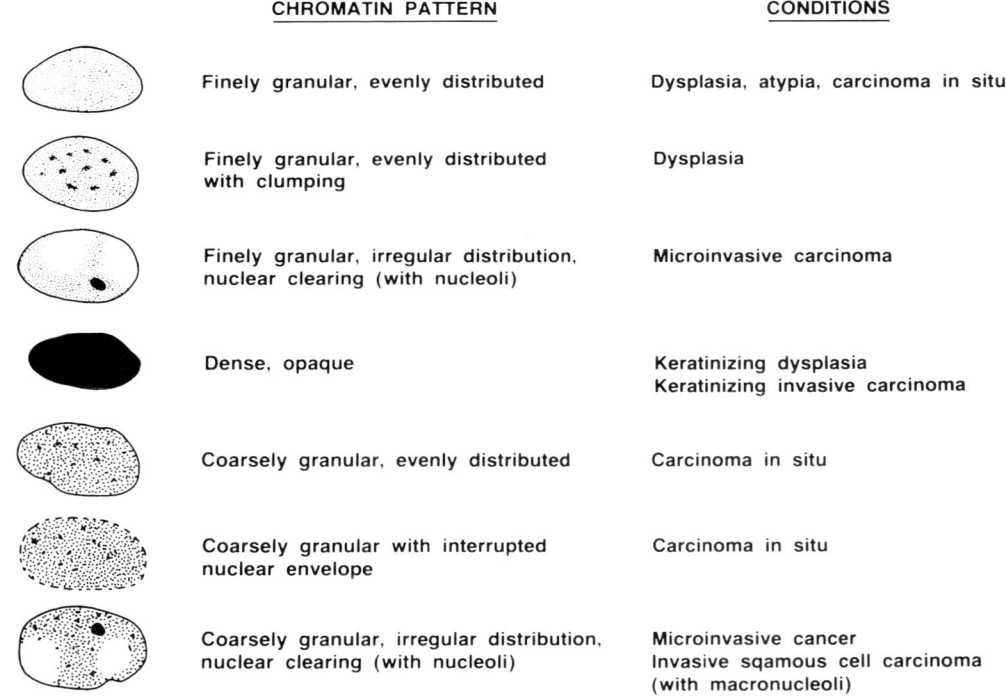

Fig. 2-50 Summary and illustration of chromatin patterns in cervical neoplasia.

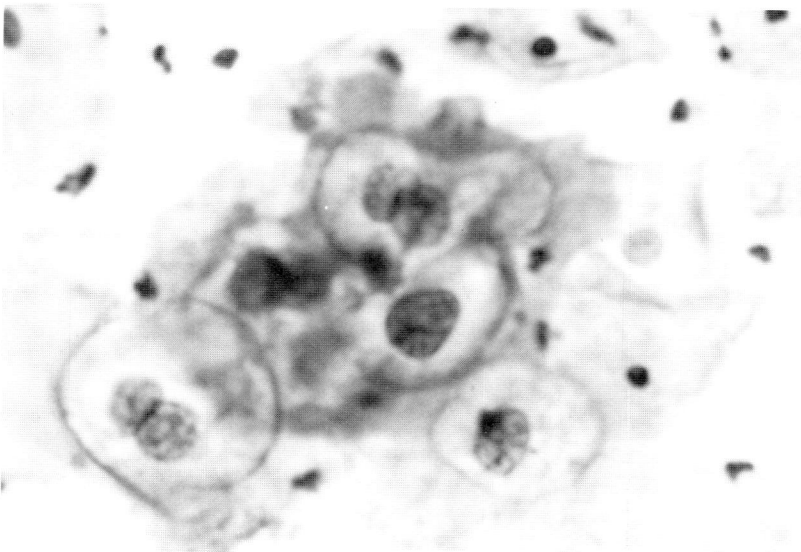

Fig. 2-51 Cells derived from slight dysplasia (CIN I) with evidence of human papillomavirus effect (koilocytosis). The degree of nuclear enlargement is evident when the nuclei of the abnormal cells are compared with normal intermediate squamous cells in the field. (Papanicolaou stain, × 200.) (See Plate 2-15.)

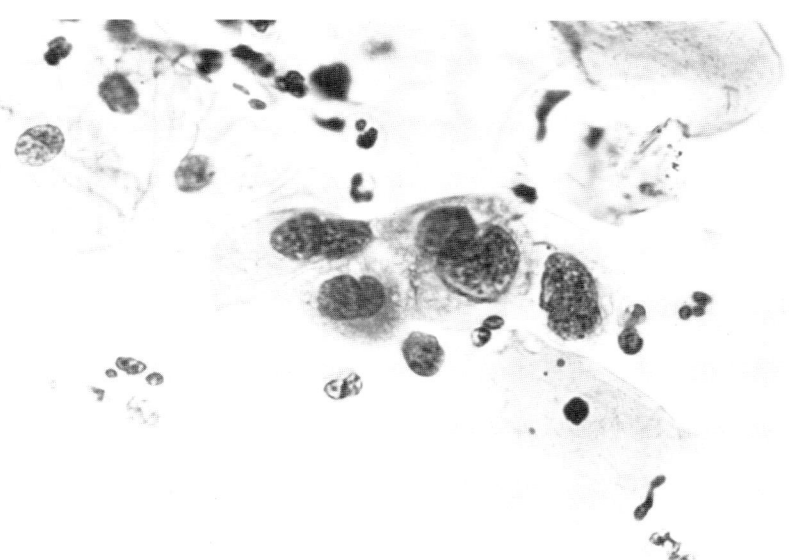

Fig. 2-52 The cells in the center of this field represent a case of moderate dysplasia (CIN II). They have a higher nuclear/cytoplasmic ratio and a more immature cytoplasm than do those in cases of slight dysplasia. (Papanicolaou stain, × 200.)

nucleocytoplasmic ratio with increasing severity. The nucleus itself reflects the severity of the process by changes that include a progressive increase in chromatin abnormalities and nuclear envelope irregularities.

There is also a relationship between the severity of a lesion and the number of abnormal cells present. Although the number of abnormal cells in a cytologic sample varies with the collection technique used, and the counts of abnormal cells vary from one case to another, in general, lesser degrees of dysplasia are associated with fewer abnormal cells per slide, whereas more severe lesions often demonstrate a markedly increased number of abnormal cells.

These criteria are most useful in relation to the common nonkeratinizing types of intraepithelial neoplastic processes. The keratinizing lesions may present difficulties for the cytopathologist in terms of predicting the degree of severity on the basis of a cytologic sample. Relatively few cells may be shed from severe intraepithelial or even invasive keratinizing processes, and although the other criteria noted are generally valid for this lesion, their application in individual cases may be difficult. This is discussed further in the sections on invasive carcinoma.

Summary of Cytologic Features of Nonkeratinizing Dysplasia/Carcinoma In Situ

Slight nonkeratinizing dysplasia of the cervix is characterized by abnormal cells that are arranged singly and in sheets, with well-defined, thin cytoplasms similar to those found in normal mature squamous cells. The nuclei, which are enlarged 5 to 6 times the size of normal intermediate nuclei, are hyperchromatic, with finely granular, evenly distributed chromatin. A small to moderate number of abnormal cells are usually present (Figs. 2-51 and 2-52).

In cases of moderate dysplasia, additional abnormal cells are usually found. Although cells similar to those just described may be present, less mature abnormal cells may also be identified. These cells have an increased nuclear/cytoplasmic ratio and a dense cytoplasm which, in texture and configuration, is similar to that found in squamous metaplastic cells. Nuclei are hyperchromatic, may exhibit increased clumping of chromatin, and may demonstrate some irregularities in the nuclear envelope. These cells, like those that are characteristic of slight dysplasia, are found singly or in sheets, and have well-defined cell borders (Figs. 2-53 and 2-54).

In marked dysplasia, abnormal cells are abundant. The nuclear/cytoplasmic ratio is higher than that seen in lesser grades of dysplasia, and the cells tend to be round to oval, with relatively little cytoplasm. The cytoplasm, however, remains well-defined, mimicking the appearance of the very immature metaplastic cell. Nuclei are large and hyperchromatic, and demonstrate increased irregularities of the nuclear envelope. The cells, when in groups, remain in the form of sheets in contrast to the syncytial type of arrangement seen in more severe reactions (Figs. 2-55 and 2-56).

Cases of CIS are also characterized by large numbers of abnormal cells. Although cells with features of dysplasia are almost always present, there are also more primitive-appearing cells that are typical of CIS. These cells may appear singly or in syncytial aggregates that are characterized by ill-defined cell borders and a disordered arrangement of nuclei in relationship to one another. The cells vary in size from case to case, and small and large cell variants, as well as intermediate types, have been recognized as subtypes of CIS. The cytoplasm in all types of CIS is scant, wispy in appearance, and ill-defined. Single cells from the process have similar cytoplasm, or they may be characterized simply by a very thin rim of cytoplasm surrounding the nucleus. The chromatin pattern varies from finely granular to coarsely granular. The nuclear envelope is irregular in configuration and may appear to be interrupted, an indication of impending cell division (Figs. 2-57 to 2-59, Plate 2-17).

Summary of Cytologic Features of Keratinizing Dysplasia

Keratinizing dysplasia is characterized by the presence of pleomorphic cellular forms. Cells similar to those described for nonkeratinizing dysplasia are present, but they are accompanied by cells that are elongated, caudate, or spindle-shaped. The cytoplasm is often orangeophilic, reflecting a high degree of keratinization, but it may also be eosinophilic or basophilic. Pleomorphic nuclear forms are identified, and these are frequently markedly hyperchromatic

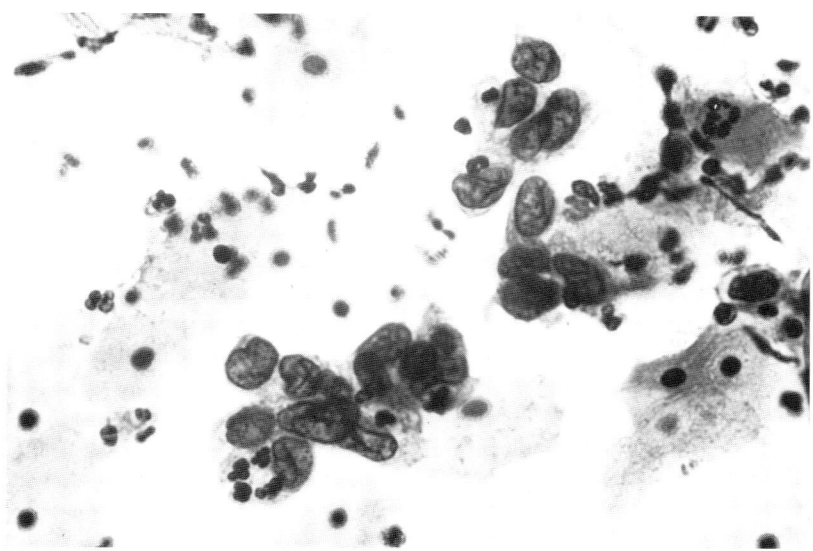

Fig. 2-57 CIS. These cells appear in syncytial aggregates and have nuclei that are arranged irregularly with respect to one another. The cytoplasm is very scanty and the nuclear envelopes are wrinkled and folded. (Papanicolaou stain, × 200.) (See Plate 2-17.)

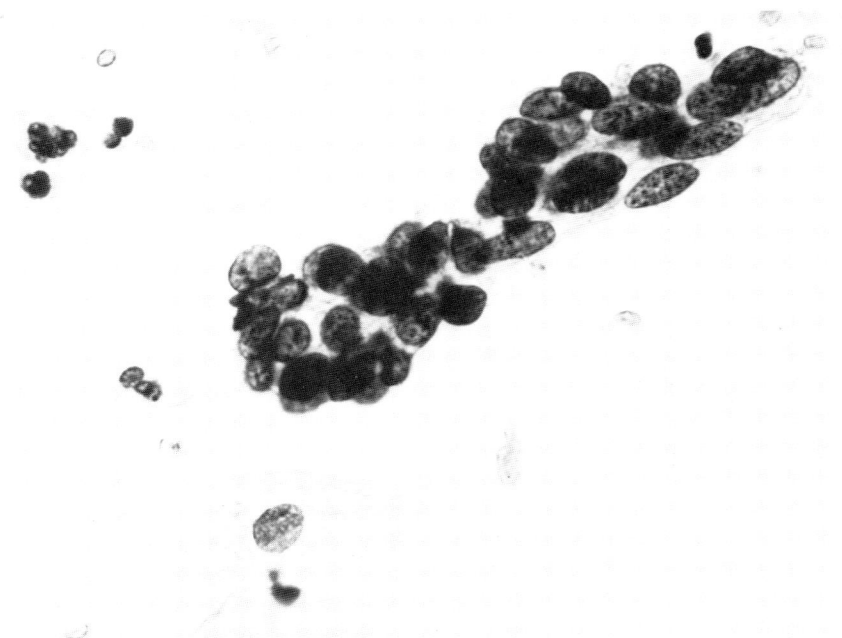

Fig. 2-58 CIS. Large syncytial aggregate of primitive-appearing cells with ill-defined, scanty cytoplasm is seen. (Papanicolaou stain, × 200.)

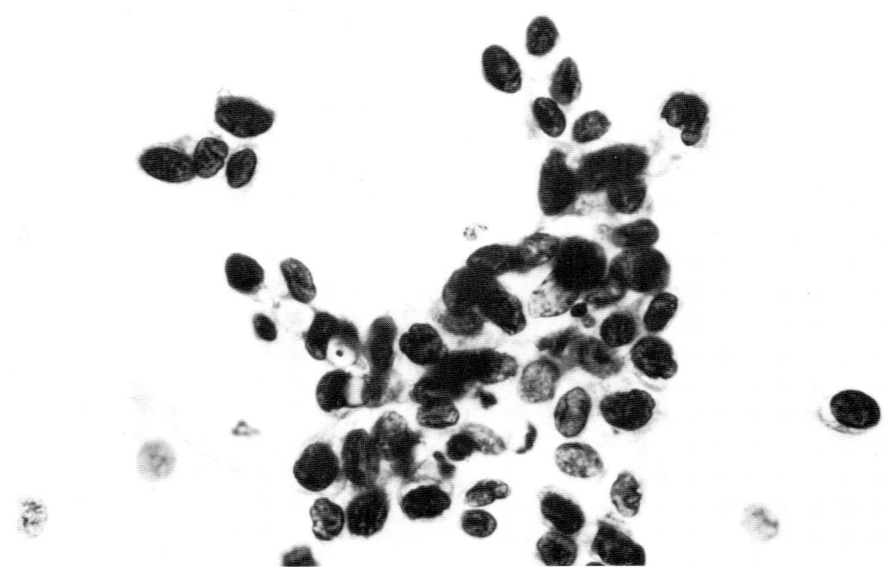

Fig. 2-59 Small cells from a case of CIS. A syncytial aggregate and single cells are present. Note the minimal amount of cytoplasm. (Papanicolaou stain, × 200.)

and opaque, with irregular nuclear membranes (Figs. 2-60 and 2-61, Plate 2-18). The number of abnormal cells present varies from few to many, and does not always correlate with the severity of the process. Evidence of hyperkeratosis or parakeratosis may be associated with these abnormal cells (Fig. 2-62).

CYTOLOGIC MANIFESTATIONS OF MICROINVASIVE CARCINOMA

Microinvasive squamous cell carcinoma of the uterine cervix is defined as a carcinoma that has in-

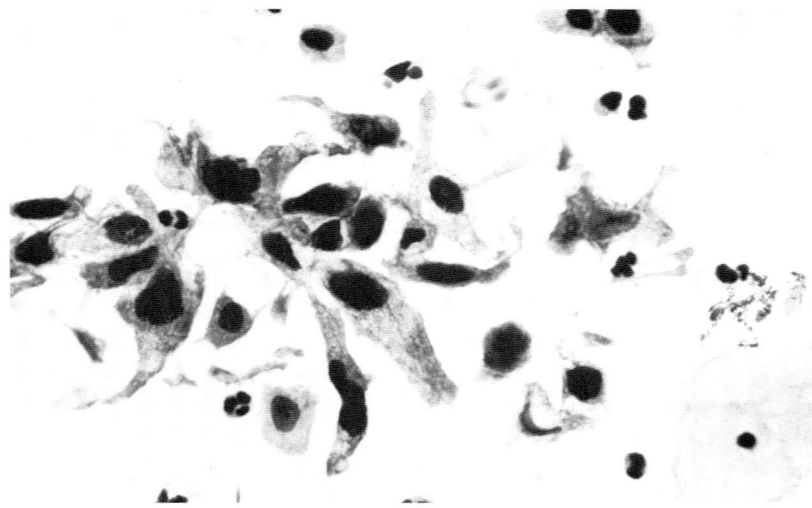

Fig. 2-60 Cells derived from a patient with keratinizing (pleomorphic) dysplasia. The cellular pleomorphism and opaque nuclear forms are characteristic of this condition. (Papanicolaou stain, × 200.) (See Plate 2-18.)

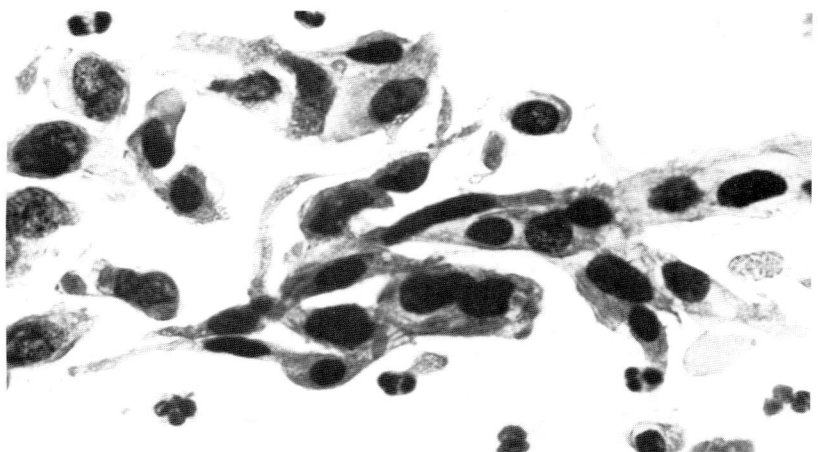

Fig. 2-61 Spindle-shaped and caudate cellular forms in a case of marked keratinizing dysplasia (keratinizing CIS). Differentiation between this and keratinizing invasive carcinoma may be difficult with this type of specimen. (Papanicolaou stain, × 200.)

vaded the cervical stroma to a depth of 3 mm or less from the site of origin and that does not demonstrate lymphatic or blood vessel invasion. Other definitions have been proposed for this entity, but this one is the one most commonly employed and is the one accepted by the Society of Gynecologic Oncologists.

In most cases, the invasive foci develop from an overlying epithelium that is involved by CIS. In the remaining instances, the overlying epithelium usually has the characteristics of marked dysplasia (Fig. 2-63).

The cytologic characteristics of microinvasive carcinoma were originally described in detail by Ng and associates in 1972.[64] They noted that the cells derived from microinvasive carcinoma varied in their appearance according to the depth of invasion. The cells

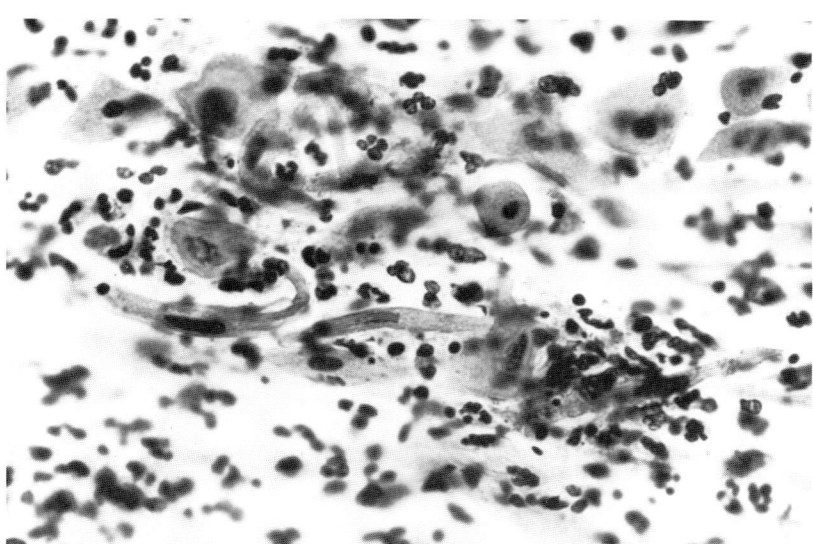

Fig. 2-62 Pleomorphic parakeratotic cellular forms from a case of keratinizing dysplasia (Papanicolaou stain, × 200.)

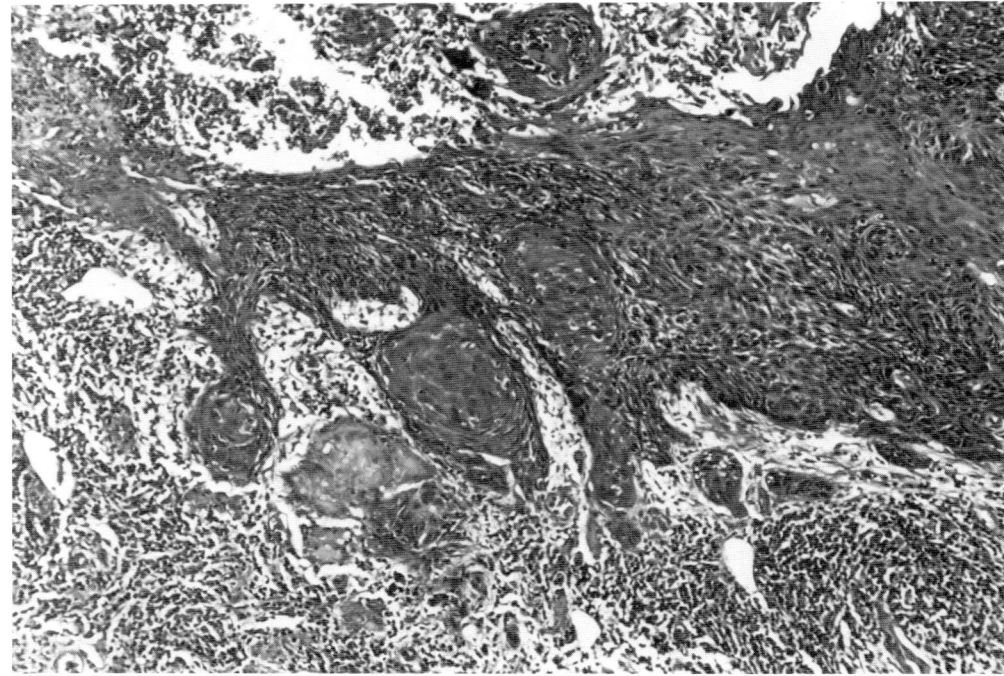

Fig. 2-63 Microinvasive squamous cell carcinoma of the uterine cervix. Several nests of invasive tumor are evident just below the epithelium in this example. (H & E stain, × 40.)

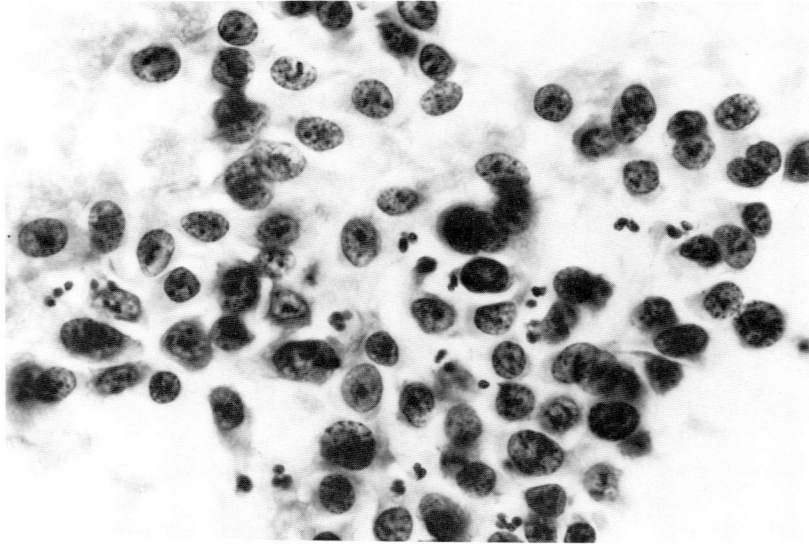

Fig. 2-64 Cytologic specimen derived from a case of microinvasive carcinoma. The presence of true nucleoli and the irregularity of the chromatin distribution distinguish these cells from those characterizing CIS. (Papanicolaou stain, × 200.) (See Plate 2-19.)

most characteristic of the microinvasive process were found in association with lesions that had invaded the stroma to a depth of 2 to 3 mm. In tumors associated with lesser degrees of invasion, the cells are less easily distinguished from those of CIS. The cells derived from microinvasive cancer occur both as isolated forms and as syncytial aggregates. The presence of true nucleoli and chromatin-clearing in some of the cells distinguishes the process from CIS (Fig. 2-64, Plate 2-19). In the study conducted by Ng's group, the abnormal cells were noted to have a mean area of 219.1 μm^2. The average area of the nucleus was found to be 88.2 μm^2. Nucleoli were observed in 16 percent of the cells, and were usually small. With increasing depth of invasion, these authors noted that the cells began to increasingly resemble those of frank, invasive carcinoma. The total number of cells displaying true nucleoli increases in such cases, as does nucleolar size. The total number of cells with irregularities of chromatin distribution, manifested as so-called chromatin-clearing, also increases. A true tumor diathesis was noted in about 40 percent of the cases involving invasion of less than 2 mm; this increased proportionately in cases characterized by a deeper level of invasion. Experience in other laboratories, including my own confirms that early invasion of the cervical stroma can often be predicted on the basis of the cytologic criteria noted, and that microinvasive carcinoma can, in many but not all cases, be distinguished from CIS and from frank, invasive carcinoma.

CYTOLOGIC MANIFESTATIONS OF INVASIVE SQUAMOUS CELL CARCINOMA

The subclassification of invasive squamous cell carcinoma of the uterine cervix is based on histologic morphology. It differs from the popular subclassification first formulated by Broder,[65] which is based on a grading system utilizing keratinization as the main index of differentiation.

The current subclassification, which has been adopted by the World Health Organization (WHO), was proposed by Wentz and Reagan in 1959.[66] It divides squamous cell carcinoma into keratinizing, large cell nonkeratinizing, and small cell types. This classification corresponds to current theories of carcinogenesis. The keratinizing type of cancer is thought to arise in the ectocervical area from preexisting keratinizing dysplasia. The nonkeratinizing variety is thought to arise in the transformation zone, developing through the dysplasia/CIS pathway, whereas small cell carcinoma is thought to be derived from small-cell CIS that has been preceded by atypical reserve cell hyperplasia, usually high in the transformation zone within the canal. Using this subclassification, correlation between histologic type and survival following radiation therapy is possible.[66] This is not the case with other subclassifications and grading systems that have been utilized.

It is probable that small cell carcinoma of the cervix actually includes a heterogeneous group of neoplasms. Some of these tumors represent true small cell variants of squamous cell carcinoma of the cervix, whereas others may represent neuroendocrine carcinomas of the cervix that are similar to the atypical carcinoid tumors and small cell carcinomas of the lung. Further studies of this relatively rare entity are necessary to determine the significance of further subclassification of these tumors.

General Cytologic Features of Invasive Carcinoma

Cellular samples from cases of nonkeratinizing and small cell types of squamous cell carcinoma almost invariably contain evidence of a tumor diathesis that is characterized by the presence of a granular, proteinaceous precipitate and broken-down blood in the slide background. Keratinizing carcinomas, because they are usually exophytic growths without evidence of ulceration, are usually not associated with a tumor diathesis (Figs. 2-65 and 2-66).

The cellular samples from cases of invasive carcinoma may contain relatively few abnormal cells compared with those derived from cases of dysplasia or CIS. This is particularly true of specimens derived from a keratinizing cancer. In some cases, cytologic recognition and correct interpretation is difficult with this type of invasive carcinoma. In general, the ectocervical sample is the most reliable single specimen for the detection of invasive carcinoma arising in the cervix, as most of the abnormal cells are found in this sample (Fig. 2-67).

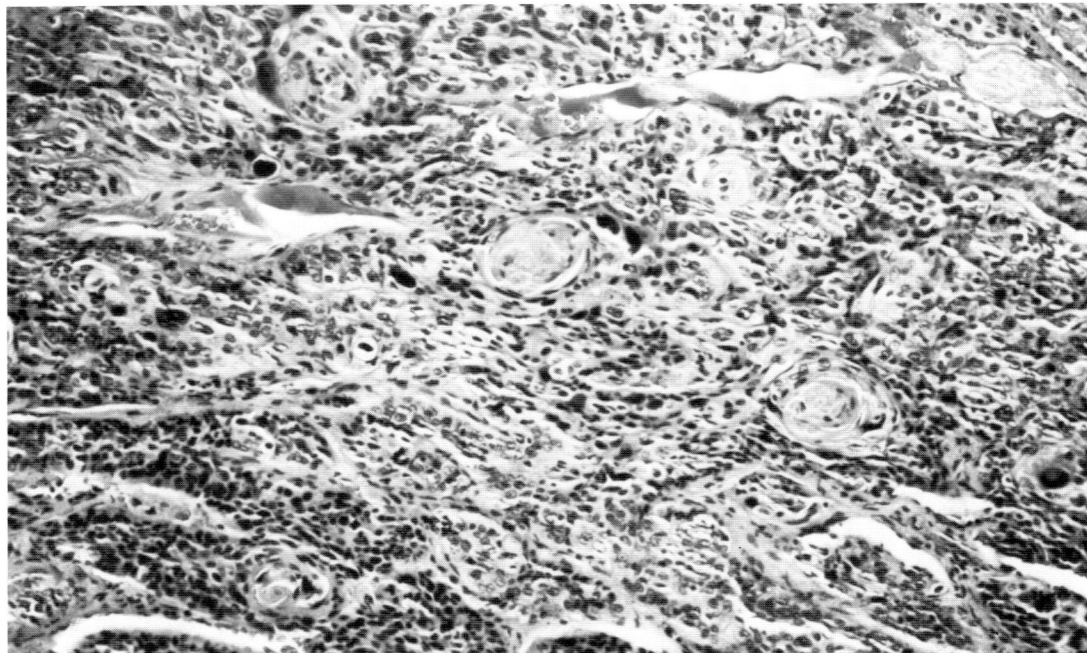

Fig. 2-65 Invasive keratinizing squamous cell carcinoma. Note the presence of the keratin pearls which distinguish this as a keratinizing carcinoma. (H & E stain, × 40.)

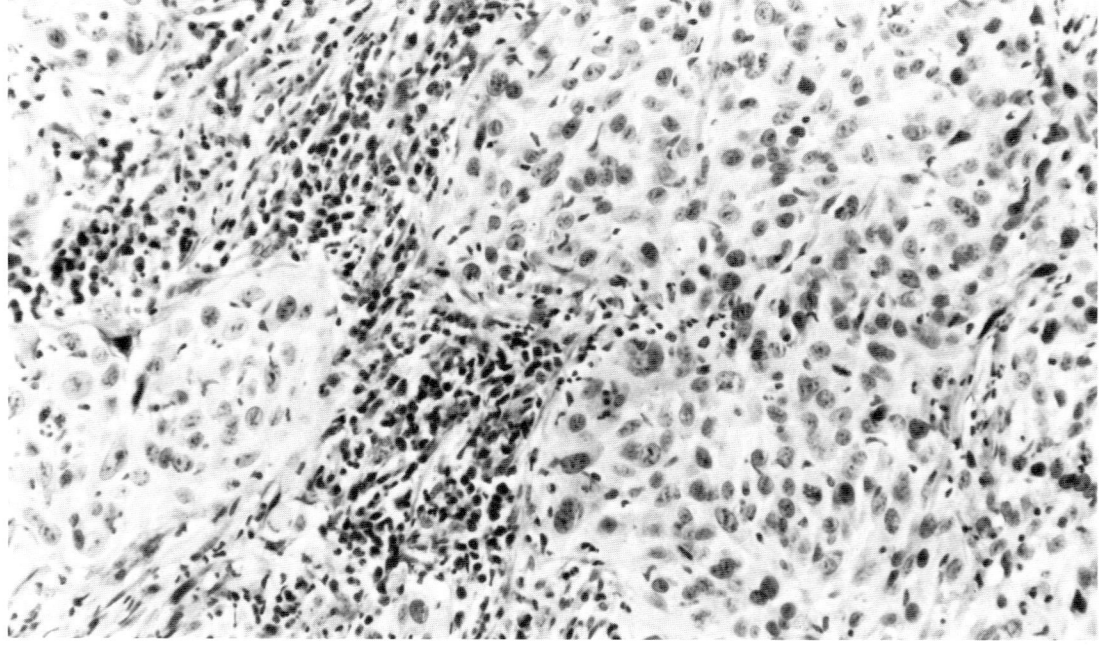

Fig. 2-66 Nonkeratinizing squamous cell carcinoma in a tissue biopsy specimen. (H & E stain, × 40.)

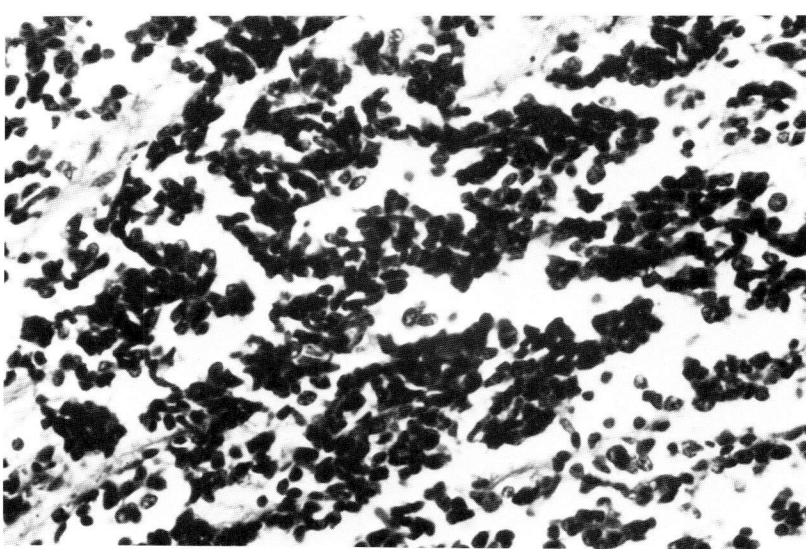

Fig. 2-67 Small cell type of invasive carcinoma of the cervix in a tissue specimen. The cervical stroma has been invaded and largely replaced by the diffuse infiltrate of small, loosely cohesive, malignant cells. (H & E stain, × 40.)

Cytologic Manifestations of Keratinizing Squamous Cell Carcinoma

The cell population in cases of keratinizing squamous carcinoma includes a variety of cellular forms of differing in size and configuration. There is often evidence of associated hyperkeratosis in the form of anucleate squames, as well as of pleomorphic parakeratosis in the form of miniature, variably shaped squamous cells with pyknotic nuclei (Fig. 2-68, Plate 2-20). The mean cellular area per case is reported to be 274.6 ± 106.8 μm^2.[67] About 15 percent or more of the abnormal cell population is characterized by elongated and caudate forms that are not seen in other varieties of squamous cell carcinoma. The cytoplasm varies from orangeophilic to cyanophilic. The nuclei have a mean area of approximately 80 μm, and are often of irregular configuration. The chromatin is darkly staining, coarsely granular, and often irregularly distributed. Many abnormal cells contain opaque nuclear masses that are indicative of degeneration. Macronucleoli are present, but they occur less commonly than in other forms of squamous cell carcinoma and are often difficult to identify in the cellular sample.

It must be stressed that differentiating between keratinizing dysplasia and keratinizing invasive carcinoma on the basis of a cytologic sample is often difficult. Differentiating features include the presence of a relatively large number of pleomorphic forms and the identification of a coarsely granular, irregularly distributed chromatin in some of the cells derived from invasive carcinoma (Fig. 2-69). The identification of macronucleoli and the presence of syncytia of abnormal cells can sometimes facilitate diagnosis. In a certain proportion of cases, a definitive differentiation cannot be accomplished, and diagnosis must await the results of a biopsy examination.

Cytologic Manifestations of Nonkeratinizing Squamous Cell Carcinoma

The cellular sample from nonkeratinizing squamous cell carcinoma is usually characterized by the presence of a tumor diathesis. Individual cells are large, with a mean nuclear area of 256 ± 37 μm^2. They are either isolated or appear in a loose, syncytial arrangement with ill-defined cell borders and a cytoplasm that ranges from cyanophilic to amphophilic.

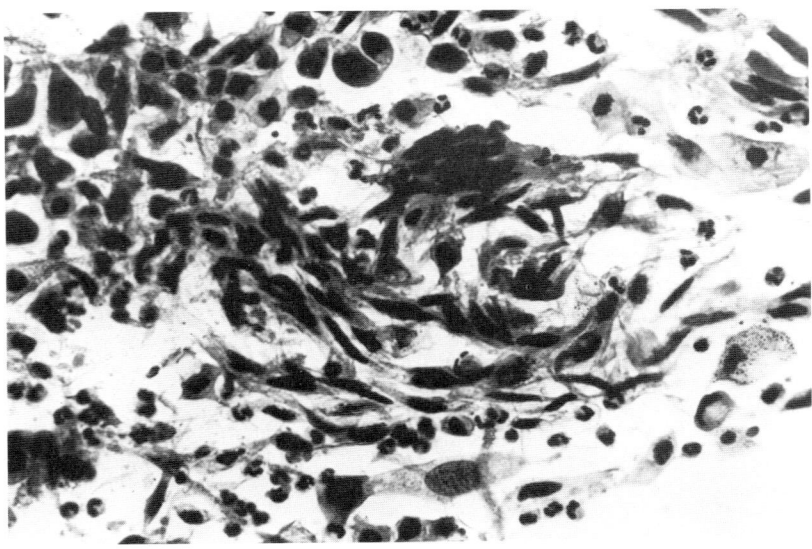

Fig. 2-68 Cells derived from a patient with keratinizing invasive carcinoma. Note the large number of pleomorphic forms. (Papanicolaou stain, × 100.) (See Plate 2-20.)

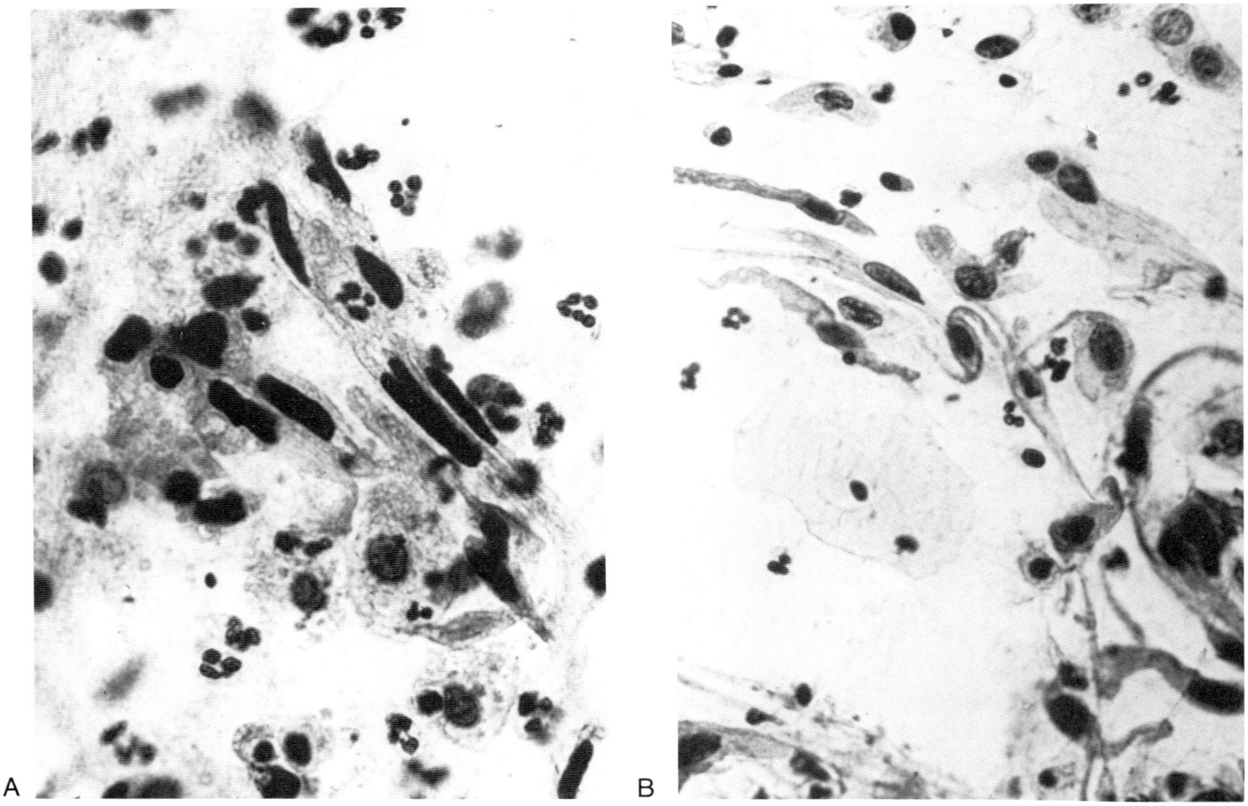

Fig. 2-69 (A & B) Pleomorphic malignant cells from a case of keratinizing invasive carcinoma. A tumor diathesis is evident in the background of Fig. B. (Papanicolaou stain, × 100.)

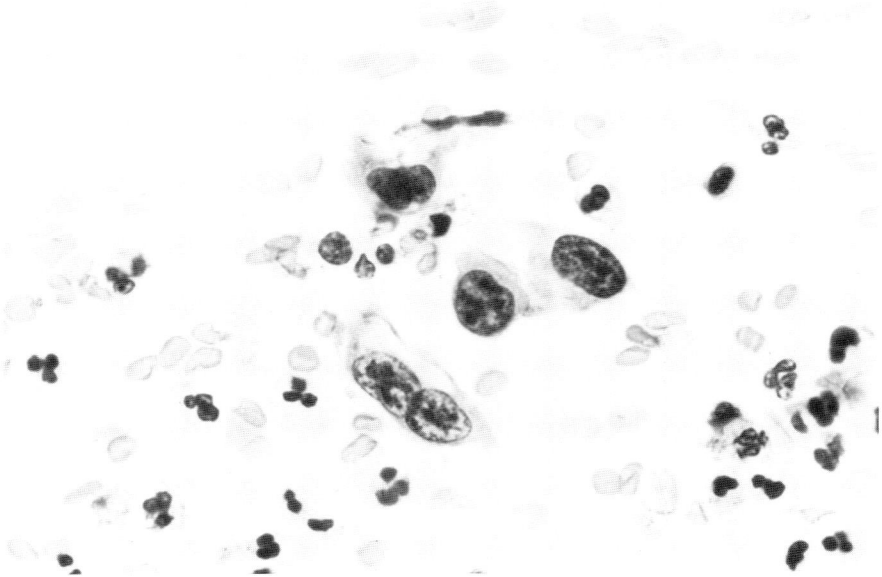

Fig. 2-70 Single tumor cells in a case of nonkeratinizing squamous cell carcinoma of the uterine cervix. (Papanicolaou stain, × 200.) (See Plate 2-21.)

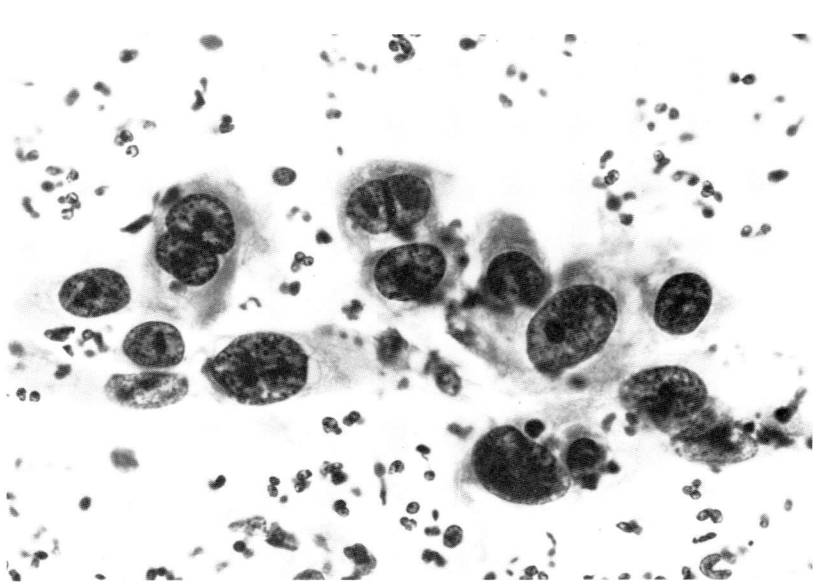

Fig. 2-71 A loose syncytial aggregate of cells from nonkeratinizing squamous cell carcinoma. (Papanicolaou stain, × 200.)

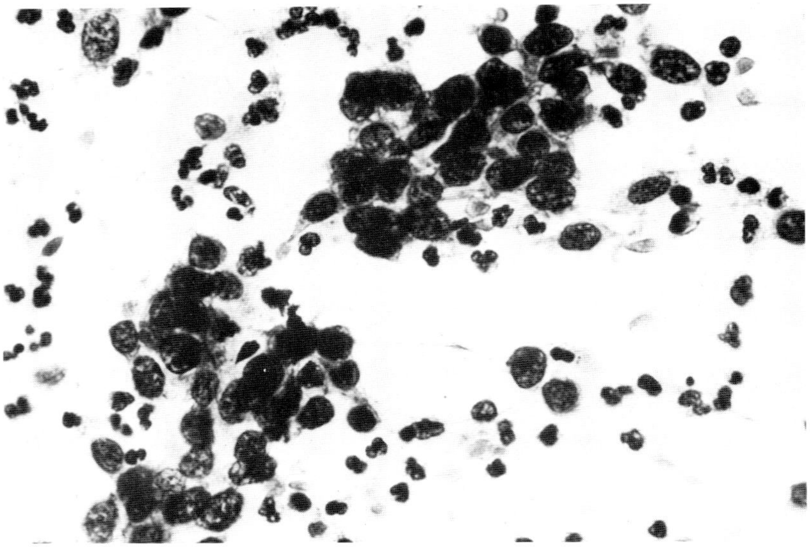

Fig. 2-72 Small cell carcinoma of the cervix (Papanicolaou stain, × 200.) (See Plate 2-22.)

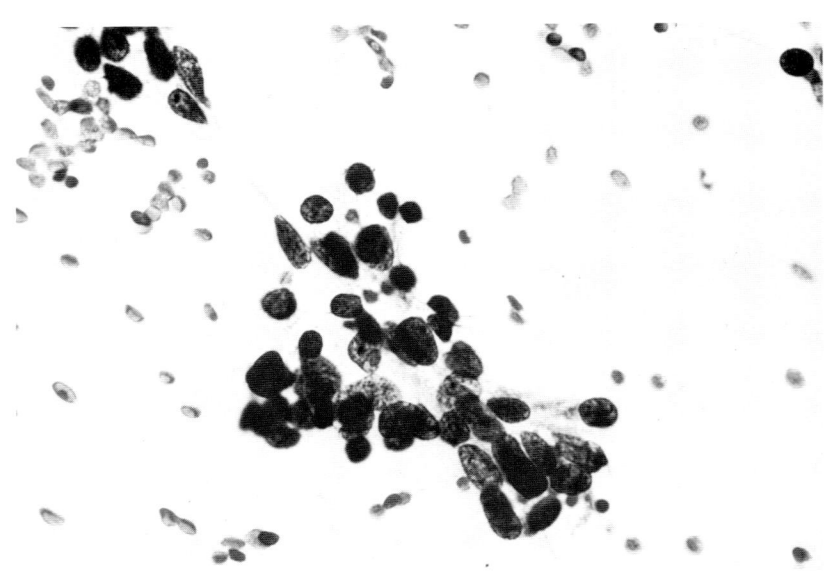

Fig. 2-73 Small cell carcinoma. The presence of nucleoli help to distinguish this from CIS. (Papanicolaou stain, × 200.) (See Plate 2-23.)

The nuclei are round to oval to irregular in configuration, averaging approximately 90 μm^2 in area.[67] The chromatin is coarsely granular, irregularly distributed, and densely stained. Macronucleoli are common and are easily identified. There is usually cellular evidence of coexisting dysplasia and CIS (Figs. 2-70 and 2-71, Plate 2-21).

Cytologic Manifestations of Small Cell Carcinoma

Small cell carcinoma is usually characterized by a large number of abnormal cells that are present in a dirty background that reflects the destructive process caused by the invading tumor. The cells are small and relatively uniform in size, with a mean area of 169 ± 37 μm^2.[67] They also are either isolated or in syncytial aggregates (Figs. 2-72 and 2-73, Plates 2-22 and 2-23). The cytoplasm is very scant and often not identifiable. The nuclei, which average 65 ± 13 μm^2 are round to oval or angulated, with densely staining, coarsely granular, irregularly distributed chromatin. Nucleoli are identifiable but are not as large as the nucleoli associated with the other variants of squamous carcinoma.

DIFFERENTIAL DIAGNOSIS OF SQUAMOUS CELL CARCINOMA

The cytologic diagnosis of squamous cell carcinoma is usually achieved with little difficulty. The differential morphologic features distinguishing invasive carcinoma from intraepithelial lesions have been discussed earlier and are summarized in Table 2-5. There are, however, a number of different entities that may mimic the changes of invasive cancer; these must be excluded when considering individual cases.

Keratinizing dysplasia has already been described as a condition often posing a diagnostic dilemma to the cytopathologist. Likewise, reparative processes involving the cervix can mimic invasive cancer. This perhaps is the entity most frequently confused cytologically with malignant disease. The distinction between reparative changes and those reflective of invasive cancer is made on the basis of three principle features of reparative reactions: (1) a lack of tumor diathesis, (2) the absence of chromatin and nuclear envelope irregularities, and (3) the presence of virtually all the abnormal cells in aggregates, with only rare, if any, isolated abnormal cells[68] (Figs. 2-74 and 2-75, Plates 2-24 and 2-25).

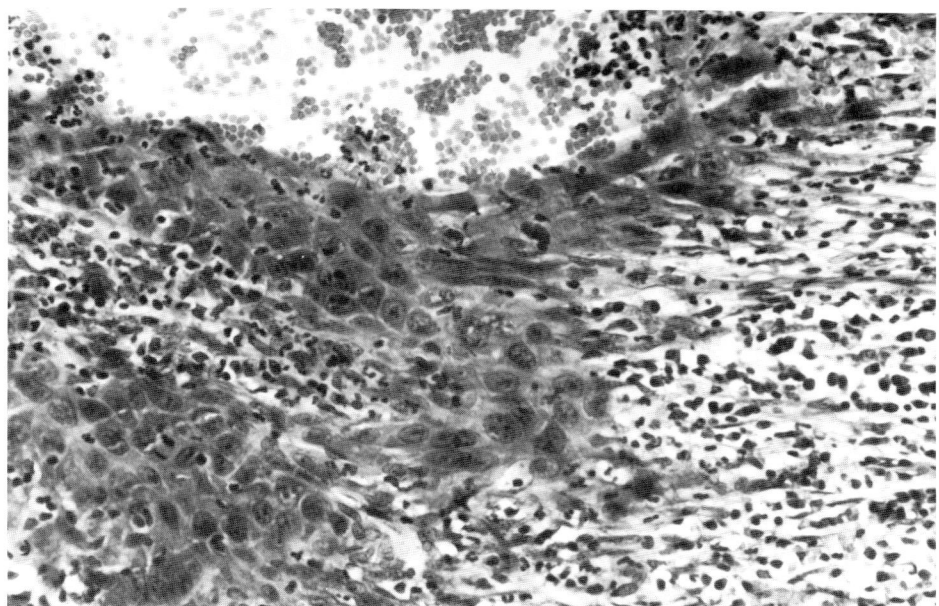

Fig. 2-74 Tissue section of the cervix showing evidence of inflammation and epithelial repair. (H & E stain, × 40.) (See Plate 2-24.)

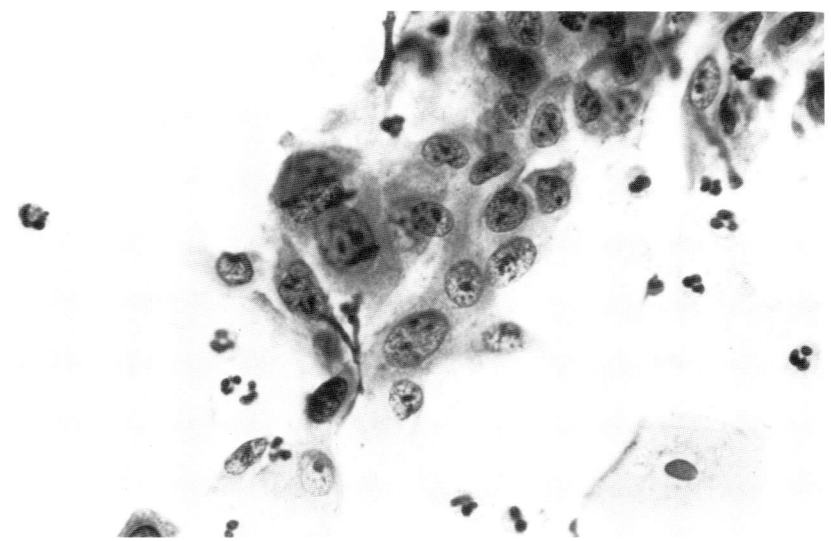

Fig. 2-75 Epithelial reparative reaction of the cervix. (Papanicolaou stain, × 200.) (See Plate 2-25.)

Other lesions that may be confused with squamous cell carcinoma of the uterine cervix in the cytologic sample include viral infections, radiation or chemotherapeutic effects, decidual reactions of the cervix, pemphigus vulgaris, and poorly differentiated adenocarcinoma (either metastatic or primary). A definitive diagnosis is usually established by a combination of a thorough clinical history and a careful, systematic approach that utilizes the outlined cytologic criteria. In those relatively rare cases in which a definitive diagnosis is impossible, it is both appropriate and necessary that the pathologist relate the diagnostic possibilities to the clinician so that appropriate additional diagnostic procedures can be performed.

Endocervical Adenocarcinoma
Darryl G. Heustis

Endocervical adenocarcinoma is a rare tumor, representing less than 10 percent of all cervical carcinomas.[69,70] This slow-growing tumor, which often remains clinically undetected in it early stages, features malignant cells that are typically shed singly or in small groups. Although papillary or rosette formations may be present, the cellular aggregates often retain their side-by-side arrangement.[71] The typical nuclear features of these cells include the following (Figs. 2-76 to 2-78):

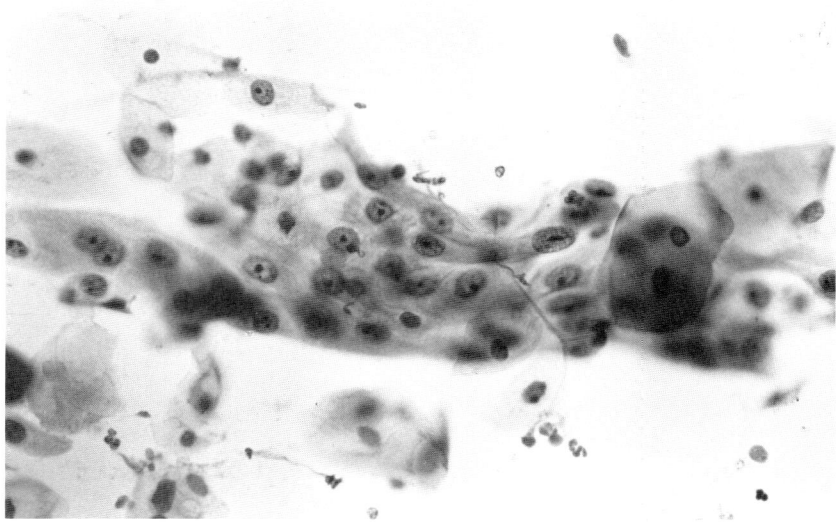

Fig. 2-76 Cluster of reparative cells showing well-defined cellular borders, finely granular chromatin, and prominent nucleoli. No single cells are present. (Papanicolaou stain, × 500.)

1. Nuclear variation and enlargement, often to two to three times the size of normal endocervical nuclei
2. Usually round or oval nuclear contours surrounded by smooth membranes
3. Prominent round or irregular nucleolus or multiple prominent nucleoli
4. Finely granular, usually evenly dispersed chromatin with some condensation at the nuclear border

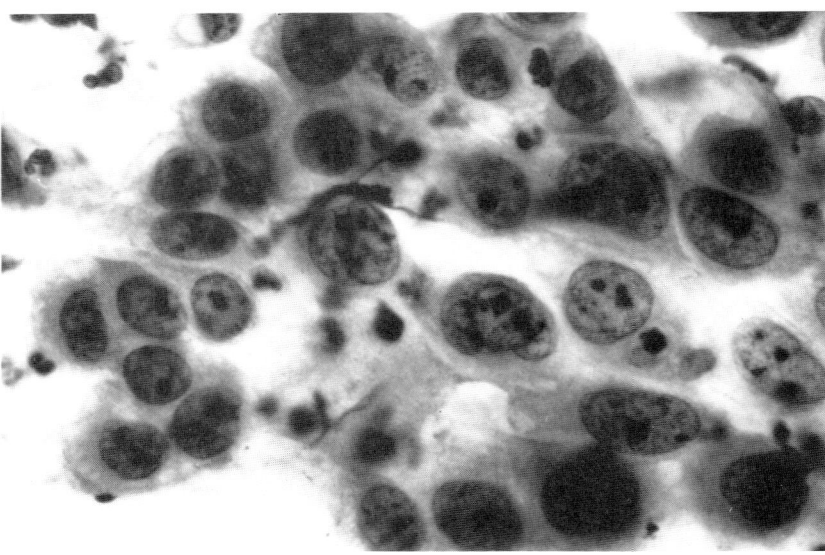

Fig. 2-77 Well-differentiated endocervical adenocarcinoma exhibiting side-by-side arrangement. Note the granular cytoplasm, finely granular chromatin, prominent nucleoli, and gland formation. (× 1000.)

84 PRACTICAL CYTOPATHOLOGY

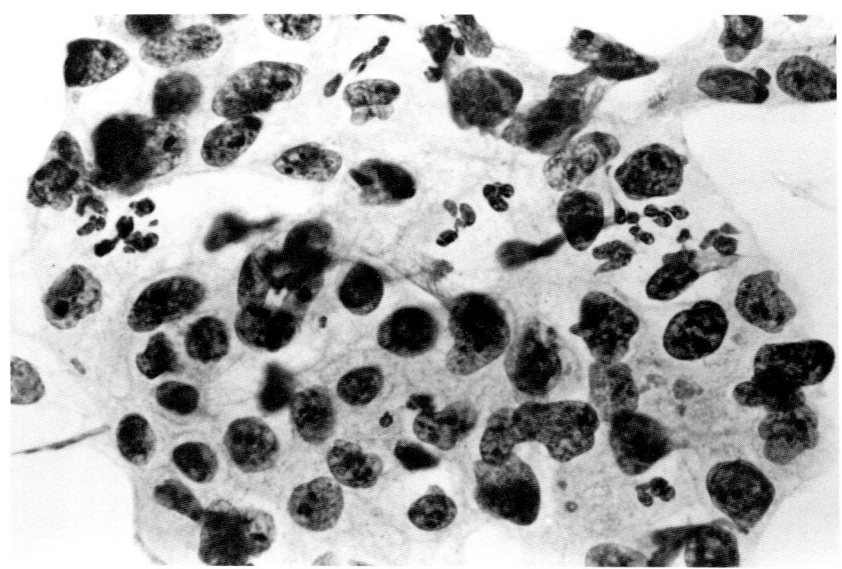

Fig. 2-78 Poorly differentiated endocervical adenocarcinoma demonstrating pleomorphic nuclei and ill-defined cytoplasmic borders, but retaining a flat sheet appearance. (Papanicolaou stain, × 1000.)

The cytoplasm is usually abundant and dense, and is more often granular than vacuolated. This is in contradistinction to endometrial carcinoma, in which vacuolization is common (Table 2-4) (Fig. 2-79).

Endocervical adenocarcinoma presents with little cellular degeneration; thus, the slide background is usually clean. The tumor is often accompanied by squamous metaplastic cells and occasional psammoma bodies (Fig. 2-80, Plates 2-26, 2-27).

Much attention is currently focused on the development of criteria for diagnosing endocervical adenocarcinoma in its earliest stages. Early endocervical adenocarcinoma generally refers to the following conditions: adenocarcinoma in situ, microinvasive adenocarcinoma, and adenocarcinoma limited to a single polypoid structure. Since the morphology of early endocervical neoplasia was first reported in 1953 by Friedell and McKay,[72] relatively few cases have been reported. Recent articles by Betsill and Clark[73] and Ayer et al.[74] have provided additional insight into the cytologic criteria necessary to establish this diagnosis, which are as follows:

1. A low cell yield featuring tissue fragments of

Table 2-4 A Comparison of Cytologic Findings in Endocervical Carcinoma and Endometrial Carcinoma

	Endocervical Carcinoma	Endometrial Carcinoma
General findings		
Cell yield	High; found mainly on cervical smear	Low; found mainly on vaginal smear
Cell groupings	Side-by-side groupings	Three-dimensional ball
Nuclear characteristics		
Chromatin	Finely granular	Moderately coarse
Nucleoli	Macronucleoli, sometimes multiple	Micronucleoli
Cytoplasmic characteristics		
	Granular	Finely vacuolated
	Columnar configuration that is often maintained	Columnar configuration that often is not apparent
	Rare ingestion of leukocytes	Abundant ingestion of leukocytes

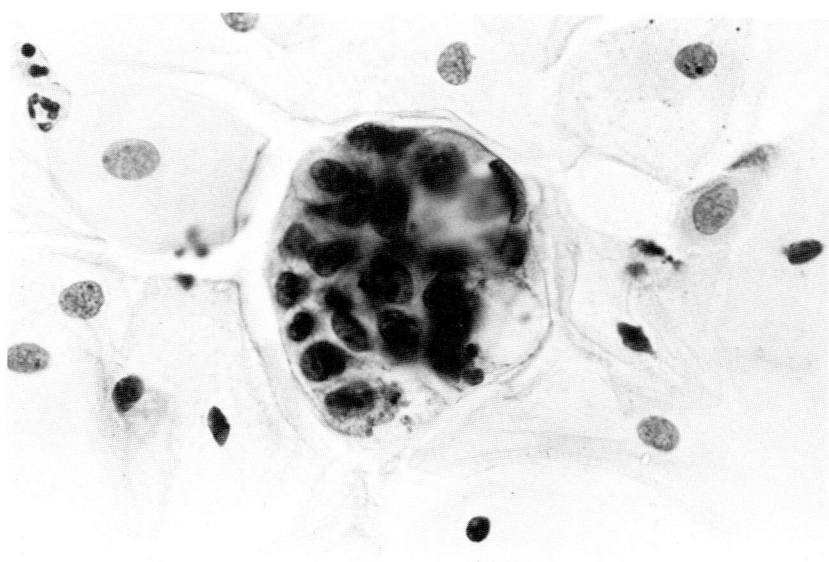

Fig. 2-79 Endometrial adenocarcinoma showing three-dimensional grouping, a vacuolated cytoplasm, and micronucleoli. (Papanicolaou stain, × 1000.)

crowded cells and only rare single cells, as well as rosettes in some cases
2. Nuclear enlargement, but without great variation in nuclear size and shape
3. Inconspicuous single nucleoli that may, in some cases, be absent
4. Moderate hyperchromasia and moderate granularity with even distribution
5. Usually, a clean background

Table 2-5 shows the cytologic differences between early and invasive endocervical adenocarcinoma as well as a common differential diagnosis, repair.

Table 2-5 A Cytologic Comparison of Repair, Early Endocervical Adenocarcinoma, and Invasive Endocervical Adenocarcinoma

	Reparative Changes	Early Endocervical Adenocarcinoma	Invasive Endocervical Adenocarcinoma
Nuclear size	Variable	Larger than normal endocervical cells	Very large
Nucleocytoplasmic ratio	Variable	Mild increase	Increased
Chromatin	Small granules	Hyperchromatic, finely granular	Hyperchromatic, finely granular
Cytoplasmic characteristics	Varied; elongated shape	Columnar shape; occasional vacuoles	Columnar shape; granular or vacuolated
Nucleoli	Prominent; may be multiple and variable in shape	Not prominent; may be absent	Prominent; may be multiple
Smear patterns			
Cell yield	Low; flat sheets	Low; tissue fragments	Moderate; tissue fragments
Single cells	Usually none	Rare	Easily seen
Background	Often dirty	Clean	Clean

86 PRACTICAL CYTOPATHOLOGY

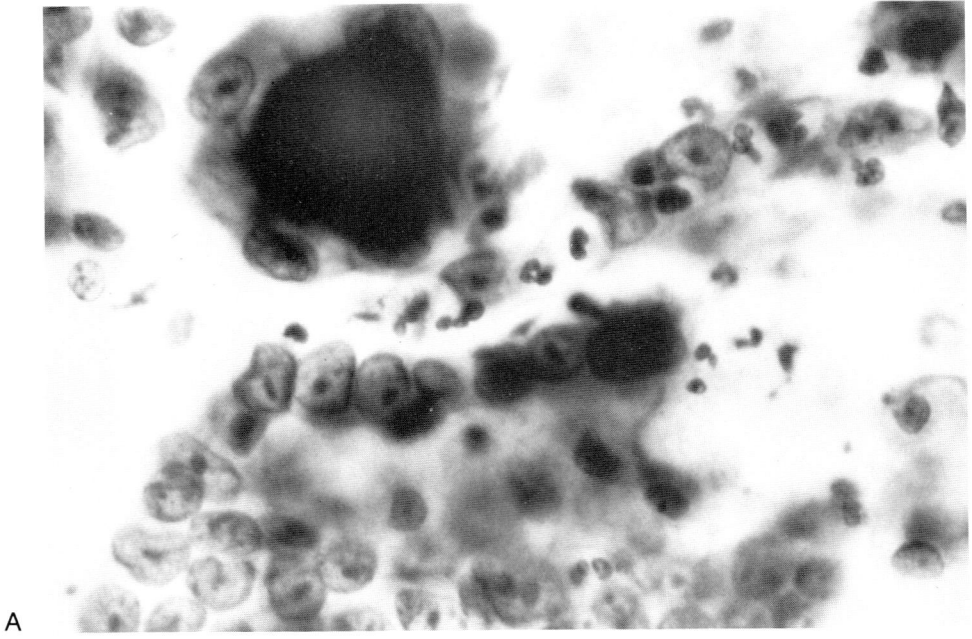

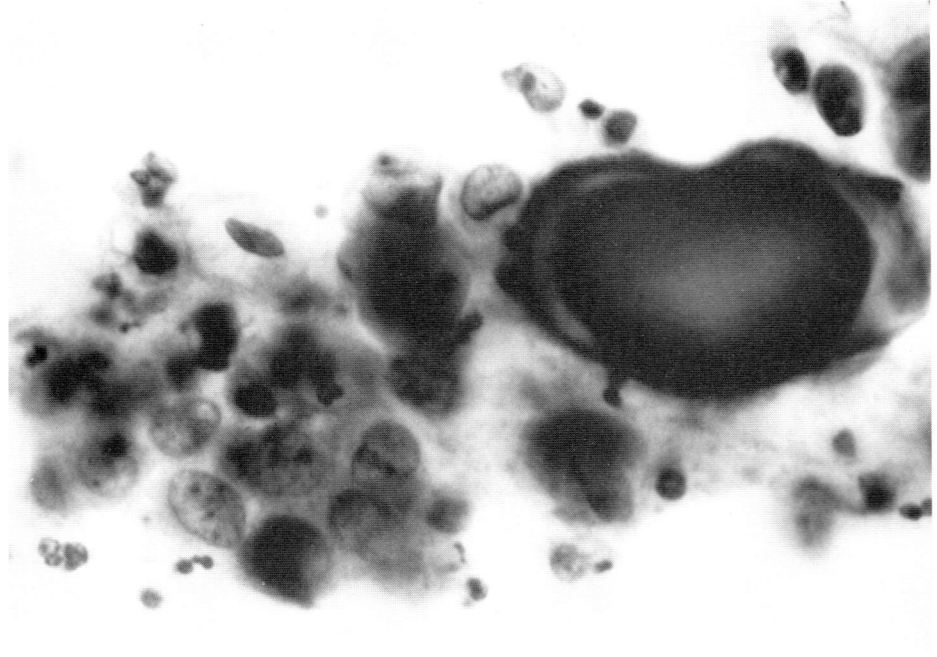

Fig. 2-80 (A,B) Two photographs of endocervical adenocarcinoma displaying prominent psammoma bodies. Note also the side-by-side arrangement of malignant cells and prominent nucleoli. (Papanicolaou stain, × 200.) (See Plates 2-26, 2-27.)

Cytology of the Endometrium
Roberta K. Nieberg

CYTOLOGY OF BENIGN ENDOMETRIAL DISORDERS

During the menstrual cycle, the endometrium is bombarded by a variety of hormonal agents to which it responds accordingly. Both the endometrial glands and the endometrial stroma exhibit the alterations of the proliferative and secretory phase. However, endometrial cells do not normally exfoliate, except during menstruation, unless there is a pathologic condition.

Sampling Techniques

Although there are several more sophisticated cytologic techniques available for evaluating the status of the endometrium, the cervical-vaginal-endocervical (CVE) smear still remains the most common noninvasive method for screening and evaluating cells from the endometrium. This is due to its relatively inexpensive cost, ease and safety of technique, and lack of discomfort to the patient. A cervical scrape alone yields minimal endometrial cells for examination. With material collected from the vaginal pool, endometrial cells may be obtained. However, Vuopala reported a similar detection rate of endometrial cells with both methods.[75] A battery of new techniques has been introduced during the past 40 years in an effort to enable more accurate sampling of the endometrium, especially in asymptomatic patients. These techniques involve the use of a metal cannula,[76] endometrial lavage,[77] brushes,[78,79] the Gravlee jet washer,[80,81] endometrial aspirators,[82-84] the Mi-mark plastic helix technique,[85] and the Isaacs endometrial cell sampler.[86-89] All of these techniques have their advocates. Other techniques have not been able to reproduce the excellent results originally shown.[90,91]

Aspiration and other instrumentation methods require special handling and an aseptic technique, as well as possible anesthesia; advanced cytologic training is necessary for proper interpretation. Thus, the CVE smear, especially in this day of cost containment and economic cutbacks, is still in demand as a routine cytologic screening test. If the patient is bleeding inappropriately, most clinicians perform endometrial tissue sampling as the initial procedure. The interpretation of benign endometrial cells obtained by routine CVE smears is discussed in this section; the following section will focus on the evaluation of malignant endometrial cells.

Diagnostic Considerations

It is absolutely essential that information concerning the patient's age, menstrual status, date of last menstrual period, method of contraception, pregnancy history, clinical history (bleeding, instrumentation, presence of other neoplasm), use of drugs (hormones or others), and course(s) of therapy (irradiation) be made available to the cytopathologist. Unfortunately, all too often, a thorough gynecologic history is unavailable; however, the importance of this information must be stressed to the clinician if a proper evaluation is to be rendered.

Interpretation of endometrial cells in a CVE smear is complicated by the presence of cells in a state of degeneration. These cells have been exfoliated, deprived of their oxygen supply, and autolyzed by enzymatic processes; moreover, they have been lying in a vaginal pool for a length of time, and have been further altered by changes in pH and bacterial decomposition. As in other fluid media, cells tend to "round up," lose their in situ cytologic features, degenerate, and exhibit artifactual profiles.

It is normal to see endometrial cells during or after menstruation, up to approximately day 12 in the menstrual cycle. The presence of endometrial cells during the latter half of the cycle, or at any time in a post menopausal patient, raises the possibility of a pathologic process in the endometrium. Such cases must be investigated by tissue sampling unless a reasonable explanation can be given.

CHANGES ASSOCIATED WITH MENSTRUATION

During menstruation, the CVE smear contains much blood, cellular debris, and endometrial cells (exodus) (Figs. 2-81 to 2-85). Averaging approximately 10 μm in diameter, endometrial cells are seen in tight clusters, irregular aggregates, streams of cells, or in wreathlike structures. The clusters show clumping and overlapping of small cells with round or slightly indented, moderately hyperchromatic nuclei containing evenly distributed chromatin with one or two chromocenters. The cytoplasm is ill-defined and cyanophilic, and may contain minute vacuoles. As the cells degenerate further, the nucleus becomes more hyperchromatic, and may vary in shape. The endometrial wreathlike appearance mimics structures seen in histologic sections of mensing endometrium, with small pyknotic stromal cells impacted within a circle of larger epithelial cells. When seen isolated or in loose linear formation, the cytologic features of the epithelial cells may be better realized. When the cytoplasm is preserved, it appears as a thin basophilic rim around the nucleus. The accompanying degenerating stromal cells may be difficult or impossible to differentiate from endometrial epithelial cells, especially during the late menstrual or postmenstrual phase. The superficial stromal cell nuclei are oval or reniform in shape, and the cytoplasm is pale, foamy, and may contain fine vacuoles. Deep stromal cells tend to be spindle-shaped, with elongated nuclei, coarse chromatin, nuclear grooving, and indistinct cytoplasm.

Accompanying the endometrial epithelial and stromal cells are histiocytes. These cells resemble superficial stromal cells, from which they may be impossible to differentiate, although they usually exhibit a greater amount of pale cytoplasm (Fig. 2-86). Histiocytes are found whenever there is a breakdown of tissue. They may be seen in association with cervical

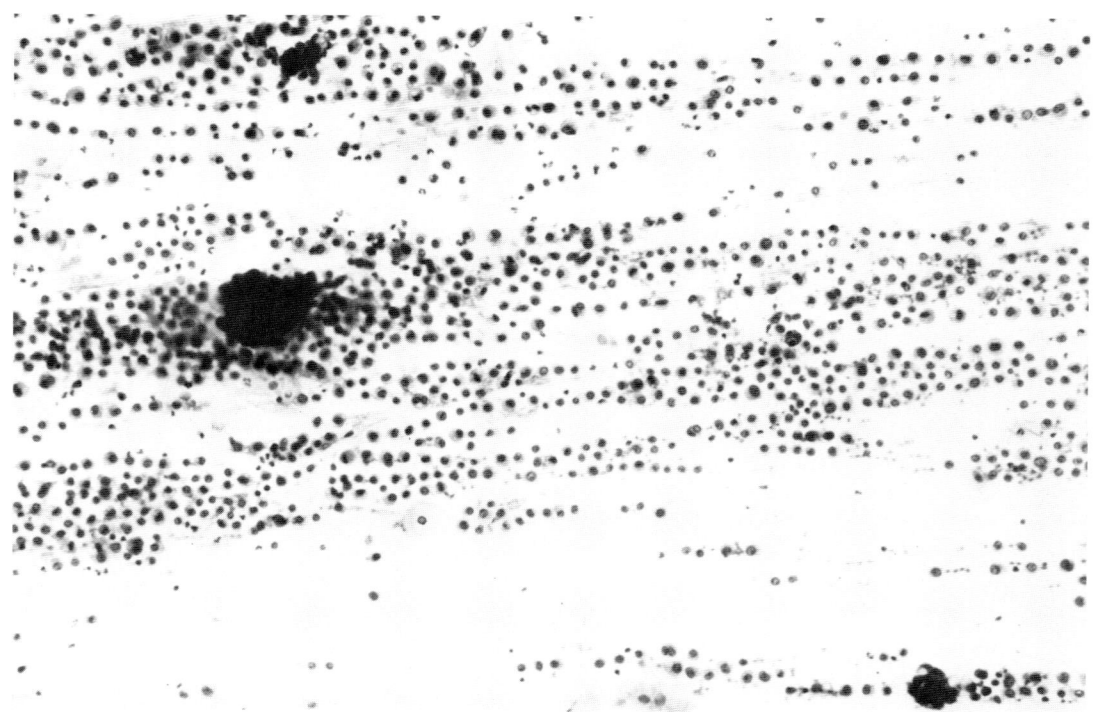

Fig. 2-81 Menstrual endometrium. Clumped and loosely dispersed endometrial cells with diathesis are evident. (CVE smear, × 120.)

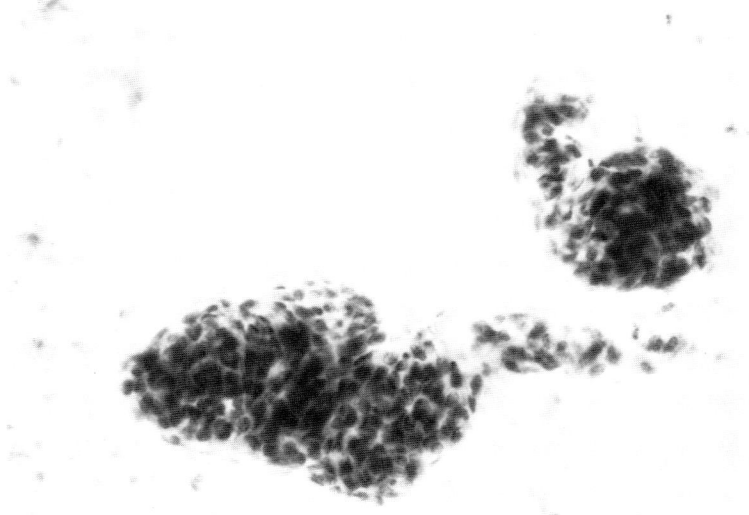

Fig. 2-82 Menstrual endometrium. Note the three-dimensional ball and glandlike clusters of overlapping small endometrial cells with uniform nuclei and finely dispersed chromatin. (CVE smear, × 310.)

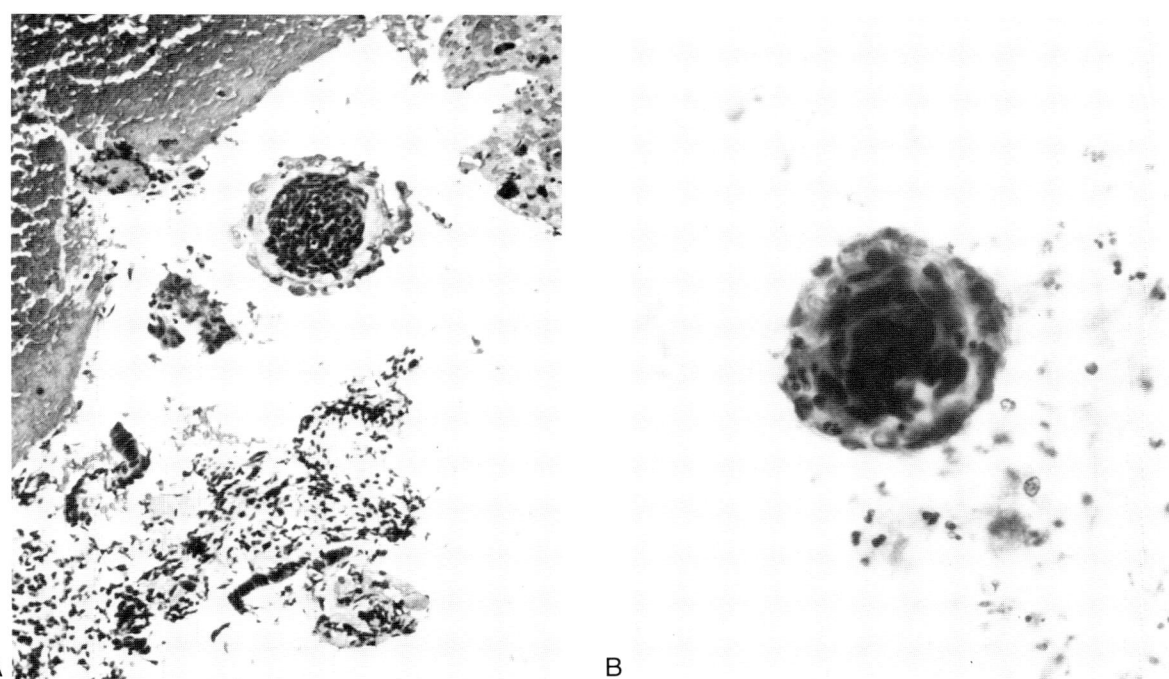

Fig. 2-83 (A) Menstrual endometrial with endometrial "wreath." Tightly packed stromal cells are seen within a rim of pale epithelial cells. (CVE smear, × 310.) **(B)** Menstrual endometrium with endometrial "wreath." (Endometrial curettage, H & E stain, × 120.)

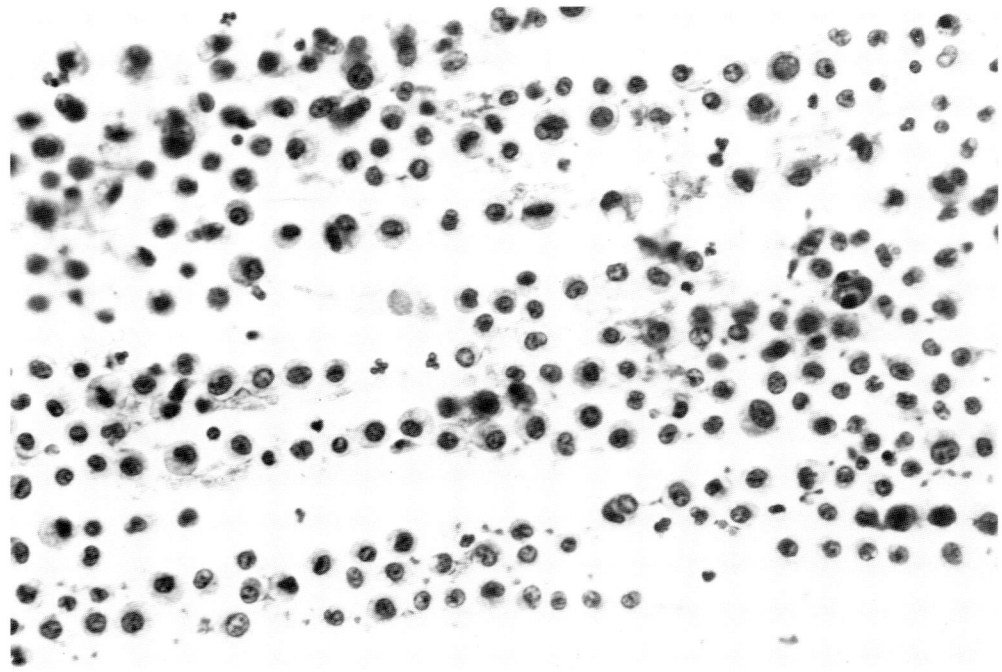

Fig. 2-84 Menstrual endometrium. Note the mixed endometrial epithelial and stromal cells that are accompanied by inflammatory cells and nuclear debris. (CVE smear, × 310.)

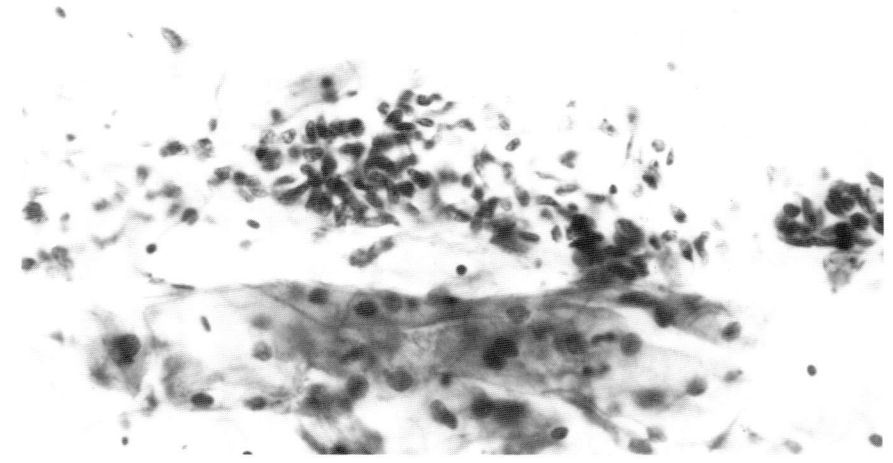

Fig. 2-85 Menstrual endometrium. The deep stromal cells are spindle-shaped and compact. (CVE smear, × 310.)

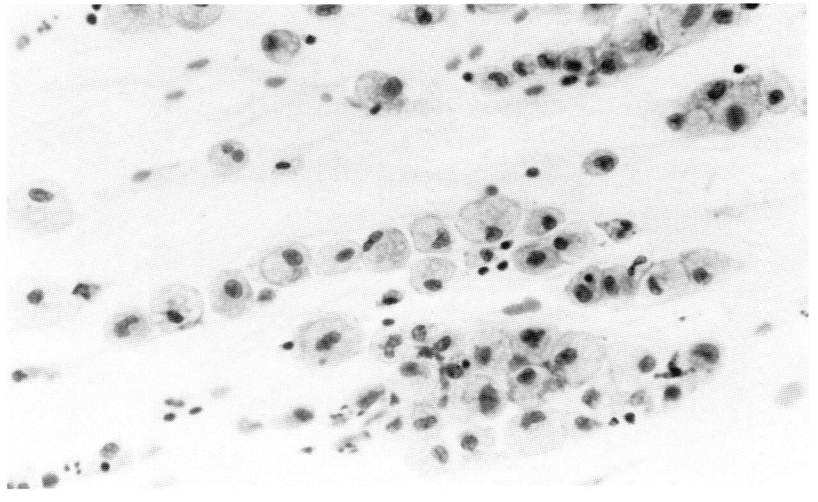

Fig. 2-86 Histiocytes. This smear was obtained 2 weeks postabortion. (CVE smear, × 310.)

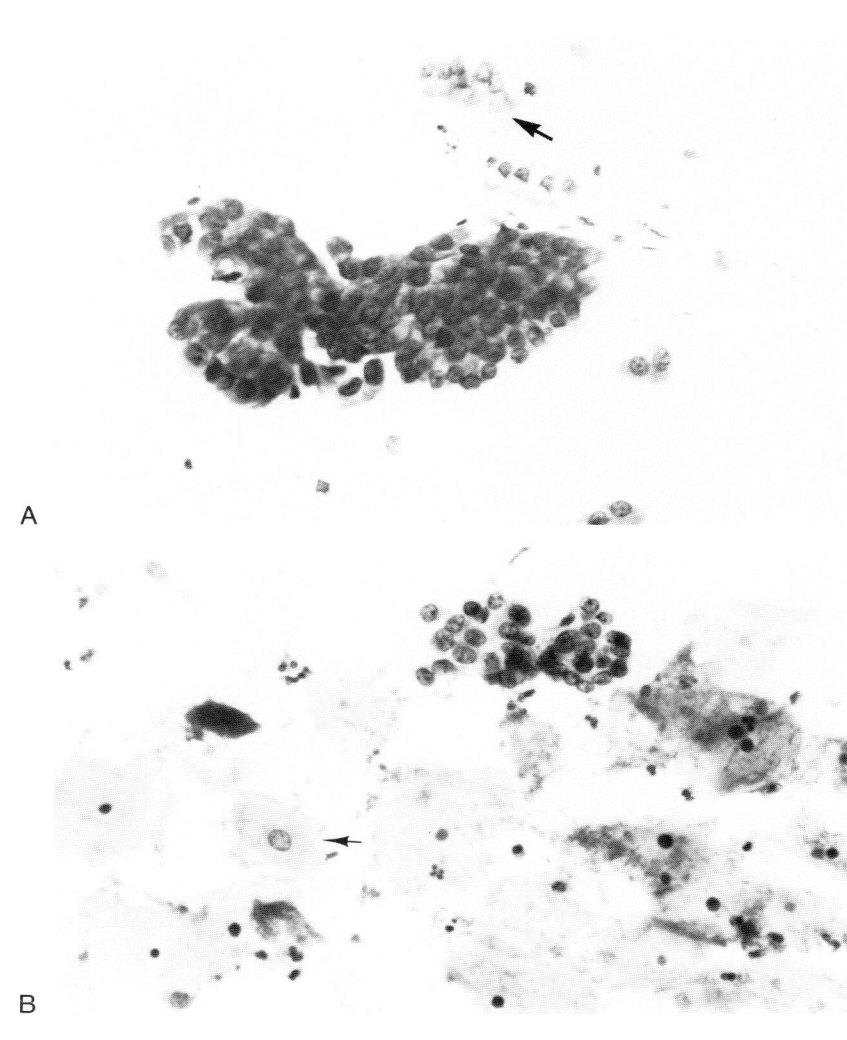

Fig. 2-87 (A) Cluster of endocervical cells with a honeycomb pattern and gland formation. The cells are larger than endometrial cells and have abundant, pale cytoplasm with a distinct border. A picket-fence formation (*arrow*) is evident. (CVE smear, × 310.) **(B)** Cluster of less cohesive endometrial cells with ill-defined cytoplasm and minor nuclear variations in shape. Compare the size of these cells to that of a squamous intermediate cell nucleus (*arrow*). (CVE smear, × 310.)

and endometrial inflammations, atrophic vaginitis, pregnancy, and neoplasia. The origin of these histiocytes is controversial, with evidence variably pointing to the circulating macrophage and to a transformation of existing stromal cells.[92]

DIFFERENTIATION BETWEEN ENDOMETRIAL AND ENDOCERVICAL CELLS

Endometrial cells must be differentiated from endocervical cells in a routine Papanicolaou smear (Fig. 2-87). The latter are larger, measuring 1.5 times the size of an endometrial epithelial cell. They may appear either in glandular clusters, with the cells exhibiting a distinct, abundant, pale cytoplasm with sharp cytoplasmic borders that form a honeycomb pattern; in strips resembling a "picket-fence" pattern; or in a loose aggregate of seminaked nuclei surrounded by wispy, pale, cyanophilic, ill-defined cytoplasm. The nuclei are uniform, oval or round, vesicular, paler than those in endometrial cells, and have finely stippled and evenly distributed chromatin and a small chromocenter.

Abnormal Shedding of Normal Endometrial Cells

Whenever normal endometrial cells are seen at an inappropriate time, an explanation is necessary. In premenopausal women, the etiology is usually benign, and cannot be determined by tissue samples. However, 20 percent of the postmenopausal women who shed normal endometrial cells will have a significant lesion.[93] In my institution, perimenopausal and postmenopausal women who shed endometrial cells inappropriately are evaluated with tissue sampling. In premenopausal women, tissue sampling is not necessary if the etiology can be clarified by clinical history. The causes of inappropriate shedding are presented in Table 2-6.

USE OF INTRAUTERINE DEVICES

Patients with an IUD in place may shed endometrial cells anytime during the menstrual cycle.[94] The cells exfoliate in two patterns. They may appear in small clusters and have slightly enlarged, hyperchromatic, round nuclei with abundant, pale cytoplasm

Table 2-6 Causes of Abnormal Shedding of Normal Endometrial Cells

Premenopausal	Postmenopausal
Presence of IUD	
Inflammation	
Anovulatory bleeding	
Pregnancy	
Immediate postpartum period	
Abortion	
Endometriosis in cervix or vagina	
Following instrumentation	
Endometrial polyp	Endometrial polyp
Hormonal therapy	Hormonal therapy
Submucous leiomyoma	
Endometrial hyperplasia	Endometrial hyperplasia
Endometrial carcinoma	Endometrial carcinoma

that is frequently associated with large vacuoles.[95–97] These vacuoles push the nucleus to an eccentric location (Fig. 2-88). In this guise, they may mimic a cluster of adenocarcinomatous cells. Other atypical cells of indeterminate type that may be seen in smears from patients using an IUD may appear as single, small to medium-sized cells with round, crenated, hyperchromatic nuclei exhibiting coarse chromatin clumping and a thin rim of cytoplasm. These may be either endometrial cells or metaplastic cells.[97] These small single cells can mimic small cell CIS of the cervix. However, in the latter condition, other larger, dysplastic cells are usually found. Actinomyces species, surrounded by debris and polymorphonuclear leukocytes, are also frequently seen in smears of patients using an IUD. If they are present, the diagnosis of IUD effect may be made more confidently. Endometrial cells may also be seen inappropriately in patients with a nonspecific, chronic endometritis or following instrumentation. It is rare to find plasma cells in vaginal smears. However, their occurrence with atypical endometrial cells suggests a diagnosis of chronic endometritis. The clinical history of the patient is especially important in the evaluation of reparative processes (Fig. 2-89).

PREGNANCY-RELATED CHANGES

A cause for alarm to the uninformed observer is the presence of the cellular changes associated with preg-

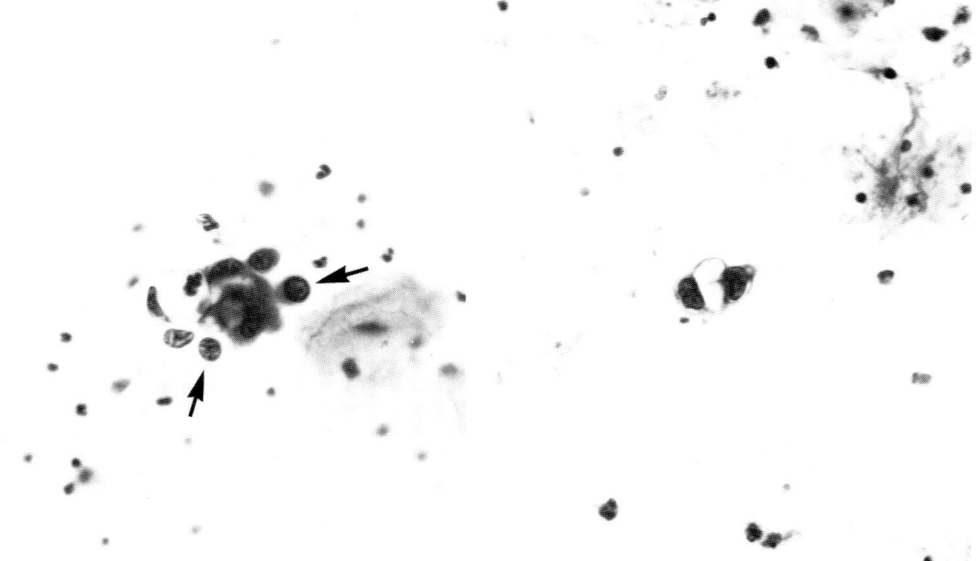

Fig. 2-88 IUD effect. Note the clusters of atypical endometrial cells with prominent vacuoles that mimic adenocarcinoma. Single, small, round cells (*arrows*) may mimic small cell squamous dysplasia. (CVE smear, × 310.)

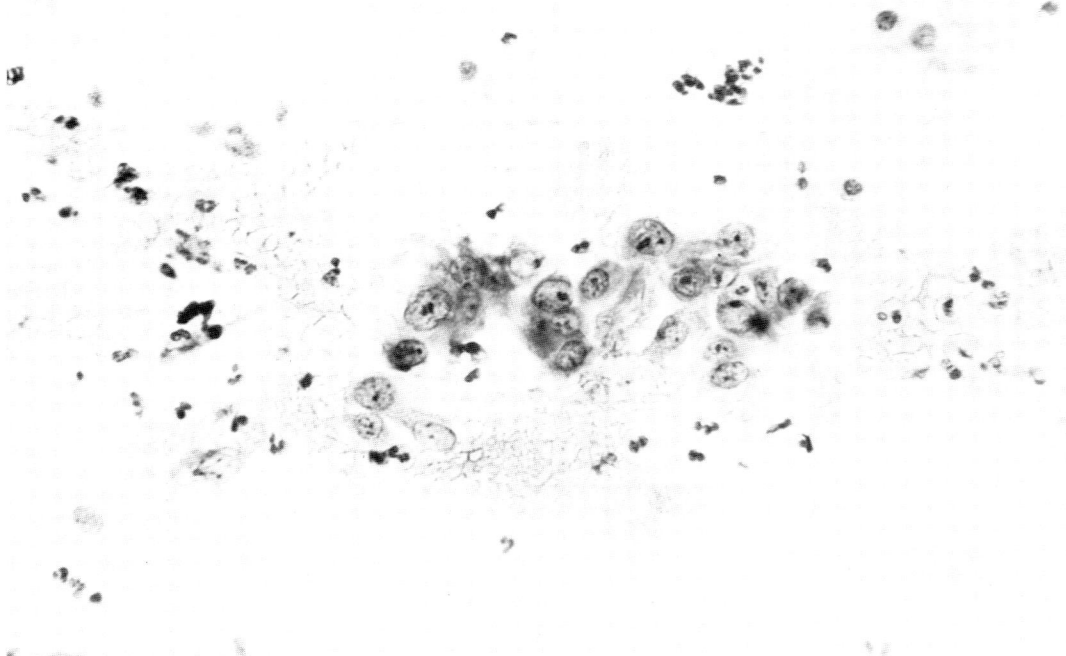

Fig. 2-89 Repair. A false-positive diagnosis of carcinoma was made on the basis of this smear, without benefit of a clinical history, in a patient who underwent endometrial curettage for benign disease. The cells are pleomorphic and exhibit irregular nuclear membranes, chromatin clearing, and prominent nucleoli. (CVE smear, × 400.)

nancy. Decidualized stromal cells from both the endometrium or endocervix may exfoliate. Decidual cells are large and have a centrally placed, vesicular nucleus and abundant, thick, cyanophilic, or basophilic cytoplasm. They occur singly or in small flat sheets (Fig. 2-90, Plates 2-28 and 2-29). Occasionally, these cells may be binucleated or have intracytoplasmic vacuoles. However, with severe degeneration in the postpartum or postabortion smear, decidual cells show relatively enlarged, bizarre, and hyperchromatic nuclei, and possibly even orangeophilic cytoplasm, especially in a partially dried smear. They may then be confused with dyskeratotic or highly atypical squamous cells.[98-100] A history of pregnancy and a lack of accompanying definitively dysplastic squamous cells should alert the observer to their benign origin.

The Arias-Stella phenomenon, first described by the famous Peruvian pathologist, refers to the changes in glandular cells associated with the elevated progesterone and human chorionic gonadotropin hormone levels seen in pregnancy. The glandular changes occur not only in the endometrium, but may also be present in the endocervix and in foci of vaginal adenosis. The columnar cells may have either large, distorted, hyperchromatic nuclei or pale nuclei with nucleoli and abundant clear cytoplasm (Fig. 2-91). They usually appear in small clusters.[101] If associated with the other cell types that occur during pregnancy, such as trophoblasts or decidual cells, and if pertinent history of pregnancy is given, a diagnosis of Arias-Stella phenomenon may be suggested. Decidual and atypical columnar cells may be shed in cases of intrauterine pregnancy as well as in ectopic pregnancy (Fig. 2-92).[102] However, without a history of pregnancy, the cells may appear sufficiently atypical to suggest the possibility of an adenocarcinoma, whereas degenerated decidual cells may suggest squamous dysplasia or a malignant squamous component.[99]

Another cell type that is associated with pregnancy is the multinucleated syncytiotrophoblastic giant cell from chorionic villi. These cells are bizarre, large, and have many dense, clustered nuclei (Fig. 2-93). "Cockleburrs" are hematoidin or orangeophilic rhomboidal crystals associated with hemorrhage and necrotic debris. They are produced in areas of decreased oxygen tension, and have been seen in association with both pregnancy and abortion (Fig. 2-94, Plate 2-30).[103,104]

BENIGN ENDOMETRIAL POLYPS

Although benign endometrial polyps are usually seen in older women, they may also occur in women who are in their reproductive years. If the polyp outgrows its blood supply, the structure may partially necrose, shedding endometrial cells along with blood and degenerating debris. However, the superficial epithelial cells of the polyp may exfoliate in an otherwise perfectly unremarkable smear. The cells may appear in small, tight clusters and may resemble normal endometrial cells (Fig. 2-95). Occasionally, upon degeneration, the cytoplasm is vacuolated and the nuclei may exhibit coarse chromatin with a prominent chromocenter or a small nucleolus. Of course, the polyp may be hyperplastic, and then the features of hyperplastic endometrial cells are observed.

ENDOMETRIAL HYPERPLASIA

The normal endometrial cell approximates the size of an intermediate squamous cell nucleus, and this is a good point of reference for comparison. Any recognizable endometrial cell that is larger than an intermediate squamous cell nucleus may be indicative of hyperplasia or carcinoma. A small percentage of patients with endometrial carcinoma and a greater percentage of patients with endometrial hyperplasia are asymptomatic and have no history of bleeding. These patients may show completely negative smears or they may shed normal or hyperplastic endometrial cells.

Endometrial hyperplasia typically occurs during the perimenopausal or postmenopausal period. The probability of this condition increases with obesity and the use of exogenous hormones, especially unopposed estrogen. In this case, the smear background shows an increased estrogenic effect. Seldom are inflammatory or necrotic debris and blood noted. Rather, normal endometrial cells, which may or may not be mixed with abnormal endometrial cells, are usually evident. Cells may be few or transient. Depending on the type of hyperplasia (e.g., cystic, adenomatous, or atypical), the endometrial cells will vary from being normal to being severely abnormal. Frequently, the only clue to a hyperplastic or neo-

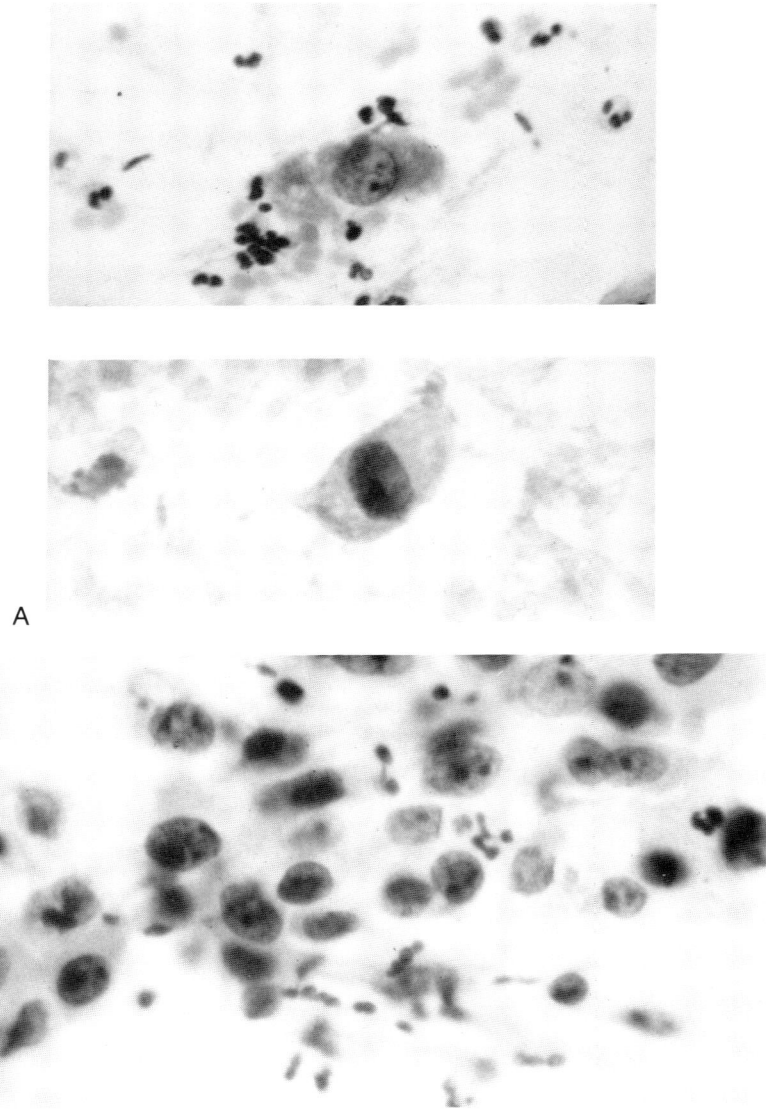

Fig. 2-90 (A) Single decidual cells in a smear obtained from a pregnant female. (See Plate 2-28.) **(B)** Sheets of decidual cells in a pregnant patient with a decidualized polyp protruding through the cervical os. (CVE smear, × 310.) (See Plate 2-29.)

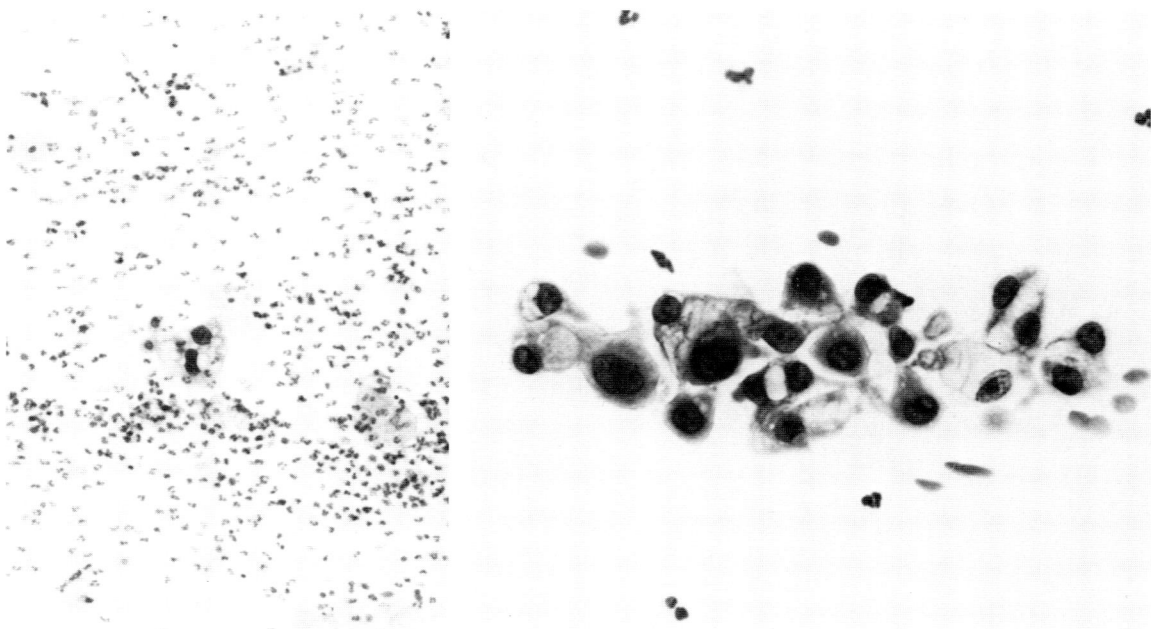

Fig. 2-91 Arias-Stella phenomenon. Atypical cells with hyperchromatic nuclei and voluminous, vacuolated cytoplasm. The patient was 3 months pregnant. (*Left,* CVE smear, × 120; *right,* CVE smear, × 310.)

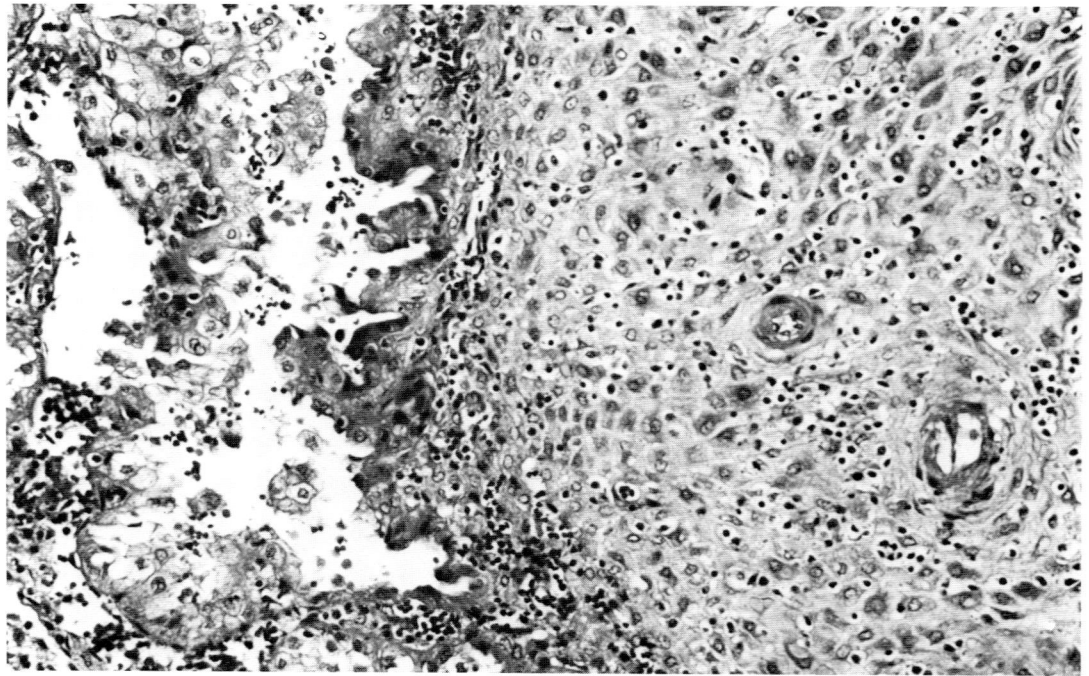

Fig. 2-92 Decidualized stroma and endometrial glands showing Arias-Stella effect. (Endometrial curettage, × 310.)

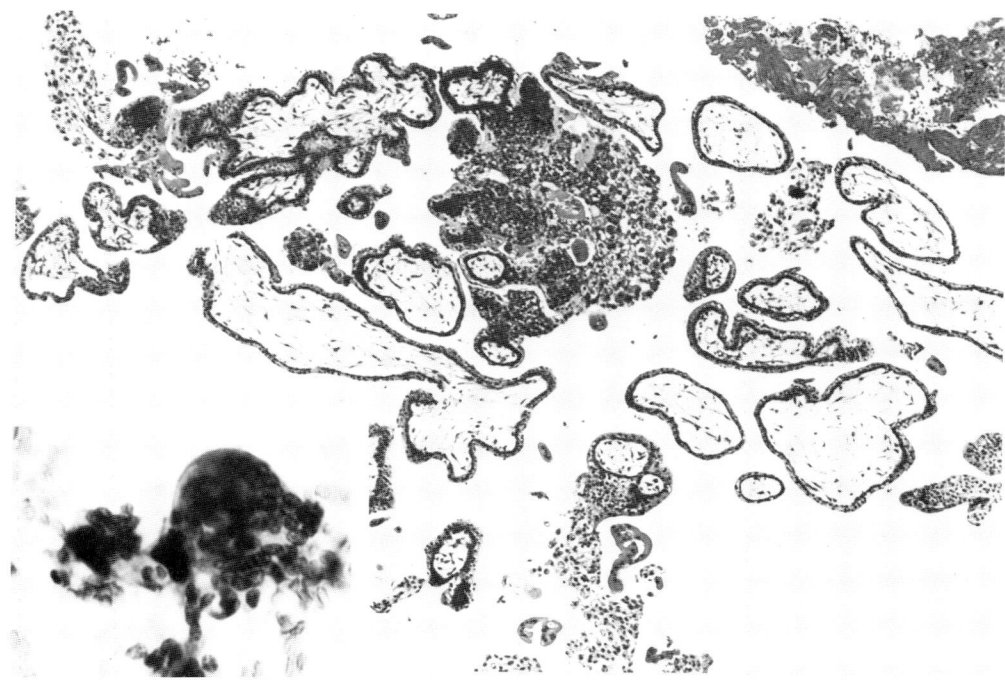

Fig. 2-93 First-trimester chorionic villi. (Endometrial curettage, × 120.) *Inset:* Multinucleated syncytiotrophoblast. (CVE smear, × 310.)

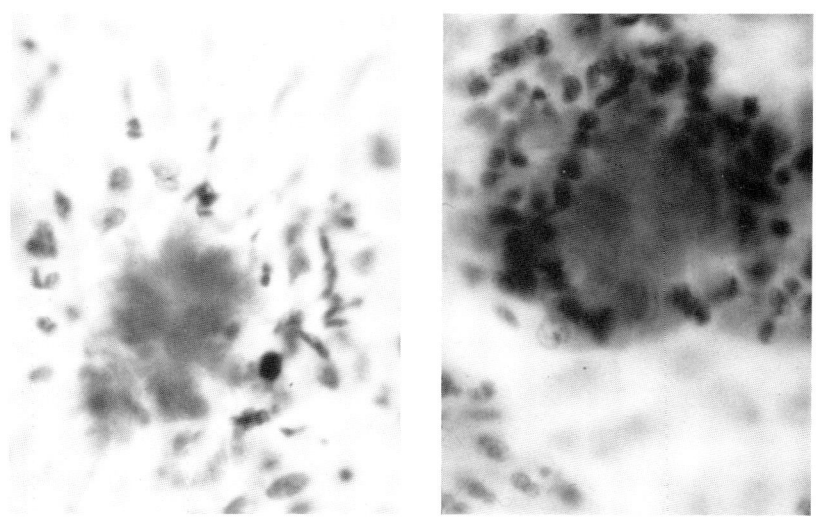

Fig. 2-94 "Cockelburrs." Hematoidin crystals in a patient who was 7 months pregnant. (CVE smear, × 310.) (See Plate 2-30.)

98 PRACTICAL CYTOPATHOLOGY

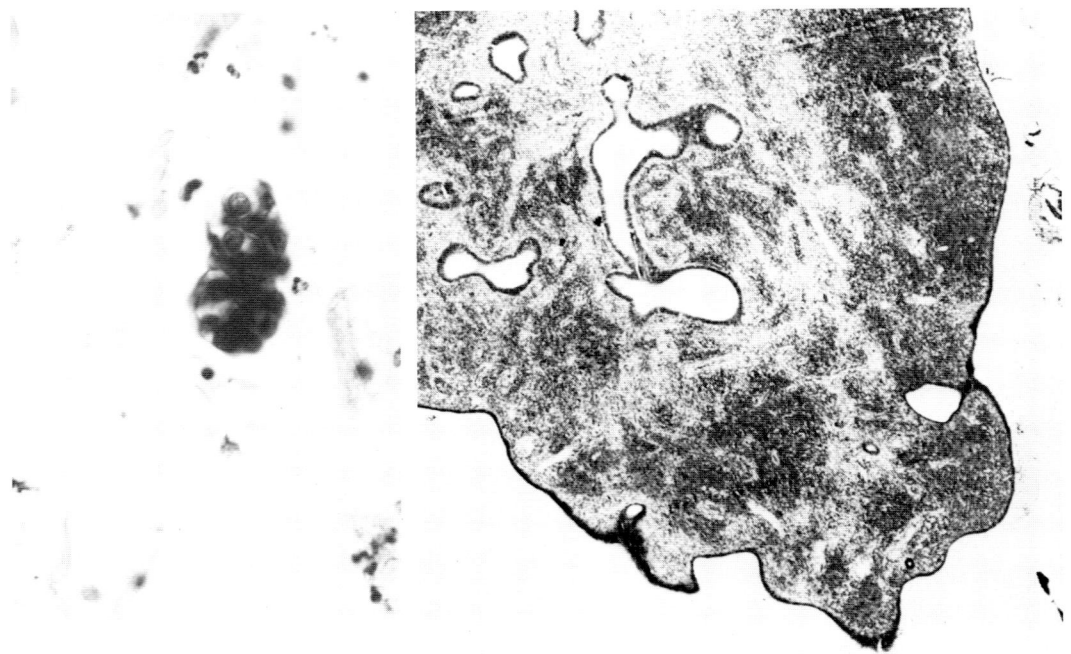

Fig. 2-95 Tight cluster of benign endometrial cells that were inappropriately shed in a patient with an endometrial polyp. (*Left*, CVE smear, × 310; *right*, endometrial curettage, × 50.)

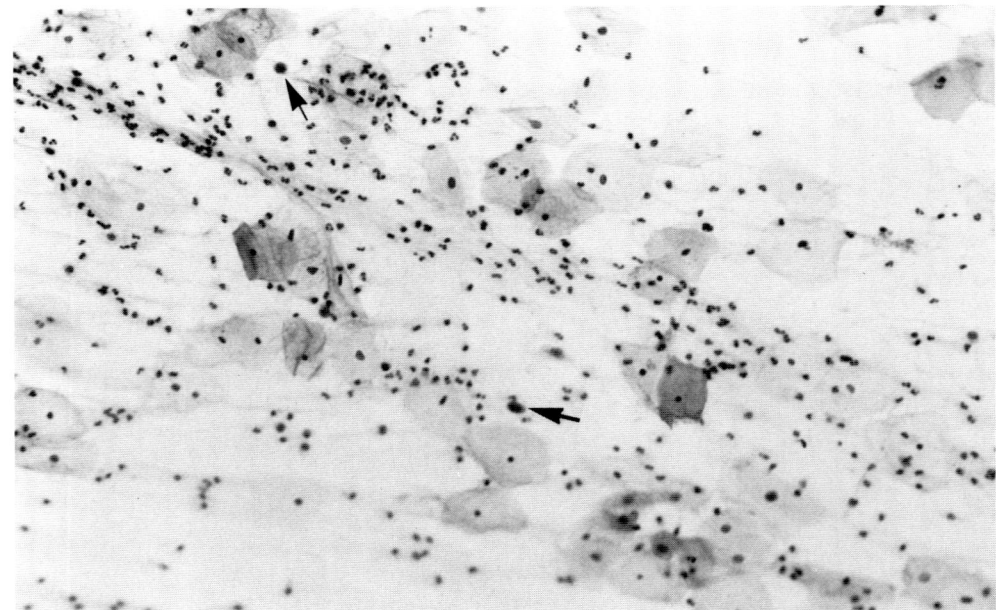

Fig. 2-96 Clean smear with elevated estrogenic effect and rare, isolated, single endometrial cells (*arrows*) in a perimenopausal patient. Subsequent curettage revealed mild adenomatous hyperplasia without atypia. (CVE smear, × 120.)

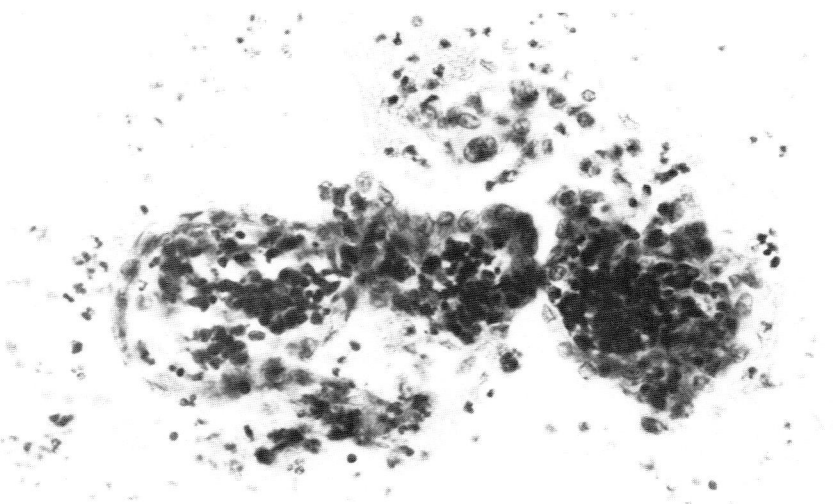

Fig. 2-97 Inappropriately shed, slightly atypical endometrial cells that appear in both isolated and glandular ball form. The patient was postmenopausal and symptomatic. Endometrial curettage revealed adenomatous hyperplasia without atypia. (CVE smear, × 310.)

plastic condition is the presence of isolated normal or atypical endometrial cells in an otherwise unremarkable smear (Fig. 2-96).[105,106] Once there is tissue necrosis, diathesis will be noted.

The exfoliated cells of cystic and adenomatous endometrial hyperplasia may show slight cellular and nuclear enlargement, with variations in cell size and shape. The hyperplastic endometrial cells may be shed singly or in tight clusters, with molding of cells, or in an acinar formation with overlapping of cells. The nuclei reveal an irregular dispersement of chromatin (Fig. 2-97). The greater the nuclear size and number of nucleoli, and the greater the degree of cytologic atypia, cellular pleomorphism, and hyperchromasia, the greater is the likelihood of progressively severe histologic findings.[107,108] In severely atypical hyperplasia, nucleoli are present, and the cells closely resemble those of a low-grade adenocarcinoma (Fig. 2-98).

In my experience, the main clue to low-grade endometrial hyperplasia is the presence of inappropriately shed endometrial cells of normal or atypical types, or both. This finding may be associated with histiocytes, blood, or an elevated estrogenic effect, but this is not necessarily so. The presence of only the latter three criteria does not increase the risk of endometrial hyperplasia or neoplasia in subsequent biopsy tissue. This finding has been reported by others,[109] although some have stressed that the presence of histiocytes alone can be a substantial clue for the diagnosis of hyperplasia or neoplasia.[110]

One reason for the faulty correlation between cytology and histology in cases of endometrial hyperplasia is the anatomy of the endometrium in some cases of endometrial hyperplasia. Frequently, the surface epithelium is unremarkable and intact, whereas the deeper endometrium may contain zones of atypical endometrial proliferations. Thus, without shedding of the deep epithelial cells, cytologic examination may yield negative results.[111] Only in the more severe cases of hyperplasia, which are accompanied by surface involvement and endometrial breakdown, are atypical endometrial cells exfoliated.

In a recent study conducted at my institution, 5 of 13 cases (38 percent) of tissue-confirmed endometrial hyperplasia were undetected on the CVE smear. Upon meticulous retrospective review, 12 (92 percent) revealed findings that were suspicious for endometrial hyperactivity. This discrepancy was caused by a failure to detect, in a clean smear and with a good estrogenic effort, single, normal endometrial cells that were inappropriately shed. This study emphasizes the necessity for careful cytologic screening. Clearly, the clues are there, and the CVE smear may not be such a poor screening test for this condition after all.

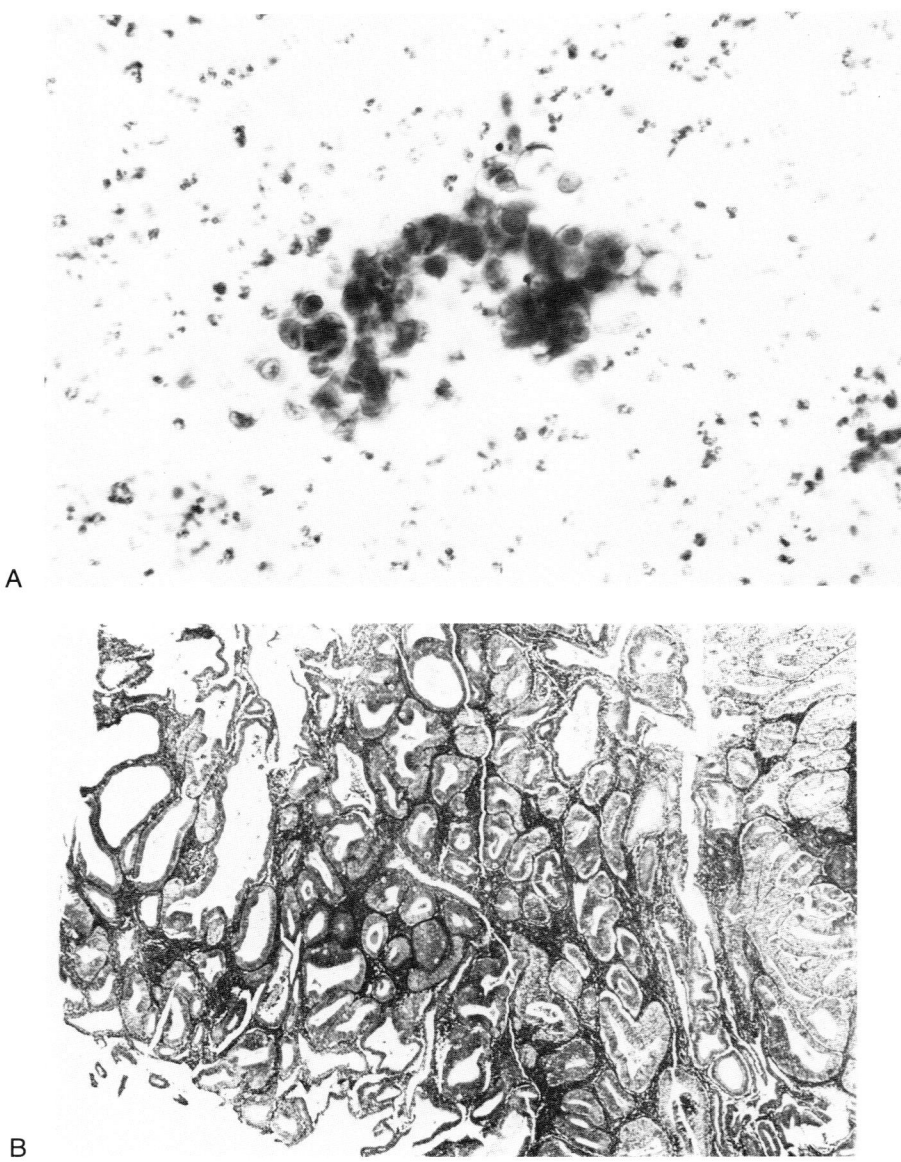

Fig. 2-98 **(A)** An irregular cluster of markedly atypical endometrial cells with diathesis, suggesting malignant disease in a patient with severely atypical adenomatous hyperplasia. (CVE smear, × 310.) **(B)** Severely atypical adenomatous hyperplasia. (Endometrial curettage, × 120.)

CYTOLOGY OF MALIGNANT NEOPLASMS

Carcinoma of the Endometrium

Adenocarcinoma of the endometrium, although less prevalent worldwide than cervical cancer, is increasing in the United States, as evidenced by a projected estimate of 35,000 new cases for 1987.[112] Although all of the conditions associated with the development of endometrial cancer have not been identified, certain risk factors that predispose women to the development of endometrial carcinoma have been recognized and accepted. These include age (more than 95 percent of affected women are 40 years of age or older); obesity (those who are 10 to 15 pounds overweight have a three times greater risk; whereas those who are more than 20 pounds overweight have a risk that is 8 to 10 times greater than that of persons who are not obese);[113,114] diabetes;[115] hypertension;[113] liver disease;[115] a history of infertility or multiparity; ovarian disease (Stein-Leventhal syndrome);[116] menstrual irregularities; late menopause; pelvic irradiation;[113] prolonged use of exogenous estrogens;[117] and a history of other hormone-related tumors (involving the breast or ovary).[118,119]

Precursor hyperplastic lesions occur in women who are 40 to 70 years old, whereas invasive cancer peaks in the sixth decade.[120] All cases of endometrial carcinoma are not symptomatic. Koss reported an incidence of 8 in 1,000 among asymptomatic females.[121,122]

DIAGNOSTIC CONSIDERATIONS

Conventional cytology is not an optimal screening method for endometrial carcinoma. Other invasive techniques, as mentioned in the previous section, may yield a greater sensitivity and specificity. However, the latter techniques have not been uniformly accepted for routine use because of a variety of reasons (cost, time, complicated procedures, patient discomfort, and training of personnel, among others). Thus, most cytopathologists and cytotechnologists use routine CVE smears to detect endometrial carcinoma and its precursors. Although a diagnostic accuracy of 40 to 50 percent is the norm reported in most studies for detection of endometrial carcinoma by this technique, rates as high as 60 percent[123] and 72.5 percent have been reached, with the highest rates being achieved with rescreening of tissue-confirmed cases of endometrial carcinoma.[124]

The reasons for false-negative smears are many. The shedding of endometrial cells may be limited and inconstant. Endometrial cells may be so degenerate by the time they are removed from the vaginal pool that they are not recognizable as such. A few patients in the older age group have cervical stenosis, so that cells from the endometrium are not present in a routine sample. Von-Ludinhausen has suggested that the surface endometrium may be unremarkable, whereas the glands in the deeper stroma may contain atypical or neoplastic cells; however, the latter do not exfoliate.[125] Factors influencing the exfoliation of malignant cells relate to the extent of surface occupied by the tumor, tumor grade, endocervical involvement, pattern of growth (papillary or polypoid versus endophytic), and the presence of a squamous component.[123]

CYTOLOGIC FINDINGS

Meticulous cytologic screening at the initial stage of examination cannot be overemphasized. As with endometrial hyperplasia, the only clue that a neoplastic process exists in the endometrium may be the presence of inappropriately shed normal or atypical endometrial cells. The literature is replete with mention of such instances.[120,126,127] Single endometrial cells may be hidden in a deceptively clean smear (Fig. 2-99, Plate 2-31). Blood, histiocytes, and an elevated estrogenic effect may not be present. Histiocytes, although usually present,[128] are also noted in a variety of benign conditions, and are especially common in atrophic smear patterns. Rather, it is the presence of atypical endometrial cells that is most reliable indicator of malignant disease.[129]

The cytologic features that may be noted in the CVE smear in endometrial adenocarcinoma are listed below

1. Elevated estrogen index
2. Old fibrinated or fresh blood
3. Cellular debris
4. Normal endometrial cells appearing singly or in groups
5. Histiocytes

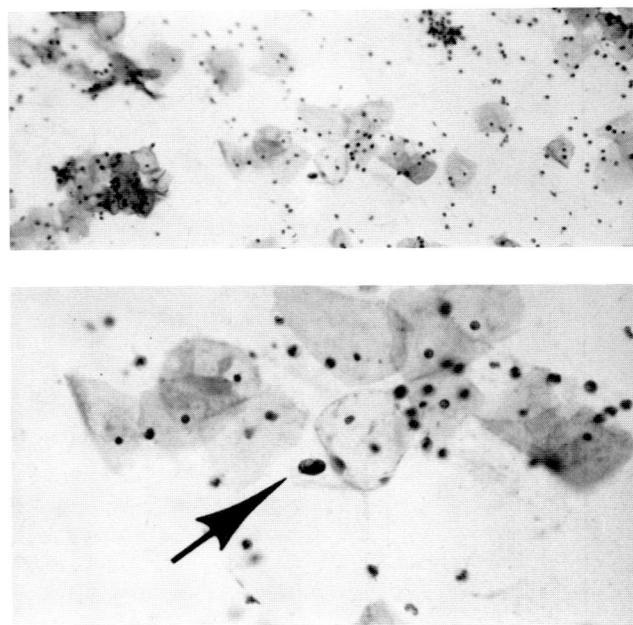

Fig. 2-99 Grade I adenocarcinoma. A single, atypical, endometrial cell (*arrow*) in a clean smear with elevated estrogenic effect. (*Upper:* CVE smear, × 120; *Lower:* CVE smear, × 310.) (See Plate 2-31.)

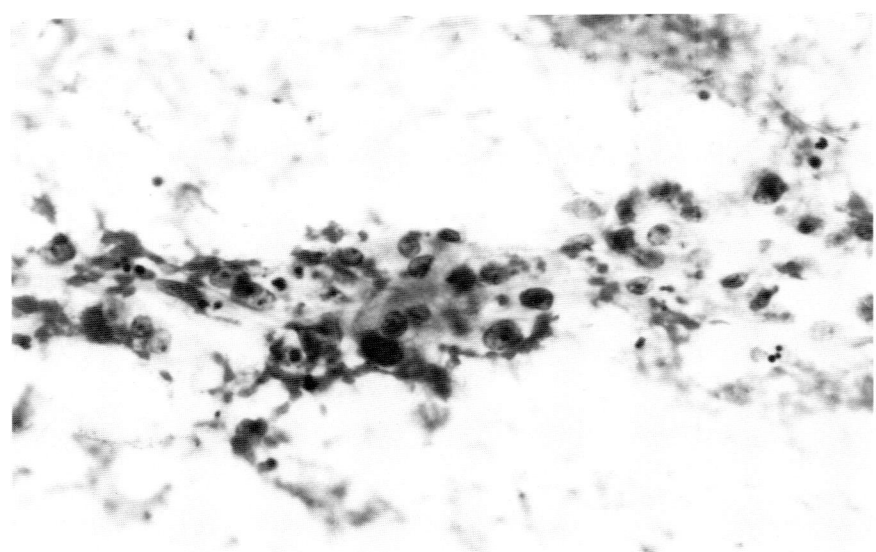

Fig. 2-100 Grade I adenocarcinoma. Malignant endometrial cells vary from one to another in size, shape, chromatin content, and presence of nucleoli. Cells are loosely cohesive and admixed with hemolyzed and fresh blood and nuclear debris. (CVE smear, × 310.)

6. Abnormal single endometrial cells or clusters of cells that range in size and nature from slightly enlarged to frankly malignant
7. Balls of polymorphonuclear leukocytes in which malignant cells are hidden

The majority of patients with endometrial carcinoma, however, will exhibit diathesis in the smear. Abnormal endometrial cells are usually present, admixed with fresh and hemolyzed blood, nuclear debris, inflammatory cells, and histiocytes (Fig. 2-100). The number of abnormal cells and the degree of cytologic atypia usually reflect the grade and histologic type of neoplasm.

Cells of grade I or well-differentiated adenocarcinoma may resemble those of atypical adenomatous hyperplasia. Usually, however, the cells of the former are larger. The cells are arranged in small clusters or balls. The nuclear chromatin pattern is irregular, differs from cell to cell, and frequently is associated with irregular clearing. Occasionally, the nuclei are hyperchromatic, and internal analysis of the chromatin pattern is impossible. However, nucleoli, which are prominent, are usually observed (Figs. 2-101 and 2-102).

As the grade of the tumor increases, the cells become more bizarre, with an increasing degree of cytomegaly and nuclear pleomorphism. The chromatin pattern becomes increasingly irregular. Nucleoli are especially conspicuous. The cytoplasm may be scanty or superabundant, and may contain vacuoles. If the cell groups are intact, the cells in the glands overlap and demonstrate a loss of polarity and a disrespect for cytoplasmic borders (Figs. 2-103 and 2-104).

As the tumor becomes less differentiated, the cellular features described earlier in this section become more exaggerated. Although ball and glandular profiles may be present, the cells may appear in irregular formations or they may be dispersed as poorly differentiated, single epithelial cells (Figs. 2-105 and 2-106). Occasionally, the diathesis may be overwhelming, and balls of polymorphonuclear leukocytes are seen in which few viable or degenerating tumor cells may be hidden (Fig. 2-107).

SEROUS PAPILLARY CARCINOMA

Serous papillary carcinoma of the endometrium is biologically a very aggressive tumor.[130] It may, by virtue of its exophytic exuberant papillary growth, exfoliate abundant, tiny, intact papillary profiles (Fig. 2-108).

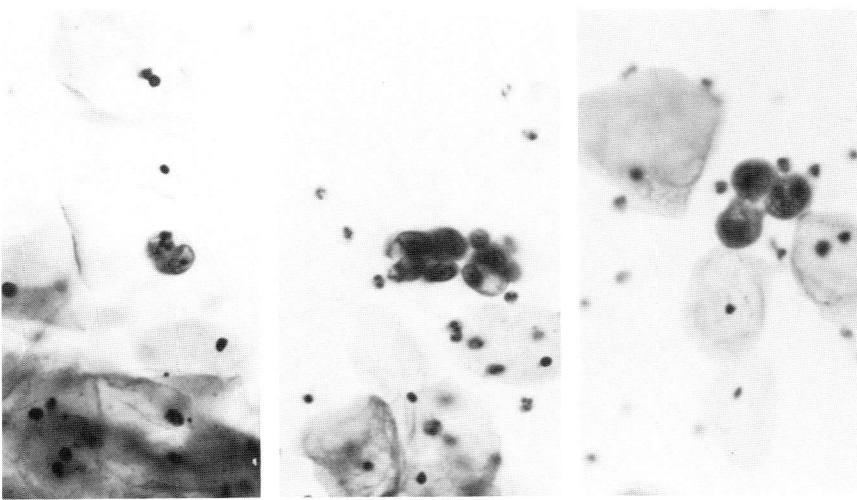

Fig. 2-101 Grade I adenocarcinoma. Small clusters of malignant endometrial cells in a relatively clean smear with elevated estrogenic effect. Tumor cells show nuclear enlargement, pleomorphism, and nucleoli. (CVE smear, × 310.)

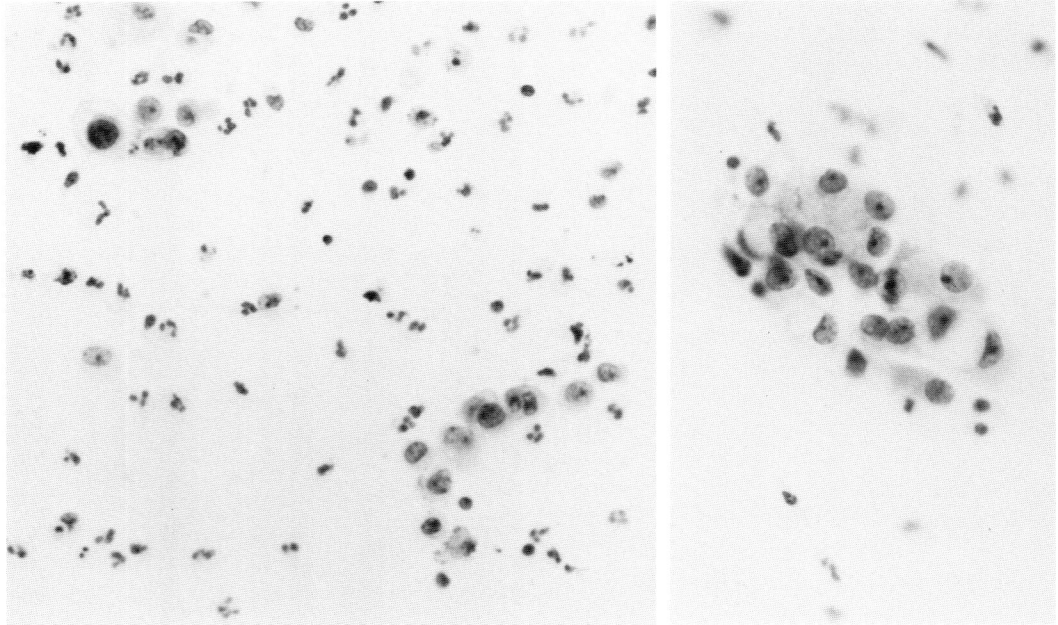

Fig. 2-102 Loosely dispersed malignant endometrial cells with a glandlike cluster. Cells show chromatin clearing and abundant pale cytoplasm. (CVE smear, × 310.)

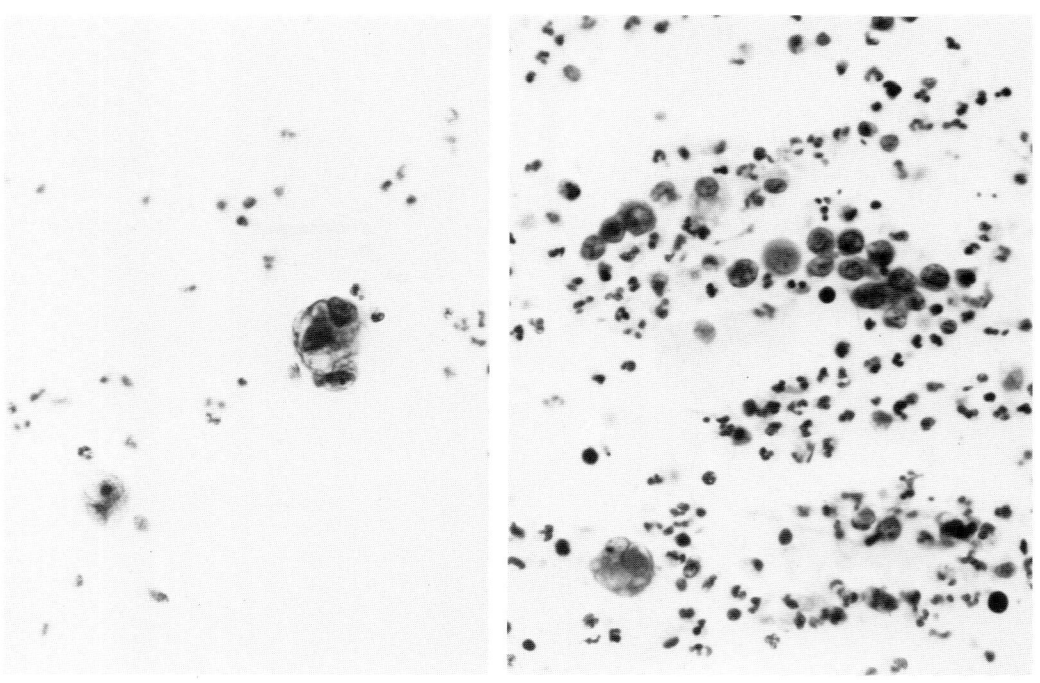

Fig. 2-103 *Left,* Cluster of hyperchromatic, pleomorphic cells with cytoplasmic vacuolization. *Right,* Grade II endometrial adenocarcinoma. Loose dispersement of malignant cells. (CVE smear, × 310.)

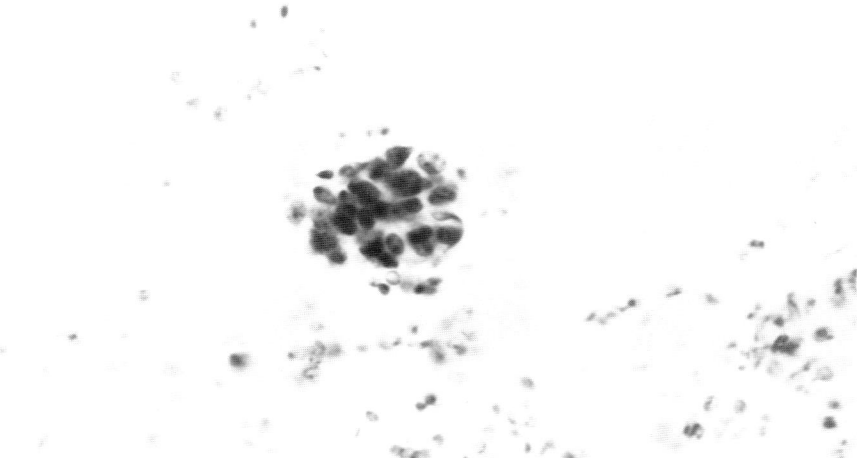

Fig. 2-104 Grade II adenocarcinoma. Three-dimensional ball of pleomorphic malignant cells with loss of cytoplasmic borders and accompanying diathesis. (CVE smear, × 310.)

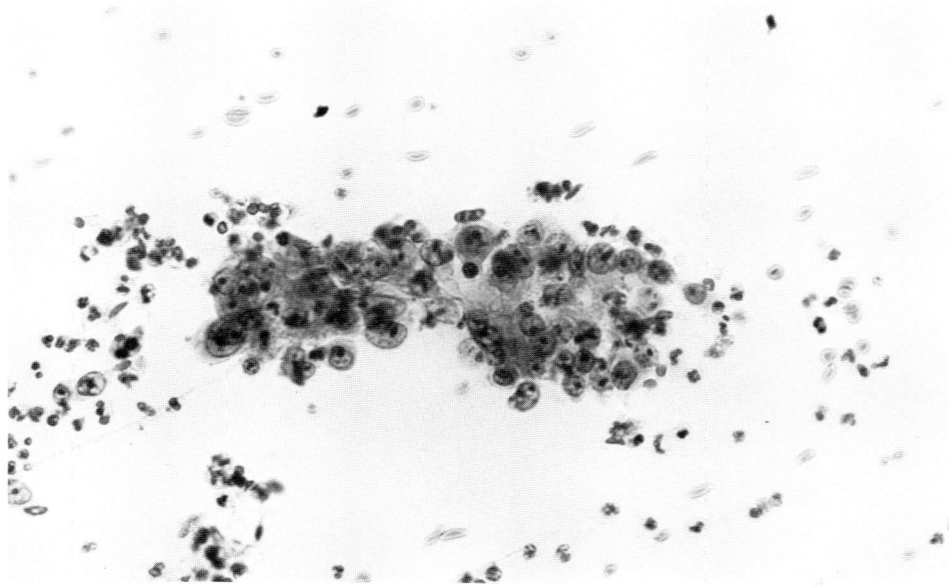

Fig. 2-105 High-grade adenocarcinoma. Glandlike profile of large malignant endometrial cells with irregular chromatin pattern and prominent nucleoli. (CVE smear, × 310.)

106 PRACTICAL CYTOPATHOLOGY

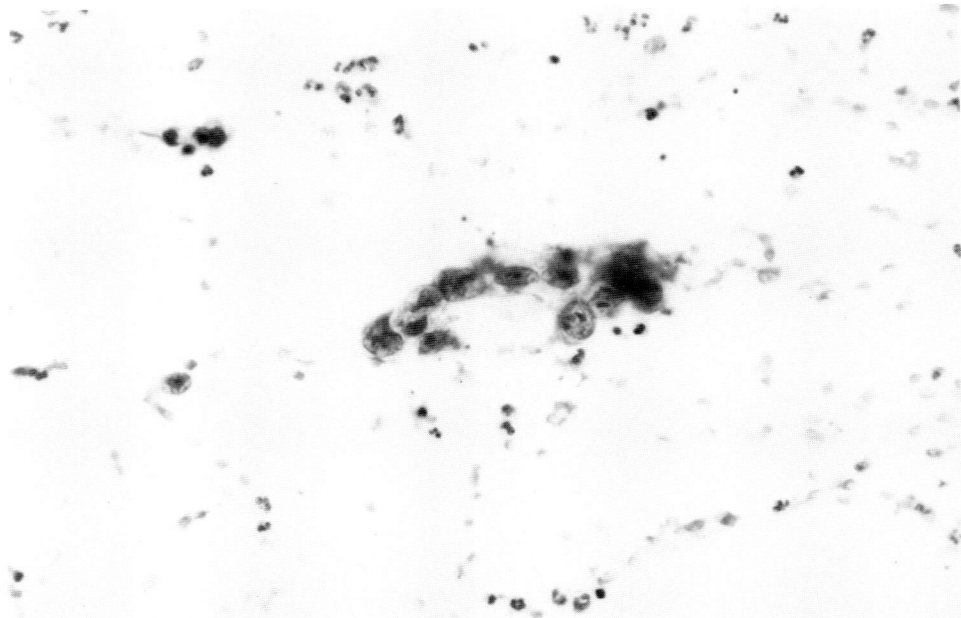

Fig. 2-106 Grade III adenocarcinoma. Large pleomorphic cells in an ill-defined configuration showing cellular molding with accompanying diathesis. (CVE smear, × 310.)

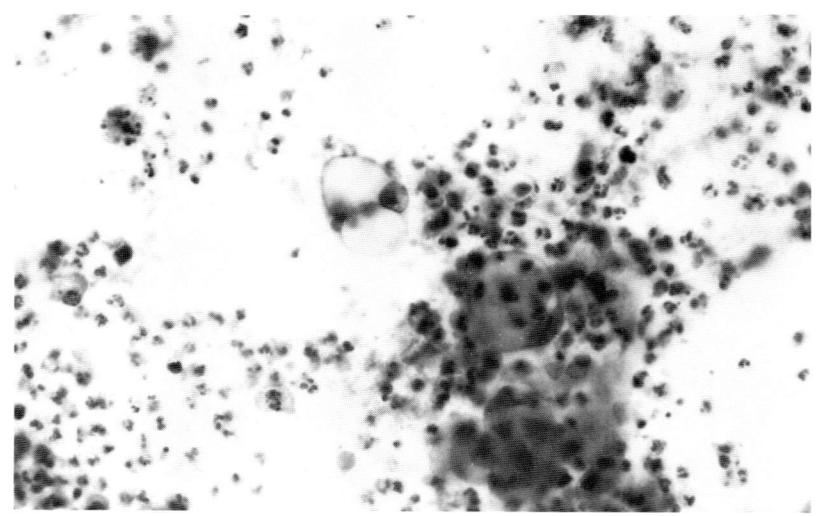

Fig. 2-107 High-grade adenocarcinoma. Overwhelming diathesis with ball-like clusters of polymorphonuclear leukocytes admixed with tumor cells. (CVE smear, × 310.)

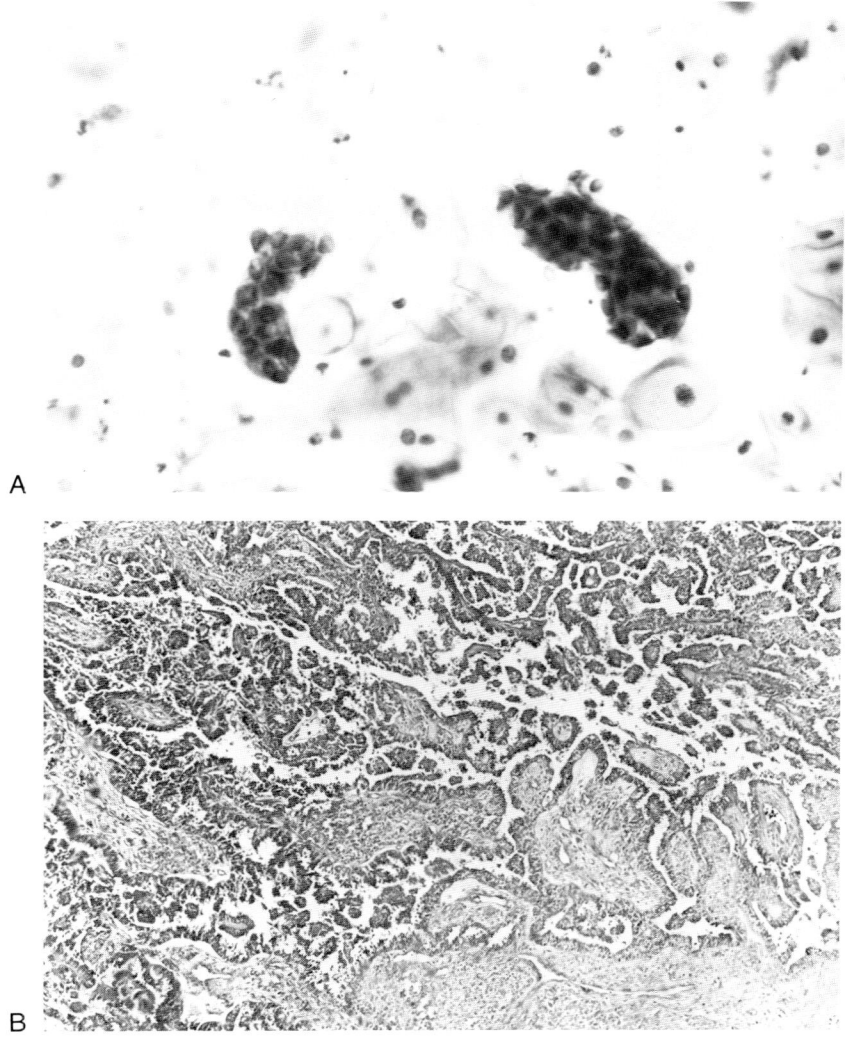

Fig. 2-108 (A) Two papillary-like clusters of malignant cells. (CVE smear, × 310.) **(B)** Papillary serous adenocarcinoma of the endometrium. (Uterus, hysterectomy, × 310.)

CLEAR CELL CARCINOMA

Clear cell carcinoma of the endometrium, a variant of adenocarcinoma, may not be definable as a typical clear cell neoplasm. Rarely, malignant cells with clear or whispy cytoplasm may be seen (Fig. 2-109, Plate 2-32). A cellular cluster with a markedly eccentric, protruding nucleus may also suggest this tumor type, and may reflect the hobnail pattern noted in clear cell tumors (Fig. 2-110).

ADENOACANTHOMA AND ADENOSQUAMOUS CARCINOMA

Endometrial carcinoma may have mixed epithelial proliferations that exhibit both glandular and squamous features. The latter may be benign (adenoacanthoma) or malignant (adenosquamous carcinoma). Although two distinct cell populations are present in both types of tumors on histologic sections, the squamous component may be misinterpreted or missed

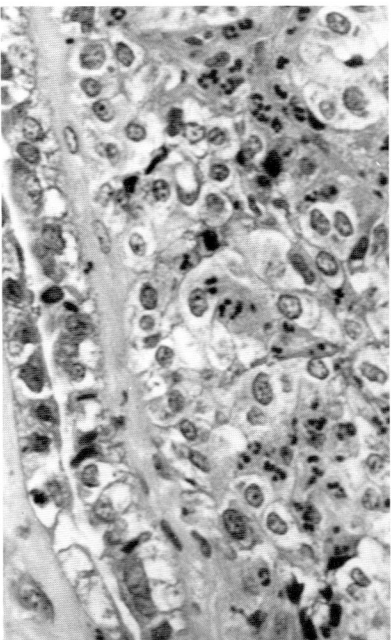
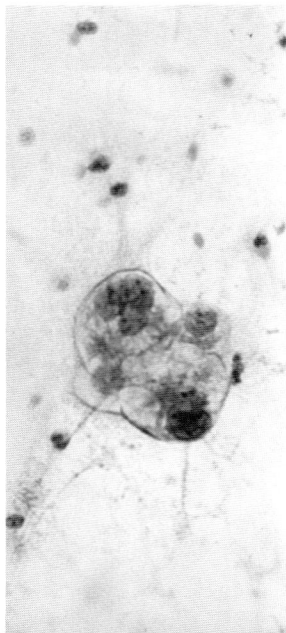

Fig. 2-109 *Right,* Cell ball from a clear cell adenocarcinoma of the endometrium. (CVE smear, × 400.) *Left,* Tissue section of the tumor. (Uterus, hysterectomy, × 400.) (See Plate 2-32.)

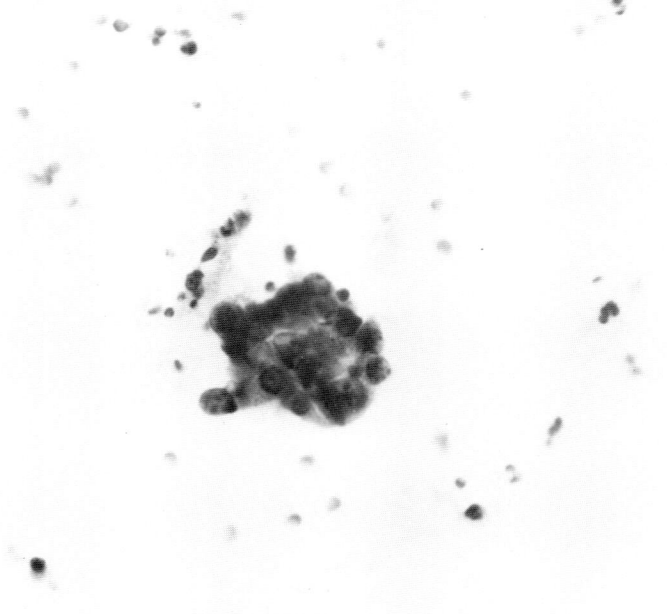

Fig. 2-110 Clear cell adenocarcinoma. Ball of malignant cells with protruding, eccentric nucleus. Possible hobnail cell. (CVE smear, × 310.)

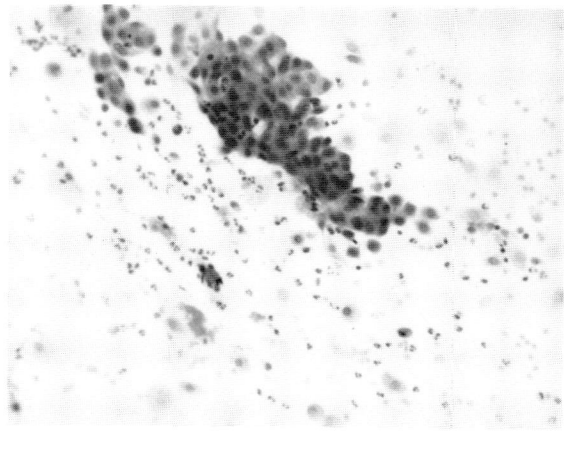

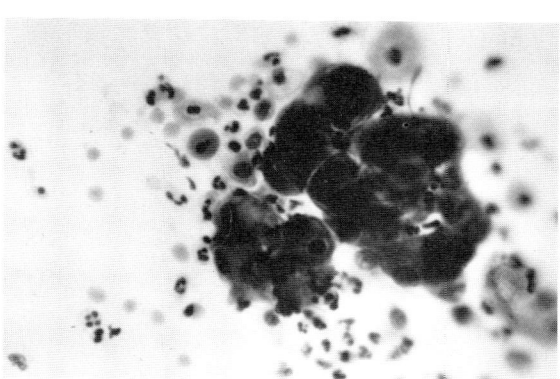

Fig. 2-111 *Bottom,* Adenoacanthoma. Irregular cluster of malignant glandular cells with entrapped, atypical, keratinizing squamous cells. (CVE smear, × 500.) *Top,* Adenoacanthoma. Benign squamous metaplastic cells with abnormal keratinization. (CVE smear, × 310.) (See Plate 2-33.)

on cytologic examination. In adenoacanthoma, low-grade malignant endometrial cells are seen admixed with or separate from immature metaplastic squamous cells or atypical keratinized cells (Fig. 2-111, Plate 2-33). Keratinaceous material, either free floating or in association with other cellular components, may be noted (Fig. 2-112, Plates 2-34, 2-35).[131] Frequently, scattered atypical squamous cells are thought to represent a separate dysplastic process in the cervix; however, if noted in close association with endometrial glandular cells, the diagnosis of adenoacanthoma may be suggested.

Adenosquamous carcinoma is a neoplasm of higher grade than adenoacanthoma and has a malignant glandular component and malignant squamous cells. The latter resemble the cells seen in cervical squamous carcinoma. Keratinized malignant cells occur less frequently than do large, nonkeratinized, malignant squamous cells (Fig. 2-113).

Malignant Müllerian Tumors

Malignant mixed müllerian tumors consist of both malignant epithelial and mesenchymal components. These neoplasms may be homologous mixed müllerian tumors (e.g., composed of malignant müllerian epithelium plus endometrial stroma or leiomyomatous elements) or heterologous (e.g., composed of malignant epithelium plus exogenous stromal elements, such as rhabdomyosarcoma, chondrosarcoma, osteosarcoma, or liposarcoma). Malignant mixed müllerian tumors are high-grade tumors, and the epithelial component is usually recognized as such on cytologic examination.[132] However, the stromal component may not be appreciated on conventional smears (Fig. 2-114), although it may be recognized by invasive endometrial techniques.[133,134] The difficulty in detecting the stromal cells may be related to the fact that epithelial cells shed more easily, and that

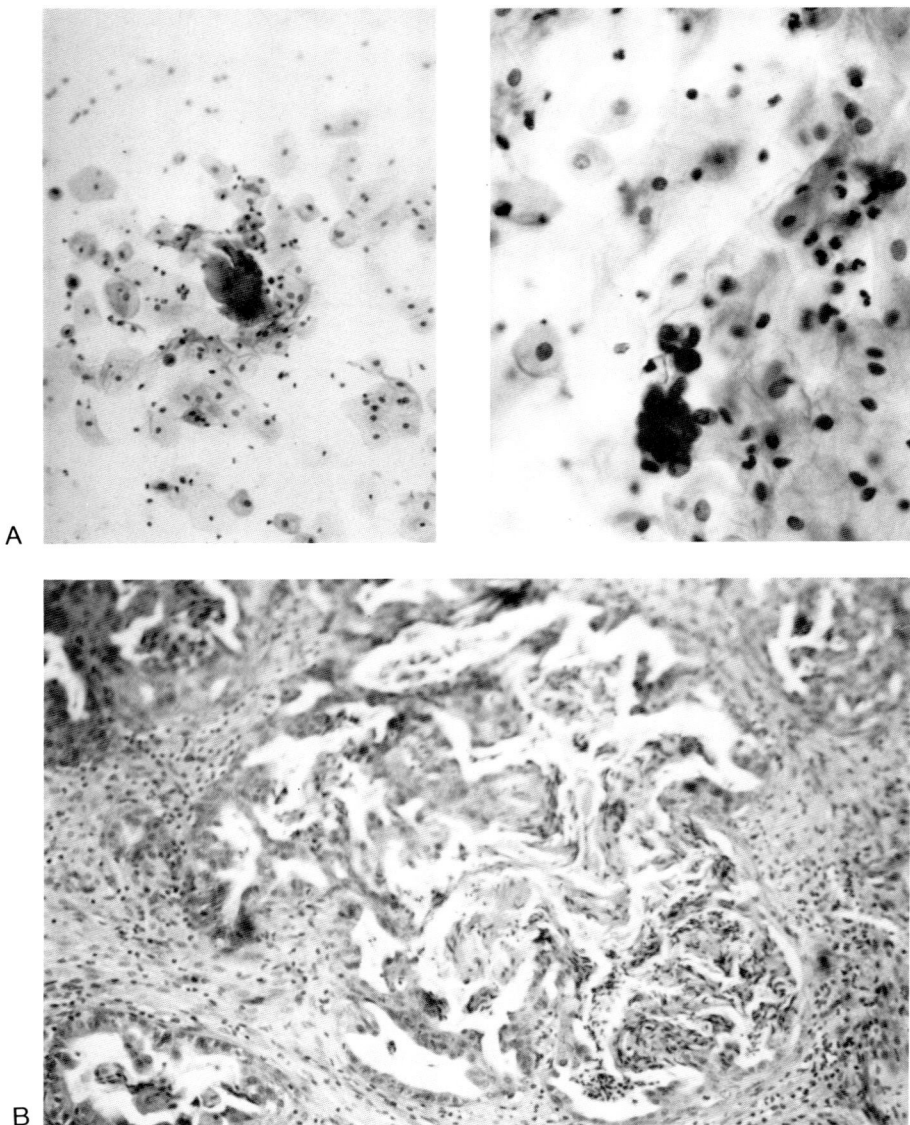

Fig. 2-112 (A) Adenoacanthoma. *Left,* Keratinaceous material floating in a clean background. (CVE smear, × 120.) *Right,* Adenoacanthoma. Tight cluster of low-grade malignant glandular cells. (CVE smear, × 310.) (See Plate 2-34.) **(B)** Adenoacanthoma with keratin production. (Uterine curettage, × 310.) (See Plate 2-35.)

Fig. 2-113 Adenosquamous carcinoma. The malignant glandular cluster on the left contrasts with the malignant squamous cells on the right. (CVE smear, × 310.)

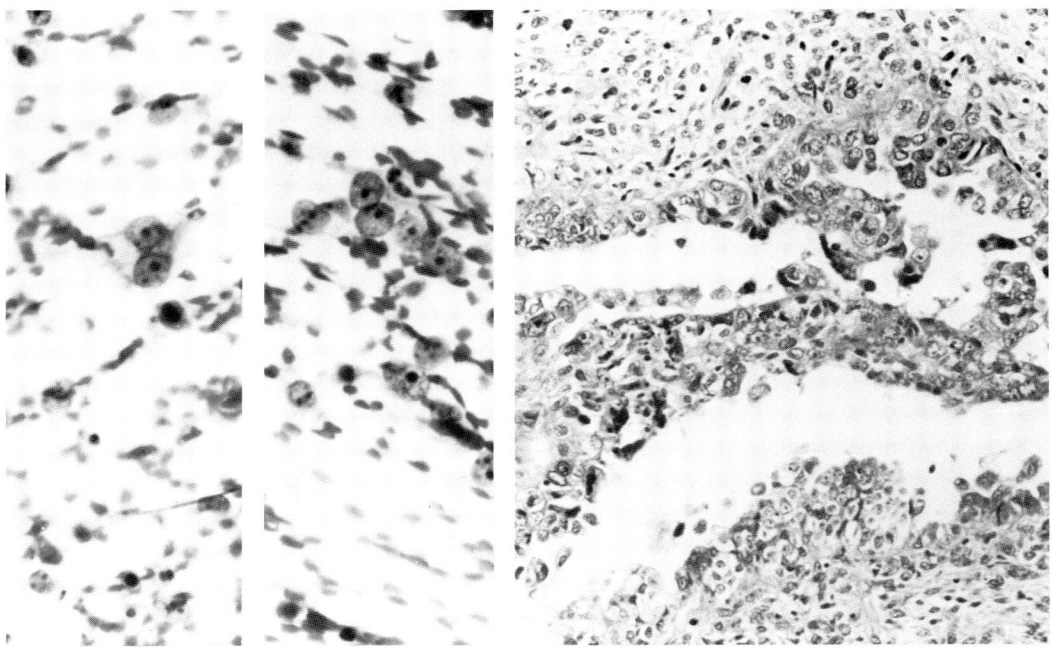

Fig. 2-114 Mixed müllerian tumor, homologous type. The poorly differentiated, large, malignant epithelial cells are seen to be loosely dispersed. (*Left* and *Middle,* CVE smear, × 310; *Right,* Uterus, hysterectomy, × 310.)

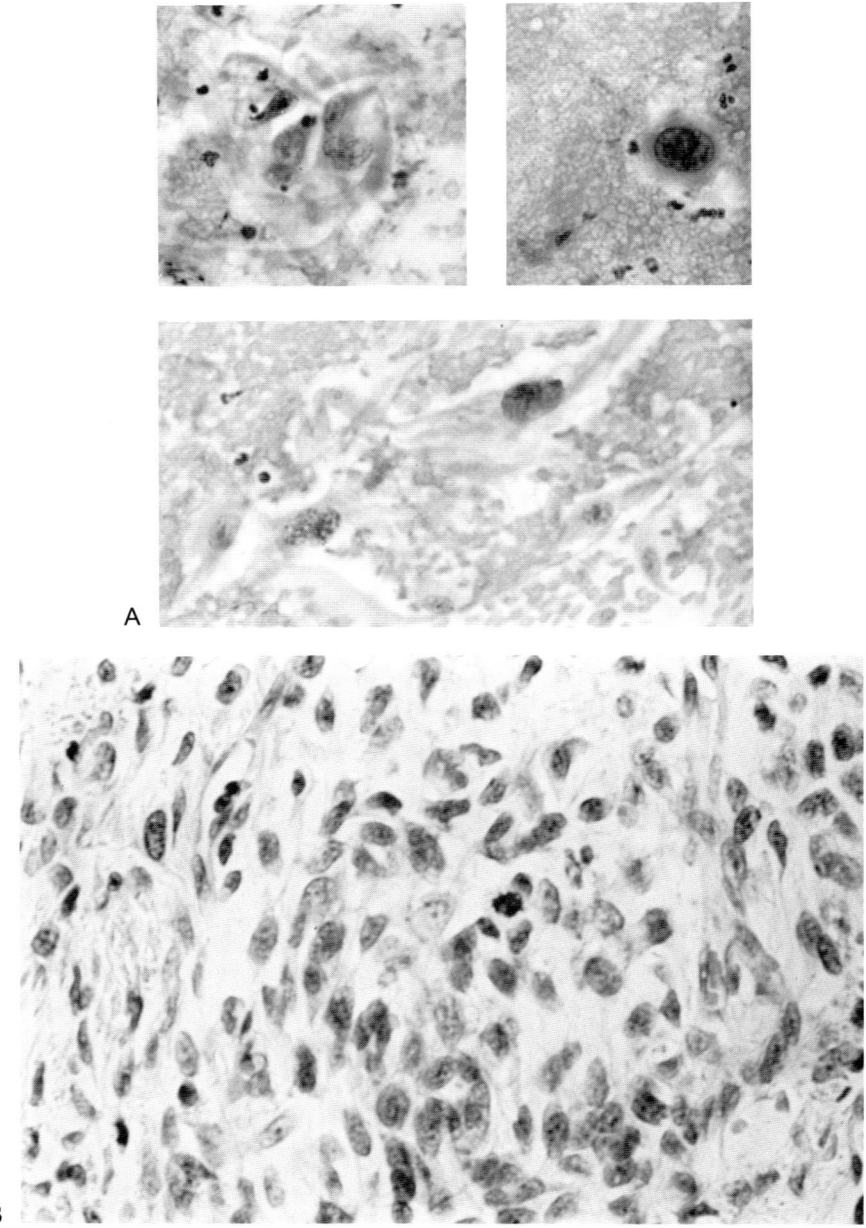

Fig. 2-115 (A) Single pleomorphic spindle cells from a stromal sarcoma. (CVE smear, × 400.) (See Plate 2-36.)
(B) Stromal sarcoma. (Uterus, hysterectomy, × 400.) (See Plate 2-37.)

with the necrosis and diathesis usually seen in these tumors, the degenerative changes render it impossible to define two malignant cell populations. A mixed tumor may be suggested if two distinct malignant cell populations are noted. In heterologous tumors, malignant rhabdomyoblasts may be appreciated by their abundant eosinophilic cytoplasm, which may be characterized by cross striations. Bizarre chondroblasts or associated osteoid material also confirm a heterologous stromal component. Immunocytochemical stains are helpful in differentiating less obvious heterologous cell types (e.g., myoglobin for rhabdomyoblasts, S100 protein for chondroblasts).

Other Endometrial Malignant Neoplasms

Pure stromal sarcomas are rare. Malignant cells tend to shed singly, without clustering or cohesion, and may appear as undifferentiated, small, round cells with minimal or whispy, tapering cytoplasm (comet cell).[135] Alternatively, the cells may be large and spindle-shaped, with abundant cytoplasm (Fig. 2-115, Plates 2-36 and 2-37). Leiomyosarcomatous cells in the CVE smear also appear as large, spindle-shaped cells with blunt nuclear poles, or as convoluted round cells with generous amounts of pale cytoplasm (Fig. 2-116). Choriocarcinoma can be identified by the presence of large, bizarre, multinucleated syncytiotrophoblastic cells with markedly hyperchromatic, irregular nuclei and abundant, basophilic cytoplasm, often occurring in a syncytium (Fig. 2-117, Plate 2-38). Malignant cytotrophoblastic cells appear as large, undifferentiated malignant cells.

Metastatic Disease

Malignant neoplasms can metastasize to the endometrium, or they may spread from the peritoneal cavity into the fallopian tube, passing through the uterus, to be detected only in the vaginal pool. CVE smears in the latter case are usually "clean" and lack a diathesis, although malignant cell clusters are present. The cells and their organization often reflect their tissue of origin. If there is a marked tissue reaction to a metastatic tumor, a diathesis may occur and the tumor may mimic an endometrial primary neoplasm. A pertinent clinical history should help to confirm the diagnosis of a metastatic tumor (Fig. 2-118).

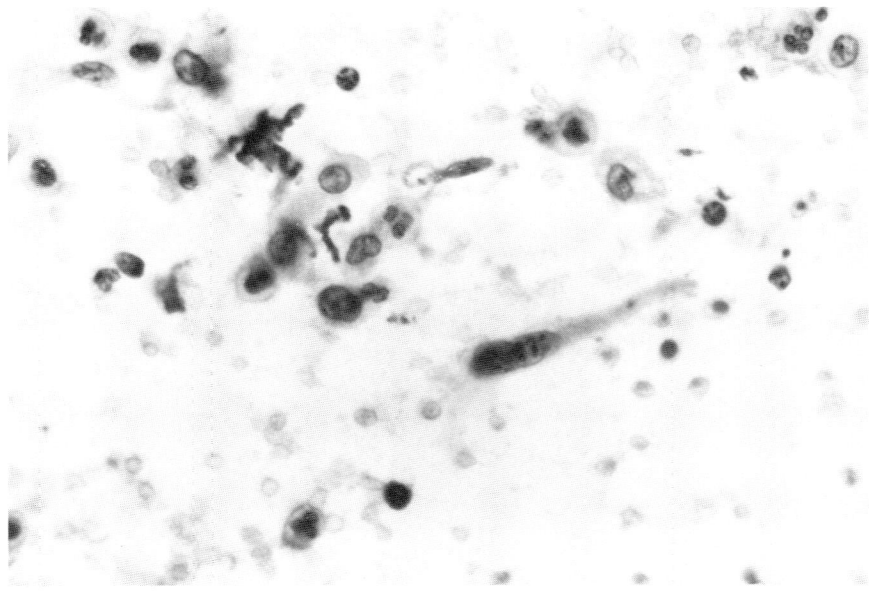

Fig. 2-116 Leiomyosarcoma. Note the large, bizarre, single, spindle-shaped cell, and the round cells with lobulated nuclei and ample cytoplasms. (CVE smear, × 310.)

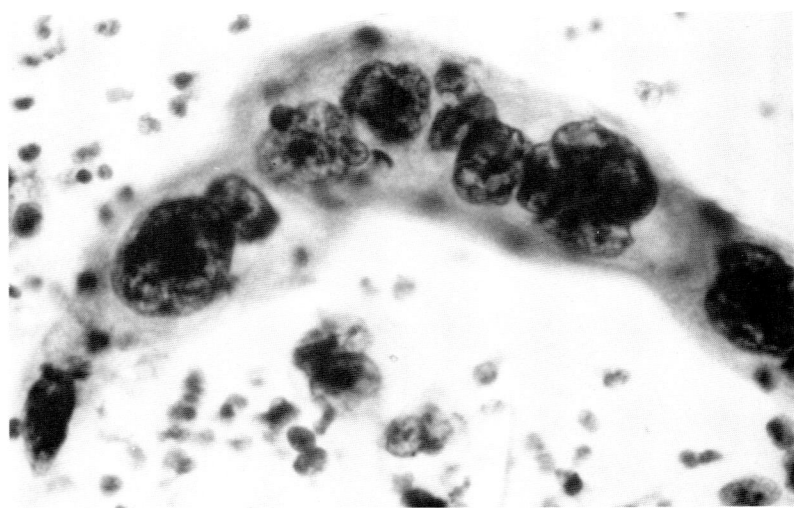

Fig. 2-117 Choriocarcinoma. Malignant syncytiotrophoblasts. (CVE smear, × 450.) (See Plate 2-38.)

DIFFERENTIAL DIAGNOSIS

Once malignant disease is suspected or identified, it is an academic exercise to define the type, as further tissue studies will quickly be performed. Adenocarcinoma of the endocervix can usually be differentiated from endometrial adenocarcinoma by cytologic features and by the increased amount of neoplastic cells and tissue fragments present in the smears. However, endometrial carcinoma may extend into the endocervical canal, and abundant tissue fragments may be seen on cytologic examination in this case also. Frac-

Fig. 2-118 Metastatic adenocarcinoma of the colon. Malignant tall columnar cells in elongated, glandular structure simulates colonic glandular origin. (CVE smear, × 310.)

Table 2-7 Changes Simulating Primary Corpus Malignant Disease

Benign	Malignant
Artifactual changes (drying)	Cervical carcinoma, both squamous and glandular
IUD effects	Metastatic tumors
Reparative or regenerative endometrium	
Reserve cell hyperplasia	
Immature squamous metaplasia with leukocytic inclusions	
Arias-Stella phenomenon	
Follicular cervicitis	
Histiocytes in infections and atrophic states	
Endometritis	
Radiation effects	
Benign polyps	
Endometrial hyperplasia	

tional curettage and tissue sampling usually help to define the tumor's origin.

Many conditions mimic the findings in uterine cancer. Before a diagnosis of endometrial carcinoma can be established, the clinical history must be studied carefully, and all of the many possible causes of benign atypia simulating malignant disease must be ruled out. Table 2-7 lists the many benign and malignant conditions that simulate endometrial adenocarcinoma.

Extrauterine Cancer
Fritz Lin

Cells from various carcinomas and their precursors that originate in the uterine cervix and corpus can be recognized with a considerable degree of accuracy in CVE cytologic preparations. However, the ability to detect cellular evidence of an extrauterine cancer is equally important. The presence or absence of extrauterine cancer not only indicates the extent of disease, but also is one of the most important criteria in determining the prognosis of and appropriate therapeutic course for patients with cancer. Furthermore, the presence of an extrauterine cancer in the CVE cytologic sample influences the mode of investigation and of confirmation of the neoplasm.

INCIDENCE

It is not an uncommon clinical experience to encounter metastatic disease in oncologic patients. The precise incidence of involvement of the uterus and vagina by extragenital neoplasms, however, is difficult to determine. Several large series presenting results of surgical pathology and autopsy studies have indicated that involvement of the uterine cervix, uterine corpus, or both, was a rare event.[136-140] Mazur et al.[141] reported 325 cases of metastatic neoplasm to the female genital tract from a total of 445,000 cases derived from surgical pathology files. In this report, 20 percent of the metastases involving the ovary and vagina that were of extragenital origin were detected before the primary lesion was found. In another study,[139] a malignant neoplasm was the first indication of an extragenital carcinoma in 25 percent of 63 cases of metastatic disease involving the uterine corpus.

The precise origin of most extragenital neoplasms is unconfirmed. On the basis of surgical pathologic and autopsy studies, several investigators[137-139] have cited mammary neoplasms as the most common source of cancers involving the female genital tract, whereas others[140,141] have reported gastrointestinal neoplasms to be the predominant source. However, of the extrauterine neoplasms that were detected on cytologic examination of CVE samples, the ovary was the most common primary site.[142-145] Regardless of the origin of the primary lesion, involvement of the female genital tract by an extrauterine cancer is an indication of advanced disease and a poor prognosis. Most importantly, extrauterine cancers have been detected in patients who are asymptomatic.[146-148] In one report,[144] the incidence of asymptomatic cases was 6.1 percent. Therefore, it is important for the cytopathologist to be able to recognize such cases.

OVARIAN NEOPLASMS

The prevalence of malignant tumor cells derived from ovarian carcinoma, as observed in CVE samples, varies according to investigators. Whereas Rubin and Frost[145] reported that 4.6 percent of the cases of ovarian carcinoma they studied had malignant tumor cells detected in CVE samples, Graham and Van Niekerk[143] reported a prevalence rate of 30 percent in their series. Takashina et al.[149] reported a comparable prevalence rate.

Although cellular evidence of ovarian carcinoma in CVE samples was reported by various authors,[142-154] it was probably French who made the first such observation in 1949.[154a] He mentioned that the malignant tumor cells bore a striking resemblance to those in the parent tissue. Other observers stated that the diagnosis of various extrauterine cancers did not seem applicable to the CVE smear technique.[147,155] Detailed cytologic descriptions were often lacking. However, Graham and Van Niekerk[143] provided a brief description of the cells derived from ovarian carcinoma, stating that macronucleoli were conspicuous and that 35 percent of the cells were arranged in clusters, whereas 62 percent appeared singly. By contrast, in their report of four cases of ovarian carcinoma detected on a CVE smear, Wachtel and Plester[154] stated that the desquamated malignant tumor cells were not arranged in clusters as seen in typical uterine carcinoma. Rather, they reported that the cells were arranged mostly singly, an observation that was confirmed by others.[148,151]

It was not until 1973 that Reagan and Ng[156] provided a detailed account of their morphologic analyses of cells derived from 28 ovarian carcinomas. Extrauterine cancer of ovarian origin could still be confused with uterine adenocarcinomas, however.[144] In my experience and that of others,[156] malignant neoplastic cells in CVE samples originating from ovarian cancers are larger than those derived from endometrial carcinoma. They are comparable to, and sometimes larger than, the cells derived from endocervical carcinoma. They are often arranged in loose aggregates with considerable overlapping, and they have a three-dimensional effect (Fig. 2-119, Plate 2-39). To a lesser degree, the cells are arranged in tight aggregates (Fig. 2-120, Plate 2-40) simulating the cellular arrangement of mammary carcinoma in CVE samples. Rarely are leukocytes seen in the malignant neoplastic cells of ovarian origin (Fig. 2-121, Plate 2-41). When malignant neoplastic cells of ovarian origin are arranged singly, they often reflect a poorly differentiated carcinoma. Occasionally, the cells exhibit marked variations in cellular and nuclear size and shape (Fig. 2-122, Plates 2-42 to 2-44).

The chromatin is frequently fine and evenly distributed in well-differentiated carcinomas. Cells with moderately coarse chromatin reflect poorly differentiated carcinoma. Nucleoli are often seen. In the poorly differentiated carcinoma, the cells often have conspicuous marconucleoli that are irregular in shape. Sometimes, they have multinucleoli (Fig. 2-122B, Plate 2-43).

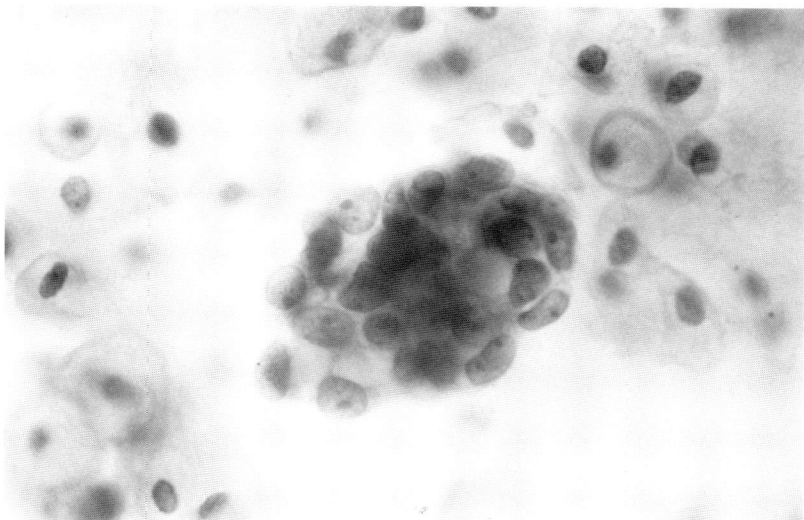

Fig. 2-119 Ovarian carcinoma. The cells are loosely arranged in a cluster, exhibiting a three-dimensional effect. Note the normal epithelial cells in the background and the absence of a tumor diathesis. (CVE smear, × 640.) (See Plate 2-39.)

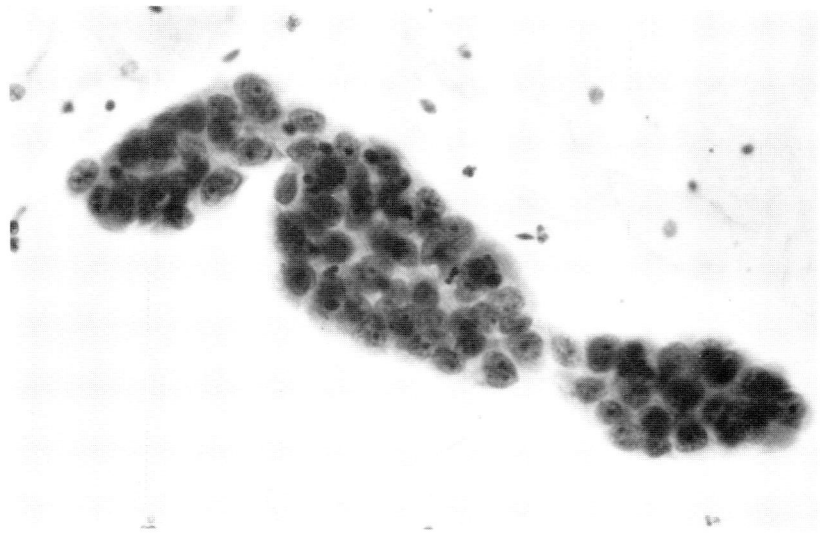

Fig. 2-120 Ovarian carcinoma. The cells are arranged in a tight cluster without a three-dimensional effect. Note that the background is clean, with normal epithelial cells. (CVE smear, × 400.) (See Plate 2-40.)

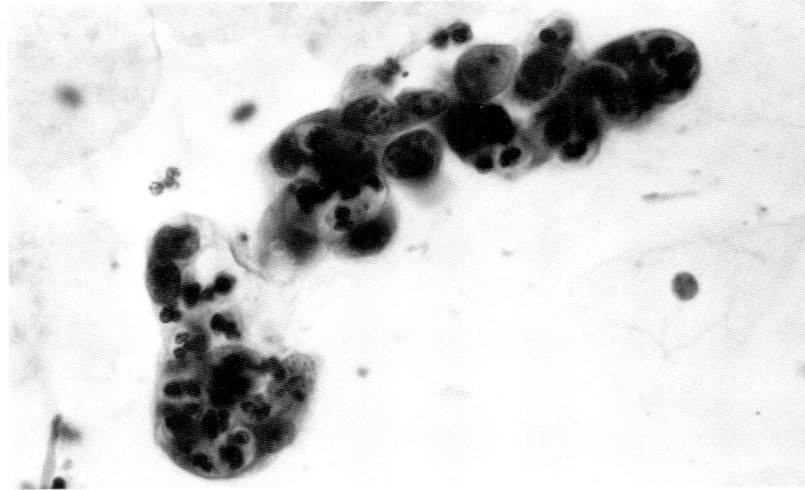

Fig. 2-121 Ovarian carcinoma. Inflammatory cells in the cytoplasm of a loosely arranged cell cluster. (CVE smear, × 640.) (See Plate 2-41.)

MAMMARY NEOPLASMS

Cells derived from mammary carcinoma of ductal origin, when observed in CVE samples, are usually smaller than those derived from ovarian carcinoma. Although cell aggregates re present more frequently than are single cells, my group has noted a pattern of compact cell groups, as have other investigators.[157] In my experience, the compact cell arrangement often lacks a three-dimensional effect, as is most often seen in ovarian carcinoma (Fig. 2-123, Plates 2-45, 2-46). The chromatin is often fine, and macronucleoli are conspicuous (Fig. 2-124, Plates 2-47, 2-48). Multinucleoli are less frequently encountered in cells derived from mammary carcinoma than in cells from ovarian carcinoma.

When malignant neoplastic cells are small, uniformly round to oval, and arranged mostly singly but sometimes in a linear fashion—a so-called Indian-file arrangement—a mammary carcinoma of lobular origin must be considered. The nuclei in these cells are often hyperchromatic and eccentric in location. Rarely, a gland structure may be evident (Fig. 2-125, Plates 2-49 to 2-51). In some cases, cells derived from a lobular carcinoma may be rather small, with a faintly eosinophilic cytoplasm and polyhedral shape (Fig. 2-126, Plates 2-52 to 2-54). Cellular cohesiveness is rarely a feature of lobular carcinoma as observed in CVE samples.

COLONIC NEOPLASMS

Cellular evidence of colonic carcinoma, as observed in the CVE samples, has been briefly mentioned.[144,158] Although no detailed description exists in the literature, malignant tumor cells derived from colonic carcinoma often have a low to tall columnar configuration and a palisading arrangement (Fig. 2-127, Plates 2-55 to 2-57). Such cellular features may be a constant feature of a metastatic colonic carcinoma, regardless of the site of metastasis (Fig. 2-128, Plate 2-58). Extracellular accumulation of mucin also may be seen in colonic carcinoma or examination of CVE samples (Fig. 2-129, Plates 2-59, 2-60). In poorly differentiated colonic carcinomas, there is greater variation in cellular size and shape (Fig. 2-130, Plates 2-61, 2-62). and columnar cells with a palisading arrangement may be discerned with difficulty. In some poorly differentiated colonic carcinomas, the desquamated cells in the CVE sample are rather small, simulating cells typical of an endometrial carcinoma. Accompanying these malignant neoplastic cells, columnar cells having a palisading ar-

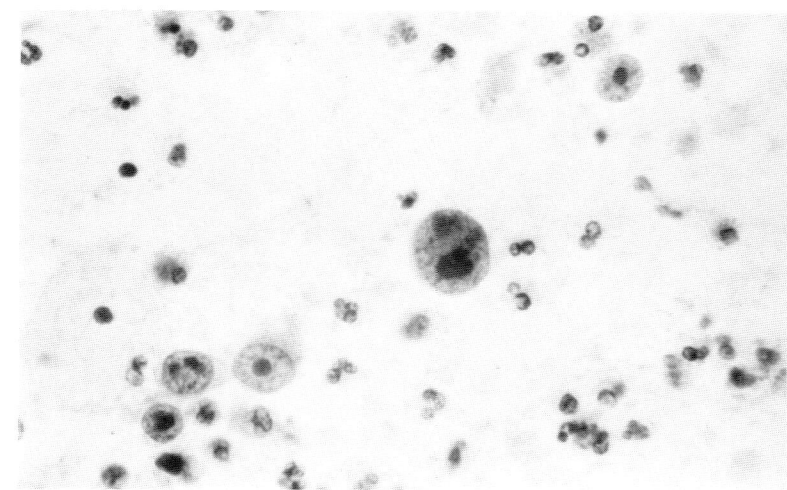

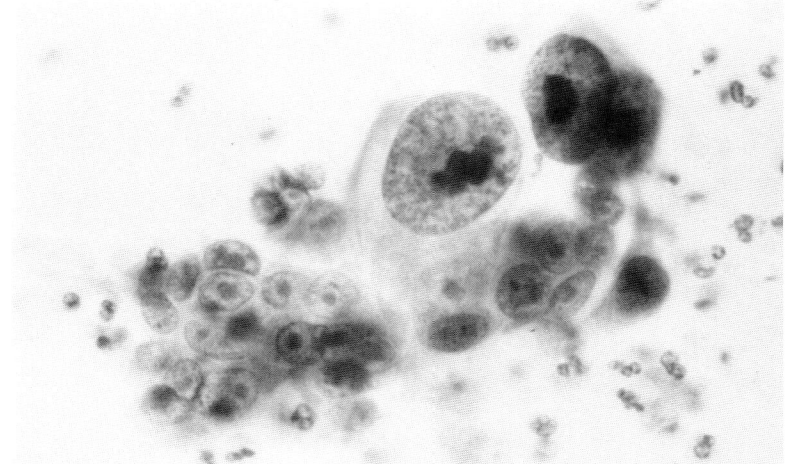

Fig. 2-122 (A) Ovarian carcinoma. Note the single cells in a poorly differentiated carcinoma (CVE smear, × 640.) (See Plate 2-42.) **(B)** Ovarian carcinoma. The cells of this poorly differentiated carcinoma exhibit marked variations in size, as well as macronucleoli. (CVE smear, × 640.) (See Plate 2-43.) **(C)** Ovarian carcinoma. Note the poor differentiation in the same carcinoma as pictured in Fig. B. (× 312.) (See Plate 2-44.)

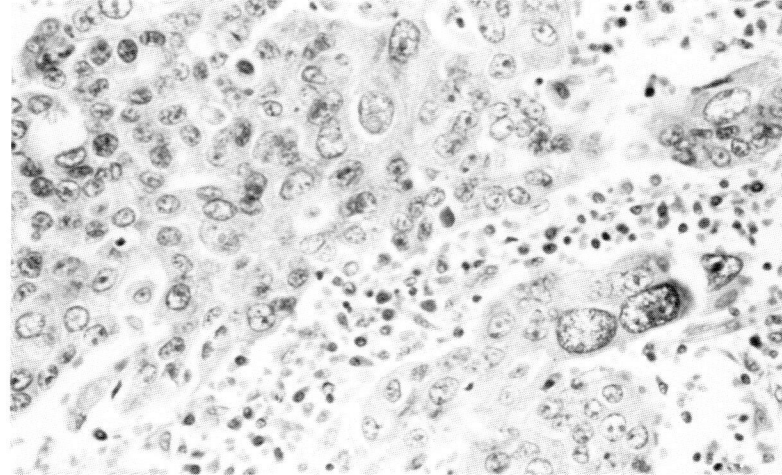

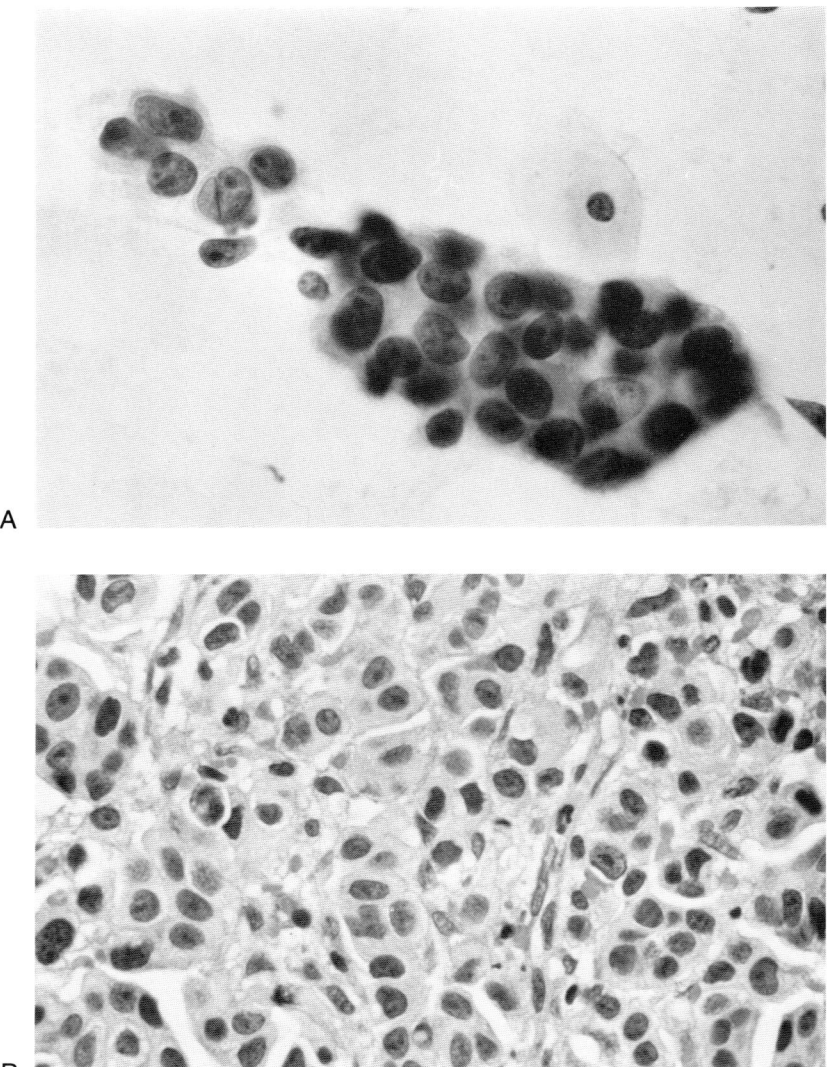

Fig. 2-123 (A) Mammary carcinoma. A cluster of cells that are compactly arranged and exhibit a three-dimensional effect. Note the absence of a tumor diathesis. (CVE smear, × 640.) (See Plate 2-45.) **(B)** Mammary carcinoma. Histomorphologic confirmation of a metastatic mammary carcinoma involving the uterine cervix. (× 500.) (See Plate 2-46.)

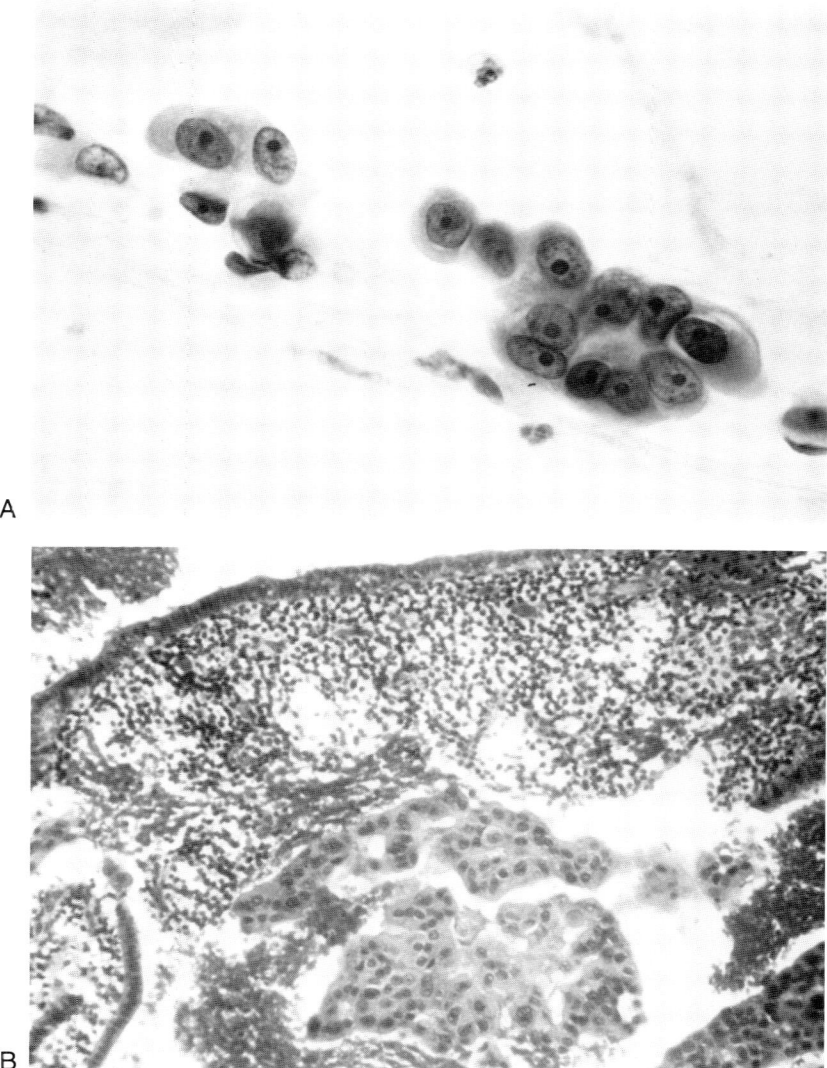

Fig. 2-124 (A) Mammary carcinoma. Note the compact cellular arrangement and clean smear background. Macronucleoli are also evident. (CVE smear, × 640.) (See Plate 2-47.) **(B)** Mammary carcinoma. Histomorphologic confirmation of a metastatic mammary carcinoma involving the endometrium. (× 160.) (See Plate 2-48.)

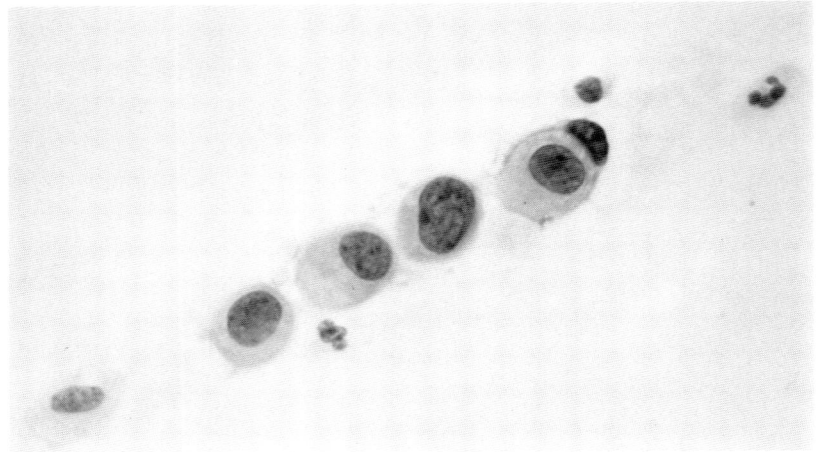
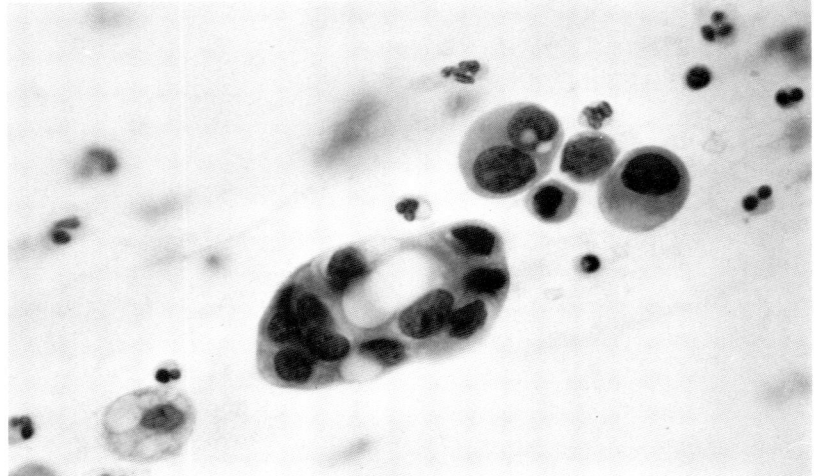
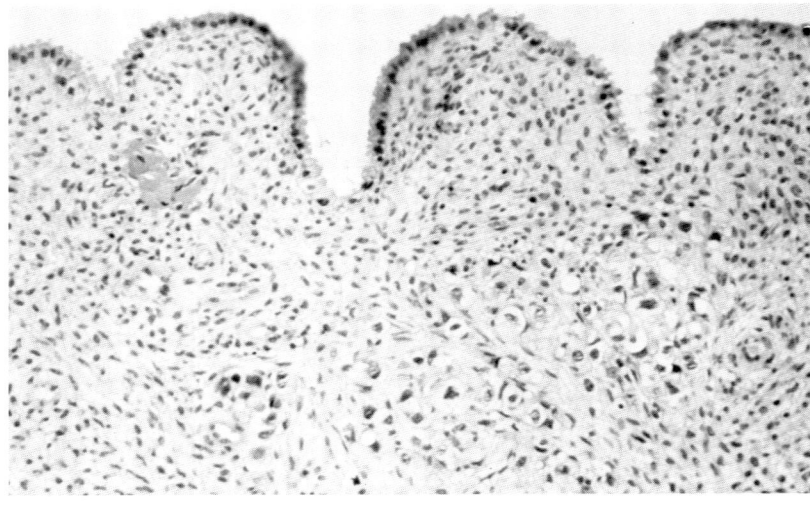

Fig. 2-125 (A) Mammary carcinoma. The small cells in this lobular carcinoma are arranged in a linear fashion. Note the absence of a tumor diathesis. (CVE smear, × 640.) (See Plate 2-49.) **(B)** Mammary carcinoma. An unusual gland-like feature in a lobular carcinoma. (CVE smear, × 640.) (See Plate 2-50.) **(C)** Mammary carcinoma. Histomorphologic confirmation of a metastatic lobular carcinoma involving the uterine cervix. (× 160.) (See Plate 2-51.)

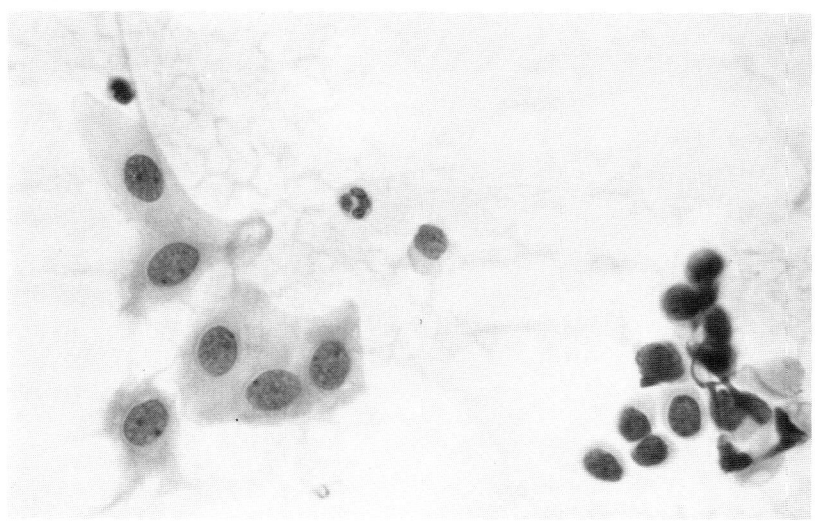

Fig. 2-126 (A) Mammary carcinoma. Cells derived from a lobular carcinoma are sometimes rather small (right) compared to the parabasal-like cells (left). (CVE smear, × 640.) (See Plate 2-52.) **(B)** Mammary carcinoma. These cells from a lobular carcinoma exhibit a lack of cohesiveness. Note the absence of a tumor diathesis. (CVE smear, × 640.) (See Plate 2-53.) **(C)** Mammary carcinoma. Histomorphologic confirmation of a lobular carcinoma involving the uterine cervix. (× 400.) (See Plate 2-54.)

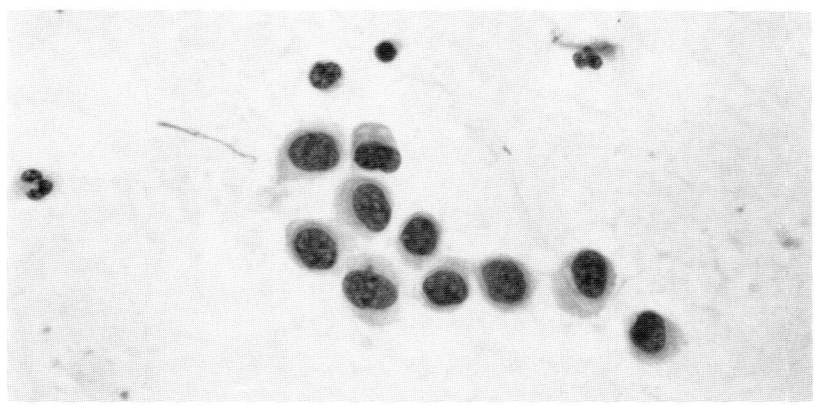

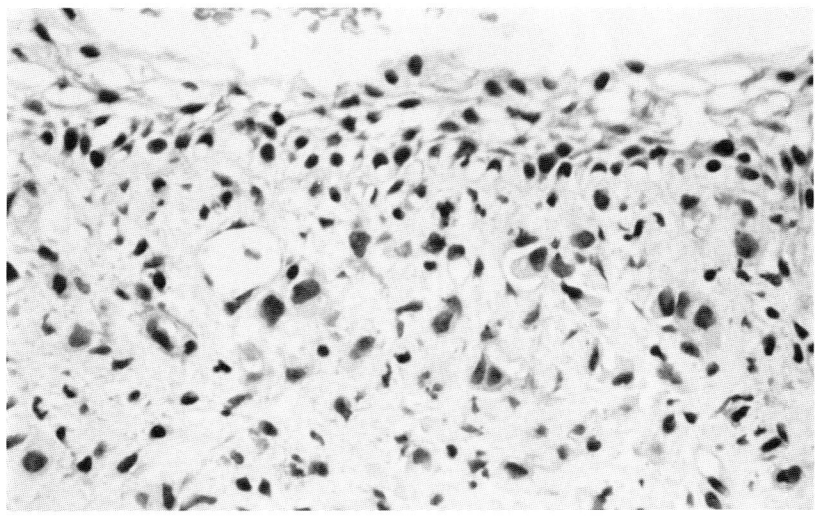

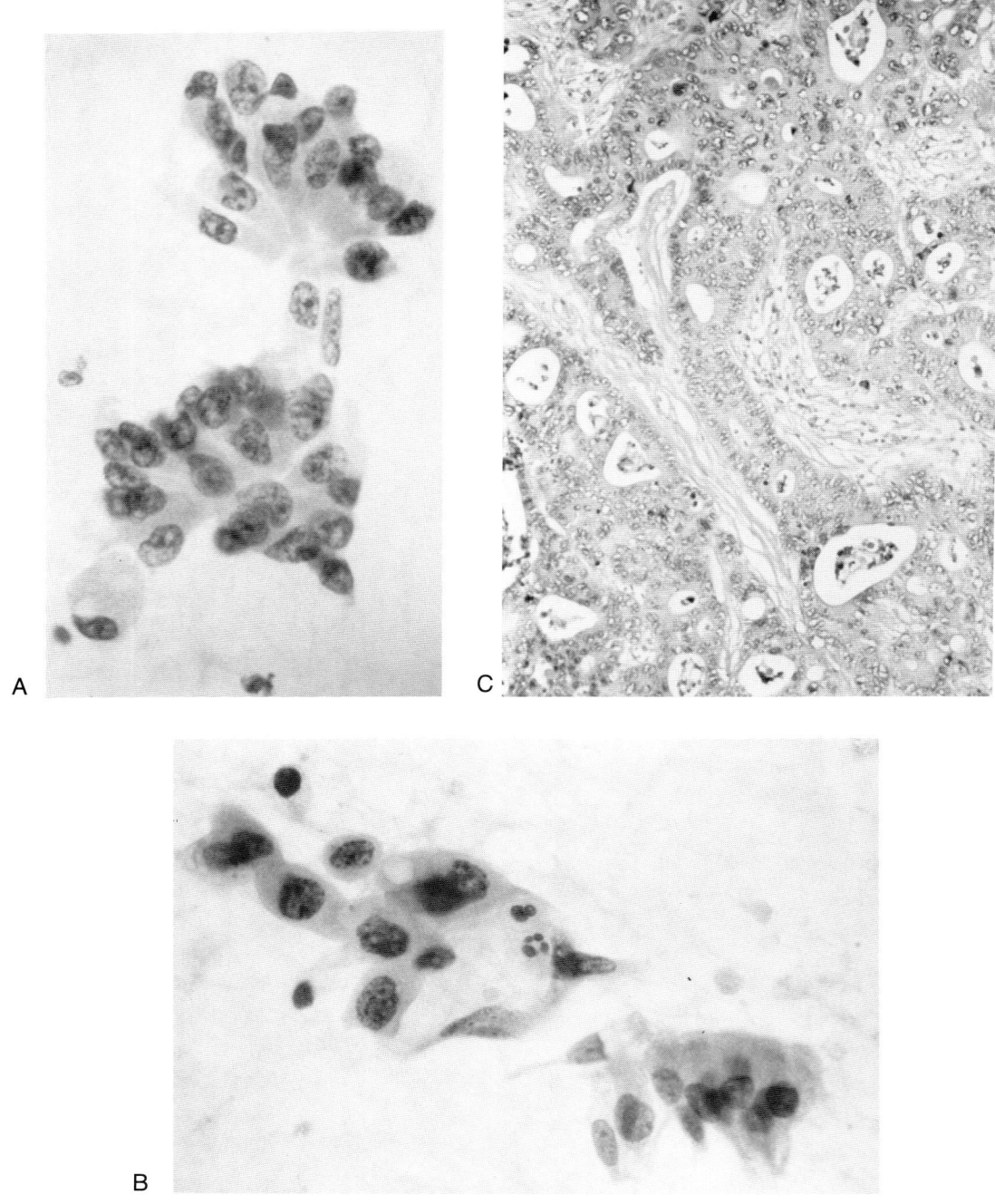

Fig. 2-127 (A) Colonic carcinoma. Low to tall columnar cells, arranged in a palisading fashion, are commonly observed. Note the absence of a tumor diathesis. (CVE smear, × 640.) (See Plate 2-55.) **(B)** Colonic carcinoma. Note the low columnar cells. A group of normal-appearing endocervical cells is apparent in the right lower corner. (CVE smear, × 640.) (See Plate 2-56.) **(C)** Colonic carcinoma. Histomorphologic confirmation of colonic carcinoma (× 125.) (See Plate 2-57.)

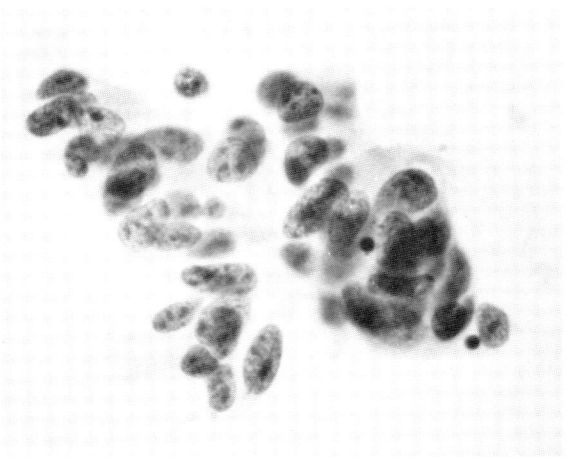

Fig. 2-128 Colonic carcinoma. Note the constant feature of columnar cells in a palisading arrangement. (Bronchial brush smear, × 640.) (See Plate 2-58.)

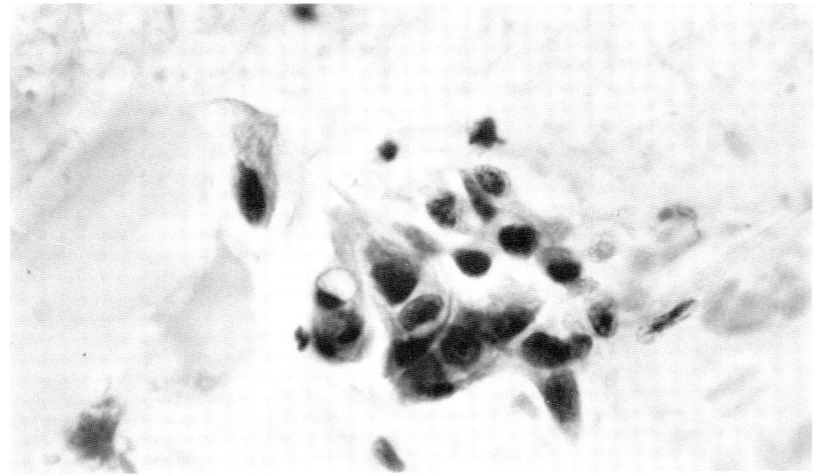

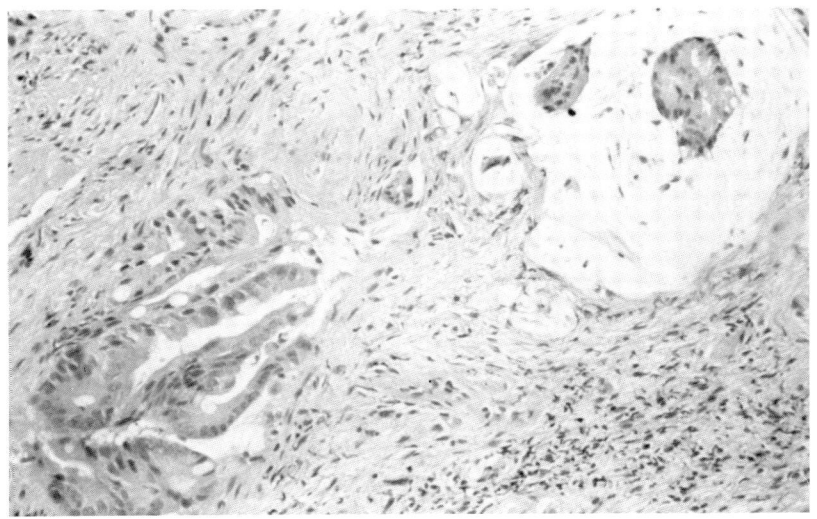

Fig. 2-129 (A) Colonic carcinoma with mucin. Note the columnar cells and tumor diathesis. (CVE smear, × 640.) (See Plate 2-59.) **(B)** Colonic carcinoma. Histomorphologic confirmation of a mucin-producing colonic carcinoma. (× 160.) (See Plate 2-60.)

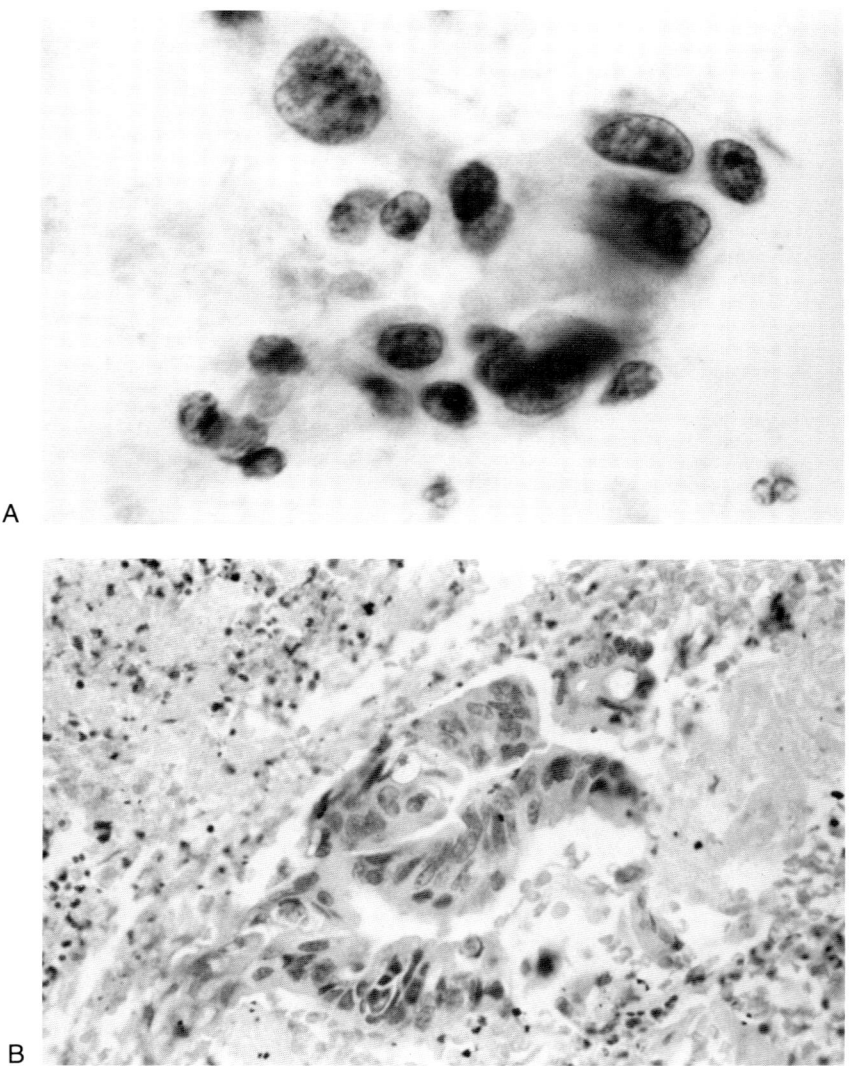

Fig. 2-130 (A) Colonic carcinoma. Variations in cellular size are apparent in this poorly differentiated carcinoma. Note the presence of a tumor diathesis. (CVE smear, × 1008.) (See Plate 2-61.) **(B)** Colonic carcinoma. Histomorphologic confirmation of a carcinoma involving the vagina. (× 312.) (See Plate 2-62.)

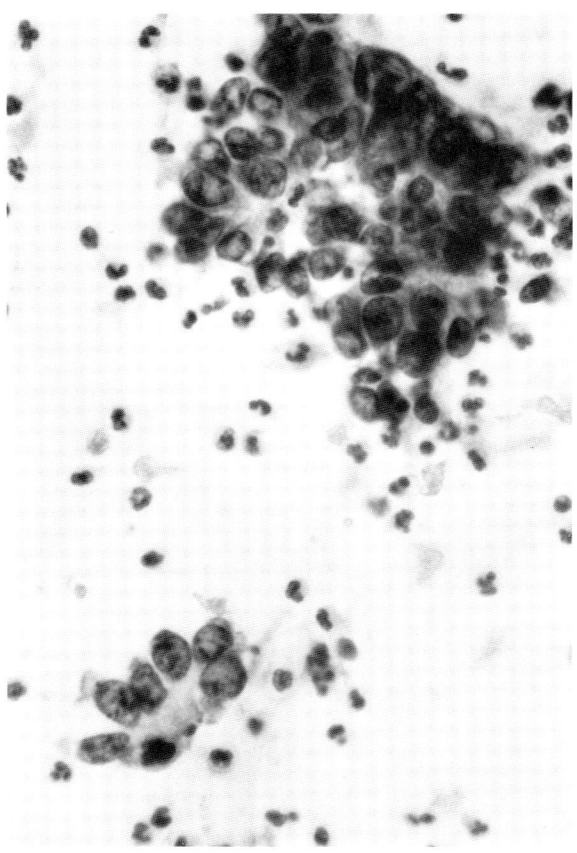

Fig. 2-131 Colonic carcinoma. Small cells derived from a poorly differentiated carcinoma are seen. Note the group of small columnar cells in the left lower corner. (CVE smear, × 500.) (See Plate 2-63.)

rangement can usually be found with a diligent search (Fig. 2-131, Plate 2-63). Koss[158] cautioned that cellular evidence of a colonic carcinoma in the CVE sample may be confused with endocervical adenocarcinoma. Indeed, a columnar cell shape is one of the cellular features of endocervical adenocarcinoma.[156]

OTHER EXTRAUTERINE NEOPLASMS

Although it is possible that the cellular features in a CVE sample may sometimes suggest the primary site of an extrauterine cancer, there are occasions when this is not the case, as some neoplastic lesions share morphologic similarities. For example, cellular evidence of adenocarcinoma of the lung, as observed in a CVE sample, may simulate the appearance of a metastatic ovarian carcinoma (Fig. 2-132, Plates 2-64, 2-65). In such instances, it is only possible to confirm the presence of an extrauterine cancer of undetermined origin (Fig. 2-133, Plate 2-66).

Malignant neoplastic cells derived from other body sites, such as the uterine tube,[144,147,155,159,160] pancreas,[144] urethra,[144,155] mesothelium,[144] urinary bladder,[142,144,155] gallbladder,[144] vulva,[155] kidney,[147] sigmoid,[159] rectum,[152] and anus,[147] also have been detected cytologically from CVE samples. A rare example of metastatic melanoma has also been recorded.[161] However, detailed morphologic descriptions of these extrauterine neoplasms, as observed in CVE samples, are lacking. Recently, Kashimura et al.[162] provided a detailed morphologic analysis of gastric carcinoma metastatic to the uterine cervix. They compared the data against that available for primary endocervical adenocarcinoma. Although the data revealed morphologic differences between these two types of carcinomas, the case load was limited,

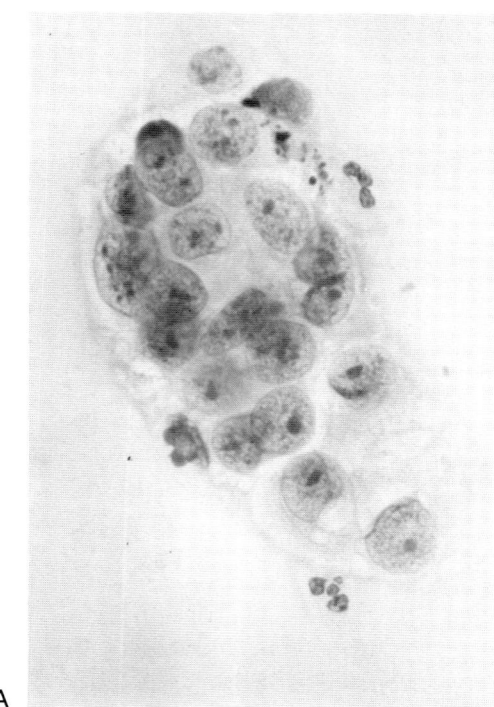 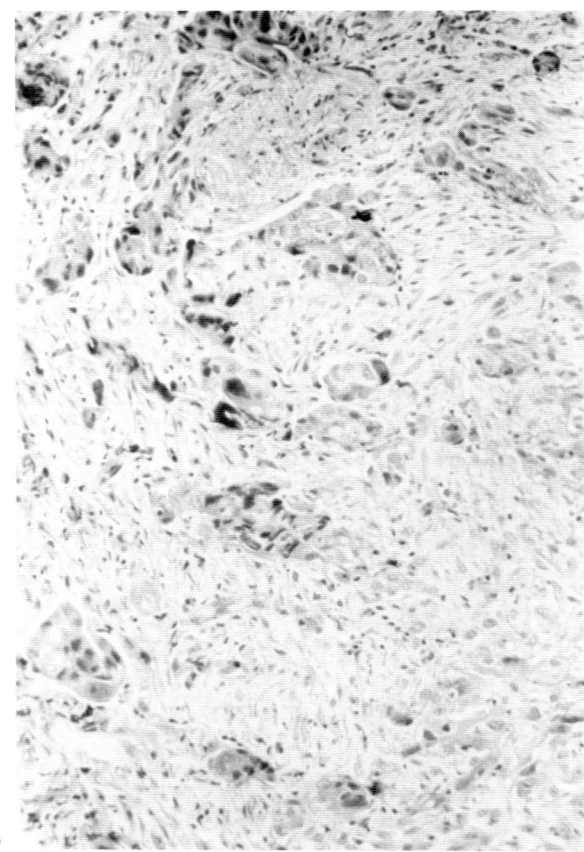

Fig. 2-132 **(A)** Lung carcinoma. Note the similarity of this carcinoma to an ovarian carcinoma. The background of the slide lacks a tumor diathesis. (CVE smear, × 640.) (See Plate 2-64.) **(B)** Lung carcinoma. Histomorphologic confirmation of a lung carcinoma. (× 160.) (See Plate 2-65.)

and the statistical significance of their comparative results was not cited.

Although most of the extrauterine cancers detected in CVE samples are of epithelial origin, a few non-epithelial malignant neoplasms have been reported. These include plasma cell tumor,[163] lymphoma[164] and leukemia.[144,165]

ASSOCIATED FINDINGS

Cellular morphology results alone are not always sufficient to arrive at an interpretation of extrauterine cancer. There are associated findings that may assist in the interpretation of an extrauterine cancer. Ng et al.[144] reported a clean smear background or a lack of tumor diathesis in 80.3 percent of the extrauterine cancers examined by CVE smear. Indeed, when the desquamated malignant neoplastic cells reach the uterus via the uterine tube, there is usually a clean smear background. (Figs. 2-119 to 2-121, 2-123A, 2-124A, 2-125A & B, 2-126A & B, 2-127A & B, 2-132A, and 2-133). However, if the metastatic deposits are large enough to produce mucosal ulcerations, a dirty background or a tumor diathesis is generally noted (Fig. 2-122A & B). Likewise, when the malignant neoplasm invades the genital tract by direct extension and destruction, as observed in rectosigmoid carcinoma, a tumor diathesis is invariably present (Figs. 2-129, 2-130A, and 2-131). It is interesting to note that, in a study by Ng et al.,[144] 15 percent and 7.5 percent of the cases of endocervical and endometrial carcinomas, respectively, were associated with a clean background in the CVE sample.

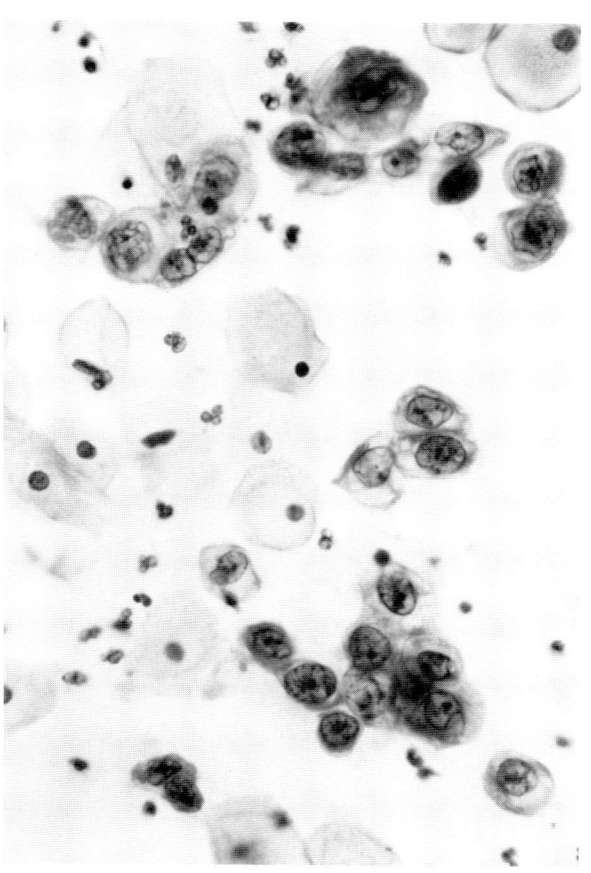

Fig. 2-133 Carcinoma of unknown origin. Note that malignant tumor cells are present in an otherwise normal cellular background that lacks a tumor diathesis. (CVE smear, × 400.) (See Plate 2-66.)

Other investigators[142,149,162] have also noted the significance of a clean background in cases of extrauterine cancer detected in CVE samples.

Because squamous cell carcinoma and adenocarcinoma originating from the uterus are often preceded by a spectrum of squamous or glandular abnormalities, tissues in proximity to these cancers may exhibit such changes before the cancer does. These changes might include squamous or glandular dysplasia or CIS. This spectrum of epithelial abnormalities is reflected in the CVE sample by cellular forms ranging from normal epithelial cells to atypical cells, and finally to cells reflecting overt cancer. The lack of such transitional forms of epithelial cells in the evolution of squamous cancer or adenocarcinoma is an associated finding of extrauterine cancer that may be observed in the CVE smears (Figs. 2-119 to 2-121, 2-123A, 2-124A, 2-125A & B, 2-126A & B, and 2-133). Therefore, when malignant neoplastic cells are present in a sample of otherwise normal epithelial cells, the presence of an extrauterine cancer must be suspected.

Psammoma bodies have been observed in the CVE sample, not only in patients with primary uterine and extrauterine cancers,[142,146,150,166–170] but also in those with a variety of benign conditions.[168,171–173] In my experience, psammoma bodies in the CVE sample are more often encountered in benign reactive processes than in malignant neoplastic lesions. In a number of cases at my institution, psammoma bodies have been seen in patients with serosal inclusion cysts of the ovary (Fig. 2-134, Plate 2-67, 2-68). They may be present in an otherwise histologically unremarkable uterine cervix (Fig. 2-135, Plate 2-69) or uterine tube (Fig. 2-136, Plate 2-70). When psammoma bodies are detected in a CVE smear without malignant neoplastic cells, one must refrain from a diagnosis of malignant disease. My group also encountered

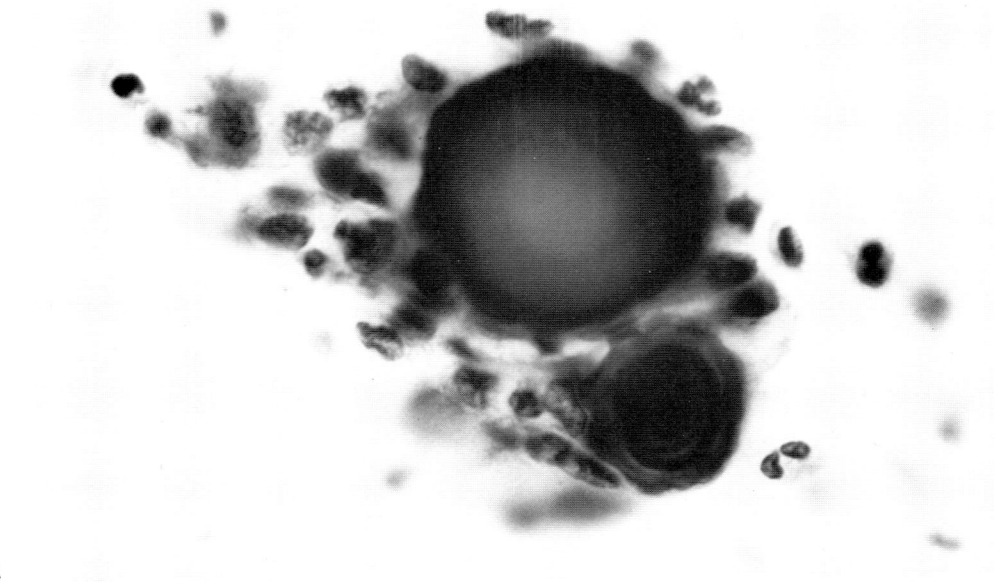

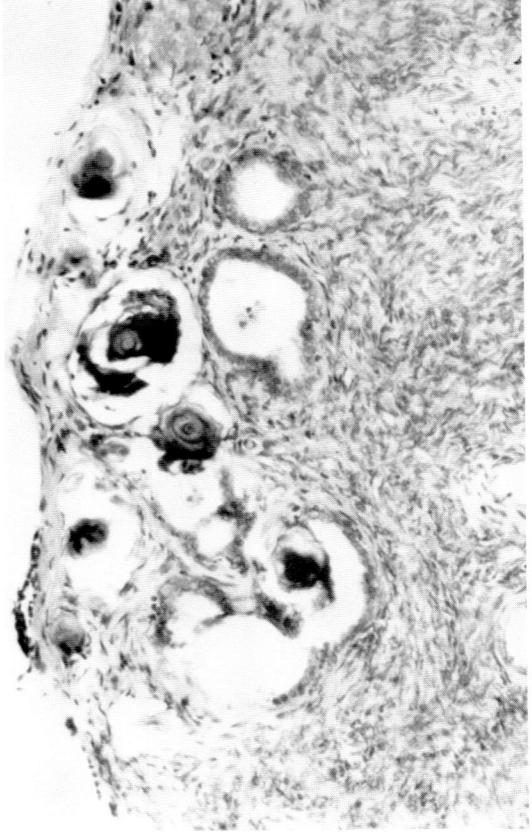

Fig. 2-134 (A) Psammoma body. Note the absence of malignant tumor cells. (CVE smear, × 800.) (See Plate 2-67.) **(B)** Histomorphologic confirmation of psammoma bodies in serosal inclusion cysts of the ovary. (× 160.) (See Plate 2-68.)

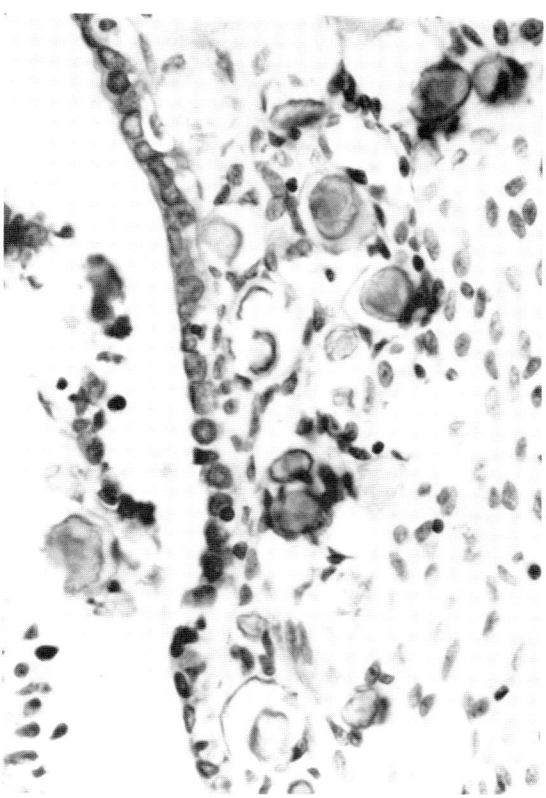

Fig. 2-135 Psammoma bodies in the uterine cervix. (× 400.) (See Plate 2-69.)

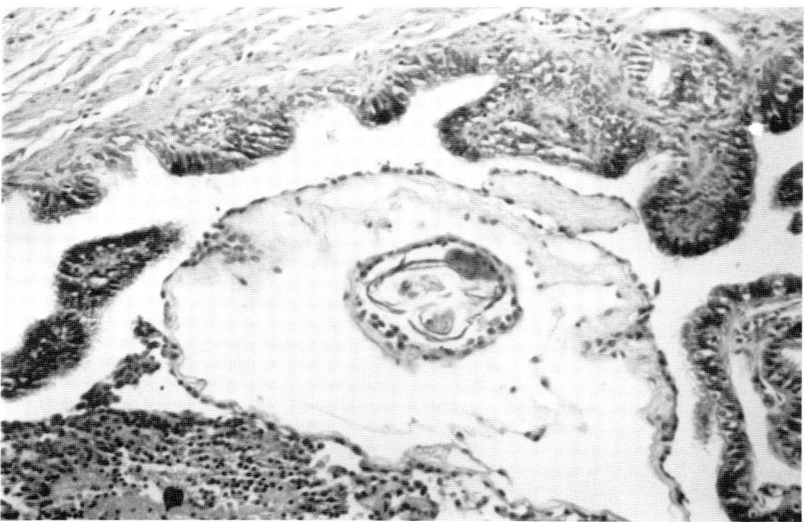

Fig. 2-136 Psammoma bodies in the uterine tube. (× 160.) (See Plate 2-70.)

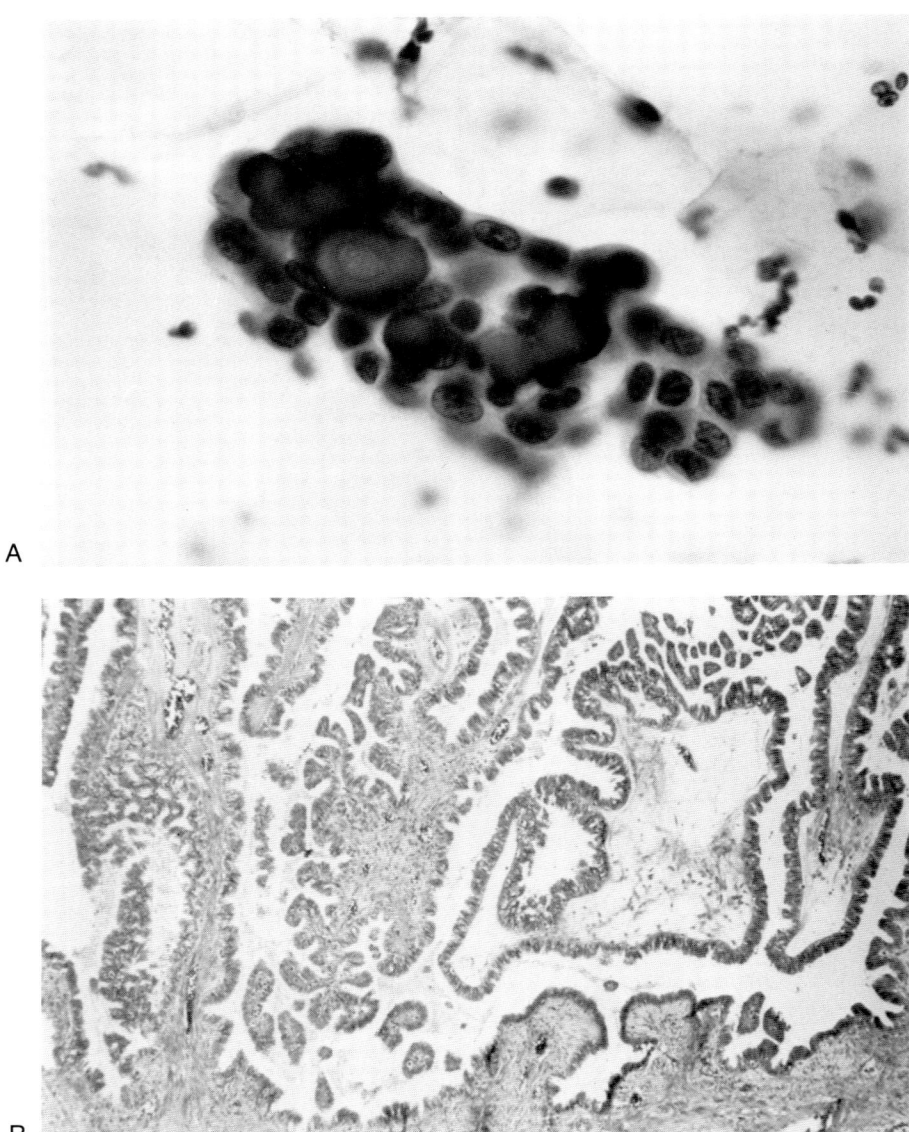

Fig. 2-137 **(A)** Psammoma bodies in an ovarian serous cystadenoma of borderline malignancy. Note that the epithelial cells do not fulfill the criteria for malignant disease. (CVE smear, × 640.) (See Plate 2-71.) **(B)** Histomorphologic confirmation of a serous cystadenoma of borderline malignancy (× 64.) (See Plate 2-72.)

an ovarian borderline lesion with psammoma bodies (Fig. 2-137, Plates 2-71, 2-72), a finding similar to that reported in another recent study.[174] A diagnosis of a serous cystadenocarcinoma of the ovary was rendered. On reviewing the case, it was clear that the epithelial cells accompanying the psammoma bodies did not met the criteria of malignant disease. Although psammoma bodies may not be an indication of a malignant neoplastic process, their mere presence warrants further clinical investigation of a possible coexistent neoplastic disease. Thus, the presence of psammoma bodies is another important associated finding in the detection of an extrauterine cancer in the CVE smear.

An altered cytohormonal pattern with respect to cellular evidence of increased[145] or diminished[143] estrogen activity has been observed in CVE samples from patients with ovarian carcinoma. Although the cytohormonal pattern is generally of limited value in the detection of an extrauterine carcinoma, an increase in the number of superficial squamous cells in postmenopausal patients should provide sufficient cause for further investigation.

FACTORS INFLUENCING DESQUAMATION OF CELLS

The incidence of desquamated cells in CVE samples obtained for the detection of extrauterine cancers depends on a number of factors. For instance, sampling techniques may influence the rate of positive findings. Takashina et al.[149,160] compared the rate of positive results derived from both endometrial aspirates and CVE samples. They reported that the endometrial aspiration technique provided a higher positive rate than did samples obtained from the cervical-vaginal-endocervical site.

Although cellular evidence of extrauterine cancer in a CVE sample has often been associated with a poorly differentiated carcinoma,[144,156] others have reported[149] that the positive rate is higher in well-differentiated serous cystadenocarcinomas than in neoplasms that are less well-differentiated. Graham and van Nickerk[143] have reported that histologic types do not influence the incidence of desquamated cells derived from extrauterine cancers.

The presence of ascites may be an important finding in relation to the incidence of cellular evidence of extrauterine cancers in CVE samples. In one report,[144] 38 of 66 patients with extrauterine cancer were found to have ascites at the time that cellular evidence of cancer was detected. In another report,[143] massive ascites was observed, but these investigators did not mention the significance of ascites in relation to the positive yield of the diagnostic cells in the CVE sample. Takashina et al.[149] did note, however, that the positive rate was related to the absence or presence of ascites rather than to the volume, and they reported that the positive rate was 2.1 times higher in patients with ascites than in those without.

In a number of instances in which metastatic deposits were not evident in the uterus and vagina, isolated malignant neoplastic cells from an extrauterine source were observed in the lumen of the uterine tube.[143,144,146,147,149,157,160] Therefore, patency of the uterine tube for transit of malignant neoplastic cells into the uterus is another factor that contributes to the positive rate of detection of extrauterine cancer in CVE samples.

Although the study by Ng et al.[144] cited the extent of extrauterine cancer at the time of malignant cell detection, no attempt was made to correlate the extent of the disease with the positive rate of cellular evidence of extrauterine cancer in the CVE sample. Research by Takashina et al.[149] does indicate that the positive rate is higher in the more advanced clinical stages of disease.

CONCLUSION

Despite the numerous published reports on secondary tumors involving the genital tract, it is still not always possible to correlate morphologic evidence of extrauterine cancer derived from CVE samples with the site of origin of the neoplasm. However, certain features can facilitate establishment of a diagnosis. Among these are the following considerations:

1. Cellular evidence of metastatic cancer differs from the usual pattern of endometrial and endocervical carcinoma.
2. The size of neoplastic cells is larger than both normal and neoplastic endometrial cells, and is comparable to (and is sometimes larger than) that of normal endocervical cells.
3. Neoplastic cells that are loosely arranged in a papillary cluster and that have a three-dimensional appearance are probably ovarian in origin.
4. Neoplastic cells that are compactly arranged in clusters, without a three-dimensional feature, are probably of mammary origin. When the cells are small, isolated, or aligned in a linear manner, they probably represent a mammary carcinoma of lobular origin.
5. Neoplastic cells that are low to tall columnar in form and that exhibit a palisading pattern are probably of colonic origin.
6. Lack of transitional forms of cells participating in

the evolution of cancer is suggestive of metastatic disease.
7. Lack of tumor diathesis is suggestive of metastatic disease.
8. The presence of psammoma bodies should signal the need for further investigation of a possible co-existing metastatic disease.

Metastases in the female genital tract, although occurring infrequently, pose diagnostic difficulties for both clinicians and cytopathologists, as these lesions can be insidious, masquerading as primary disease at the metastatic site. The recognition of extrauterine cancer in CVE samples is directly related to the experience of cytopathologists as well as of cytotechnologists, and its detection is important in the clinical evaluation of oncologic patients. Its presence in CVE samples allows determination of the extent of the disease, helps to elucidate the appropriate mode for further investigation, and serves as a guide for selecting an optimal therapeutic regimen for patient management.

REFERENCES

BASIC PRINCIPLES

1. Vooijs GP, van der Graaf Y, Elias AG: Cellular composition of cervical smears in relation to the day of the menstrual cycle and the method of contraception. Acta Cytol 31:417, 1987
2. Reagan JW, Ng AB: The Cells of Uterine Adenocarcinoma. 2nd Ed. Monograms in Clinical Cytology. Vol. 1. S Karger AG, Basel, 1973
3. Frost JK: Gynecologic and obstetric clinical cytopathology. In Novak ER, Woodruff JD (eds): Novak's Gynecologic and Obstetric Pathology. WB Saunders, Philadelphia, 1979
4. Wied GL, Bahr GF: Vaginal, cervical and endocervical cytologic smears on a single slide. Obstet Gynecol 14:362, 1959
5. Koch F, Stakemann G: Irrigation smear: Accuracy in gynecologic cancer detection. Dan Med Bull 9:127, 1962
6. Davis HJ: The irrigation smear. A cytologic method for mass population screening by mail. Am J Obstet Gynecol 84:1017, 1962
7. Gravlee LC Jr: The Gravlee jet washer: Detection of adenocarcinoma of the endometrium. Prog Gynecol 6:185, 1975
8. Wied GL, Bibbo M, Harris MJ, Rao C: Endometrial jet wash technique. In Koss AG et al (eds): Compendium on Diagnostic Cytology. 5th Ed. Tutorials of Cytology. Vol. 4. International Acad Pathology, Chicago, 1983
9. Wied GL (ed): Symposium on hormonal cytology. Acta Cytol 12:87, 1968
10. Naib ZM: Exfoliative Cytopathology. 3rd Ed. Little, Brown, Boston, 1985
11. Gardner HZ, Dukes CD: Hemophilus vaginalis vaginitis. Ann NY Acad Sci 83:280, 1959
12. Gupta PK: Intrauterine contraceptive device: Vaginal cytology, pathologic changes and their clinical implications. Acta Cytol 26:571, 1982
13. Hager WD, Majmudar B: Pelvic actinomycosis in women using intrauterine contraceptive devices. Am J Obstet Gynecol 133:60, 1979
14. Monif GRG: Infectious diseases. In Obstetrics and Gynecology. 2nd Ed. Harper and Row, Philadelphia, 1982
15. Luff RD, Gupta PK, Spence MR et al: Pelvic actinomycosis and the intrauterine contraceptive device: A cytohistomorphologic study. Am J Clin Pathol 69:581, 1978
16. de la Monte SM, Gupta PK, White CL: Systemic actinomyces infection: A potential complication of intrauterine contraceptive device (IUD). JAMA 248:1876, 1982
17. Shurbaji MS, Newman MM, Gupta PK: Hepatic actinomycosis diagnosis by fine needle aspiration. Acta Cytol 31:751, 1987
18. Kiviat NB, Peterson M, Kinney-Thomas E, et al: Cytologic manifestations of cervical and vaginal infections. II. Confirmation of Chlamydia trachomatis infection by direct imunofluorescence using monoclonal antibodies. JAMA 253:977, 1985
19. Gupta PK, Lee EF, Erozan YS, et al: Cytologic investigations in Chlamydia infection. Acta Cytol 23:315, 1979
20. Meisels A, Fortin R: Condylomatous lesions of the cervix and vagina. I. Cytologic patterns. Acta Cytol 20:505, 1970
21. Purola E, Savia E: Cytology of gynecologic condyloma accuminatum. Acta Cytol 21:26, 1977
22. Gupta JW, Gupta PK, Shah KV, et al: Distribution of human papillomavirus antigen in cervical smears and cervical tissues. Int J Gynecol Pathol 2:160, 1983
23. Gupta JW, Gupta PK, Rosenshein N, et al: Detection of human papillomavirus in cervical smears: A comparison of in situ hybridization, immunocytochemistry and cytopathology. Acta Cytol 31:387, 1987
24. Koss LG: Diagnostic Cytology and Its Histopathologic Bases. 3rd Ed. JB Lippincott, Philadelphia, 1979

25. Gupta PK, Frost JK: Cytopathology and histopathology of female genital tract in Trichomonas vaginalis infection. Ch. 14. In Honigberg BM (ed): Trichomonads Parasitic In Humans. Springer-Verlag, New York, 1987

VAGINAL AND VULVAR CYTOLOGY

26. Koss LG: Diagnostic Cytology and Its Histopathologic Bases. JB Lippincott, Philadelphia, 1979
27. Bhambhani S, Milner A, Pant J, Luthra UK: Ova of Taenia and Enterobius vermicularis in cervicovaginal smears. Acta Cytol 29:913, 1985
28. Mali BN, Joshi JV: Vaginal parasitosis: An unusual finding in routine cervical smears. Acta Cytol 31:866, 1987
29. Naib ZM: Exfoliative Cytopathology. Little, Brown, Boston, 1985
30. Grönroos M, Tyrkkö J, Siiteri PK, et al: Cytolysis and karyopyknosis in postmenopausal vaginal smears as markers of endometrial cancer, diabetes, and obesity. Acta Cytol 30:628, 1986
31. Kanbour AI, Klionsky B, Murphy AI: Carcinoma of the vagina following cervical cancer. Cancer 34:1838, 1974
32. Murad TM, Durant JR, Maddox WA, Dowling EA: The pathologic behavior of primary vaginal carcinoma and its relationship to cervical cancer. Cancer 35:787, 1975
33. Kurman RJ, Scully RE: The incidence and histogenesis of vaginal adenosis. Hum Pathol 5:265, 1975
34. Clark AH, Betsill WL Jr: A morphometric study of primary adenocarcinoma of the vagina. Acta Cytol 30:323, 1986
35. Lang WR: Female genital tract—Diseases of the vulva and vagina. p. 137. In Keebler M, Reagan JM (eds): A Manual of Cytotechnology. American Society of Clinical Pathologists Press, Chicago, 1983
36. Holmquist ND, Torres J: Malignant melanoma of the cervix. Report of a case. Acta Cytol 32:252, 1988

BENIGN DISORDERS OF THE CERVIX

37. Naib ZM: Exfoliative Cytopathology. Little, Brown, Boston, 1985
38. Siapco BJ, Kaplan BJ, Bernstein GS, Moyer DL: Cytodiagnosis of candida organisms in cervical smears. Acta Cytol 30:477, 1986
39. Ng ABP, Reagan JW, Lindner E: The cellular manifestations of primary and recurrent herpes genitalis. Acta Cytol 14:124, 1970
40. Vesterinen E, Purola E, Saksela E, Leinikki P: Clinical and virological findings in patients with cytologically diagnosed gynecologic herpes simplex infections. Acta Cytol 21:199, 1977
41. Meisels A, Fortin R: Condylomatous lesions of the cervix and vagina. I. Cytologic patterns. Acta Cytol 20:505, 1976
42. Meisels A, Roy M, Morin C, et al: Human papillomavirus infection of the cervix: The atypical condyloma. Acta Cytol 25:7, 1981
43. Kitay DZ, Wentz WB: Cervical pathology in folic acid deficiency of pregnancy. Am J Obstet Gynecol 104:931, 1969

CYTOPATHOLOGY OF DYSPLASIA, CARCINOMA IN SITU, AND INVASIVE CARCINOMA OF THE UTERINE CERVIX

44. Patten SF: Diagnostic Cytopathology of the Uterine Cervix. 2nd Ed. S Karger, AG Basel, 1978
45. Reagan JW, Patten SF: Dysplasia, a basic reaction to injury in the uterine cervix. Ann NY Acad Sci 97:662, 1962
46. Reagan JW: Dysplasia of the uterine cervix. In Gray LA (ed): Dysplasia, Carcinoma in Situ and Microinvasive Carcinoma. Charles C Thomas, Springfield, IL, 1965
47. Richart RM: Cervical Intraepithelial Neoplasia. Pathol Ann 7:301, 1973
48. Fu YS, Reagan JW, Richart RW: Definition of precursors. Gynecol Oncol 12:s220, 1981
49. Jenson AB, Lancaster WD, Kurman RJ: Uterine Cervix. p. 249. In Albores-Saavedra J (ed): The Pathology of Incipient Neoplasia. WB Saunders, Philadelphia, 1986
50. Koss LG, Durfee GR: Unusual patterns of squamous epithelium of the uterine cervix: Cytologic and pathologic study of koilocytotic atypia. Ann NY Acad Sci 63:1245, 1961
51. Meisels A, Fortin R: Condylomatous lesions of the cervix and vagina. I. Cytologic patterns. Acta Cytol 20:505, 1976
52. Purola E, Savia E: Cytology of gynecologic condyloma acuminatum. Acta Cytol 21:26, 1977
53. Reid R: Papilloma virus and cervical neoplasia. Modern implications and future prospects. Col Gynecol Laser Surg 1:3, 1984
54. zur Hausen H: Human genital cancer: Synergism between two virus infections or synergism between a virus infection and initiating events? Lancet 11:1370, 1983
55. zur Hausen HJ: Human papillomaviruses and their possible role in squamous carcinomas. p. 1. In Arber W (ed): Current Topics in Microbiology and Immunology. Springer-Verlag, New York, 1977

56. Stoler MH, Broker TR: In situ hybridization detection of human papillomavirus DNAs and messenger RNAs in genital condylomas and a cervical carcinoma. Hum Pathol 17:1250, 1986
57. Durst M, Kleinhanheinz A, Hotz M, Gissman L: The physical state of human papillomavirus type 16 DNA in benign and malignant genital tumors. J Gen Virol 66:1515, 1985
58. Lorincz A, Lancaster WD, Temple GF: Cloning and characterization of the DNA of a new human papilloma virus from a woman with dysplasia of the uterine cervix. J Virol 58:225, 1985
59. Editorial: Statement of caution in the interpretation of papillomarivus-associated lesions of the epithelium of the uterine cervix. Acta Cytol 27:107, 1983
60. Reagan JW, Bell BA, Neuman JL, et al: Dysplasia in the uterine cervix during pregnancy: An analytic study of the cells. Acta Cytol 5:17, 1961
61. Reagan JW, Harmonic MJ: Dysplasia of the uterine cervix. Ann NY Acad Sci 63:1236, 1956
62. Reagan JW, Seideman IL, Saracusa Y: The cellular morphology of carcinoma in situ and dysplasia or atypical hyperplasia of the uterine cervix. Cancer 6:224, 1953
63. Weid GL, Legorreta G, Mohr D, Rauzy A: Cytology of invasive cervical carcinoma and carcinoma in situ. Ann NY Acad Sci 97:759, 1962
64. Ng ABP, Reagan JW, Lindner E: The cellular manifestations of microinvasive squamous cell carcinoma of the uterine cervix. Acta Cytol 16:5, 1972
65. Broders AC: Carcinoma grading and practical application. Arch Pathol 2:376, 1926
66. Wentz WB, Reagan JW: Survival in cervical cancer with respect to cell type. Cancer 12:384, 1959
67. Reagan JW, Harmonic MJ, Wentz WB: Analytic study of the cells in cervical squamous-cell cancer. Lab Invest 6:241, 1957
68. Giersson G, Woodworth FE, Patten SF, Bonfiglio TA: Epithelial repair and regeneration in the uterine cervix. Acta Cytol 21:371, 1977

ENDOCERVICAL ADENOCARCINOMA

69. Abel MR, Gosling JGP: Gland cell carcinoma (adenocarcinoma) of the uterine cervix. Am J Obstet Gynecol 83:729, 1962
70. Menczner J, Modan B, Oelsner G, et al: Adenocarcinoma of the uterine cervix in Jewish women. Cancer 41:2464, 1978
71. Ng AB: Female genital tract—Diseases of the uterine corpus. p. 117. In Keebler M, Reagan JM (eds): A Manual of Cytotechnology. American Society of Clinical Pathologists Press, Chicago, 1983
72. Friedell GH, McKay DG: Adenocarcinoma in situ of the endocervix. Cancer 6:887, 1953
73. Betsill W, Clark AH: Early endocervical glandular neoplasia. I. Histomorphology of cytomorphology. Acta Cytol 30:115, 1986
74. Ayer B, Pacey F, Greenberg M, Bousfield L: The cytologic diagnosis of adenocarcinoma in situ of the cervix uteri and related lesions: I. Adenocarcinoma in situ. Acta Cytol 31:397, 1987

CYTOLOGY OF BENIGN ENDOMETRIAL DISORDERS

75. Vuopala S: Diagnostic accuracy and clinical applicability of cytological and histological methods for investigating endometrial cancer. Acta Obstet Gynecol Scand (Suppl) 70(8):1, 1977
76. Cary W: A method of obtaining endometrial smears for study of their cellular content. Am J Obstet Gynecol 46:422, 1943
77. Torres J, Holmquist N, Danos M: The endometrial irrigation smear in the detection of adenocarcinoma of the endometrium. Acta Cytol 13:163, 1969
78. Johnson J, Stormby N: Cytological brush technique in a malignant disease of the endometrium. Acta Obstet Gynecol Scand 47:38, 1968
79. Ayer J: Rotating endometrial brush: New technique for the diagnosis of fundal carcinoma. Obstet Gynecol 5:137, 1955
80. Henderson S, Roxburg D, Bobrow L, et al: Endometrial washings. Histological and cytological assessment of material obtained with an intrauterine jet washing device. Br J Obstet Gynecol 82:976, 1975
81. Dowling E, Gravelee L, Hutchins K: A new technique for the detection of adenocarcinoma of the endometrium. Acta Cytol 13:496, 1969
82. Bibbo M, Kluskens L, Azizi F, et al: Accuracy of 3 sampling techniques for the diagnosis of endometrial carcinoma and hyperplasia. Acta Cytol 27:622, 1982
83. Inglis R, Weir J: Endometrial suction biopsy: Appraisal of a new instrument. Am J Obstet Gynecol 125:1070, 1976
84. Inone Y, Ikeda M, Kimura K, et al: Accuracy of endometrial aspiration in the diagnosis of the endometrial cancer. Acta Cytol 27:477, 1983
85. Milan A, Markley R: Endometrial cytology by a new technique. Obstet Gynecol 42:469, 1973
86. Bamford D, Hall E, Newman M: The Isaacs endometrial cell sampler. Acta Cytol 28:101, 1984
87. Isaacs J, Wilhoitte R: Aspiration cytology of the endometrium: Office and hospital sampling procedures. Obstet Gynecol 108:679, 1974
88. Morse A: The value of endometrial aspiration in

gynecological practice. In Koss L, Coleman D (eds): Advances in Clinical Cytology. p. 44. Butterworth, London, 1981
89. Veneti S, Kyrkou K, Kitlas C, Perides A: Efficacy of the Isaacs endometrial cell sampler in the cytologic detection of endometrial abnormalities. Acta Cytol 28:546, 1984
90. Crow J, Gordon H, Hudson E: An assessment of the Mi-Mark endometrial sampling technique. J Clin Pathol 33:72, 1980
91. Afonso J: Value of the Gravlee jet washer in the diagnosis of endometrial cancer. Obstet Gynecol 46:141, 1975
92. Fechner R, Bossart M, Spjut H: Ultrastructure of endometrial stromal foam cells. Am J Clin Pathol 72:628, 1979
93. Richart R (moderator): Endometrial Cancer Symposium. Contemp Obstet Gynecol 14:100, 1979
94. Kobayashi T, Casslin B, Stormby N: Cytologic atypias in the uterine fluid of intrauterine contraceptive device users. Acta Cytol 27:38, 1983
95. Czernobilsky B, Rotenstreich L, Mass N, Lancet M: Effect of intrauterine device on the histology of the endometrium. Obstet Gynecol 45:64, 1974
96. Fornari M: Cellular changes in the glandular epithelium of patients using IUCD—A source of cytologic error. Acta Cytol 18:341, 1974
97. Gupta P, Burroughs F, Luff R. et al: Epithelial atypias associated with intrauterine contraceptive devices (IUD). Acta Cytol 22:286, 1978
98. Danos M, Holmquist N: Cytologic evaluation of decidual cells: A report of 2 cases with false abnormal cytology. Acta Cytol 11:325, 1967
99. Murad T, Terhart K, Flint A: Atypical cells in pregnancy and postpartum smears. Acta Cytol 25:623, 1981
100. Kobayashi T, Yuasa M, Fujimoto T, et al: Cytologic findings in postpartum and postabortal smears. Acta Cytol 24:328, 1980
101. Shrago S: The Arias-Stella Reaction: A case report of a cytologic presentation. Acta Cytol 21:310, 1977
102. Kobayashi T, Fujimoto T, Okamoto H, et al: Cytologic evaluation of atypical cells in cervicovaginal smears from women with tubal pregnancies. Acta Cytol 27:28, 1983
103. Capaldo G, Le Galvan D, Dramczyk J: Hematoidin crystals in cervicovaginal smears. Acta Cytol 27:237, 1983
104. Hollander D, Gupta P: Hematoidin cockleburrs in cervicovaginal smears. Acta Cytol 18:268, 1974
105. Gondos B, King E: Significance of endometrial cells in cervicovaginal smears. Ann Clin Lab Sci 7:486, 490, 1977
106. Ng A, Reagan J, Hawliczek S, Wentz B: Significance of endometrial cells in the detection of endometrial carcinoma and its precursors. Acta Cytol 18:356, 1974
107. Ng A: The cellular detection of endometrial cancer and its precursors. Gynecol Oncol 2:162, 1974
108. Ng A, Reagan J, Cechner R: The precursors of endometrial cancer: A study of their cellular manifestations. Acta Cytol 17:439, 1973
109. Zucker P, Kasdan D, Feldstein M: The validity of Pap smear parameters as predictors of endometrial pathology in menopausal women. Cancer 56:2256, 1985
110. Blumenfeld W, Holly E, Manuar D, King E: Histiocytes and the detection of endometrial adenocarcinoma. Acta Cytol 29:317, 1985
111. Von Ludinhausen M, Anastasiadis P: Anatomic bases of endometrial cytology. Acta Cytol 28:555, 1984
112. The American Cancer Society: A Cancer Journal for Clinicians. Ca 36(1): 16, 1986
113. MacMahon B: Risk factors of endometrial carcinoma. Gynecol Oncol 2:122, 1974
114. Wynder E, Escher G, Mantel N: An epidemiological investigation of cancer of the endometrium. Cancer 19:489, 1966
115. Spect H: Endometrial cancer and hepatic cirrhosis. Cancer 2:597, 1949
116. DeVere R, Dempter K: A case of the Stein Leventhal syndrome associated with cancer of the endometrium. J Obstet Gynecol Br Emp 60:865, 1953
117. Cramer DW, Knapp RC: Review of epidemiologic studies of endometrial cancer and exogenous estrogens. Obstet Gynecol 54:521, 1979
118. Schoenberg BS, Greenberg RH, Eisenberg H: Occurrence of certain multiple primary cancers in females. J Natl Cancer Instit 43:15, 1969
119. Salerno L: Feminizing mesenchymomas of the ovary: An analysis of 28 granulosa-theca cell tumors and their relationship to co-existent carcinoma. Am J Obstet Gynecol 84:731, 1962
120. Ng A, Reagan J: Normal endometrial cells and their significance in the detection of benign and malignant endometrial lesions. p. 164. In Wied GL (ed): Compendium on Diagnostic Cytology. 5th ed. International Academy of Pathologists, Chicago, 1983
121. Koss L, Cramer D, Ferenczy A, et al: Recent advances in endometrial neoplasia. Acta Cytol 24:478, 1979
122. Koss LG, Schreuber K, Oberlander SG, et al: Screening of asymptomatic women for endometrial cancer. Obstet Gynecol 57:681, 1981
123. Lozowski M, Meshriki Y, Solitare G: Factors determining the degree of endometrial exfoliation and

their diagnostic implications in endometrial adenocarcinoma. Acta Cytol 30:624, 1986
124. Vuopala S: Diagnostic accuracy and clinical applicability of cytological and histological methods for investigating endometrial cancer. Acta Obstet Gynecol Scand (Suppl) 70(8):1, 1977
125. Von-Ludinghausen M, Anastasiadis P: Anatomic basis of endometrial cytology. Acta Cytol 28:555, 1984
126. Gondos B, King E: Significance of endometrial cells in cervical vaginal smears. Ann Clin Lab Sci 7:486, 1977
127. Ng A, Reagan J, Hawliczek S, Wentz B: Significance of endometrial cells in the detection of endometrial carcinoma and its precursors. Acta Cytol 18:356, 1974
128. Blumenfeld W, Holly E, Mauser D, King E: Histiocytes and the detection of endometrial adenocarcinoma. Acta Cytol 29:317, 1985
129. Zucker P, Kasdan E, Feldstein M: The validity of Pap smear parameters as predictors of endometrial pathology in menopausal women. Cancer 56:2256, 1985
130. Walker A, Mills S: Serous papillary carcinoma of the endometrium. Diagn Gynecol Obstet 4:261, 1982
131. Buschmann C, Hergenrader M, Porter D: Keratin bodies. A clue in the cytologic detection of endometrial adenocanthoma. Acta Cytol 18:297, 1974
132. Nguyen G: Cytologic aspects of a metastatic malignant mixed müllerian tumor of the uterus. Acta Cytol 26:521, 1982
133. An-Foraker S, Kawada C: Cytodiagnosis of endometrial malignant mixed mesodermal tumor. Acta Cytol 29:137, 1985
134. Mitchard P, Swingler G, Cave D: Cytologic features of a mixed müllerian tumor of the uterus demonstrated by cells obtained with the Mimark endometrial sampler. Acta Cytol 24:363, 365, 1980
135. Becker S, Wong J: Detection of endometrial stromal sarcoma in cervicovaginal smears. Acta Cytol 25:272, 1980

EXTRAUTERINE CANCER

136. Abrams HL, Spiro R, Goldstein, A: Metastasis in carcinoma: Analysis of 1000 autopsied cases. Cancer 3:74, 1950
137. Charache H: Metastatic carcinoma in the uterus. Am J Surg 53:152, 1941
138. Esposito JM, Zarou DM, Zarou GS: Extragenital adenocarcinoma metastatic to the cervix uteri. Am J Obstet Gynecol 92:792, 1965
139. Kumar NB, Hart WR: Metastases to the uterine corpus from extragenital cancers: A clinicopathologic study of 63 cases. Cancer 50:2163, 1982
140. Lemoine NR, Hall PA: Epithelial tumors metastatic to the uterine cervix. Cancer 57:2002, 1986
141. Mazur MT, Hsueh S, Gersell DJ: Metastase to the female genital tract. Cancer 53:1978, 1984
142. Dance EF, Fullmer CD: Extrauterine carcinoma cells observed in cervicovaginal smears. Acta Cytol 14:187, 1970
143. Graham RM, van Niekerk WA: Vaginal cytology in cancer of the ovary. Acta Cytol 6:496, 1962
144. Ng ABP, Teeple D, Lindner E, Reagan JW: The cellular manifestations of extrauterine cancer. Acta Cytol 18:108, 1973
145. Rubin DK, Frost JK: The cytologic detection of ovarian cancer. Acta Cytol 75:191, 1963
146. Benson PA: Psammoma bodies found in cervicovaginal smears. Case report. Acta Cytol 17:64, 1973
147. Song YS: The significance of positive vaginal smears in extrauterine carcinomas. Am J Obstet Gynecol 73:341, 1957
148. Umiker W, Skeen M: Carcinoma of the ovary with malignant cells in the vaginal smear of an asymptomatic patient. Am J Obstet Gynecol 66:674, 1953
149. Takashina T, Ono M, Kanda Y, et al: Cervicovaginal and endometrial cytology in ovarian cancer. Acta Cytol 32:159, 1988
150. Differding JT: Psammoma bodies in vaginal smear. Acta Cytol 11:199, 1967
151. Figge DC, de Alvarez RR: Diagnosis of ovarian carcinoma by vaginal cytology. Obstet Gynecol 8:655, 1956
152. Kranshaar OF, Bradbury JT, Brown WE: The vaginal smear in population screening for uterine carcinoma. Am J Obstet Gynecol 58:447, 1949
153. McGarvey RN: Cytologic diagnosis of ovarian cancer: Report of a case; review of literature. Obstet Gynecol 5:257, 1955
154. Wachtel E, Plester JA: The vaginal smear as an aid to diagnosis of genital tract malignancy in women. J Obstet Gynecol Br Emp 59:323, 1952
154a. French HC: Adenocarcinoma of the ovary diagnosed by vaginal smear. Am J Obstet 57:802, 1949
155. Isbell NP, Jewett JF, Allan MS, Hertig AT: A correlation between vaginal smear and tissue diagnosis in 1045 operated gynecologic cases. Am J Obstet Gynecol 54:576, 1947
156. Reagan JW, Ng ABP: The Cells of Uterine Adenocarcinoma. 2nd rev. ed. Monographs in Clinical Cytology. Vol. 1. S Karger AG, Basel, 1973
157. Bhagavan BS, Weinberg T: Cytopathologic diagnosis

of mestastatic cancer by cervical and vaginal smears with report of a case. Acta Cytol 13:377, 1969
158. Koss LG: Diagnostic Cytology. 3rd ed. pp. 502. JB Lippincott, Philadelphia, 1979
159. Garrett R: Extrauterine tumor cells in vaginal and cervical smears. Obstet Gynecol 14:21, 1959
160. Takashina T, Ito E, Kudo R: Cytologic diagnosis of primary tubal cancer. Acta Cytol 29:367, 1985
161. Takeda M, Diamond SM, DeMarco M, Quinn DM: Cytologic diagnosis of malignant melanoma metastatic to the endometrium. Acta Cytol 22:503, 1978
162. Kashimura M, Kashimura Y, Matsuyama T, et al: Adenocarcinoma of the uterine cervix metastatic from primary stomach cancer. Acta Cytol 27:54, 1981
163. Figueroa JM, Huffaker AK, Diehl EJ: Malignant plasma cells in cervical smear. Acta Cytol 22:43, 1978
164. Uyeda CK, Stephens SR, Bridger WM: Cervical smear diagnosis of Hodgkin's disease. Report of a case. Acta Cytol 13:652, 1969
165. Ceelen GH, Sakurai M: Vaginal cytology in leukemia. Acta Cytol 6:370, 1962
166. Beyer-Boon, ME: Psammoma bodies in cervicovaginal smears: An indicator of the presence of ovarian carcinoma. Acta Cytol 18:41, 1974
167. Fox CH: Adnexal malignancy detected by cervical cytology. Am J Obstet Gynecol 132:148, 1978
168. Jenkins DM, Goulden R: Psammoma bodies in cervical cytology smears. Acta Cytol 21:112, 1977
169. Spjut HJ, Kaufman RH, Carrig SS: Psammoma bodies in the cervicovaginal smear. Acta Cytol 8:352, 1964
170. Weaver R, Wilson R: Endometrial carcinoma with psammoma bodies in the vaginal smear. Am J Obstet Gynecol 97:869, 1967
171. Highman WJ: Calcified bodies in the intrauterine device. Acta Cytol 15:473, 1971
172. Picoff RC, Meeker CI: Psammoma bodies in the cervicovaginal smear in association with benign papillary structures of the ovary. Acta Cytol 14:45, 1970
173. Tutschka BG, Lauchlan SC: Psammoma bodies in cervicovaginal smears. Case report and review of the literature. Acta Cytol 22:507, 1978
174. Qazi FM, Geisinger KR, Barrett RJ, et al: Cervicovaginal psammoma bodies. Arch Pathol Lab Med 112:564, 1988

3
Cytopathology of Irradiation and Chemotherapy

Parviz Haghighi

This chapter will discuss and illustrate the cytomorphology of radiation therapy and chemotherapy in humans. For a detailed presentation of the histopathology and pathobiology of irradiation, the reader is referred to selected excellent publications on these subjects.[1-6] Radiation cytopathology has been studied most extensively in terms of carcinoma of the uterine cervix, but the available data indicate similar cytopathology may be expected elsewhere in the body. During the course of radiation therapy, normal cells of the cancerous organ and, to some extent, those of adjacent noncancerous organs are also affected. The cytomorphology of irradiated benign and malignant cells is essentially similar, although morphologic alterations appear to be more intense in the nuclei of malignant cells.[7] Although we are still awaiting further investigations and the availability of additional data (owing to an increasing number of new drugs), the cytologic changes that are associated with the use of chemotherapeutic agents appear to be basically similar to those resulting from irradiation. Finally, various types of therapeutic irradiation seem to lead to similar cytologic alterations.

It should be emphasized that cytologic changes associated with irradiation, although often characteristic, are not absolutely specific. For this reason, certain conditions, such as an estrogen or folic acid deficiency (Fig. 3-1), as well as chemotherapeutic effects (Fig. 3-2) and inflammatory conditions, should be considered in the differential diagnosis. Adequate clinical information is of paramount importance.

Because most of the available information on radiation cytopathology has been derived from the study of cervicovaginal mucosa, cytopathologic changes in this area will be described in detail. Additional changes occurring outside the cervicovaginal mucosa will be noted briefly whenever applicable.

RADIATION CYTOPATHOLOGY OF CERVICOVAGINAL MUCOSA

Acute Radiation Reaction

Changes of acute radiation reaction affect both the nucleus and the cytoplasm of benign and malignant cells. Radiation changes are usually manifested 13 to 14 days after treatment is begun.[8]

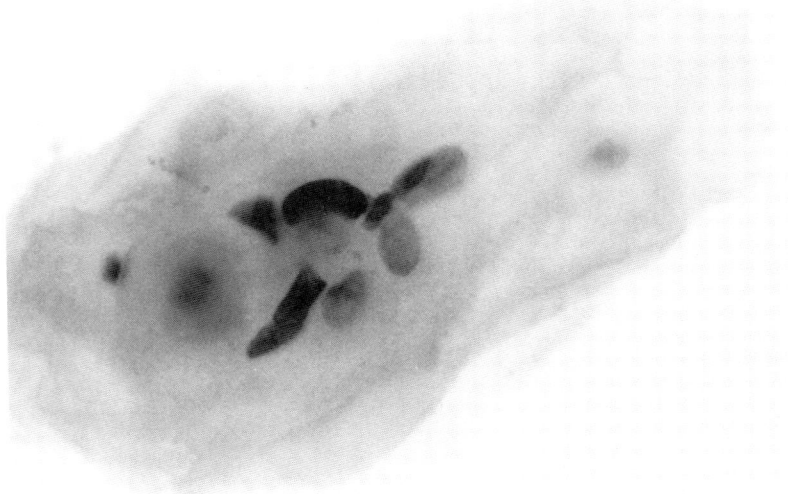

Fig. 3-1 Sputum. Chemotherapeutic effect from methotrexate, squamous cell. Note that the alterations are morphologically indistinguishable from folic acid deficiency. (× 160.)

CYTOPLASMIC CHANGES

Cytoplasmic changes, which usually precede nuclear changes by 1 to 14 days, may involve vacuolation; changes in staining characteristics; cytoplasmic "autolysis"; phagocytosis; leukocytic invasion; or cytoplasmic "deposits".[9]

Vacuolation

Vacuolation is one of the earliest changes seen at the light microscopic level. Vacuoles may be single, double, or multiple (Figs. 3-3 to 3-5). They are discrete, often large, and are randomly distributed, whereas the vacuoles associated with inflammatory

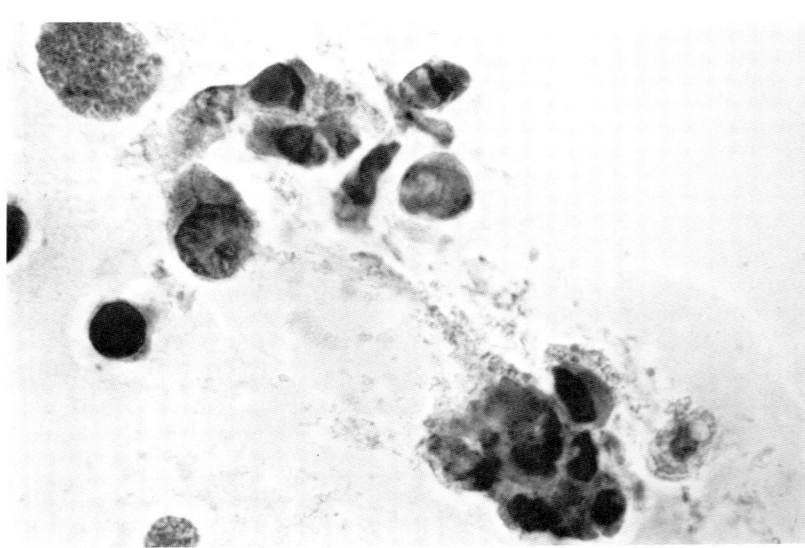

Fig. 3-2 Voided urine specimen showing cyclophosphamide effect. Note the highly bizarre urothelial cells with hypechromatic nuclei. (× 160.) (See Plate 3-1.)

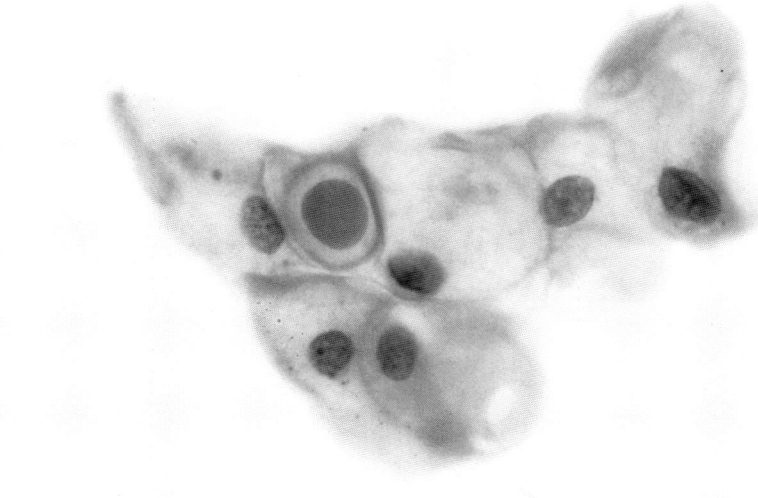

Fig. 3-3 CVE smear obtained 2 weeks post-irradiation. Intermediate cell showing a large, single, discrete cytoplasmic vacuole with inclusion. (× 160.)

conditions are usually seen around the nucleus. They are not empty vacuoles (Figs. 3-5 to 3-8), and may contain an eosinophilic center that exhibits lamination. In such cases, they are considered by some observers to be characteristic of or even specific for irradiation, especially in the early phase of acute radiation reaction. They usually do not stain for lipid. On electron microscopic examination, the vacuoles correspond to dilated cisternae of endoplasmic reticulum.[10] Although vacuolization may be seen in nonirradiated cells, extreme cytoplasmic vacuolation and very large, discrete vacuoles are considered to be

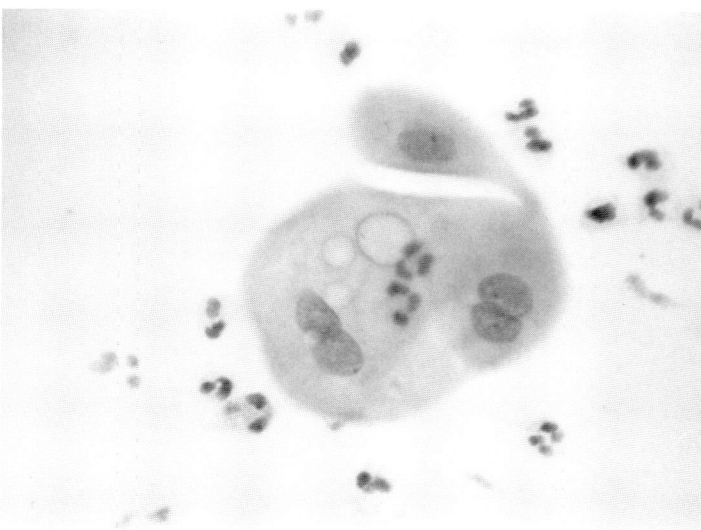

Fig. 3-4 Radiation effect. Multinucleated intermediate cell with bizarre cell shape. A discrete cytoplasmic vacuole is also seen. (× 160.) (See Plate 3-2.)

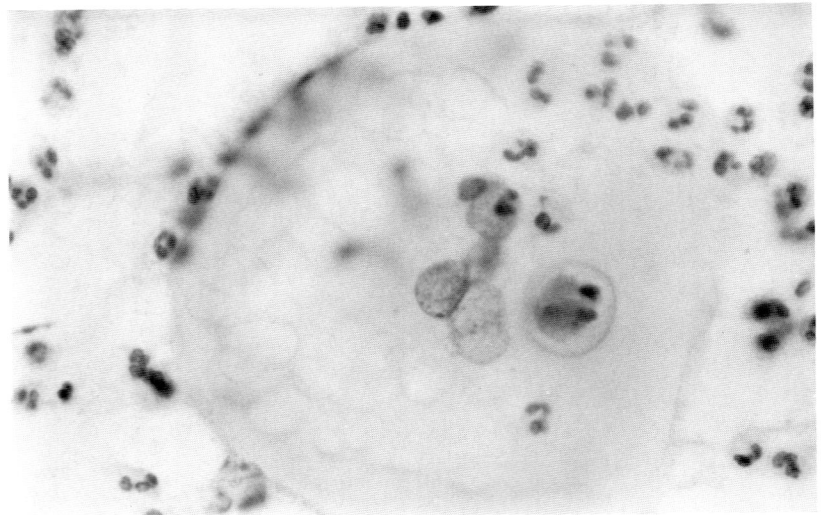

Fig. 3-5 Radiation effect. This intermediate cell shows multinucleation, multiple cytoplasmic vacuoles with one discrete vacuole containing a polymorphonuclear leukocyte nucleus, and polymorphonuclear "superimposition." (× 160.) (See Plate 3-3.)

characteristic of a radiation effect.[11] The vacuoles may be so large as to displace and compress the nucleus to the periphery of the cell, thus creating the so-called signet ring cell appearance. A paranuclear vacuole may also occur, and this must be distinguished from the perinuclear halo that is related to shrinkage of the nucleus. Although present in acute radiation reaction, vacuolation may also be observed months or years after cessation of therapy.

In cervicovaginal material, vacuoles are most com-

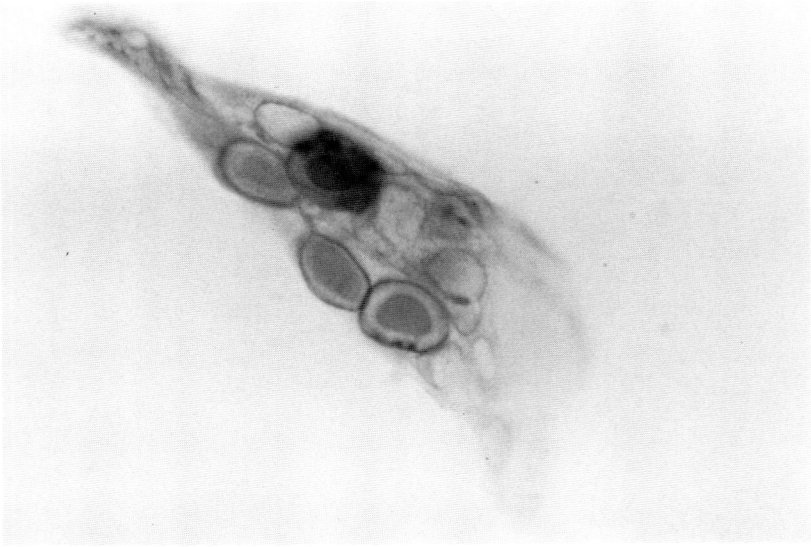

Fig. 3-6 Same case as Fig. 3-3. Abnormally shaped intermediate cell with pyknotic nucleus and multiple, discrete, cytoplasmic vacuoles containing inclusions. (× 160.)

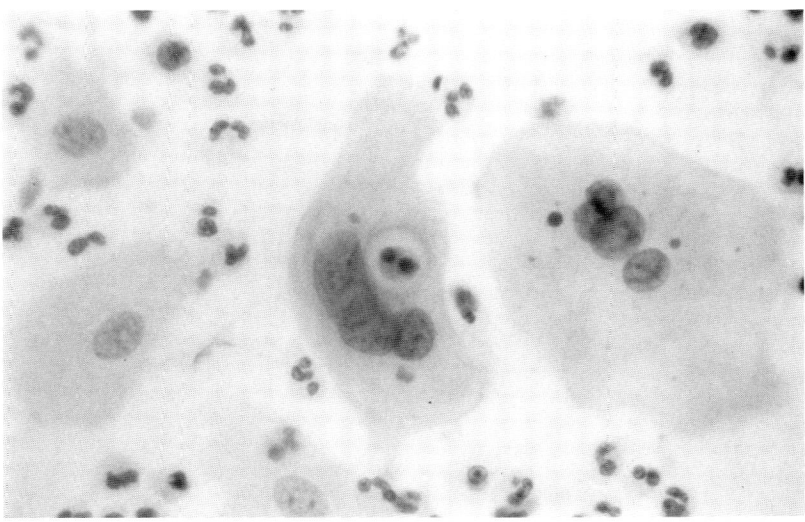

Fig. 3-7 Radiation effect, intermediate cells. Note the binucleation and nuclear enlargement, as well as the nucleus of a polymorphonuclear leukocyte within the discrete cytoplasmic vacuole. (× 160.) (See Plate 3-4.)

monly seen in parabasal cells, and sometimes appear in intermediate cells. Vacuolation is first observed in basal cells, later in intermediate cells, and rarely in superficial cells. Pretreatment vacuolization in basal cells or *sensitization response* (SR),[12] correlates with a significant increase in the presence of cells showing vacuolization after initiation of radiation therapy. A favorable tumor response to radiation treatment was considered more likely when more than 10 percent of the basal cells showed vacuolization prior to therapy. Fine vacuolization in parabasal cells may be observed as early as 2 days, but usually about 9 days, after radiation therapy is begun.[9,11]

It may be difficult to differentiate between vacuo-

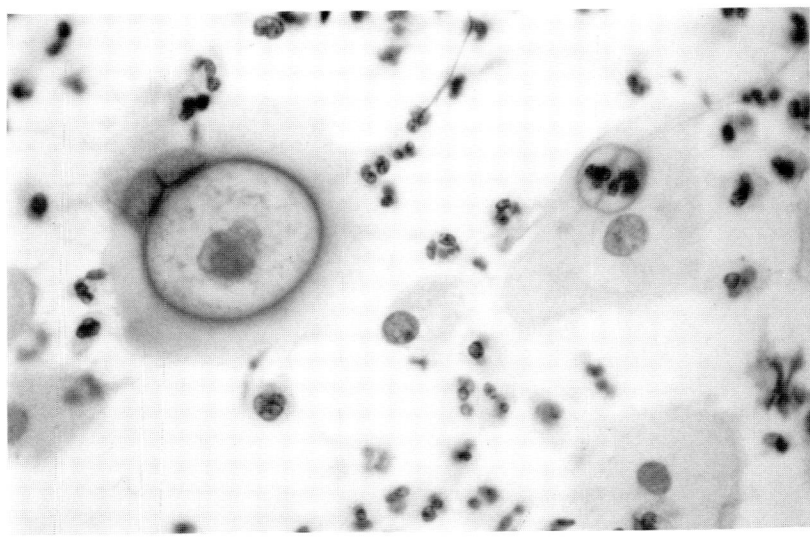

Fig. 3-8 Radiation effect. The intermediate cell on the left shows a single, discrete, cytoplasmic vacuole pushing the double nuclei to one side and containing nuclear material. (× 160.) (See Plate 3-5.)

lated parabasal cells and histiocytes. However, an indefinite cytoplasmic border, a bean-shaped and eccentrically located nucleus, and a *finely* vacuolated and transparent-appearing cytoplasm are usually indicative of histiocytes.

Change in Staining Characteristics

A change in staining characteristics, often manifested by diffuse and sometimes patchy lavender to eosinophilic cytoplasmic discoloration, is considered by some to be specific for radiation effect.[10] The term *pseudoeosinophilia* has been used by some authors to describe this change.[11] Granular and hyalinized eosinophilic-appearing cytoplasm is usually seen in acute radiation damage, although it may occasionally be observed as a late effect of irradiation. It correlates well with the presence of lysosomes on electron microscopy.[11] Central eosinophilia and peripheral cyanophilia of the cytoplasm, sometimes termed cytoplasmic amphophilia,[11] may be seen (Fig. 3-9).

Cytoplasmic "Autolysis"

In post-irradiation cervical smears, cytoplasmic disintegration occurs in the absence of Döderlein bacilli. This particularly effects the intermediate cells. If advanced, this disintegration results in the appearance of free nuclei in the smear.[11]

Phagocytosis

Although a nonspecific phenomenon, phagocytosis commonly occurs in the surface squamous cells after irradiation. The phagocytosed material may present simply as nuclear debris, or it may be identifiable as a remnant of polymorphonuclear leukocytes or even other epithelial cells. The term "birds-eye cell" has sometimes been used in this instance.[11]

Leukocytic "Invasion"

A common phenomenon in post-irradiation smears is the close association of polymorphonuclear neutrophils with the squamous cells. This is seen more frequently in intermediate and superficial cells than in parabasal cells. These neutrophils can form dense aggregates that appear to be superimposed on the epithelial cells (*superimposition*) (Fig. 3-5) or they may actually be seen within the cytoplasm of epithelial cells, sometimes inside cytoplasmic vacuoles (*immigration*) (Figs. 3-5 and 3-7). Superimposition is most often observed 10 to 31 days after initiation of radiation therapy, and precedes immigration.[11] Polymorphonuclear cells may be so numerous as to ob-

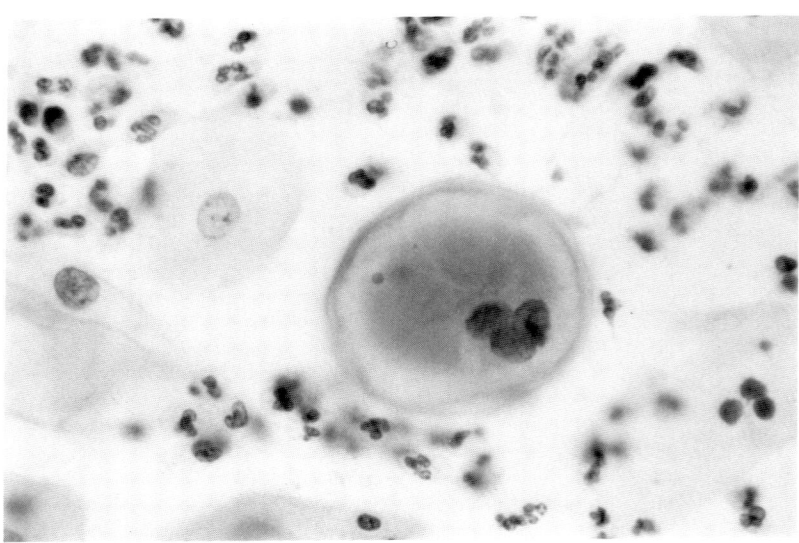

Fig. 3-9 Radiation effect. The intermediate cell in the center, in addition to trinucleation, shows a "two-tone" cytoplasm. (× 160.) (See Plate 3-6.)

scure the true nature of the underlying cell. This phenomenon can also involve histiocytes in addition to the epithelial cells.

Cytoplasmic Deposits

Dense deposits with histochemical reactions similar to those of glycogen may be seen within the cytoplasmic vacuoles. The deposits may appear to be granular, predominantly eosinophilic, and may be separated from the vacuolar wall by a clear zone, imparting a laminated appearance to the vacuole. This laminated type of deposit is considered by some to be specific for radiation change, and correlates with the lightly osmiophilic material seen on electron microscopy.[11]

NUCLEAR CHANGES

Vacuolation

Single and occasionally double vacuoles may be identified in the nuclei of irradiated epithelial cells. These vacuoles have well-defined borders and may even contain nuclear remnants of leukocytes. By electron microscopy, they appear to correlate with invagination of the cytoplasm into the nucleus and chromatin dissolution with margination.[10]

Binucleation or Multinucleation

The binucleation or multinucleation that is apparent in some cervicovaginal-endocervical (CVE) smears can involve parabasal, intermediate, and superficial cells, as well as histiocytes, although it has also been observed in other locations (Figs. 3-4 and 3-7 to 3-11).[10] The nuclei are usually vesicular but they may show vacuolation. Although variable, there may be a large number of nuclei within a mass of cytoplasm, probably indicating incoordinated nuclear and cytoplasmic maturation. The cytoplasm may exhibit radiation-associated changes, such as vacuolation and altered staining characteristics. These cells are often quite large and may qualify as giant cells. Their epithelial derivation is not always apparent, although absence of foamy cytoplasm and well-defined cell border may help to identify them as epithelial in origin. The nuclear aggregate is often eccentrically located. Giant cells can be numerous in some smears, in which case they may correlate with a favorable radiation response.[13,14]

Wrinkling of the Nuclear Membrane

A wrinkled nuclear membrane is considered to be an important, albeit nonspecific, finding, and is often associated with the late stages of irradiation.[8] Some observers believe that it is the result of nuclear swelling,[12] whereas others have suggested that it is more likely to be attributable to dehydration secondary to ionic imbalance.[10] In any case, it should be differentiated from condensed chromatin.[12]

Nuclear Enlargement

An enlarged nucleus is a common finding in radiation injury and may be related to nuclear swelling (Figs. 3-7 and 3-12). At first glance, it may mimic nuclear enlargement of malignant cells. However, in radiation injury, there is a concomitant increase in cytoplasmic volume with general maintenance of a normal or near-normal nucleocytoplasmic ratio.

Regressive Changes

Regressive changes may include chromatolysis, karyopyknosis (Fig. 3-6), and karyolysis, in that order of severity. Degenerative nuclear changes may be so advanced as to make the distinction between benign and malignant cells difficult.[11] Karyolysis commonly affects parabasal cells, as well as intermediate cells to a lesser degree.

CELL MEMBRANE

Disintegration of the cell membrane secondary to irradiation is reflected in the presence of fuzzy cell borders. Strands of cytoplasm resembling pseudopodia, stretching from the cells across the smear and creating a netlike appearance in the background, are often seen (Fig. 3-12).[11]

CHANGES IN CELL SIZE AND SHAPE

As mentioned previously, irradiated cells enlarge, sometimes enormously, but this enlargement usually involves proportionate increases in nuclear and cytoplasmic size.

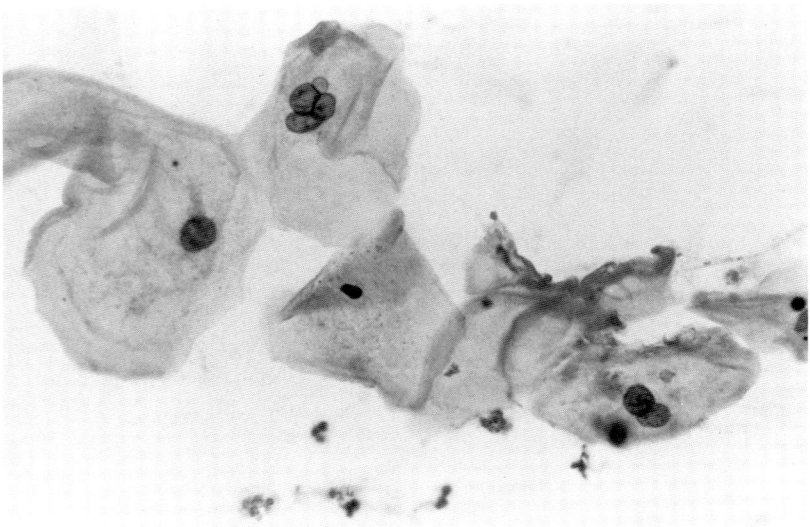

Fig. 3-10 Same case as Fig. 3-3. Binucleated and multinucleated intermediate cell. (× 100.)

Bizarre cell forms constitute one of the most reliable criteria for documenting radiation effect (Figs. 3-4, 3-6, 3-11, and 3-13).[11] Many unusual cell shapes, including monstrous forms, have been described (tadpole, cuttle-fish, tulip, and others). Such changes in cell shape can involve any of the cell constituents of surface stratified squamous epithelium. Nonepithelial cells, such as histiocytes, may also be affected. The appearance of chromatin and a normal or near-normal nucleocytoplasmic ratio help to differentiate these cells from malignant cells. Bizarre cell forms are usually characteristic of late radiation effect. They constitute approximately 1 percent of the smear cell population.[12]

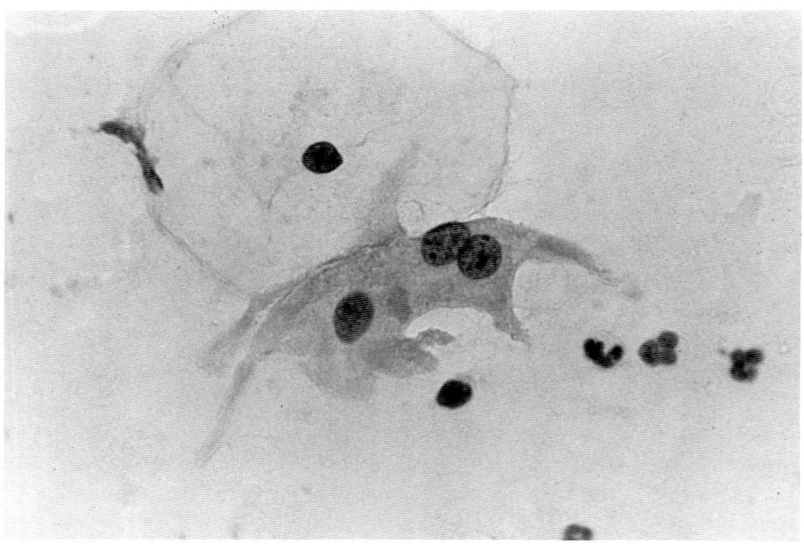

Fig. 3-11 Bizarre cell forms (intermediate cells). Also note the binucleation. (× 160.)

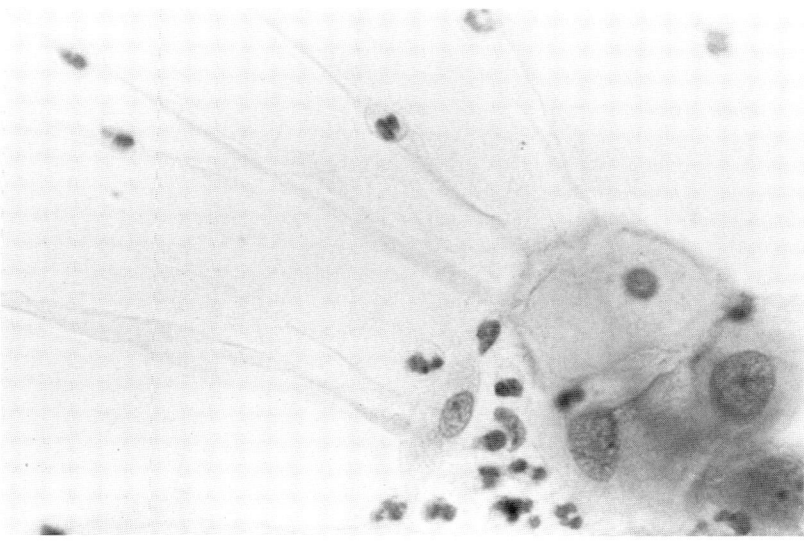

Fig. 3-12 This photograph shows "strings" of cytoplasm of intermediate cells smeared across the slide, characteristically seen in post-irradiation smears. Also note the nuclear enlargement of at least two of the intermediate cells. (× 160.)

Intermediate Radiation Reaction

According to Murad and August, an intermediate[10] reaction typifies repair and is cytologically reflected in a sheetlike arrangement of cells (Figs. 3-14 and 3-15). Spiderlike cells showing cytoplasmic extensions may be present. Mohr regards the presence of phagocytosis as the most important element in the intermediate reaction.[11]

Chronic (Late, Persistent) Radiation Changes

In most patients, acute radiation changes disappear and subsequent smears are normal. However, in a few, highly bizarre cells persist. In these patients, nuclear or cytoplasmic enlargement, hazy cell borders, atrophic "dry" smear, and occasionally, nuclear hyperchromasia often may be observed.[15] Bizarre cells, multinucleated histiocytes, and cells with altered staining characteristics are particularly characteristic of chronic radiation effects.[16] These alterations may persist indefinitely; there are, for instance, examples of changes persisting for as long as 35 years after completion of radiation therapy (and perhaps even longer).[12]

Smear Background

In irradiated patients, the smear background should be examined carefully in addition to assessing the cells on the smear. In most instances, the background is either clean or shows acute inflammatory cells, often arranged in aggregates referred to as "pus balls" (Fig. 3-14).[10] Occasionally, however, one may find hemolyzed blood and necrotic debris. In such cases the slide should be examined carefully for the presence of rare tumor cells. The mere presence of this type of background, even in the absence of malignant cells, may portend a poor prognosis with later development of recurrent carcinoma.[10] A lacy background has been considered by some to be specific for radiation injury,[10] and may reflect alteration(s) in the mucus. It is usually seen in intermediate and chronic radiation reactions.

Host Response

Cancer cells show radiation changes much earlier than do benign cells. Usually, malignant cells start to disappear from the smear within 1 week of the onset of irradiation and should be absent within 1 month after completion of the radiation regimen. Aside from radiation effect on malignant cells, the mor-

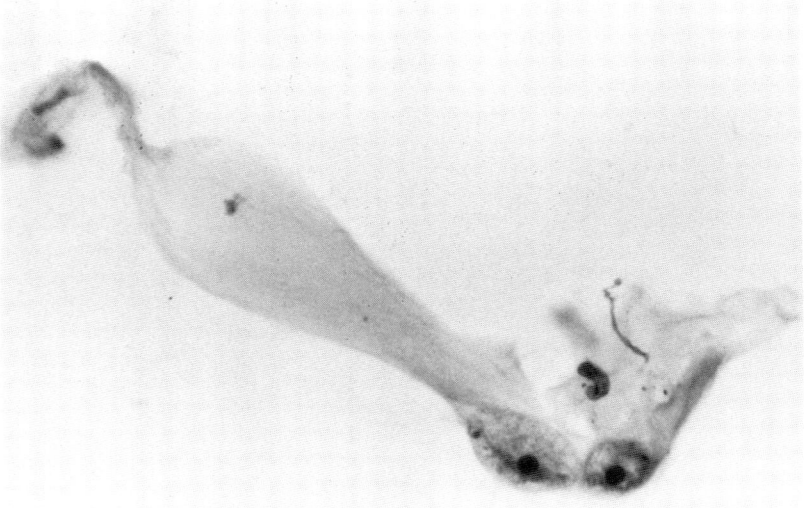

Fig. 3-13 Post-irradiation smear. Bizarre cell forms (probable intermediate cell). (× 160.)

phology of nonmalignant components has long been suspected to have some bearing on (1) the outcome of the patient's tissue response to radiation injury (namely, the chances of failure of wound healing to take place) and (2) the ultimate tumor response to radiation therapy. Within a short time (i.e., a few days to a week) of onset of irradiation, there may be a profuse outpouring of acute inflammatory cells. Sometimes these cells break down with no further tissue response apparent, so that the smear background shows only necrotic and hemolyzed blood. This finding indicates a poor host response, and in such cases, the chances of poor wound healing and tissue breakdown are high. However, this type of reaction may be supplanted, in time, by the presence of lymphocytes and endothelial cells. This indicates satisfactory host response and good healing.[16] It is interesting and yet puzzling that, in some patients, profound changes are seen in the benign cells of the smear after irradiation, whereas in others, this does not occur.

The percentage of superficial squamous cells displaying cytoplasmic vacuolization was considered by Graham to correlate with the patient's tumor response or so-called radiation response (RR). A figure of 68 percent was empirically suggested as the cut-off point between those designated as responders and those considered to be nonresponders.[15]

Radiation Changes in the Endometrium and Endocervix

The same principles mentioned earlier apply to radiation-induced changes in the endometrium and endocervix. Multinucleated cells are most commonly seen in CVE smears.[10] Endocervical cells often react to radiation by excessive shedding and less commonly exhibit the other cytologic alterations that were described previously.[11]

Post-Irradiation Smears (General Appearance)

Post-irradiation CVE smears may vary somewhat from patient to patient, but they often show an atrophic pattern in which parabasal and even basal cells may be seen. Some of these cells appear as bare nuclei which, at times, are arranged in clusters; others show cytoplasmic or nuclear vacuolation. Other cells that occur in variable combinations include epithelial cells with bizarre forms and enlarged or multiple nuclei, some of which exhibit degenerative changes, and histiocytes, including multinucleated and bizarre forms. Not all multinucleated cells seen in post-irradiation smears are necessarily of histiocytic origin. In fact, the exact nature of such cells is not entirely clear.[10] The number of histiocytes may correlate with

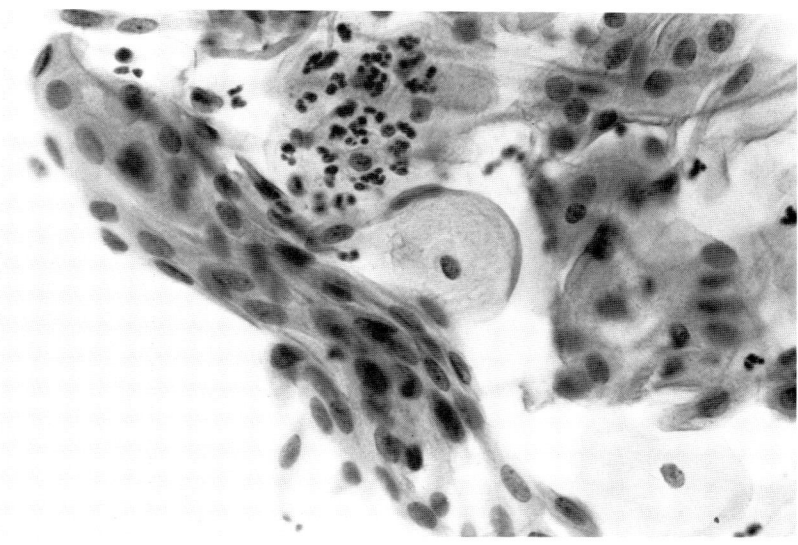

Fig. 3-14 Repair in irradiated cervicovaginal mucosa. Note the typically elongated squamous cells with vesicular nuclei. A "poly ball" is also present. (× 100.)

the patient's tumor response to irradiation. Rarely, fibroblasts exhibiting radiation-type changes may be seen.

Postradiotherapy vaginal smear cytology in cervical cancer not only can detect cancer cells, but may also be helpful in identifying responders and nonresponders.[17] Various aspects of smear cytology have been correlated with clinical outcome, including karotypic index,[18] percentage of histiocytes and superficial cells in pretreatment smears,[19] percentage of

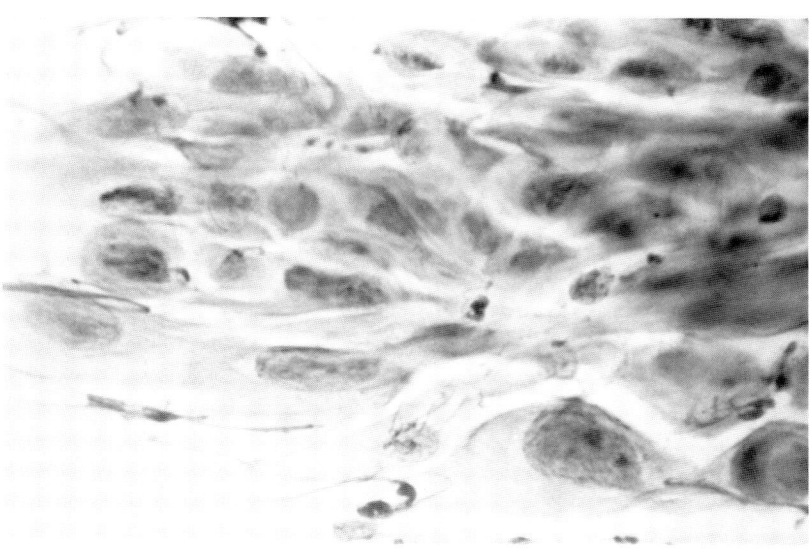

Fig. 3-15 Radiation repair. Note the typical repair arrangement of the keratinocytes, as well as the nuclear enlargement that is consistent with radiation effect. (× 160.) (See Plate 3-7.)

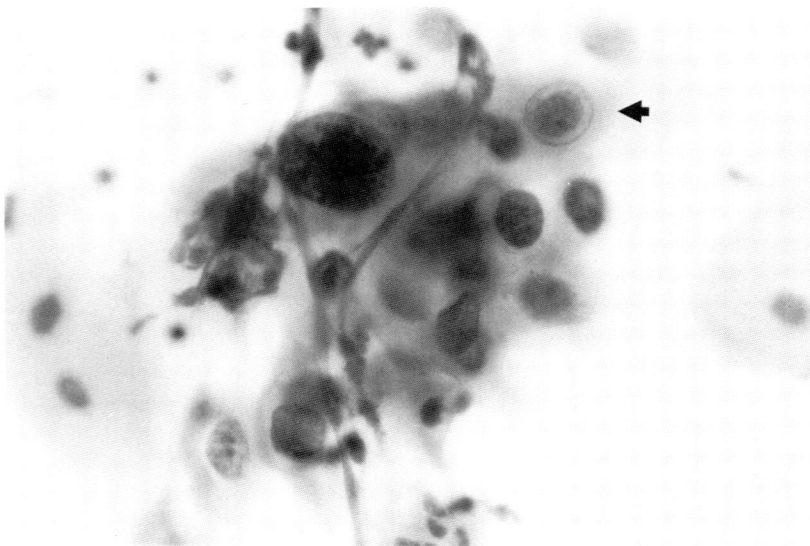

Fig. 3-16 Post-irradiation dysplasia. Note the marked nuclear abnormalities, including parachromatin clearing and clumping and nuclear enlargement. However, there is abundant cytoplasm present, and the nuclear/cytoplasmic ratio is relatively maintained. To the right of the dysplastic keratinocyte is a cell that is probably an intermediate cell with an ill-defined nucleus but a well-defined cytoplasmic vacuole (*arrowhead*). (× 160.)

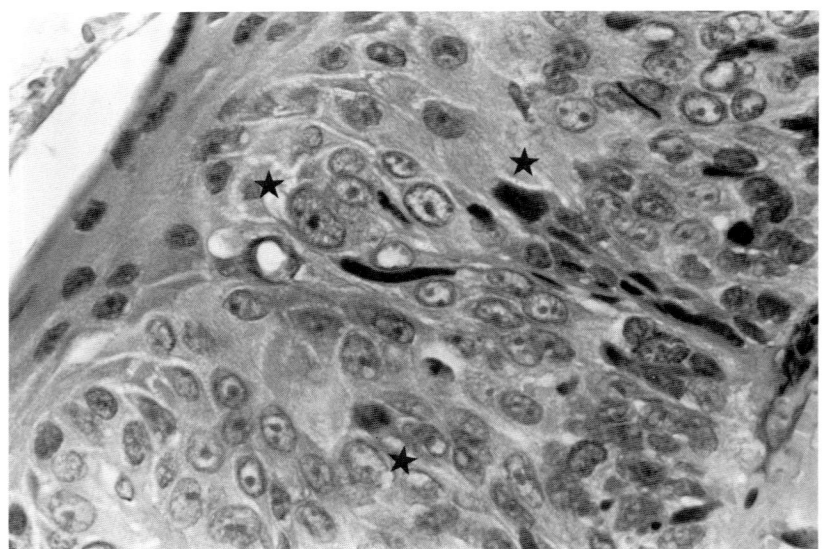

Fig. 3-17 Post-irradiation dysplasia of the cervical mucosa evident on biopsy. This photograph shows the entire thickness of the epithelium with the surface toward the left upper corner. The area bordered by asterisks shows dysplastic keratinocytes occupying approximately the lower three-quarters of the epithelial thickness. (× 100.)

CYTOPATHOLOGY OF IRRADIATION AND CHEMOTHERAPY   153

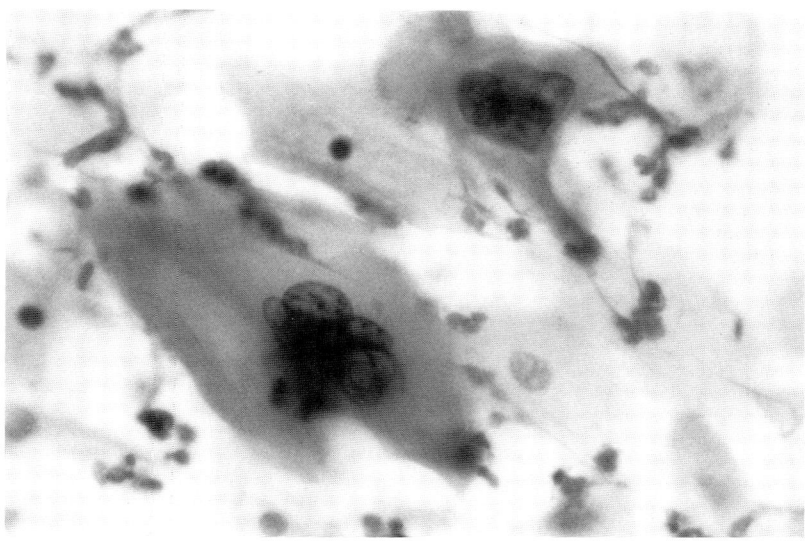

Fig. 3-18 Post-irradiation dysplasia (same case as in Fig. 3-16). Multinucleated, dysplastic keratinocytes are evident. Note the chromatin-clumping and parachromatin-clearing with proportionate nuclear enlargement. (× 160.)

basal cells showing finely vacuolated cytoplasm after treatment (an indication of SR)[19,20] and the appearance of smear background (i.e., hemolyzed erythrocytes, necrosis).[21] At various times during and after completion of therapy, the RR has also been correlated with prognosis.[13,14,21,22]

Post-Irradiation Dysplasia

Post-irradiation dysplasia should be distinguished cytologically from residual, recurrent, as well as persistent carcinoma (Figs. 3-16 to 3-20, Plates 3-1 to 3-5). Features indicating post-irradiation dysplasia

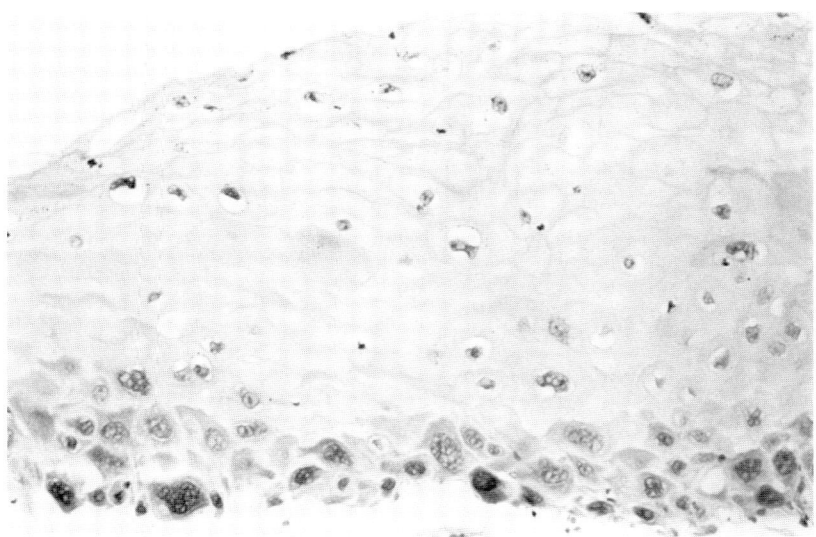

Fig. 3-19 Post-irradiation dysplasia evident on biopsy. Note the highly abnormal keratinocytes near the basement membrane. (× 50.) (See Plate 3-8.)

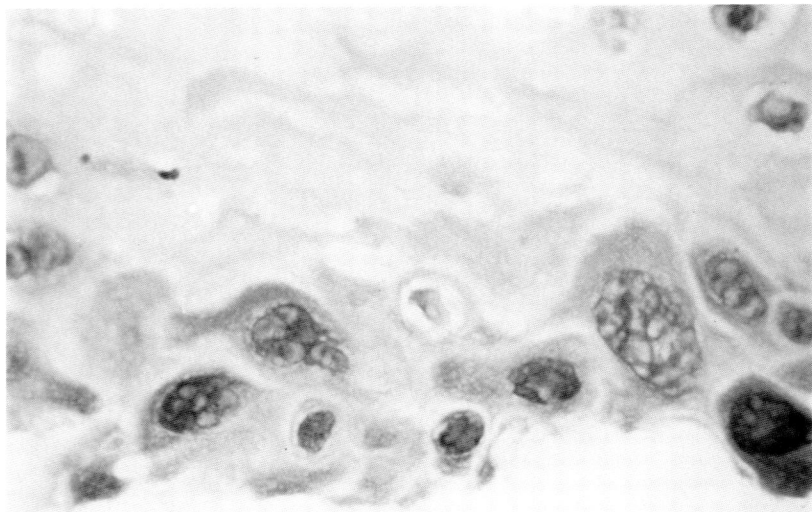

Fig. 3-20 Higher magnification of Fig. 3-19 shows markedly bizarre cells. (× 160.) (See Plate 3-9.)

include disposition of abnormal cells in groups rather than singly, a smudgy eosinophilic appearance of the cell cytoplasm, indistinct cell borders, and generally evenly distributed granular chromatin. Cytologic features of radiation effect, such as intranuclear/intracytoplasmic vacuoles, which are particularly evident at the periphery of the cell groups, may help to diagnose post-irradiation dysplasia.[10] Post-irradiation dysplasia may be observed at any time from 6 months to 21 years after completion of a course of

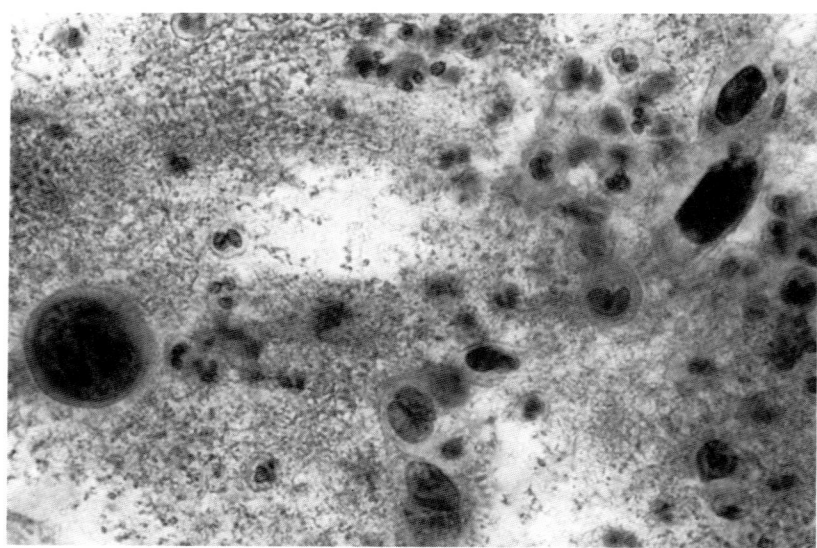

Fig. 3-21 CVE Smear. Irradiated carcinoma cells. Note the extremely high nucleocytoplasmic ratio in the cell near the left border of the photograph and the "dirty" granular background. (× 160.)

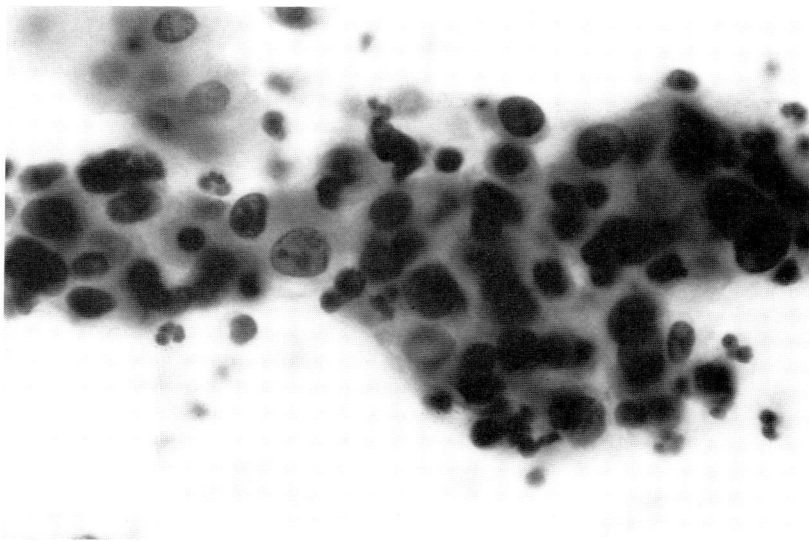

Fig. 3-22 Recurrent squamous carcinoma of the cervix after a previous course of irradiation. Note the generally "healthy" appearance of the cancer cells. (× 160.)

radiation therapy for cervical cancer. The first clue to its occurrence may be the presence of superficial squamous cells in the smear (namely, an estrogen-like effect) 6 months after completion of radiation therapy. Some observers have established a minimum disease-free interval of 18 months to 2 years between onset of irradiation and the appearance of abnormal cells as a requisite for diagnosing post-irradiation dysplasia. Several studies point to the ominous nature of post-irradiation dysplasia in terms of

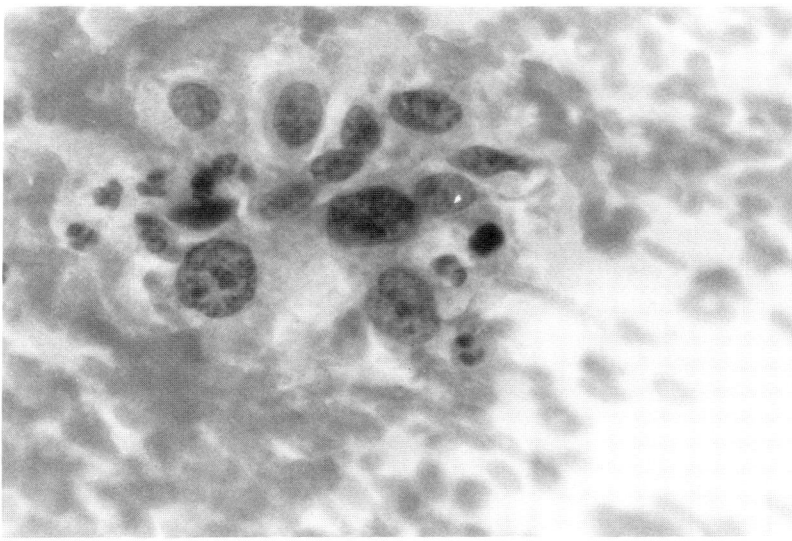

Fig. 3-23 Irradiated squamous carcinoma. Note the bloody and necrotic background, markedly increased nuclear/cytoplasmic ratio, and the coarse chromatin with parachromatin-clearing. (Papanicolaou stain, × 160.)

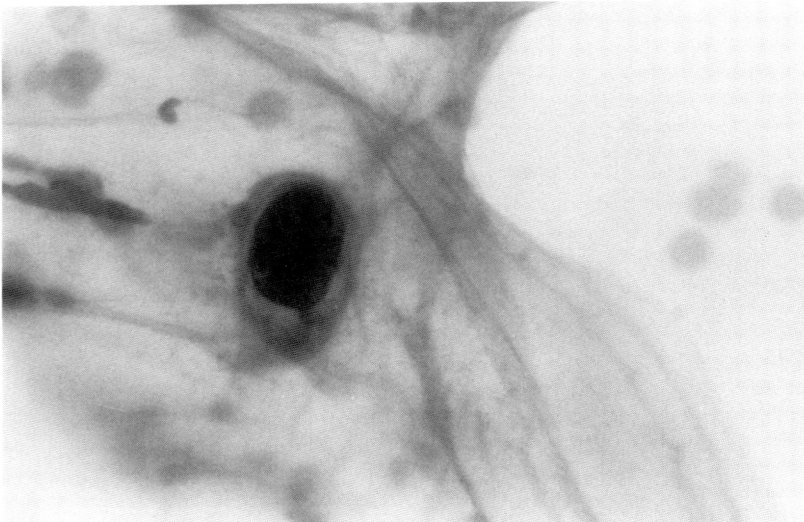

Fig. 3-24 Irradiated squamous carcinoma. Note the perinuclear halo in the carcinoma cell. (× 160.)

its high rate of progression to invasive carcinoma, as well as its association with residual or recurrent cancer elsewhere in the pelvis (e.g., the lymph nodes) or with distant metastases.[15,23,24] The chances of these adverse findings is even greater when post-irradiation dysplasia occurs within the first 3 years after irradiation.[24]

The presence of cancer cells in cervicovaginal smears within the first 4 months after beginning irradiation or 1 month after completion of radiotherapy

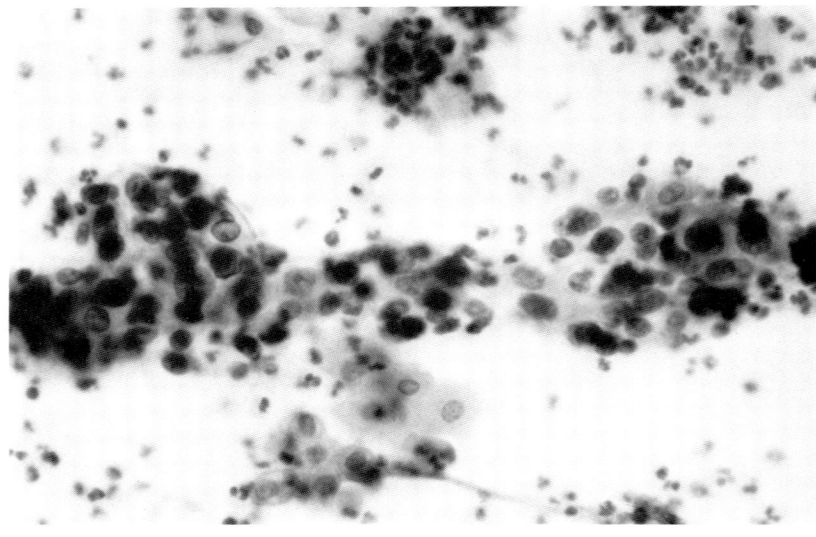

Fig. 3-25 Irradiated squamous carcinoma, recurrent. Note the "healthy" appearance of the unaffected cancer cells. (× 100.) (See Plate 3-10.)

has no implications with regard to success of treatment. However, persistence of tumor cells in the smears beyond this period indicates recurrent cancer (Figs. 3-21 to 3-25, Plates 3-6 to 3-10).[25] If there is no period during which cancer cells are absent in the smear, the condition is sometimes referred to as "radiation-persistent cancer." In such cases, the cells on the smear do not show detectable radiation changes. A few cells, however, may show nuclear/cytoplasmic enlargement.[10] Recurrent carcinomas have been classified into early and late forms, depending on the length of the cancer-cell-free interval (at least 1 month after completion of irradiation for early recurrent carcinoma and 5 years in the case of late recurrent carcinoma). In cases of recurrent cancer, radiation changes are often absent, both in cancer cells and in benign cells on the smear. In early recurrent carcinomas, the tumor cells either present at syncytia with ill-defined cell borders and prominent nucleoli (similar to microinvasive carcinoma) or as small lymphocyte-like cells arranged singly and in small groups.[10] The smears show variable but at times marked tumor diathesis. A predominant estrogen pattern is sometimes seen at or before the appearance of tumor cells.[26,27] In late recurrent carcinoma, a two-cell population, composed of distinctly keratinizing cells as well as rounded discohesive cells with cyanophilic cytoplasm and well-defined cell borders, is encountered.[10]

EFFECTS OF IRRADIATION ON EXTRAGENITAL TISSUES

Overall, the cytopathology of radiation effect in extragenital organs is basically similar to that described for cervicovaginal mucosa.[16] Normal parenchymal or neoplastic cells within an organ may be affected primarily because of irradiation of that particular organ, or secondarily as a result of irradiation directed to a different organ (e.g., radiation-induced changes occurring in the lung during or after radiotherapy for breast cancer or Hodgkin's disease involving the mediastinum).

Lower Respiratory Tract

Irradiation can affect bronchial respiratory epithelium, as well as alveolar cells.[15,28] The histopathology of pulmonary radiation injury will not be described here, but there are excellent references available on this subject.[1,3,6,29] Cytologic changes occur in both acute and chronic radiation injury.[15] In either case, extra care should be taken not to confuse irradiated benign respiratory epithelium with cancer cells. Changes in the acute phase include multinucleation of ciliated cells, proportionate nuclear and cytoplasmic enlargement, granular chromatin, prominent nucleoli, cytoplasmic vacuolation, and cellular elongation.[28] In acute radiation-induced pneumonitis, cell necrosis and "smeared" nuclear material may be prominent. Chronic changes range from mild to extreme atypia, and may include cytoplasmic eosinophilia or polychromasia, karyopyknosis, atypical cell forms, and apparent exfoliation of epithelial cells in cell ribbons. Squamous metaplasia, at times bizarre, may be present.[16,28] Fibroblasts may be seen in addition to bronchoalveolar cells in fine needle aspirates of the lung.[28] Carcinomatous cells may exhibit changes that are qualitatively similar to those described for benign cells. These changes may be more pronounced in squamous carcinoma than in other types of carcinoma.[16]

Oral Cavity

Irradiation changes are basically similar to those described for cervicovaginal epithelium.[15,16,30,31] The morphologic changes involving the nontumor cell population in the acute phase include cytoplasmic vacuolization, granularity, and polymorphonuclear leukocyte "invasion"; karyopyknosis and karyorrhexis; necrosis; and histiocytes.[32] Multinucleated epithelial cells and histiocytes may be present. Regenerated epithelial cells may have a bizarre appearance, suggesting cancer on initial examination. Tumor cells also exhibit changes, including nuclear and cytoplasmic swelling, multinucleation, and necrosis.[32]

Esophagus

Radiation-induced changes can occur as a result of radiotherapy to extra-esophageal chest organs or to the esophagus itself in patients with esophageal carcinoma, and may be demonstrated both in benign surface epithelium as well as in cells from esophageal squamous carcinoma. Radiation cytomorphology is similar to that described for the female genital tract,[15,33,34] and includes cellular enlargement with a proportionate increase in nuclear size, smudgy chromatin, pale nuclei, a disrupted nuclear membrane, multiple cytoplasmic vacuoles and polychromasia, intracytoplasmic neutrophilic migration, and necrosis.[33] Persistent or residual carcinoma may be diagnosed by examination of cytologic material, but this diagnosis should be made only on the basis of cells unaffected by radiation changes.[15]

Stomach, Small and Large Intestine, and Pancreas

The cytopathology of radiation changes in the stomach, small and large intestine, and pancreas has not been studied as extensively as that in the esophagus, perhaps because radiation therapy is often not the sole therapeutic modality used to treat cancer involving these organs.[16]

Urinary Tract

Urothelial changes reflecting radiation effect may be seen in urinary sediment. These changes can occur secondary to pelvic irradiation for extravesical cancers, such as cervical or rectal carcinoma, or in the urothelium adjacent to urothelial carcinoma. Likewise, cancer cells shed from urothelial carcinoma may exhibit radiation changes. Histologic examination may reveal radiation-induced lesions both in the urothelium as well as in the subjacent connective tissue stroma.[3]

Diagnosis of cervical carcinoma that has metastasized to the bladder in a patient who has undergone previous irradiation for primary cervical cancer may be difficult because the radiation effect on benign bladder epithelium may include nuclear hyperchromasia.[15] Urinary cytology has been helpful in the follow-up of patients with urothelial cancer treated with radiation as persistent or recurrent carcinoma may thus be diagnosed.[35] Radiation may eradicate invasive urothelial carcinoma, but carcinoma in situ (CIS) may prove to be radioresistant, and this may be the only type of carcinoma present in cystectomy specimens from patients with irradiated invasive bladder cancers.[15] It should be noted, however, that differentiation between radiation effect on benign urothelial cells and urothelial CIS may pose problems. Koss states that "if a significant epithelial lesion is observed three months after completion of radiotherapy, the odds are very much in favor of a radioresistant carcinoma in situ."[35] This applies particularly to small biopsy specimens. Indeed, histologic confirmation of cytologically diagnosed cancer in an irradiated bladder may be difficult because of marked scarring. Radiation effect on benign urothelium in cytologic material is basically similar to that found in other epithelia, and includes nuclear swelling or breakdown, as well as cytoplasmic vacuolation and eosinophilia.[15] "Blown-up" nuclei and karyopyknosis may be observed in irradiated urothelial cancer cells. A favorable response to radiotherapy may be indicated by a marked decrease in the number of cancer cells in urinary sediment over a period of time.[15,36]

Serous Cavities

Although literature on radiation cytopathology of serous membranes and effusions is relatively scarce, the changes described are generally similar to those observed in epithelial cells of mucous membranes. Such changes include proportionate cellular and nuclear enlargement; cytoplasmic vacuolation; abnormal mesothelial cell shapes (such as spindle forms); nuclear hyperchromasia (simulating cancer cells); and binucleation.[15,16] Rosette formation and nuclear vacuolation of mesothelial cells have also been described.[37] Morphologic alterations of irradiated cancer cells in effusions are variable, and may include extensive karyorrhexis of tumor cells in such neoplasms as lymphomas.

EFFECTS OF CHEMOTHERAPY

Increasing use of chemotherapeutic agents, often in multiple-agent regimens and rather complex protocols, has afforded cytopathologists and histopathologists the opportunity to observe morphologic alterations in various cells. Because these agents are often administered intravenously, the morphologic changes may affect cells of different organs. These effects most often involve epithelial cells.[15,38] Furthermore, multiple chemotherapeutic agents are often administered to patients with cancer, and it may not be easy or even possible to determine the effect(s) of an individual drug in this setting. The therapy-induced atypias (TIAs) that are reported to occur with commonly used chemotherapeutic agents (Figs. 3-1 and 3-2) are discussed in the following sections.

Adriamycin

Besides the effect of Adriamycin on normal urothelium in experimental situations,[39] human esophageal epithelial atypia has also been described.[40]

Bleomycin

The cytologic alterations caused by the use of bleomycin in humans have been debated. This is partly because the agent has often been used in conjunction with other chemotherapeutic agents, with and without irradiation.[38] The main pathology has been in the lung, where increases in the number of type II pneumocytes and bronchial squamous metaplasia have been noted.[41,42] A high frequency of ciliary loss in the bronchial cells; an increased nuclear/cytoplasmic ratio of alveolar epithelial cells; and changes in buccal squamous cells, such as binucleation, nuclear hyperchromasia, and koilocytosis, have been described.[41] These patients had received other chemotherapeutic drugs in addition to bleomycin. Histologic examination may reveal diffuse alveolar damage and interstitial fibrosis,[43] and the picture may thus simulate busulfan-induced changes in the lung.[15]

Bischloroethylnitrosourea

Enlargement of alveolar cells, probable type II pneumocytes, and pulmonary interstitial fibrosis have been reported to occur with the use of bischloroethylnitrosourea (BCNU).[38,44]

Busulfan

Busulfan (Myleran) is well known for producing profound cytologic abnormalities in the epithelia of various organs.[15,45–47] These abnormalities are particularly evident in the lung, cervix, vagina, and urinary bladder, although changes elsewhere in the urinary tract and pancreas have also been described.[46] In essence, the alterations mimic those seen with irradiation but are more pronounced.[40] Bizarrely shaped cells, nuclear enlargement and hyperchromasia which may be extreme, coarsened chromatin, single or multiple large nucleoli, variations in nuclear size and shape, cytomegaly, and cytoplasmic vacuolization may be observed. The affected cells in the lung include type II pneumocytes[48,49] and, probably, terminal bronchiolar epithelium.[28,38] In the uterine cervix, the changes are observed in the squamous epithelium, and may resemble koilocytotic atypia, dysplasia, or in situ carcinoma. The smear pattern is usually atrophic. These abnormalities may persist even after therapy is discontinued.

Chlorambucil

The use of chlorambucil has been associated with various pulmonary effects, including increased nuclear size and prominent nucleoli in bronchial cells.[28] In addition, atypical and proliferated alveolar lining cells with pulmonary fibrosis mimicking busulfan lung[50] have been described.

Cyclophosphamide

The primary cytologic abnormalities associated with cyclophosphamide involve the urinary bladder epithelium, although endothelial and smooth muscle damage has also been described in experimental situations.[15] The effects of cyclophosphamide were first reported by Koss and colleagues in experiment with the rat bladder.[51,52] Cyclophosphamide-induced hemorrhagic cystitis in humans is also a well-recognized phenomenon. Bladder epithelial changes may include nuclear enlargement, hyperchromasia, and multinucleation (Fig. 3-2). At times, cyclophosphamide-induced cytologic abnormalities may be indistinguishable from carcinoma. With cessation of therapy, however, these changes tend to regress. In a few instances, carcinoma of the bladder or ureter, and fibrosis of the bladder wall have been thought to be associated with cyclophosphamide use.[15] Changes in esophageal epithelium have also been described, including cellular enlargement, nuclear hyperchromasia, pyknosis, multinucleation, large and irregular nucleoli, and cytoplasmic vacuolation.[40] Lung changes secondary to the use of this agent include cytologic alterations of type II pneumocytes—namely, anisocytosis, poikilocytosis, nuclear hyperchromasia, pyknosis, karyorrhexis, and multinucleation—as well as severe cytoplasmic vacuolization, eosinophilia, and phagocytosis of nuclear material.[38,43,53,54] Interstitial fibrosis has also been observed.

Melphalan

Fatal pulmonary fibrosis and atypical epithelial proliferation (presumably of alveolar type II pneumocytes) have been reported to occur as a result of the use of melphalan.[55] However, the study in which these changes were reported involved examination of histologic material only.

Methotrexate

Methotrexate, a folic acid antagonist, may produce cytologic abnormalities usually observed with folic acid deficiency.[38,43] Bronchial and intestinal epithelial changes include cell enlargement, variation in cell shape, nuclear hyperchromasia, and chromatin-clumping.[56] Atypia of alveolar pneumocytes has also been described.[57,58]

Mitomycin C

Degeneration and vacuolization, chromatin clumping and nucleoli in superficial cells, and excessive shedding of normal, as well as papillary, urothelium are among the changes that have been described following intravesical administration of mitomycin C in humans.[59,60]

Thiotepa (Triethylenethiophosphoramide)

Thiotepa, also known as triethylenethiophosphoramide, is basically used as a topical chemotherapeutic medication in the treatment of bladder carcinoma. Its effects on normal and abnormal urothelium have been studied by various investigators.[61-64] Changes similar to those associated with irradiation, such as cellular and nuclear enlargement, abnormal cell shapes, multinucleation, extensive degenerative changes, karyorrhexis, cytoplasmic vacuolization, and cytoplasmic granules that stain brownish on Papanicolaou stain and purple on May-Grünwald-Giemsa (MGG) stain, have been described.[65] Multinucleation, marked nuclear enlargement, altered cytoplasmic staining, and cytoplasmic granulation (so-called freckles) have been observed in malignant urothelial cells following administration of thiotepa.[65] Several studies of this agent by Murphy et al. have revealed degenerative changes, excessive exfoliation, multinucleation, and cytoplasmic vacuolization of urothelial cells without significant atypia.[38,61-64]

ACKNOWLEDGMENTS

I wish to express my appreciation for the valuable assistance offered by the staff of the Department of Pathology at (LAC)-USC Medical Center in Los Angeles (particularly C.P. Schwinn, M.D., P.T. Chandrasoma, M.D., and Carol Carriere, C.T. [A.S.C.P.], C.M.I.A.C.) in preparing the photomicrographs used in this chapter. I also wish to thank Sue Harris, and Sarah Witherby for superb secretarial assistance.

REFERENCES

1. Ackerman LV: The pathology of radiation effect on normal and neoplastic tissue. AJR 114:447, 1972
2. Casarett GW: Radiation Histopathology. Vols. 1 and 2. CRC Press, Boca Raton, FL, 1980
3. Fajardo LF, Berthrong M: Radiation injury in surgical pathology. Am J Surg Pathol 2:159, 1978 (part 1); 5:153, 1981 (part 2): 5:273, 1981 (part 3)
4. Hall EJ: Radiobiology for the Radiologist. 3rd Ed. JB Lippincott, Philadelphia, 1988
5. Rubin P. Casarett GW: Clinical Radiation Pathology. Vol. 1, WB Saunders, Philadelphia, 1968
6. White DC: An Atlas of Radiation Histopathology. Technical Information Center, Office of Public Affairs, U.S. Energy Research and Development Administration, Washington, DC, 1975
7. Giantoli RL, Atkinson BF, Ernst CS et al: Atkinson's Correlative Atlas of Colposcopy, Cytology and Histopathology. JB Lippincott, Philadelphia, 1987
8. King E: University of California–San Francisco Cytology Training Manual
9. Boschann HW: Radiation changes in benign cells of the female reproductive tract. p. 254. In Wied GL, Koss LG, Reagan JW (eds): The Tutorials of Cytology.

Compendium on Diagnostic Cytology. 6th Ed. Vol. IV. International Academy of Pathology, Chicago, 1988
10. Murad TM, August C: Radiation-induced atypia. A review. Diagn Cytopathol 1:137, 1985
11. Boschann HW: Cytology and histology of effect of ionizing radiation on the female genital tract. In Tutorials on Cytology, International Cytology Slide Sets. Vol. XVII. 1974
12. Graham RM: The Cytologic Diagnosis of Cancer. 3rd Ed. WB Saunders, Philadelphia, 1972
13. Ceelen GH: Persistent radiation changes in vaginal smears and their meaning for the prognosis of squamous cell carcinoma of the cervix. Acta Cytol 10:350, 1966
14. Moore JG, Chang NH, Scott E et al: The early assessment of irradiation therapy in cervical cancer. Am J Obstet Gynecol 86:677, 1963
15. Koss LG: Diagnostic Cytology and its Histopathologic Bases. 2nd Ed. JB Lippincott, Philadelphia, 1979
16. Von Haam E: Radiation cell changes. p. 239. In Wied GL, Koss LG, Reagan JW (eds): The Tutorials of Cytology. Compendium on Diagnostic Cytology. 6th Ed. Vol. IV. International Academy of Pathology, Chicago, 1988
17. Von Haam E, Alber R: Recurrent carcinoma and presence of radiation cell changes. Acta Cytol 3:415, 1959
18. Rubio CA, Hralec S, Pareja A: The value of cytohormonal studies (karyotypic index) for detecting recurrence of carcinoma. Acta Cytol 11:176, 1967
19. Graham RM: Cytologic prognosis in cancer of the cervix. Am J Obstet Gynecol 79:700, 1960
20. Masabuchi K, Kubo H, Tenjin Y et al: Follow-up studies by cytology in cancer of the cervix uteri after treatment. Acta Cytol 13;323, 1969
21. Yannopoulos K, Gusberg SB: Radiosensitivity testing, virulence indices and stromal reaction in carcinoma of the cervix uteri. p. 131. In Sommers SC, Rosen PP (eds): Pathology Annual. Vol. 12. Appleton-Century-Crofts, East Norwalk, CT, 1977
22. Agnew AM, Fidler HK, Boyes DA: Evaluation of radiation response. Am J Obstet Gynecol 79:698, 1960
23. Koss LG, Melamed MR, Daniel WW: In situ epidermoid carcinoma of cervix and vagina following radiotherapy for cervix cancer. Cancer 14:353, 1961
24. Patten SF: Postradiation dysplasia of the uterine cervix: Cytopathology and clinical significance. p. 261. In Wied GL, Koss LG, Reagan JW (eds): The Tutorials of Cytology. Compendium on Diagnostic Cytology. 5th Ed. Vol. IV. International Academy of Pathology, Chicago, 1983
25. Marcial VA, Blanco MS, Delon E: Persistent tumor cells in the vaginal smear during the first year after radiation therapy of carcinoma of the uterine cervix. Prognostic significance. AJR 102:170, 1963
26. McLellan MT, McLellan CE: Prognostic value of the cornification index in patients treated for gynecologic cancer. Obstet Gynecol 18:131, 1962
27. Wachtel E: The prognostic significance of the karyotypic index after radical treatment for cancer of the female genital tract. Acta Cytol 11:35, 1962
28. Johnston WW, Frable WJ: Diagnostic Respiratory Cytopathology. Monographs in Diagnostic Cytopathology. Vol. 1 Masson Publishing, New York, 1979
29. Warren S, Spencer J: Radiation reaction in the lung. AJR 43:682. 1940
30. Umiker W: Cytology in the radiotherapy of carcinoma of the oral cavity. Acta Cytol 9:296, 1965
31. Umiker W, Lampe I, Rapp R et al: Oral smears in the diagnosis of carcinoma and premalignant lesions. Oral Surg 13:897, 1960
32. Medar H, McGrew EA, Bulakow P et al: Atlas of Oral Cytology. USPHS Publication No. 1949, US Government Printing Office, Washington, DC
33. Takeda M: Atlas of Diagnostic Gastrointestinal Cytology. Igaku-Shoin, New York, 1983
34. Drake M: P. 82, In Wied GL (ed): Gastroesophageal Cytology. Monographs in Clinical Cytology. Vol. 10 S Karger AG, Basel, 1985
35. Koss LG: Tumors of the Bladder. Fascicle XI (new series). In Atlas of Tumor Pathology. Armed Forces Institute of Pathology, Washington, DC 1975
36. O'Morchoe PJ, Riad W, Cowles LT et al: Urinary cytologic changes after radiotherapy of renal transplants. Acta Cytol 20:132, 1976
37. Fentanes de Torres E, Guevara E: Pleuritis by radiation: Report of two cases. Acta Cytol 25:427, 1981
38. Buhang JN: Therapy-induced atypias (TIA) of benign pulmonary cells. In Common Problems in Cytology. American Society of Cytology, 1983
39. Rasmussen K, Peterson BL, Jacobo E et al: Cytologic effects of Thiotepa and adriamycin on normal urothelium. Acta Cytol 24:237, 1980
40. O'Morchoe PJ, Lee DC, Kozak CA: Esophageal cytology in patients receiving cytotoxic drug therapy. Acta Cytol 27:630, 1983
41. Bedrossian CWM, Carey BJ: Abnormal sputum cytopathology during chemotherapy with bleomycin. Acta Cytol 22:202, 1978
42. Simosato V, Baba K, Watanabe S: Pulmonary lesions produced by antitumor drugs. Studies on autopsy cases. Jap J Can Clin 17:21, 1971
43. Riddell RH: Pathology of Drug-induced and Toxic Diseases. Churchill Livingstone, New York, 1982
44. Bellot PA, Valdiserri RO: Multiple pulmonary lesions in a patient treated with BCNU (1, 3-Bis(2-Chloro-

ethyl)-1-Nitrosourea) for glioblastoma multiforme. Cancer 43:46, 1979
45. Koss LG, Melamed MR, Mayer K: The effect of busulfan on human epithelia. Am J Clin Pathol 44:385, 1965
46. Nelson BM, Andrews GA: Breast cancer and cytologic dysplasia in many organs after busulfan (Myleran). Am J Clin Pathol 42:37, 1964
47. Min KW, Gyorkey F: Interstitial pulmonary fibrosis, atypical epithelial changes and bronchiolar cell carcinoma following busulfan therapy. Cancer 22;1027, 1968
48. Rosenow EC: The spectrum of drug-induced pulmonary disease. Ann Intern Med 77:977, 1972
49. Sostman HD, Matthay RA, Putman CE: Cytotoxic drug-induced lung disease. Am J Med 62:608, 1977
50. Rose MS: Busulfan toxicity syndrome caused by chlorambucil. Br Med J. 2:123, 1975
51. Forni AM, Koss LG, Geller W: Cytological study of the effect of cyclophosphamide on the epithelium of the urinary bladder in man. Cancer 17:1348, 1964
52. Koss LG: A light and electron microscopic study of the effects of a single dose of cyclophosphamide on various organs in the rat. I. The urinary bladder. Lab Invest 16:44, 1967
53. Mark GJ, Lehimgar-Zadeh A, Ragsdale BD: Cyclophosphamide pneumonitis. Thorax 33:89, 1978
54. Patel AR, Shah PC, Rhee HR, et al: Cyclophosphamide therapy and interstitial fibrosis. Cancer 38:1542, 1976
55. Taetle R, Dickman PS, Feldman PS: Pulmonary histopathologic changes associated with melphalan therapy. Cancer 42:1239, 1978
56. Weston JT, Guin GH: Epithelial atypias with chemotherapy in 100 acute childhood leukemias. Cancer 8:168, 1955
57. Sostman HD, Matthay RA, Putman CE et al: Methotrexate-induced pneumonitis. Medicine 55:371, 1976
58. Sostman HD, Matthay RA, Putman CE: Cytotoxic drug-induced lung disease. Am J Med 62:608, 1977
59. Murphy WM, Saloway MS, Finebaum PJ: Pathological changes associated with topical chemotherapy for superficial bladder cancer. J Urol 126:461, 1981
60. Soloway MS, Murphy WM, Defuria MD et al: The effect of mitomycin C on superficial bladder cancer. J Urol 125:646, 1981
61. Murphy WM, Soloway MS, Lin CJ: Morphologic effects of Thiotepa on mouse urothelium. Acta Cytol 21:701, 1977
62. Murphy WM, Soloway MS, Lin CJ: Morphologic effects of Thiotepa on mammalian urothelium: Changes in abnormal cells. Acta Cytol 22:550, 1978
63. Murphy WM, Soloway MS: The effect of Thiotepa on developing and established mammalian bladder tumors. Cancer 45:870, 1980
64. Murphy WM, Soloway MS, Finebaum PJ: Pathological changes associated with topical chemotherapy for superficial bladder cancer. J Urol 126:461, 1981
65. DeVoogt HJ, Rathert P, Beyer-Boon ME: Urinary Cytology. Springer-Verlag, Berlin, 1977

4
Fine Needle Aspiration Cytology of the Breast

Britt-Marie Ljung

The interpretation of specimens obtained by fine needle aspiration (FNA) from the breast (and from most other organs) is based on the light microscopic appearance of single cells, cell clusters, and background material, and combines the approaches of exfoliative cytology and histology. If used correctly, fine needles (22-to 25-gauge) can collect abundant clusters of cells whose architecture can then be studied. On smears, the clusters appear to be three-dimensional; hence, the cell pattern is very different from the two-dimensional image produced by histologic methods. Although a fundamental knowledge of exfoliative cytology and histology is essential to FNA interpretation, FNA material also contains many unique features that cannot be appreciated with other preparations or deduced from previous experience in exfoliative cytology or surgical pathology. Therefore, these features must be studied specifically.[1] Furthermore, diagnostic criteria may differ markedly from one body site to another.

In order to achieve proper diagnostic accuracy, there must be abundant cell clusters and single cells available for interpretation. A diagnostic impression should be confirmed in numerous areas on one or several well-prepared slides. If it is necessary to search for cells, the material is most likely nondiagnostic, and repeat FNA or some other diagnostic procedure should be performed. It is also critical that the FNA findings be consistent with the clinical impression.

The FNA sampling technique has been described frequently,[2] and the literature often states how easy it is to perform. However, in my experience, shortcomings in the sampling technique are the most common reasons for failure to reach the correct diagnosis. One study by Barrows et al.[3] showed that the single most important factor for success was the level of experience of the clinician performing the biopsy. As with any procedure, FNA requires a certain amount of effort to master, and it is best to train with someone who is well acquainted with the technique. Simply reading about it frequently results in serious inadequacies. One of the most common misconceptions regarding the procedure is that cells are "sucked" from the biopsy site by pulling back on the syringe plunger. In truth, cells are collected by moving the sharp beveled needle tip back and forth within the target, dislodging tiny fragments of tissue. The suction merely helps to transport these already separated cell clusters further up into the needle.

The Papanicolaou stain is, by tradition, the most widely used stain, and is readily available in all cytology laboratories. Histopathologists are more accustomed to hematoxylin and eosin (H & E) stains, and may therefore prefer them to Papanicolaou stains; both stains, however, provide excellent nuclear detail. The Papanicolaou stain is specific for keratin, whereas H & E stains compare well to corresponding histologic tissue sections. The other main stain group is composed of the Romanowsky stains—the May-Grünwald-Giemsa (MGG), Wright-Giemsa, and Diff-Quick stains, among others—which require that the material be air-dried prior to processing. These stains enhance preservation of the cytoplasmic features and background material (mucin, proteinaceous fluid, colloid, etc.). Air-drying also retains a larger number of cells on the slides than does immersion in alcohol. The combination of alcohol-fixed and air-dried material is complementary, and provides optimal information.

The following material on the interpretation of breast FNA includes a description of the findings in normal breast tissue and benign lesions. Malignant tumors, both primary and metastatic, are then described. Finally, atypical lesions, for which a specific diagnosis frequently cannot be rendered by FNA, are discussed.

NORMAL BREAST TISSUE

Normal breast is composed of large amounts of adipose tissue, scant fibrous stroma, scattered ducts, and lobular units. FNA easily allows extraction of fairly large clusters of fat cells (Fig. 4-1) and usually, scant mammary epithelium, which is represented by single cells and small cell clusters (Fig. 4-2). The single cells often consist of bare nuclei that are about 1.5 to 2 times larger than a red cell. The clusters are generally small and monolayered, with intact cytoplasm. The chromatin pattern is even and bland, the stromal component is scant or absent, and the smear background is clean.

BENIGN BREAST LESIONS

Fibrocystic Change

Fibrocystic change encompasses a wide spectrum of disease that includes cyst formation, fibrosis, adenosis, epitheliosis, sclerosing adenosis, and areas with a fibroadenomatous pattern; one or several of these components may be present. Clinically, these lesions are classically ill-defined, with a nodular surface and a consistency varying from markedly firm to just slightly firmer than normal breast tissue. In cases in which there is a large amount of dense stroma, it may be difficult to move the needle back and forth within the target area. In this situation, a thinner needle (25-gauge) will usually slide more easily and collect more cells than the standard 22- or 23-gauge nee-

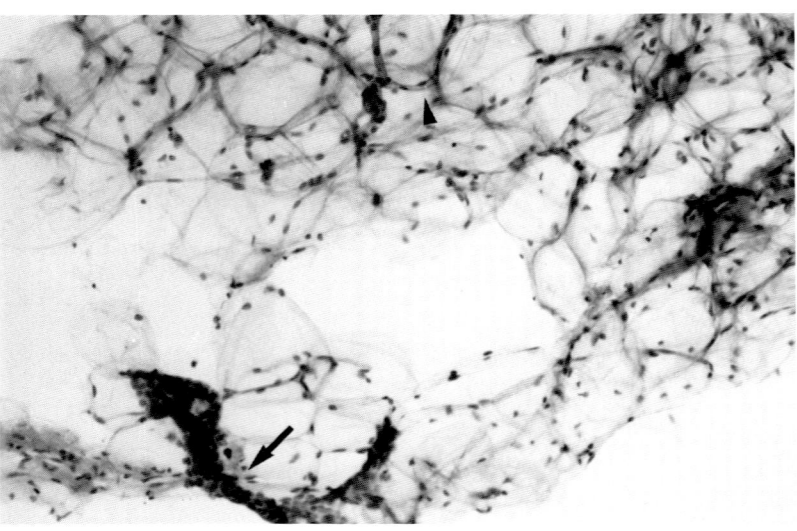

Fig. 4-1 Fragment of fat from normal breast tissue. A cluster of benign epithelium (*arrow*) and a branching capillary (*arrowhead*) are evident. (Papanicolaou stain, × 40.)

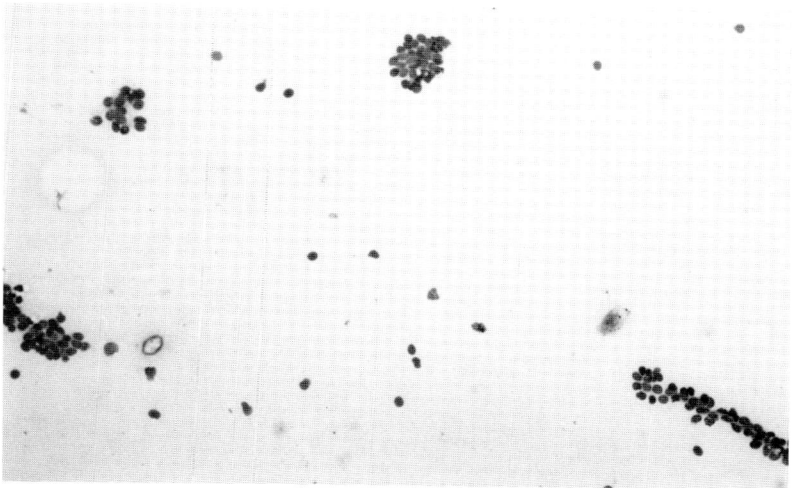

Fig. 4-2 Epithelium from normal breast tissue. Scant small cells without atypia appear singly and in small clusters. (MGG stain, × 40.)

dle. As always, when performing FNA, the lesion must be stabilized with one hand so that the needle can travel back and forth within the tissue instead of moving the lesion up and down under the skin.

The smears are usually scantly to moderately cellular, although occasionally, highly cellular smears may be obtained. Most clusters will be composed of small, bland, monotonous cells organized in monolayered sheets resembling a honeycomb (Fig. 4-3). Focally, the clusters may have two layers of cells, and may appear less organized than the typical honeycomb. Single cells are usually scant to moderate in number, but may be numerous. These cells, with their fine and even chromatin, tend to lose their cytoplasm when separated from each other during smearing, and thus appear as naked nuclei (Fig. 4-4). These cells

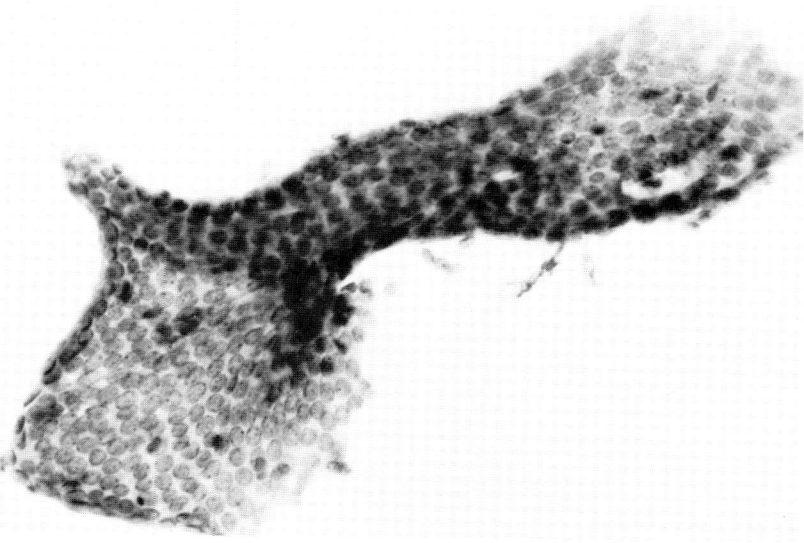

Fig. 4-3 Fibrocystic change. The regularly arranged sheet of epithelial cells is reminiscent of a honeycomb. (H & E stain, × 40.)

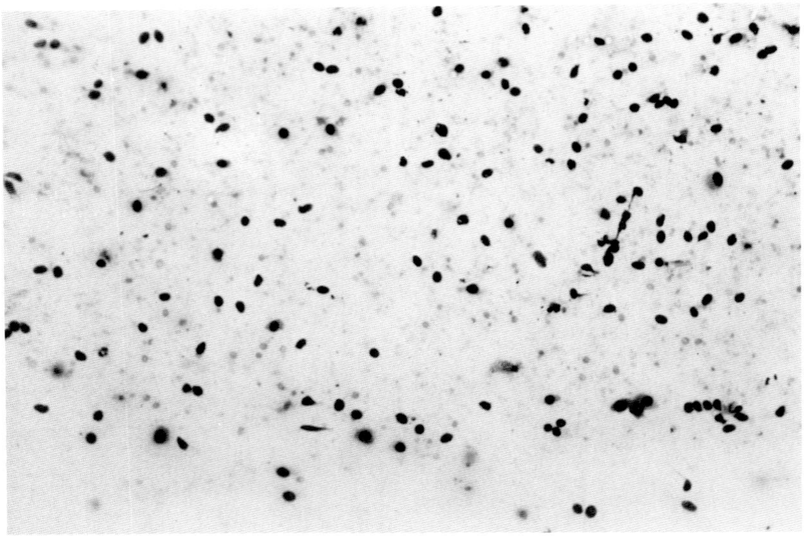

Fig. 4-4 Fibrocystic change. An area consisting of numerous small cells that have been stripped of their cytoplasm is shown. These naked, oval nuclei are present in virtually all benign breast lesions. (MGG stain, × 40.)

are round to oval and about 1.5 to 2 times the size of a red cell. Naked nuclei appear in virtually all benign lesions of the breast, but are usually absent in malignant neoplasms; hence, a definitive diagnosis of breast cancer should not be made when these cells are present. This phenomenon of naked nuclei is not generally seen in other organs, so this rule applies specifically to breast material. Of course, the presence of these naked, oval nuclei does not entirely rule out cancer, as the needle could conceivably traverse more than one lesion, collecting both benign and malignant cells. However, this circumstance is quite unusual in the breast (in contrast, for example, to the prostate gland).

The presence of apocrine cells indicates a cystic component. These cells are markedly larger than normal breast epithelium, mostly because of their abundant, well-defined, often granular cytoplasm (Fig. 4-5, Plate 4-1). When in clusters, apocrine cells usually appear in monolayered sheets, but occasionally, small papillations may be seen. Apocrine cells do not appear to be very cohesive, and therefore single cells often retain their cytoplasm; they should not, however, be confused with the single cells observed in smears from malignant lesions.

Occasionally, macrophages or stromal fragments, or both, are present in fibrocystic change. Neither finding is specific for any mammary lesion. The presence of an occasional mitotic figure is consistent with benign disease.

Cysts

Clinically, most cysts appear as well-defined, round masses. If there is a residual mass after removal of cyst fluid, a second aspiration should be performed. In most cases, the aspirated fluid will be clear to opaque, and will vary in color from yellow to dark green. Presence of cancer, then, is highly unlikely. If, however, the cyst contains blood that is not secondary to the procedure, or if the tissue fragments are visible to the naked eye, neoplasia is likely. Caution is advised in rendering a definitive diagnosis of cancer in cystic lesions as apocrine cells with degenerative features can appear to be markedly atypical, and clusters of histiocytes may mimic cancer (see the section on inflammation).

Fibroadenoma

Clinically, a fibroadenoma is a well-defined, rounded, movable mass in the breast. The mass may feel hard when palpated, but when aspirated, the needle will usually slide more easily than it does in

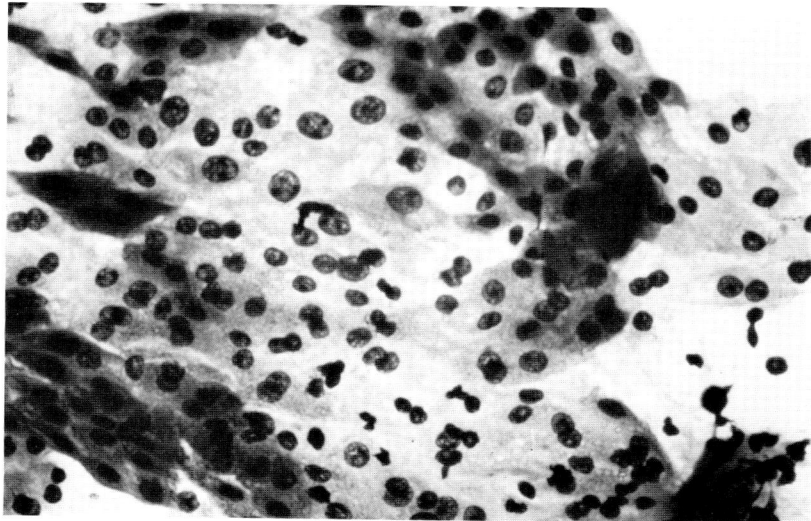

Fig. 4-5 Benign breast epithelium with apocrine change. Note the arrangement in a monolayered sheet, the abundant cytoplasm, and the enlarged nuclei in some cells. (MGG stain, × 100.) (See Plate 4-1.)

fibrocystic change because the stroma tends to be less dense. Generally, fibroadenomas are fairly easy to sample due to their abundant, easily dislodged epithelium. They produce cellular smears composed of both epithelium and stromal fragments.

There is considerable overlap in the FNA appearance of fibroadenomas and fibrocystic change, therefore, the clinical impression is important in differentiating between the two entities. There are certain differences, however, the most striking of which is that fibroadenomas often have numerous stromal fragments. These are most easily appreciated in the air-dried Romanowsky-stained smear, where they are a bright purple (Fig. 4-6, Plate 4-2). Because of

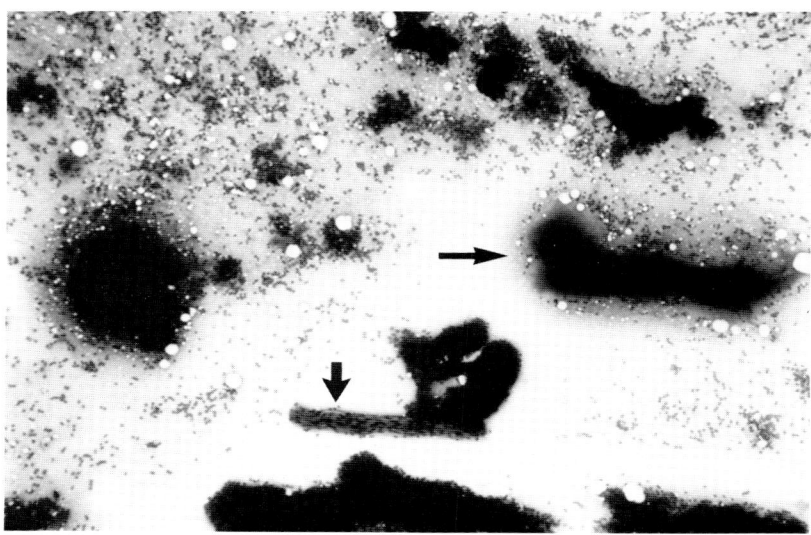

Fig. 4-6 Fibroadenoma, low-power magnification. Marked cellularity, cohesive epithelial clusters, metachromatic stroma (*thin arrow*), and a portion of a small vessel (*thick arrow*) are visible. (MGG stain, × 16.) (See Plate 4-2.)

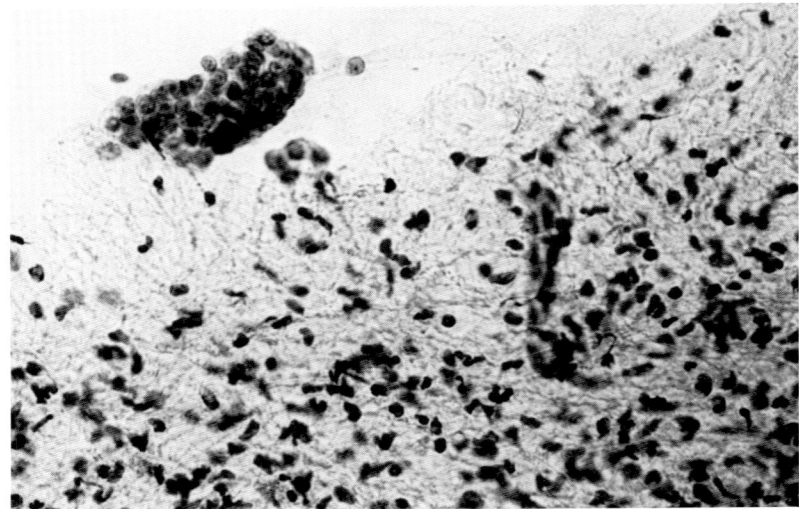

Fig. 4-7 Fibroadenoma. A small epithelial cluster is adjacent to a stromal fragment with oval to spindly cells that are loosely arranged on a fibrillary matrix. (Papanicolaou stain, × 100.)

the intense metachromatic stain, it may be difficult to study the stromal cells in the air-dried smears. The Papanicolaou stain provides better detail of these cells, which are oval and spindly, irregularly arranged, and several layers thick (Fig. 4-7). The stroma contrasts sharply with the epithelial component, which is seen in well-organized monolayered or bilayered sheets. Papillary formations occur, sometimes branching and resembling stag horns. A large proportion of the single cells are small, naked nuclei (Fig. 4-8).

Some fibroadenomas may contain clusters of larger cells with prominent nucleoli and coarse chromatin. Occasionally, these changes are prominent,

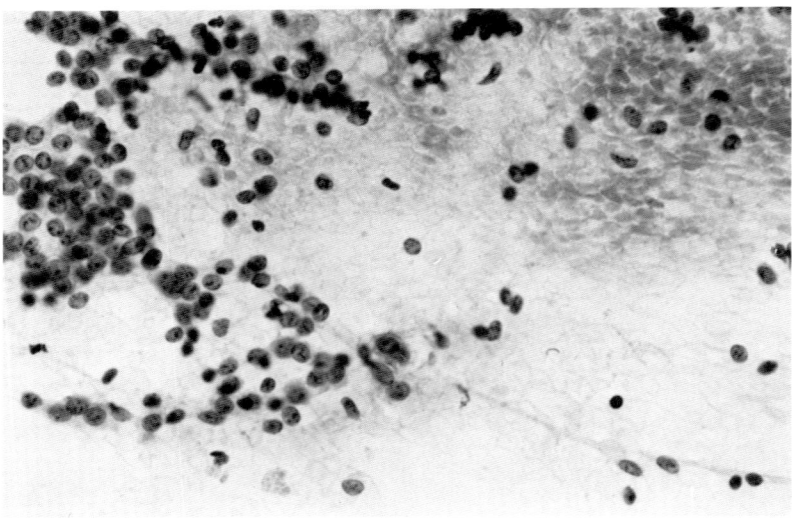

Fig. 4-8 Fibroadenoma. Epithelial cells without atypia are seen in a few clusters and also scattered singly. Numerous small, naked, oval nuclei are present. (Papanicolaou stain, × 40.)

and it may be very difficult to rule out carcinoma; however it is important to be cautious and not overcall these lesions. In such situations, an open biopsy should be requested. The presence of the naked nuclei is a very helpful feature.

Paget's Disease of the Nipple versus Benign Papilloma

Both Paget's disease of the nipple and benign papilloma may clinically appear as ulcerated areas on the nipple surface. Sampling for cytologic study can be accomplished by gently scraping the skin with a sharp edge until slight bleeding occurs. If a crust is present, it should be soaked and removed before sampling. The scraped material is then smeared onto a slide and air-dried or fixed in alcohol before staining. Specimens from patients with Paget's disease will typically show highly abnormal tumor cells that are easily recognizable as being malignant. The cells are large discohesive and have abnormal chromatin (Fig. 4-9A, Plate 4-3). The cells from the benign papilloma are cohesive, occurring almost exclusively in clusters. The individual cells are mostly small and the

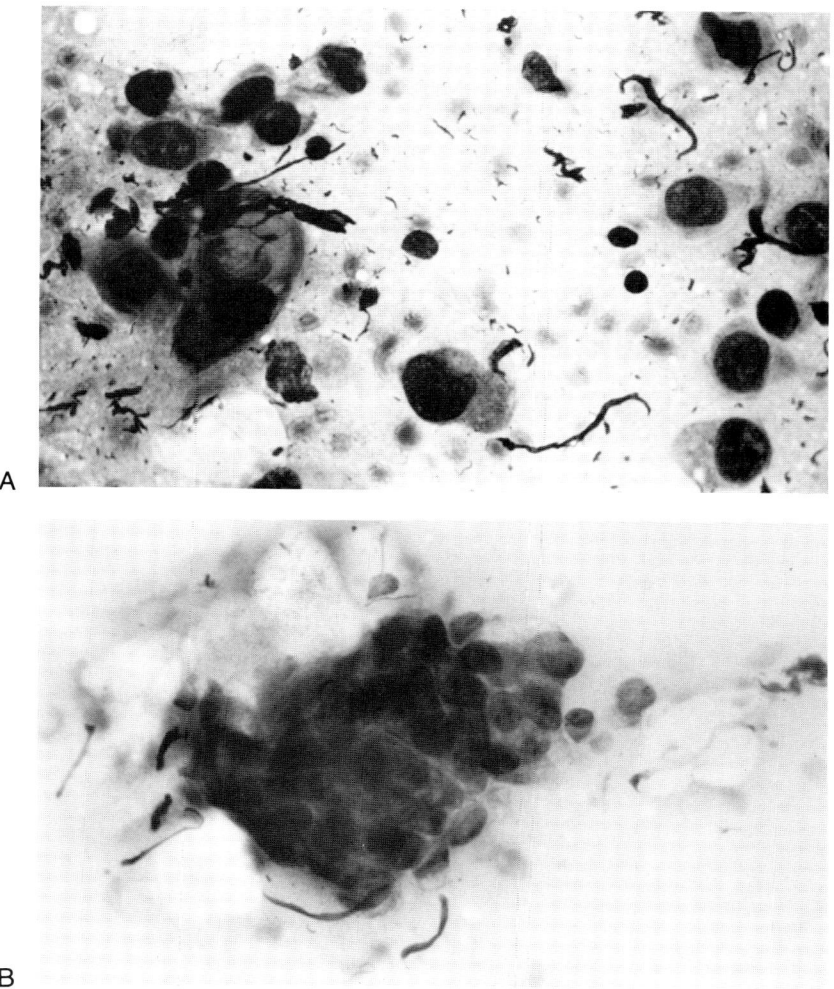

Fig. 4-9 **(A)** Paget's disease of the nipple. Discohesive, markedly atypical, and large tumor cells are seen. **(B)** Papilloma of the nipple. A cohesive cluster of epithelial cells with mild atypia is evident. Both specimens were harvested by gently scraping the surface of the nipple. (MGG stain, × 160.) (See Plates 4-3, 4-4.)

chromatin pattern is generally bland (Fig. 4-9B, Plate 4-4). However, occasional cells may be markedly large and may display prominent nucleoli.

Papillary Lesions

Papillomas usually manifest themselves as palpable masses in the central portion of the breast. When aspirated, these masses are occasionally characterized by an appreciable fluid component, in addition to numerous minute fragments of tissue. The smears often show a striking proteinaceous background with numerous macrophages. This fluid component is seldom seen on histologic examination because it drains out during dissection of the gross specimen. The epithelium appears singly and in clusters, may be monolayered, but also may be multilayered and irregularly arranged. Most papillomas contain columnar cells which, although not necessarily pathognomonic for a papillary lesion, should strongly indicate serious consideration of a papilloma in the differential diagnosis (Fig. 4-10). Papillary formations may or may not be present even when the material is strikingly abundant.

Well-differentiated papillary carcinoma is very similar to papilloma on cytologic examination. In my experience, the two are often indistinguishable. Therefore, it is recommended that all papillary lesions be excised for histologic confirmation. Fortunately, papillary lesions represent only a small fraction of all breast masses. The presence of apocrine metaplasia, as in histologic preparations, favors the diagnosis of a benign papilloma.

Diffuse papillomatosis can occur anywhere in the breast. It is less likely to cause a palpable mass and hence, is not frequently aspirated. Columnar cells are frequently present, as is benign epithelium, as seen in fibrocystic change.

The Breast in Pregnancy and Lactation

The breasts of pregnant and lactating women show identical features. Breast cells from pregnant women may often cause problems for the novice. Naturally, a complete history indicating whether or not the woman is pregnant is helpful; however, this may not be known early in gestation when cytologic changes may already have occurred. Atypical features in FNA smears should raise the possibility of gravidity.

The changes seen in pregnancy are quite specific, and are not difficult to recognize if one is alert to this condition. There is often increased cellularity compared to the usual benign breast lesion. Two cell populations are typically present; the one that may cause a diagnostic quandary consists of moderately large

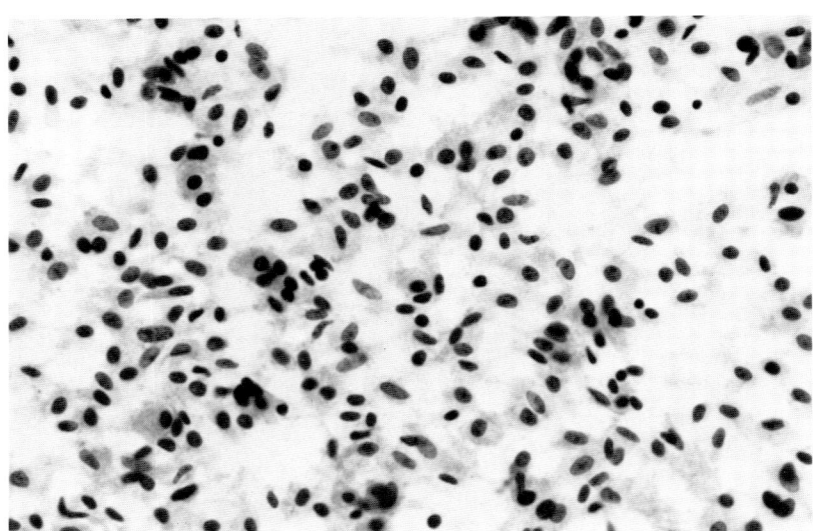

Fig. 4-10 Papilloma. Abundant single cells, most of which are columnar in shape, are pictured. Well-differentiated papillary carcinoma may yield similar material. Histologic examination is usually required for differentiation between these two entities. (Papanicolaou stain, × 40.)

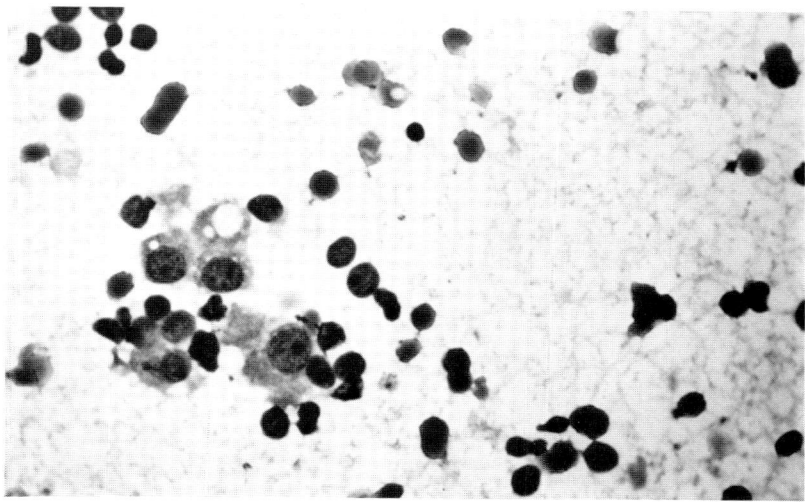

Fig. 4-11 Breast in pregnancy. High-power magnification. Small, oval, naked nuclei, as well as larger epithelial cells with a prominent nucleolus and abundant granular to vacuolated cytoplasm, are seen in a proteinaceous background. (MGG stain, × 160.) (See Plate 4-5.)

cells with round nuclei; a prominent, usually single nucleolus; and abundant, finely vacuolated or granular cytoplasm (Fig. 4-11, Plate 4-5). These cells are very monotonous and occur both singly and in cohesive clusters. The second cell component is the familiar, singly occurring, small, naked, round to oval nucleus (Fig. 4-11). (Refer to the description provided in earlier sections on mammary dysplasia and fibroadenoma.) The cellular background frequently exhibits proteinaceous material (milk), which is most easily appreciated in air-dried smears. Occasionally, large numbers of cells may be present in large, multilayered groups. On closer examination, these grape-like clusters consist of evenly sized acini connected to terminal ducts (Fig. 4-12, Plate 4-6). Even though the smears are extremely cellular and the clusters contain

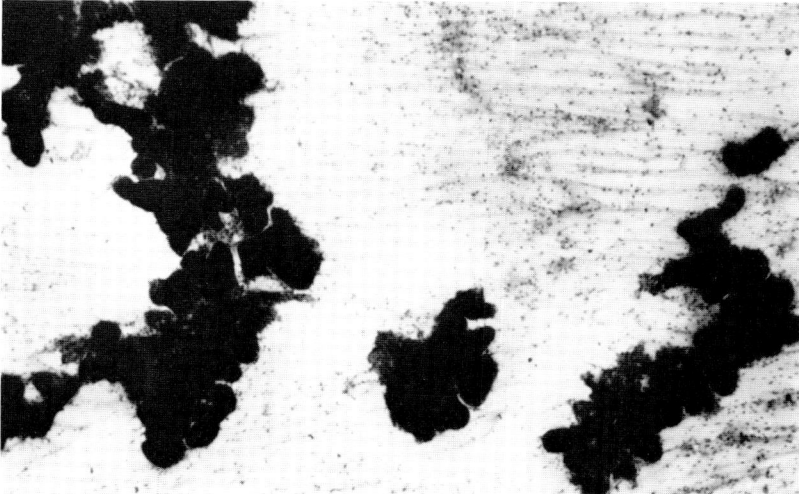

Fig. 4-12 Breast in pregnancy, low-power magnification. Extremely high cellularity is evident. However, note the scalloped outline of the clusters, which is composed of orderly, organized lobules and distal ducts. (Papanicolaou stain, × 16.) (See Plate 4-6.)

many layers of cells, these specimens, because of their characteristic architecture, are easily distinguishable from cancer.

Gynecomastia

Clinically, gynecomastia usually appears as a movable disk-shaped mass that symmetrically fills the subareolar space. The mass can be felt directly under the areolar skin but is not attached to it. Cancers in the male breast are usually asymmetrically placed and very quickly invade both the underlying muscle and the overlying skin. Cytologically, gynecomastia is very similar to benign fibrocystic change. Apocrine change, however, does not occur.

The main features of gynecomastia are monolayered, well-organized sheets of small, monotonous cells and single, small, naked nuclei. As in fibrocystic change, there may be an occasional focus of slightly overlapping cells, disorganized clusters, and some slightly enlarged cells.

Fat Necrosis

Clinically, fat necrosis may closely mimic breast carcinoma. The former usually appears as an ill-defined, moderately firm mass. There may be retraction of the overlying skin, and frequently, a "gritty" sensation is noted when the sampling needle is advanced into the lesion. All of these signs are often characteristic of cancerous lesions.

Fortunately, the cytologic appearance is straightforward in most cases. The typical cells have small, bland, round nuclei, which are usually centrally placed in very abundant, vacuolated, and sometimes granular cytoplasm. Binucleated and multinucleated forms are common. These lipophages may be mixed with stromal fragments that contain immature-appearing fibroblasts. Occasionally, highly atypical cells may be seen (Fig. 4-13, Plate 4-7). However, these atypical cells usually appear singly or in small clusters and are in the minority. Most of the cells on the slide will exhibit the above-mentioned typical features of fat necrosis. It is crucial not to base a diagnosis of malignant disease on a few atypical cells. Therefore it follows that adequate material with ample cells is a prerequisite for accurate diagnostic work.

Fat necrosis and cancer sometimes coexist. Patients with fat necrosis should be sampled carefully and then either followed very closely or encouraged to undergo an open biopsy to confirm the diagnosis.

Radiation Change

Following irradiation of breast tissue, there is dense fibrous tissue with scattered residual ducts and

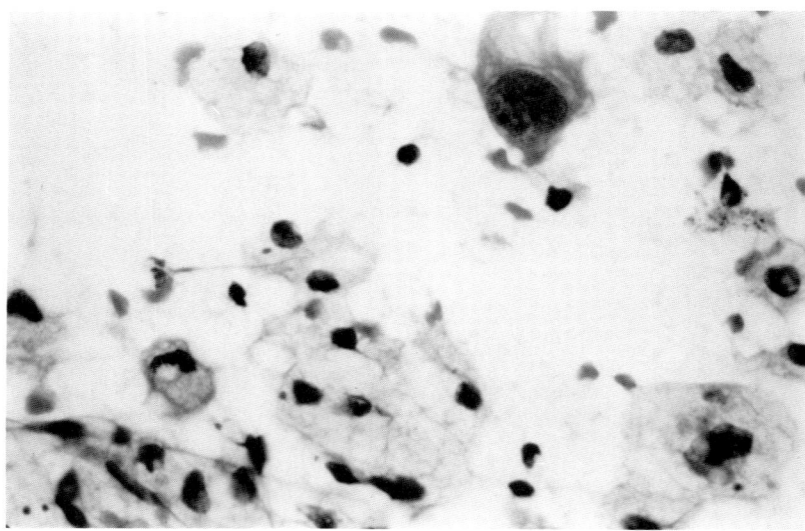

Fig. 4-13 Fat necrosis. There is one markedly atypical cell with a large nucleus and several prominent nucleoli located next to lipophages with abundant, vacuolated cytoplasm and small nuclei without significant atypia. (Papanicolaou stain, × 160.) (See Plate 4-7.)

structures that are reminiscent of lobules. Although the basic architecture of the epithelial component is preserved, the cells themselves may appear extremely atypical. This is reflected in FNA material by scant clusters of markedly large cells, often up to 30 μ in diameter. Multiple nucleoli may occur, and the chromatin pattern is often abnormal. Without a history of irradiation, the cells could easily pass for malignant cells. Because of these atypical features and a lack of extensive experience, there may be minimal, if any, indication for FNA after irradiation.

Inflammation

Cysts sometimes contain large numbers of inflammatory cells, including polymorphonuclear leukocytes, plasma cells, or lymphocytes, all of which are easily recognizable and pose no diagnostic problems. However, abundant histiocytes with atypical nuclear features, such as clumped chromatin and prominent nucleoli, may also be present, and may mimic epithelial cells, especially when they occur in clusters. Clues to their true nature are a low nuclear/cytoplasmic ratio, a foamy or vacuolated cytoplasm, and usually, small nucleoli. Anytime there is a background of acute inflammation, great caution in making a diagnosis of cancer is in order. Cancer is very seldom seen in this setting.

Inflammatory cancer is a clinical term. When cancer infiltrates extensively in cutaneous lymphatics, the skin appears warm, red, and puckered—similar to an orange peel-hence the term *peau d'orange*. Clinically, this resembles mastitis. The presence of cancer cells can be confirmed with FNA or an open biopsy; the cytologic picture will be similar to that of a non-inflammatory breast cancer. The same is true histologically, unless the cutaneous lymphatic vessels are specifically examined. Inflammatory cells are usually not seen in inflammatory cancer.

Mastitis is characterized by vast numbers of polymorphonuclear leukocytes, possibly granulation tissue, and lymphocytes, depending on the duration of the disease.

Subareolar Abscess

Subareolar abscess is a recurrent and chronic condition that appears as a subcutaneous, often tender lump in the areolar area. The skin may be red and edematous. If left untreated, the abscess will usually perforate the skin and drain. FNA material consists of inflammatory cells, most often polymorphonuclear leukocytes, granulation tissue, and squamous cells in many cases.

These abscesses are not related to lactation but rather to squamous metaplasia of the lactiferous ducts and obstruction of these ducts by squamous debris. Until the affected ducts are dissected and excised, the abscess formation will recur. Simple incision and drainage, even in combination with antibiotics, will not yield satisfactory long-term results.

Nipple Secretions

Several clinical variants of nipple secretions may be encountered. The most common is an opaque, milklike, white, yellow, or sometimes green secretion that drains from several ducts and can be extracted from both nipples. This is attributable to hormonal influence and not a sign of an underlying neoplastic condition. Cytologic examination will reveal foam cells only.

The second variant is that of one specific duct consistently or intermittently producing fluid. The secretion may be clear and colorless, brown, or show fresh blood. The latter may be associated with a papilloma or cancer and should be investigated. The fluid may or may not contain neoplastic cells on microscopic examination. Exploratory surgery of the affected duct is in order.

The third clinical variant involves a comedolike material that fills the distal ends of the ducts and is visible on examination of the nipple. The material consists of squamous debris and is produced by metaplastic squamous cells present within the ducts. This condition is the same as that which causes subareolar abscesses (see the preceding section).

CANCER

The main reason for performing FNA on breast masses is to distinguish benign from malignant lesions. Subclassification of these two categories is sometimes possible, but this is a secondary concern. In this section, features essential to the differential diagnosis of adenocarcinoma and various benign conditions are discussed. Different types of cancerous and metastatic lesions are discussed briefly.

The diagnosis of cancer is based on a combination

of several criteria. One feature alone is not sufficient, and the diagnostic impression should be reconfirmed in several fields. If there is doubt about the diagnosis, either because of the unusual appearance of a specimen, the availability of only scant material, or limited experience on the part of the interpreter, it is always best either to consult an experienced colleague or to request tissue confirmation of the diagnosis.

Cytologic Features of Ductal Carcinoma

CELLULARITY

General cellularity tends to be higher in cancer than in benign lesions; however, there are exceptions. Breast cancer with extensive sclerosis and a scant epithelial component on histologic examination will yield scant epithelium on FNA. In extreme cases, it may be impossible, despite good biopsy technique, to obtain adequate numbers of cells for a definitive diagnosis. Such cases account for 1 to 2 percent of all cancers, and are unable to be diagnosed by FNA. Fortunately, these cases are clinically highly suspicious for cancer, as they present as very firm masses secondary to the extreme sclerosis. Diagnosis can readily be established on the basis of an open biopsy or frozen section study before definitive therapy is begun.

Various benign lesions, such as fibroadenoma, pregnant breast, and mammary dysplasia, may yield abundant cells. Thus, high cellularity alone is not diagnostic of cancer.

PATTERN

Cell clusters from breast cancer show considerable crowding, cell overlap, and often, several layers of cells (Fig. 4-14). In invasive tumors, the malignant cells are frequently seen in close association with fat vacuoles, and even within fragments of adipose tissue.

CHARACTERISTICS OF INDIVIDUAL CELLS

Cancer cells have a tendency to be less cohesive than are those of benign breast epithelium, producing a smear with relatively more single cells and small clusters. Furthermore, a much greater percentage of the single tumor cells retain their cytoplasm compared to benign cells (Fig. 4-15). The presence of intact single cells is not pathognomonic for cancer, and should never be taken out of context or constitute the sole criteria for making a diagnosis of malignant disease. Certain benign cells, such as apocrine cells, histiocytes, and lipophages, may appear singly and intact in large numbers. However, these cells have distinguishing features, such as a very low nuclear/cytoplasmic ratio, cytoplasmic granulation or vacuolization, and a distinct architectural arrangement (monolayered sheets for apocrine cells), that favor a benign diagnosis.

The nuclei of cancer cells are usually large (the equivalent of four erythrocytes or greater), whereas benign breast nuclei are about the size of two erythrocytes. Again, there are exceptions; some lobular and tubular carcinomas have small nuclei. Occasionally, fibroadenomas and other benign lesions have a subpopulation consisting of relatively large cells. The presence of small, oval, naked nuclei seen throughout benign lesions, then, becomes an extremely helpful criterion (see above).

The chromatin pattern in cancer may be coarse and irregularly distributed, but this feature is absent in many tumors. Similarly, nucleoli are present in some breast cancers but not in others. To further complicate matters, nucleoli are a regular feature in pregnant and lactating breasts and are not unusual findings in fibroadenomas.

Cancer cells within one tumor usually vary considerably in size and shape, and it is difficult to find two identical cells. Despite this, the cells usually appear to make up one population. Benign lesions, particularly those with atypical features, usually have at least two recognizable cell populations—that is, atypical cells and small, single, naked nuclei. These latter cells appear quite monotonous and many will look identical. Table 4-1 provides a summary of criteria for benign and malignant lesions of breast.

A small portion of breast cancers are composed of markedly large and atypical cells. Whenever this pleomorphic picture is encountered, metastatic disease should be considered. One of the most common secondary tumors is melanoma. Pigment is not always present, but other features, such as intranuclear cytoplasmic inclusions, extreme discohesion, and binucleation and multinucleation, are usually seen. Lym-

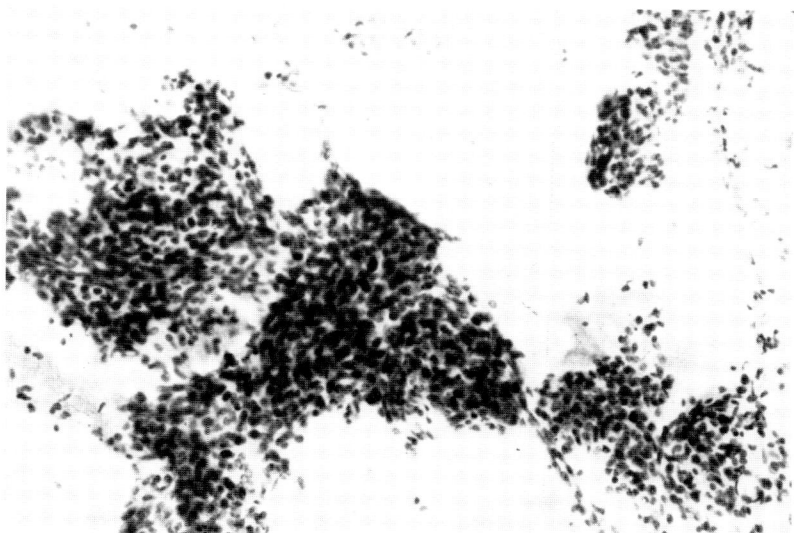

Fig. 4-14 Ductal carcinoma, low-power magnification. Irregularly arranged, multilayered clusters of tumor cells. (Papanicolaou stain, × 16.)

phoma is occasionally aspirated from breast tissue. In such cases, the often characteristic chromatin pattern and lymphoglandular bodies are helpful in establishing the diagnosis.[4] Lymphoglandular bodies are rounded fragments of cytoplasm, seen in the background of benign or malignant smears, which contain large numbers of lymphocytes. These bodies can be observed with any of the commonly used stains, but are most easily appreciated with air-dried Romanowsky-stained smears.

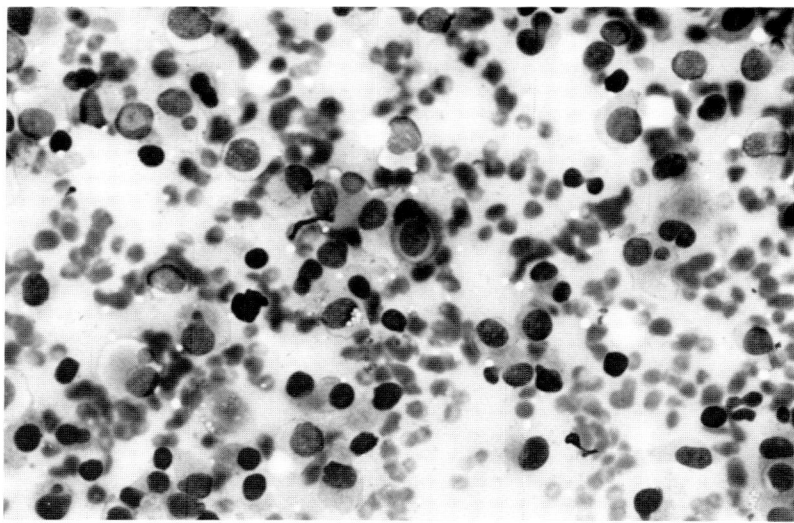

Fig. 4-15 Ductal carcinoma, high-power magnification. Most of these single tumor cells have a preserved cytoplasm. The nuclei are large and often eccentrically placed. (MGG stain, × 100.)

Table 4-1 FNA of Breast Lesions Smear Characteristics

	Benign	Malignant
Pattern	Monolayered, regularly arranged clusters; few single cells	Multilayered, irregular clusters; many single cells
Single cells	Monomorphous, oval, naked, small	Polymorphous, round or polygonal; preserved cytoplasm; large
Chromatin	Evenly distributed and light	Coarse and heavy
Nucleoli	Usually not present, but may occur in fibroadenomas and during pregnancy and lactation	Present in a moderate number of cases

Subclassification of Carcinoma

COLLOID CARCINOMA

The presence of mucus in specimens of colloid carcinoma is a prominent feature of this well-differentiated breast cancer. The mucus is stringy, brightly metachromatic on Romanowsky stains (Fig. 4-16, Plate 4-8), and pale green to yellow on Papanicolaou stain. The tumor cells are often relatively small and monotonous, occasionally appearing in monolayered sheets similar to those seen in benign breast disease. The chromatin pattern is often remarkably bland. Despite these bland features, the diagnosis is usually easy to establish. The presence of mucus is a very important clue. One of the differential diagnoses is fibroadenoma with myxoid stroma that may simulate the appearance of mucus. However, colloid cancer has only one cell population, whereas fibroadenomas have naked oval nuclei, epithelial cells in clusters with cytoplasm, and spindly stromal cells. Single tumor cells will frequently have preserved cytoplasm. Another feature of colloid cancer may be rounded, smooth, three-dimensional clusters of tumor cells in a background of mucus.

Mucocele of the breast, a very rare benign condition affecting premenopausal women,[5] has an FNA appearance that may mimic colloid carcinoma. Most colloid carcinoma occur in postmenopausal women.[6] Caution should be exercised when consid-

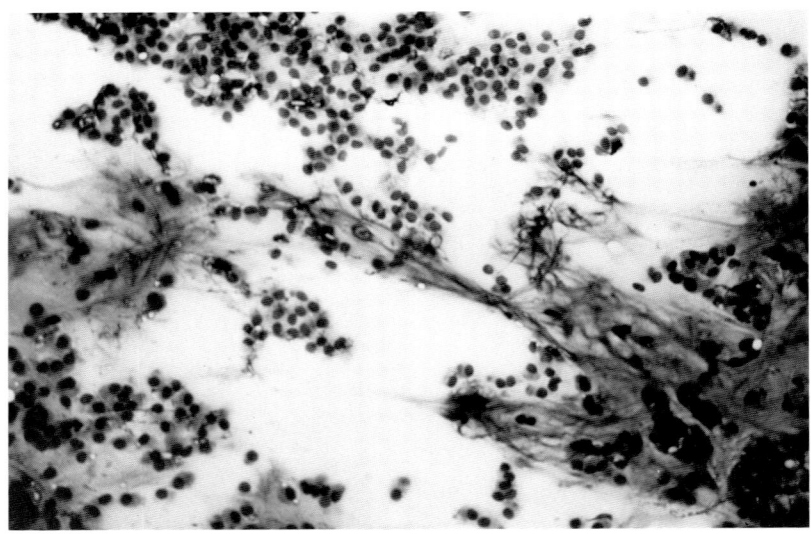

Fig. 4-16 Colloid carcinoma. Abundant metachromatic, stringy, mucinous material is mixed with cancer cells. (MGG stain, × 40.) (See Plate 4-8.)

ering colloid cancer in a premenopausal woman, especially if the cellularity is scant and there is not significant cellular atypia.

MEDULLARY CARCINOMA

Medullary carcinoma is composed of markedly large tumor cells with prominent nucleoli mixed with significant numbers of small, mature-appearing lymphocytes (Fig. 4-17). The tumor cells often have very fragile cytoplasm, resulting in many naked nuclei. Because the tumor cells are so atypical, the presence of malignancy is not the diagnostic issue. Rather, it is the differential diagnosis that is important, as one must distinguish between a medullary carcinoma with a relatively good prognosis (at least when the tumor is limited to the breast) and a poorly differentiated aggressive tumor with a poor prognosis. This distinction cannot be made accurately by cytologic methods because a well-defined tumor boundary is a requisite for diagnosing medullary carcinoma, and this feature can only be established by histologic examination upon excision of the lesion.

LOBULAR CARCINOMA

Tumor cells in lobular carcinoma tend to be small and bland. Intracytoplasmic vacuoles displacing the nucleus have been described. However, this feature may also be seen in "garden variety" ductal tumors, and thus is not pathognomonic for the lobular subtype of cancer. The general features described earlier for carcinoma, with the exception of cell size in some cases, apply to lobular carcinoma. Thus, a diagnosis of cancer based on cytologic material can usually be made despite the small cell size.

TUBULAR CANCER

Tubular carcinoma is another lesion that is challenging to diagnose, again because of generally small cell size and a tendency for cells to appear in monolayered sheets. On close examination, however, hollow, elongated tubules can be seen within large and small clusters (Fig. 4-18). When focusing up and down, two cell layers and an empty lumen can be observed. The single cells vary significantly in size and shape and often retain their cytoplasm. There are times when a definitive cytologic diagnosis of cancer is difficult. It is important to recognize the atypia and to advocate further work-up in order to avoid a false-negative diagnosis.

MISCELLANEOUS BREAST NEOPLASMS

Well-differentiated papillary cancer is composed of cells with little atypia; often, at least part of the popu-

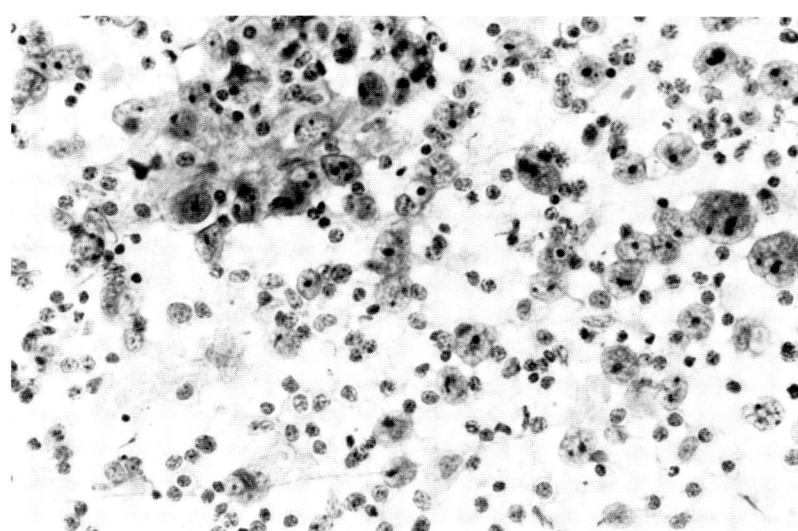

Fig. 4-17 Medullary carcinoma. Large tumor cells with prominent nucleoli are mixed with numerous small lymphocytes. (H & E stain, × 40.)

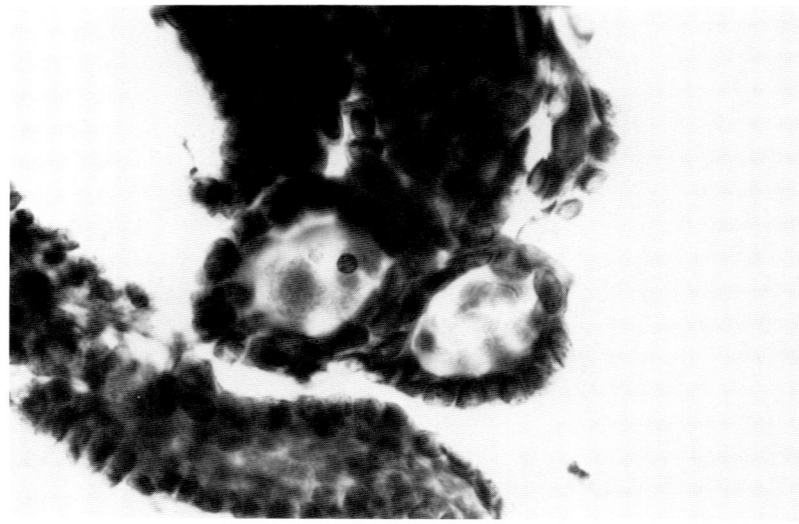

Fig. 4-18 Tubular carcinoma. Open-ended, hollow fragments of tubular structures are seen. (Papanicolaou stain, × 100.) (Courtesy of Dr. Theodore R. Miller.)

lation consists of columnar cells. This neoplasm is often indistinguishable from ductal papilloma. An open biopsy will resolve the question of invasion and reveal other architectural features that may be helpful in establishing the diagnosis.

Apocrine cancer exhibits all of the features mentioned earlier for ductal carcinoma. However, apocrine cancer has more abundant and possibly more granular cytoplasm than does the ductal form.

Phylloides sarcomas are usually large (several centimeters) at the time of diagnosis. The cytologic appearance of these tumors can range from resembling fibroadenoma to mimicking a high-grade sarcoma. One of the key features of the high-grade lesions is malignant cells in close association with stromal material. Rarely, other types of sarcoma may occur as primary tumors of the breast. The differential diagnosis between a high-grade phylloides tumor and other sarcomas, such as malignant fibrous histiocytoma, may be extremely difficult. However, from a clinical standpoint, this is not a major issue as the treatment would be similar.

Carcinoma in situ

Most cases of carcinoma in situ (CIS) involve nonpalpable lesions that are not conducive to examination by FNA unless stereotaxic techniques are employed.[7] Occasionally, CIS may coexist with adjacent fibrocystic change, causing a palpable lump. In this setting, FNA may yield cancer cells in varying amounts, often admixed with benign breast epithelium. In this situation, a descriptive diagnosis, describing both components and alerting the referring physician to the possibility of a limited in situ tumor, is in order. Another clue that CIS is present, even without this admixture of benign epithelium, is the presence of necrotic debris originating from the central portion of the distended ducts in the comedo variant of CIS.

Atypia

Most FNA specimens from breast lesions (more than 90 percent) will be obviously benign or malignant (Table 4-1). Occasionally, however, atypical cells that are difficult to classify may be present. This is most commonly the case when the overwhelming majority of cells on the smears are unremarkable, but scattered single cells or clusters exhibit atypical features, such as increased size, prominent nucleoli, irregular nuclear outline, or abnormal chromatin pattern (Fig. 4-19). Under these circumstances, a diagnosis of cancer should not be rendered based on the cytologic material, but an open biopsy should be requested. Most of these masses will prove to be benign, revealing focal lesions, such as apocrine cells with an unusual appearance, atypical hyperplasia of

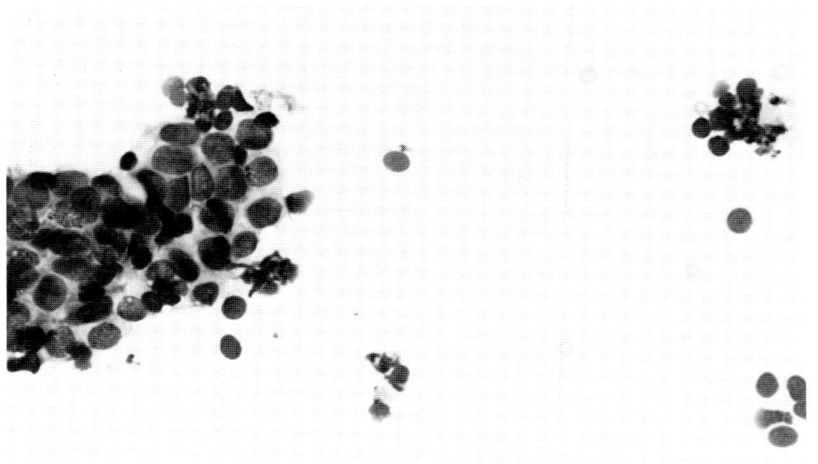

Fig. 4-19 A cluster of moderately enlarged cells adjacent to unremarkable, benign epithelium, including single, naked, oval nuclei. In this case, focal atypical ductal hyperplasia was diagnosed on the basis of histologic examination. (MGG stain, × 100.)

varying degree, or fibroadenomas with focal atypia, to mention a few possibilities. In some cases, no abnormalities will be found on histologic examination.

Occasionally, foci of CIS are found. If a substantial invasive carcinoma is documented by histologic means, scant atypical cells mixed with many benign cells on the smear may indicate a sampling problem. Certain cancers composed of small cells without much atypia, such as lobular and tubular cancer, will yield a single population of cells. These cells will have some features that are consistent with cancer, but it may be difficult to render a definitive diagnosis of malignant disease in all cases. If there is doubt about a diagnosis, an open biopsy is always in order.

REFERENCES

1. Cohen MB, Channing Rodgers RP, Hales MS et al: Influence of training and experience in fine needle aspiration biopsy of breast: Receiver operating characteristics curve analysis. Arch Pathol Lab Med 111:518, 1987
2. Löwhagen T, Willems JS, Lundell G et al: Aspiration biopsy cytology in diagnosis of thyroid cancer. World J Surg 5:61, 1981
3. Barrows GH, Anderson TJ, Lamb JL et al: Fine needle aspiration of breast cancer. Relationship of clinical factors to cytology results in 689 primary malignancies. Cancer 58:1493, 1986
4. Linsk JA, Franzen S: Clinical Aspiration Cytology. JB Lippincott, Philadelphia, 1983
5. Rosen PP: Mucocele-like tumors of the breast. Am J Surg Pathol 10:464, 1986
6. Rosen PP, Lesser ML, Kinne DW: Breast carcinoma at the extremes of age: A comparison of patients younger than 35 years and older than 75 years. J Surg Oncol 28:90, 1985
7. Svane G, Silversward C: Stereotaxic needle biopsy of nonpalpable breast lesions. Cytologic and histologic findings. Acta Radiol [Diagn] [Stockh] 24 (Fasc. 4):283, 1983

5
Cytologic Diagnosis of Respiratory Diseases

Dorothy L. Rosenthal

Respiratory cytology has assumed a position of primary diagnostic importance in the work-up for the patient with pulmonary disease. The importance placed upon the cytologic diagnosis results from the cumulative experience of the last 20 years.[1-6] The coincidence of the now obvious worldwide epidemic of carcinoma of the lung, and the development of the fiberoptic bronchoscope,[7] accelerated the experience of cytopathologists with samples from the lower respiratory tract. Today the lung represents the second most popular body site for cytologic sampling in most cytopathology laboratories that deal with both gynecologic and nongynecologic samples.

Current practice has established the immediate use of fiberoptic bronchoscopic diagnosis when a patient with evidence of pulmonary disease, either benign or neoplastic, presents to the pulmonologist.[8] The overall diagnostic yield of fiberoptic bronchoscopy is too great to justify delaying the procedure to wait for a diagnostic sputum sample. With cost-effectiveness being the key to medical survival, this technique is indispensable.

Although cancer diagnosis automatically comes to mind when considering respiratory cytodiagnosis, numerous infectious diseases can be either diagnosed definitively or strongly suspected based on samples recovered by fiberoptic bronchoscopy or transthoracic needle aspiration. As the patient population becomes more complex, including the increase in the number of immunocompromised patients from whatever cause, the need for astute diagnosis of non-neoplastic or infectious disease becomes increasingly important. Although special stains are classic "crutches", much information, which frequently is definitive, can be gained from Papanicolaou-stained material. This allows treatment to begin within a few hours of sample collection, with minimal expense.

When all factors are considered, the role of the cytotechnologist and cytopathologist in the management of patients with respiratory disease is key to the successful outcome of patient treatment. The high diagnostic yield of pulmonary cytodiagnosis is without question the result of a team approach. Based on our experience at UCLA, we strongly and enthusiastically emphasize the importance of the close collaboration of the cytology staff with the bronchoscopy team and the thoracic radiologists.

CELL CHANGES CURRENTLY NOT ASSOCIATED WITH NEOPLASIA

The cellular components of the lung, like all other biologic entities, react to stimuli in a limited variety of ways in order to restore homeostasis. Frost et al.[9]

summarize responses of the lung "resulting from chronic inflammation and irritation, hypersensitivity, irradiation, drug therapy or chemotherapy, and viral diseases. Although lung tissues react to their environment in only a few basic ways, combinations of changes can produce a wide range of morphologic abnormalities that may be mistaken for cancer."

Cytologic Changes Specific to Cell Types

BENIGN SQUAMOUS CELLS

Squamous cells from the mouth respond to irritants in the same manner that squamous cells from the female vaginal tract respond to infection and irritation—that is, with accelerated maturation. Therefore, if dentures or other appliances irritate a squamous focus, hyperkeratinization will occur and will be reflected by true keratin formation in large squamoid cells. Since there is no squamocolumnar junction in the same sense as in the uterine cervix, smaller metaplastic cells are usually not encountered in the mouth unless ulceration with healing has occurred, and basal cells have become dyskeratotic.

Fungi, especially Candida, become pathogenic under certain circumstances, grow in the squamous epithelium, and produce a dramatic hyperkeratosis. Such lesions should be investigated thoroughly, including a full-thickness biopsy, to exclude squamous carcinoma. These squamous cells can contaminate sputum specimens, but their large size indicates their origin in the mouth rather than the lower respiratory tract.

"Repair" Cells

Cousins to large squamous cells, so-called repair cells in the respiratory tract are similar to the repair cells seen in the female genital tract. They are characterized by cohesive sheets of polyhedral cells, and have attenuated cytoplasmic connections, semiopaque cytoplasm, enlarged nuclei with delicate nuclear chromatin, and usually prominent and sometimes irregular nucleoli (Fig. 5-1). Multinucleation is occasionally seen. Such cells can exfoliate from the mouth following a mucosal ulceration, but can be diagnostically treacherous when they actually come from the lower respiratory tract. They are a frequent consequence of respiratory epithelial abrasion secondary to therapeutic or diagnostic instrumentation, and can be

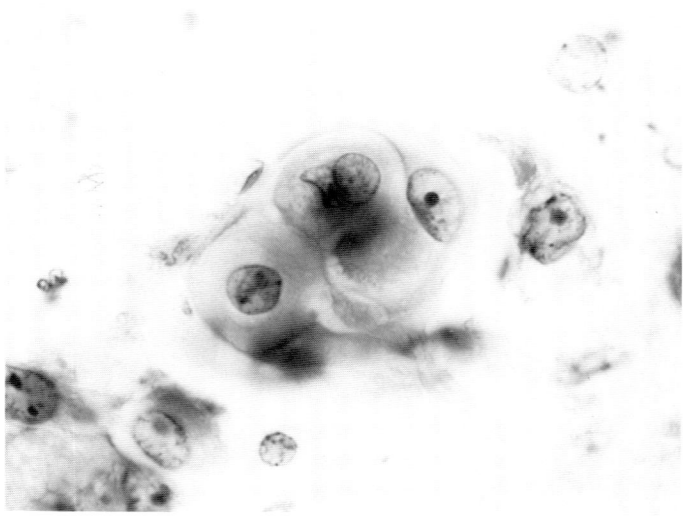

Fig. 5-1 Reparative process (bronchial brushing). Large fragments of squamous epithelium from the lower respiratory tract indicate either a metaplasia/reparative process or squamous carcinoma. The cohesion of the cells and the fine chromatin pattern indicate a benign diagnosis. Also, no single tumor cells are noted. The patient had recently undergone bronchial biopsy, resulting in this healing pattern. (Papanicolaou stain, × 1,000.)

confused with squamous carcinoma cells. Careful attention to the cohesiveness of the cell groups (absence of single cells), uniform thinness of the nuclear membrane, and delicacy of the nuclear chromatin will attest to their benign nature. When in doubt, a careful history to document prior instrumentation, biopsy, or both, and a period of watchful waiting with repeat studies will usually clarify the issue.

Benign Metaplastic Cells

When a columnar epithelium, including the respiratory type, becomes sufficiently irritated, as by pneumonia, cigarette smoke, or other toxic inhalants, squamous metaplasia is the unavoidable result. These cells are smaller than those from the mouth or those that characterize a reparative process, they have a mosaic appearance, and are essentially the same as those found in the uterine cervix (Fig. 5-2). To be considered totally benign, they should have uniform nuclear size, delicate chromatin, and small, round nucleoli. Nuclear/cytoplasmic ratios should be constant. They can be confused with plant cells; however, the double refractile wall in the latter identify them as inanimate.

COLUMNAR CELLS

Columnar cells respond to stress either by individual nuclear enlargement or by multinucleation in response to the need to increase the cell population, unless the stem cells undergo squamous metaplasia. The pattern of cell change seen will depend upon the specific cell type that is needed (e.g., columnar cells for mucus production or metaplastic cells for protection).

Ciliated Columnar Cells

Ciliated columnar cells usually respond by an overall increase in cell size, an increase in nuclear size with some coarsening of the chromatin, and accentuation of nucleoli. If the need for more cells is present, then multinucleation of cell groups will result.

When such hyperplastic cell groups exfoliate and are recovered in sputum, they can appear curled, like

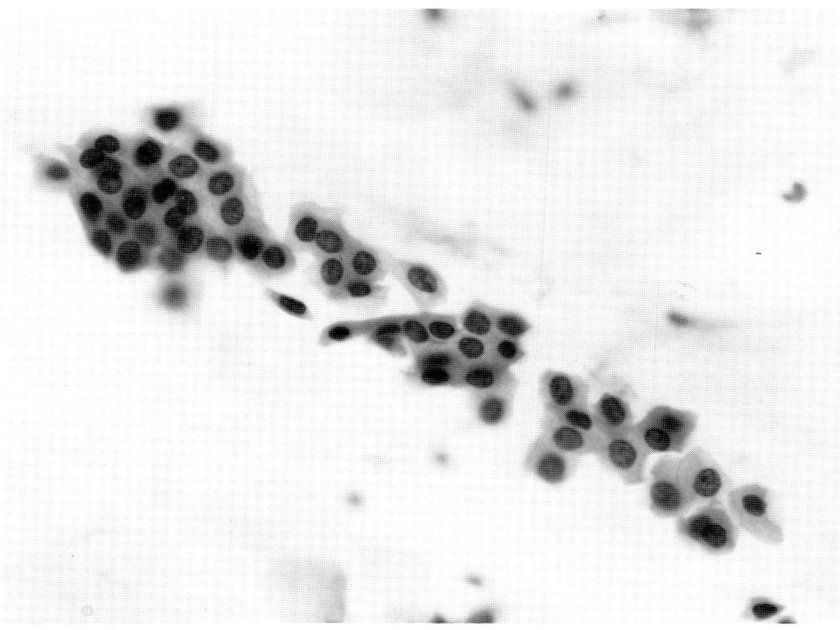

Fig. 5-2 Squamous metaplasia (sputum). Groups of uniformly sized metaplastic cells are frequently seen in benign lung diseases, such as pneumonia, bronchiectasis, and asthma. The uniform nuclear size and chromatin distribution attest to their benign nature. A careful search for more severe changes is imperative. (Papanicolaou stain, × 400.)

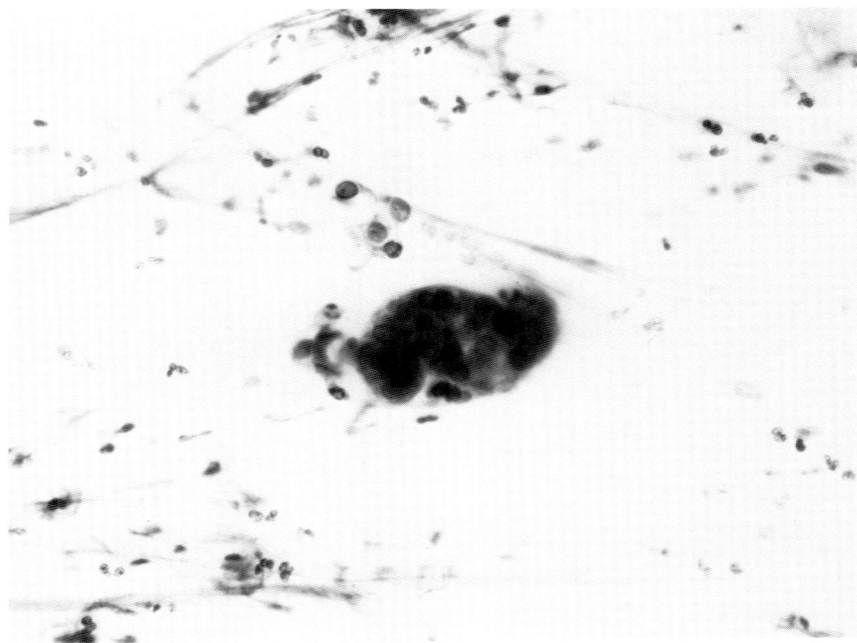

Fig. 5-3 Creola body (sputum). A typical Creola body, this curled fragment of benign respiratory epithelium is covered with cilia. (Papanicolaou stain, × 400.)

a caterpillar, and may be mistaken for a fragment of an adenocarcinoma (Fig. 5-3). The benign nature of these so-called Creola bodies is verified by the presence of cilia. These groups are most abundant in patients with asthma and other chronic bronchial diseases.

In all cases, cilia are retained if the specimen is fresh, and the benign nature of the cells is thus assured. Degenerative changes can mimic reactive coarsening of chromatin, but the nuclear membrane in a degenerated cell will be interrupted, providing evidence that the changes are degenerative and not reactive.

Nonciliated Goblet Cells

If the cells are nonciliated goblet cells, the response to irritants is one of increasing mucus within single cells, as well as an increase in the number of mucus-containing cells. Goblet cell hyperplasia commonly results from cigarette smoke, and reflects chronic obstructive pulmonary disease, emphysema, and chronic bronchitis.[10] Especially in a brushing, goblet cell hyperplasia can be seen by focusing through groups of epithelial cells and appreciating the increased number of "holes" within the epithelial sheet (Fig. 5-4). Remember that the usual ratio of goblet cells to ciliated respiratory epithelial cells is approximately 1:5 or 1:6. The nuclear changes in such cells are similar to the ciliated cell changes.

Clara Cells

Clara cells are nonciliated, mucus-producing cells of the bronchioles. Like the goblet cells, they respond to stimuli by becoming hyperplastic. If such proliferation involves the immature mucus-secreting cells, which are precursors of both goblet and Clara cells, glandular hyperplasia can result, perhaps heralding the development of bronchioloalveolar carcinoma. If such a proliferative process is accompanied by diffuse fibrosis, the end result may be Hamman-Rich syndrome. If a localized fibrous nodule is produced, this may represent the groundwork for a "scar" adenocarcinoma. None of these cancer precursor states has been proven.

Additional causes of atypical epithelial hyperplasia, as compiled by Bedrossian,[10] are listed in Table 5-1.

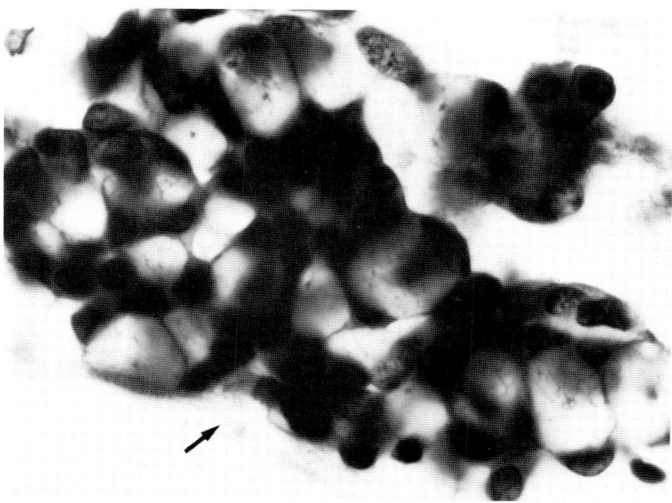

Fig. 5-4 Glandular cell atypia. An increased number of goblet cells is present in this fragment of benign respiratory epithelium (the ratio of normal respiratory epithelium is 1 goblet cell:5 to 6 ciliated cells). The "holes" correspond to the mucous vacuoles in the cytoplasm of goblet cells. Note the small nuclear size and cilia (arrow). (Papanicolaou stain, × 1,000.)

TABLE 5-1 Causes of Cytologic Atypia Affecting Distal Air Spaces

Infections
  Viruses
  Mycoplasma
  Pneumocystis
Inhalants
  Oxygen
  Nitrogen dioxide
  Smoke (from fire)
Chemotherapy
  Bleomycin
  Busulfan
  Methotrexate
  Cytoxan
  BCNU
  Melphalan
  Chlorambucil
Radiation Therapy
Miscellaneous
  Hamman-Rich syndrome
  Scleroderma
  Rheumatoid arthritis
  Old granulomas
  Asbestosis

(From Rosenthal,[6] with permission.)

BASAL CELL OR RESERVE CELLS

Basal cells, or reserve cells, are germinal cells that respond to stimuli, as do germinal cells throughout the body, by an increase in mitotic activity in order to increase the number of second and third generation cells. These cells are usually shed in groups, and are seen in dense aggregates in a brushing specimen or an aspirate. Their hyperchromasia may suggest neoplasia, but careful attention to their usual small size, cohesiveness, and visible cytoplasm, as well as to their regular, fine chromatin, should convince the observer that they are benign (Fig. 5-5). The most common pitfall is to mistake them for oat cell carcinoma. The latter can be distinguished by cellular characteristics that include an almost invisible cytoplasm, a coarser "salt and pepper" chromatin, and clearly discernible molding, despite a disconnected appearance.

PNEUMOCYTES

Pneumocytes are commonly divided into two types. Type I pneumocytes are so fragile that they are rarely seen in any preparations for light microscopy.

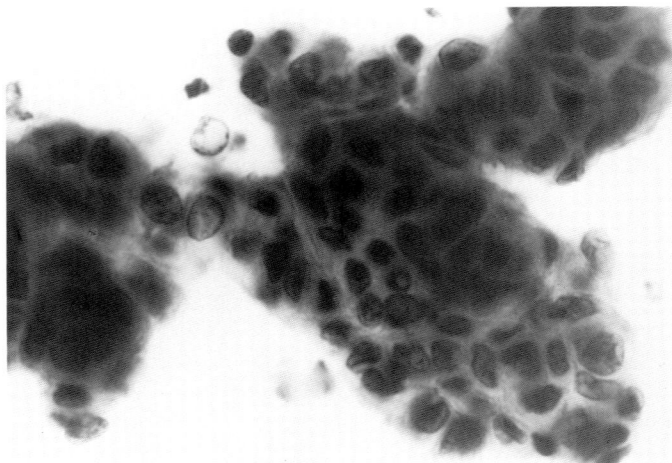

Fig. 5-5 Reserve cell hyperplasia (bronchial brushing). A large fragment of small, tightly clustered, columnar cells should not be mistaken for an adenocarcinoma or small cell carcinoma. The cohesion of the cells, the obvious cytoplasm, and the small size of the cells when compared with nearby inflammatory cells indicate their benign nature. (Papanicolaou stain, × 1,000.)

Type II pneumocytes are hardy and respond dramatically to stimuli, especially toxic or viral injury. They are characteristically large epithelial cells, with squamoid cytoplasm, large nuclei, and huge nucleoli, often indistinguishable from viral inclusions (which they frequently are). Electron microscopy is necessary to identify definitively the type of pneumocyte and the presence and kind of viral particles.

NONCELLULAR ELEMENTS

Curschmann's spirals are produced when inspissated mucus accumulates in the terminal bronchioles, partially solidifies, and then is coughed up (Fig. 5-6). The central stringlike axis stains purple with hematoxylin and eosin (H&E) and is often covered by an outer, semitransparent sheath in which a helix is ap-

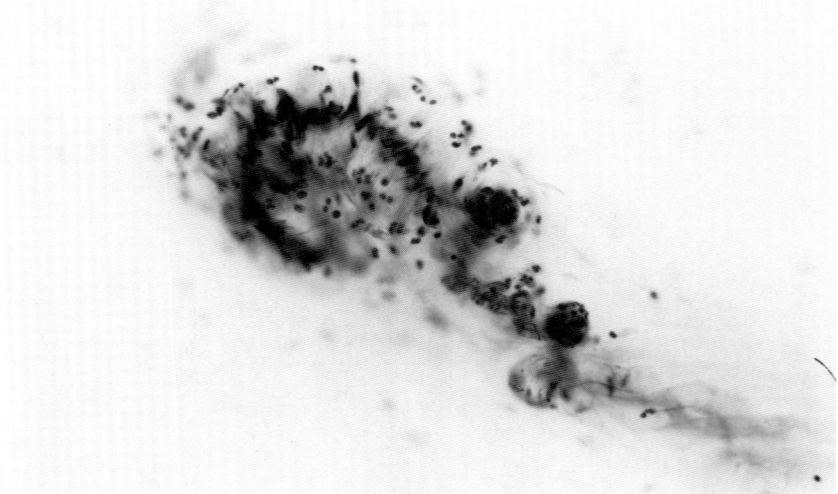

Fig. 5-6 Curschmann's spiral (sputum). Note the coiling, the mucoid sheath, and the association of inflammatory cells. Such spirals are usually seen in patients with chronic lung disease. (Papanicolaou stain, × 200.)

preciated. Such spirals can be only a few millimeters long or as long as several centimeters. Their presence indicates some form of obstructive lung disease.

Charcot-Leyden crystals are most frequently seen in the sputum of patients with asthma, and are thought to be derived from crystallized fragments of degenerated eosinophils. They are difficult to appreciate on Papanicolaou stain; toluidine blue stain demonstrates them well in a fresh specimen.

Asbestos bodies, or more properly, *ferruginous bodies,* result from the impregnation of a filament of asbestos or other mineral fiber by iron-protein pigment (Fig. 5-7). Generally, the central fiber itself cannot be recognized unless oil immersion is used or the fiber is especially thick. Ferruginous bodies usually measure between 5 and 200 μm in length, and will appear either yellow, gold, or black. The ends of the bodies can assume a branching, attenuated, or rounded appearance, and the intervening rod usually is segmented, resembling a string of beads or segments of bamboo. Ferruginous bodies can be recovered from approximately 80 percent of the population, so their presence is pathogenically significant in only a small percentage of the population. Their association with mesothelioma and bronchogenic carcinoma is now well established.[1,3]

Concretions of both amorphous mucus and accumulations of edematous fluid proteins—so-called *corpora amylacea*—may occasionally be observed in sputum. These concretions stain medium to dark purple.

Calcific concretions may be seen in patients with chronic pulmonary diseases, such as tuberculosis. A rare entity, *alveolar microcalcinosis,* may also be indicated by such concretions, especially if they are present in significant numbers.[3]

Psammoma bodies should alert the microscopist to the strong possibility of a pulmonary adenocarcinoma, either primary or derived from thyroid or ovary, or other adenocarcinoma.

INFECTIOUS DISEASES

Disease entities previously seen only in the surgical pathology laboratory are now frequently encountered in the cytology laboratory owing to the accessibility of all lesions by fine needle aspiration (FNA)[11-13] and bronchoalveolar lavage.[14] Until a

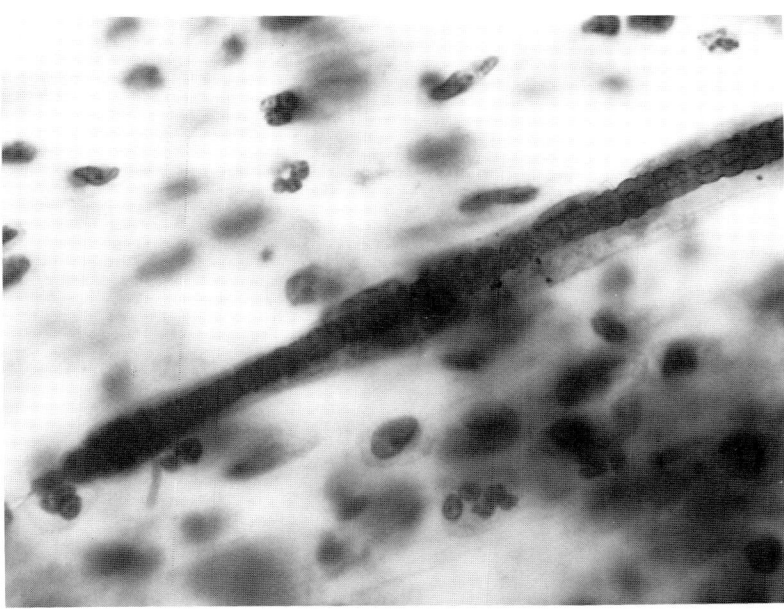

Fig. 5-7 Ferruginous ("asbestos") body (sputum). These ferruginous bodies are usually formed by asbestos, but any inert mineral can become coated with iron (hence, the name). The irregular layer of iron over the thin mineral filament produces the bamboo or string-of-beads effect. (Papanicolaou stain, × 1,000.)

short time ago only bronchial and peribronchial infections concerned the cytologist. Now the pattern of parenchymal lesions is of vital interest in attempting to identify the diagnostic possibilities.[15,16] The diseases in the next few sections are therefore grouped not only according to the type of infectious organism, but also according to the disease pattern that the organism produces. The incidence of such diseases varies depending upon the geographic location of the receiving laboratory; however, given the transience of the world populations, the unexpected should be anticipated. Such diagnostic surprises have changed the once banal "benign" specimens into fascinating challenges.[6,17]

The infectious organisms whose hallmarks can be recognized by Papanicolaou stain or inferred by cytologic features can be divided into two categories: those creating a pneumonic process and those resulting in a granulomatous infection. Of the latter, tuberculosis, the prototype of granulomatous infections, and sarcoidosis have no pathognomonic features that are recognizable in Papanicolaou-stained material. However, these diseases can be identified by the patterns of their cellular and noncellular material.

Tuberculosis and Sarcoidosis

TUBERCULOSIS

Tuberculosis (TB), a disease of historic significance and protean manifestations, is still to be found worldwide. Although classically an infection of the impoverished, TB is not a respecter of class or caste; it should be considered a ubiquitous disease, and should always be part of the differential diagnosis of pulmonary lesions.

TB has not been a common diagnostic consideration for the cytologist because of the paucity of diagnostic material retrievable in routine cytologic specimens (e.g., from sputa, bronchial washings, and brushings). Occasionally, Langhans type giant cells are recovered in these specimens; in such instances, TB should be high on the list of possible diagnoses.[18,19] However, pulmonary FNA provides material directly from the granuloma. The infecting organism of TB cannot be identified by Papanicolaou stain, but the contents of the granulomatous complex is sufficiently characteristic to prompt a search for visible organisms—that is, fungi (described later)—or to destain and restain for mycobacteria.

The cytologic features of all aspirated granulomas, regardless of the infectious organism, are similar; however, more amorphous debris can be expected from caseous centers of tuberculous granulomas. Clusters or confluent sheets of epithelial cells, necrotic debris, calcified particles, lymphocytes, and multinucleated Langhans type giant cells[20,21] are sufficiently strong clues to suggest the diagnosis. Special stains (Fite's or auramine-rhodamine) are necessary to locate and tentatively identify the mycobacteria. As is illustrated in a later section, the granuloma-producing fungi are readily seen on Papanicolaou-stained material.

SARCOIDOSIS

Sarcoidosis has always been diagnosed by exclusion, as no causative agent has been associated with this multisystem disease. The pulmonary diagnosis has traditionally been made by open lung biopsy and more recently, by transbronchial biopsy via the fiberoptic bronchoscope. Rare reports have documented the appearance of classic Schaumann or asteroid bodies in multinucleated histiocytes recovered in sputa.[3] We recently reviewed bronchoscopic specimens from a patient with suspected sarcoidosis, in which the transbronchial biopsy and brushing samples contained noncaseating granulomas (Fig. 5-8). Although the retrieval of diagnostic material by transbronchial biopsy was expected, the cytologic features of a noncaseating granuloma in a bronchial brushing were a surprise.

Major Fungi Causing Granulomatous Inflammation in the Lung

Table 5-2 characterizes the four most common fungi to produce significant granulomatous disease in the lung. Their incidence varies depending upon geographic location; blastomyces is commonly found in southeastern United States, Histoplasma is prevalent in the Midwest, Coccidioides is found primarily in the southwest, and Cryptococcus is a ubiquitous and frequent second invader following another debilitating disease.

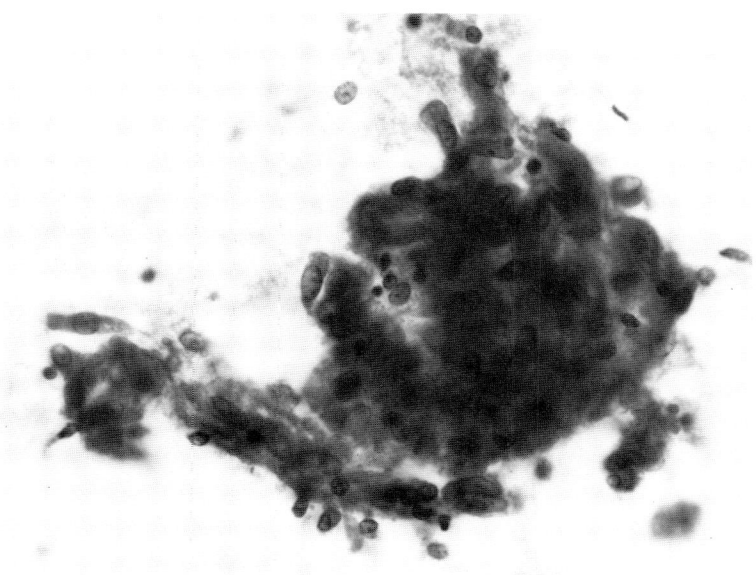

Fig. 5-8 Sarcoidosis (bronchial brushing). Note the tangle of monocytes, fibroblasts, and macrophages mixed with chronic inflammatory cells in this unusual and excellent cytologic sample of granulomatous inflammation. If caseation is present, then a diagnosis of tuberculosis or fungal infection should be considered over sarcoidosis, in which there is no necrosis. (Papanicolaou stain, × 400.)

HISTOPLASMOSIS

Histoplasma capsulatum is found in the soil throughout the midwestern United States, especially in areas with large amounts of bird droppings. The mycelial form in nature is transformed to the yeast phase at body temperature. The clinical syndrome of histoplasmosis is quite variable, and is usually benign in its outcome, affecting only the lung. Disseminated histoplasmosis can occur in both healthy and immuno-

Table 5-2 Contrasting Morphologic Features of Major Fungi Causing Granulomatous Inflammation in the Lung

	Histoplasma	Coccidioides	Cryptococcus	Blastomyces
Average size	3 μm (range of 1–5 μm)	30–60 μm (spherules); 2–5 μm (endospores)	4–7 μm (range of 2–15 μm)	8–15 μm (range of 2–30 μm)
Morphologic features	Oval, budding yeast	Spherules, endospores; no budding forms	Round, budding yeast; fragmented forms	Round, broad based budding yeast
Distinguishing structural features (H&E stain)	Single nucleus; perinuclear clear zone (intracellular organisms only[a])	Thick wall; central basophilic endospores (spherule only)	Pale, thin cell wall; extracellular clear zone	Thick cell wall; basophilic protoplasm; multiple nuclei
Mucicarmine staining	−	−	+	−
Type of granulomas	Caseating	Caseating; early lesions, suppuration	Caseating, noncaseating	Necrotizing with suppuration

[a] Intracellular organisms are seen only in disseminated histoplasmosis. Histoplasma cannot be visualized within caseous necrosis in lung granulomas on sections stained with H&E.
(From Rosenthal,[6] with permission.)

compromised people, with approximately one third of affected patients being younger than 1 year old. This form of the disease affects not only the lung but multiple organs, in which marked histiocytic proliferation is the predominant finding. Necrotizing granulomas are usually absent, but interstitial lung infiltrates are apparent on radiographic examination.

Chronic histoplasmosis occurs in patients with long-standing lung disease; for years, it was the confusing mimic of tuberculosis. In fact, many midwestern tuberculosis sanitariums admitted a significant percentage of patients with histoplasmosis or tuberculosis, or both. Both infiltrative and cavitary lesions characterize the chest radiograph. Sputum culture for the infecting organisms is the definitive test, although lung biopsies may be necessary if the culture is negative.

Histoplasmomas are the lesions most likely to be misinterpreted as neoplasms, for they appear on radiographic examination as well-circumscribed lesions that may enlarge gradually. They are usually found on chest x-ray studies in otherwise healthy individuals. The lesions are traditionally excised to exclude the possibility of neoplasm, although the diagnosis could well be made by FNA.[16] On visual inspection, the amorphous center of histoplasmomas is the same as that in caseating granulomas caused by mycobacteria.

Of the four fungi discussed in this section, Histoplasma is the one for which the Papanicolaou stain is the least helpful. However, these small (2 to 5 m) intracytoplasmic yeasts may be suggested in the cytoplasm of multinucleated histiocytes (Fig. 5-9), and can be demonstrated by silver stains.

COCCIDIOIDOMYCOSIS

Coccidioides immitis is a saprophytic fungus that also occurs in the soil. A dimorphic fungus, the natural growth form is a mold, but in humans, the spherule contains the endospores, which are the infective components. Lung involvement is usually asymptomatic or mildly symptomatic, with chest radiography revealing patchy, hazy infiltrates. Usually self-limited, the disease clears within 2 to 3 weeks. If the disease persists for more than 6 to 8 weeks, persistent pneumonia and miliary dissemination may ensue. A less common form—chronic progressive pneumonia—closely resembles tuberculosis. Occasionally, a cavity or coccidioidoma, detected on routine chest x-ray

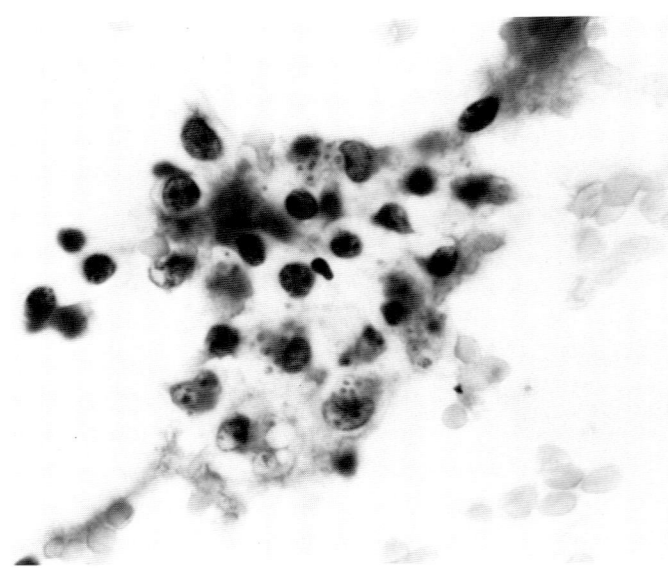

Fig. 5-9 Histoplasmosis (FNA of cervical lymph node). These organisms were aspirated from the cervical lymph node of a patient with pulmonary histoplasmosis. The organisms are quite small, and are invariably found within the cytoplasm of macrophages. Giemsa or PAS stains are usually preferred, but the Papanicolaou stain can reveal these organisms. (Papanicolaou stain, × 1,000.)

studies, may result, the lining of which resembles "repair" or metaplastic epithelium (Fig. 5-10). Disseminated disease is rare, but is most common in immunocompromised patients, pregnant women, blacks, Mexicans, and Filipinos.[16]

The cytologic features of coccidioidomycosis are best appreciated on FNA of a lung lesion, which may be cystic. The pink-staining round spherules (measuring 30 to 60 μm) are readily identified by Papanicolaou staining, and the endospores, if present within the spherules, are also easy to recognize, as they also stain pink[3] (Fig. 5-11). Empty, sometimes collapsed spherules are also apparent. Small endospores (2 to 5 μm) can be distinguished from Histoplasma and Cryptococci because the endospores of cocci do not bud. Not only will the granulomatous reaction be obvious, but an acute inflammatory reaction is thought to be provoked by the endospores, so the pattern will be a combined granulomatous and acute inflammatory response. According to Johnston and Frable, and in our experience, the spherules of cocci may be seen frequently in the sputum of infected patients.[1]

CRYPTOCOCCOSIS

Cryptococcus neoformans is a ubiquitous yeast found in soils, especially those rich in pigeon droppings. The organism can produce primary disease, but is frequently a secondary invader in an immunocompromised host. The disease can be found not only in bronchial material but in urine and cerebrospinal fluid (CSF).

The infectious pattern varies depending upon the patient's immune status, with granulomatous reaction occurring in otherwise healthy individuals. These granulomas contain numerous intracellular organisms, and can be caseating or noncaseating.[22,23]

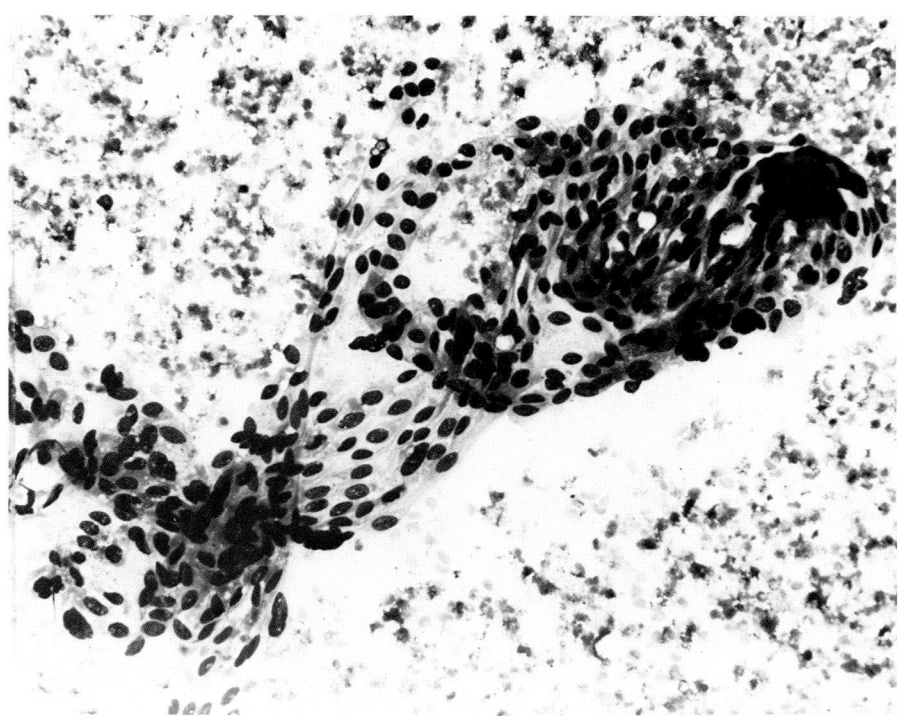

Fig. 5-10 Coccidioidomycosis (FNA). This squamous epithelium was aspirated from the lining of a mycetoma cavity containing coccidioides. The amorphous debris in the background and the uniform pattern of the epithelium indicate the benign diagnosis. Be aware that squamous carcinomas can be found in benign cavity linings. A careful examination of the entire specimen is mandatory. (MGG stain, × 200.)

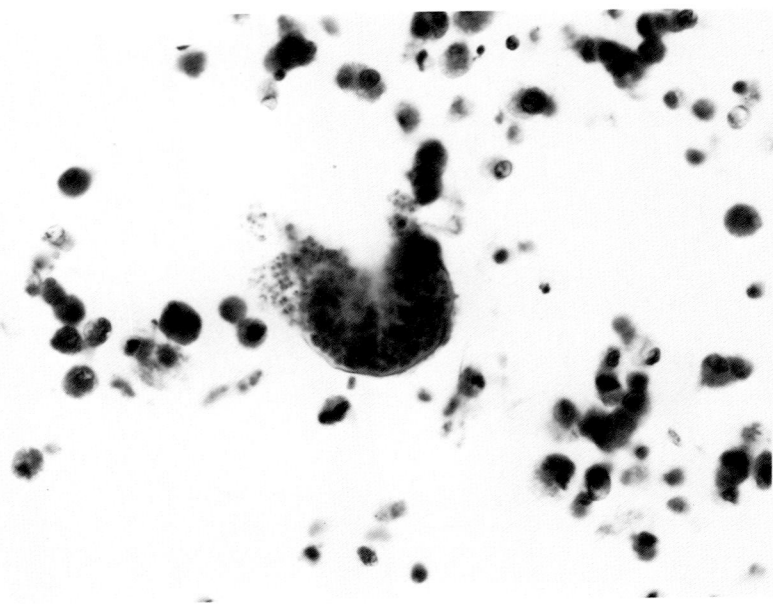

Fig. 5-11 Coccidioidomycosis (bronchoalveolar lavage). Scattered throughout the specimen and containing predominantly macrophages are large spherules containing the endospores of coccidioides. Note the thick wall of the spherule and the small nuclei of the organisms. Empty spherules can also be seen in such specimens. (Papanicolaou stain, × 400.)

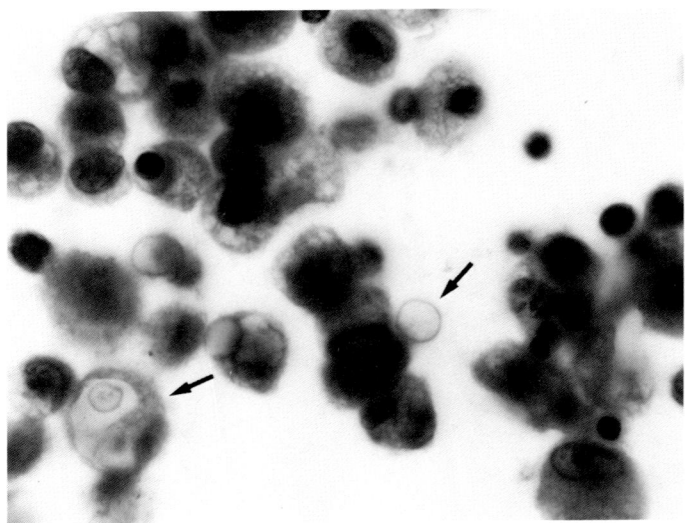

Fig. 5-12 Cryptococcosis (bronchoalveolar lavage). The organisms (*arrows*) can be found both within the cytoplasm of macrophages and free-floating. Their size is approximately that of a macrophage nucleus, and the characteristic capsule is best seen when the organism is contained within cytoplasm. Because of its thick cell wall, a birefringent center is often noted, and should not be confused with mounting medium artifact. (Papanicolaou stain, × 1,000.)

Most patients who are immunocompromised do not manifest a granulomatous pattern, but will exhibit sheets of organisms within the alveolar spaces, with little cellular response. This is similar to the nonresponse seen in CSF.

The budding organism has a thick, mucinous capsule and a widely variable size, averaging 4 to 7 μm, with a range of 2 to 15 μm.[24] Cryptococcus can be distinguished from Histoplasma by its larger size, thicker cell wall, and budding. The thin isthmus of the bud distinguishes Cryptococcus from the broader-based bud of Blastomyces. On cytologic examination of a Papanicolaou-stained specimen, the budding yeast may have a darkened, birefringent center resembling a mounting-medium artifact, or it may appear simply as a pale, pink, round or budding structure with a thick outer rim and central density[25,26] (Fig. 5-12).

Organisms can be identified using H&E or Papanicolaou stains, but are most characteristically developed by silver stain and the periodic acid-Schiff (PAS) stain. India ink preparation is another diagnostic method that can clearly demonstrate the thick capsule.

NORTH AMERICAN BLASTOMYCOSIS

Blastomycosis is caused by *Blastomyces dermatitidis*, a dimorphic fungus that grows as mycelia at room temperature and as yeasts (the usual infectious form) at body temperature. The source of the fungus is not clearly defined, but endemic areas include the south, south-central, and Great Lakes areas of the United States, and parts of Canada; scattered cases have also been reported in Africa and South America. The lung is the primary target of blastomycosis, which affects young to middle-aged adults with greater frequency than other age groups.

The microscopic pattern of the pneumonia progresses from an acute inflammatory stage to a histiocytic response with granulomatous formation. Necrotizing granulomas are constructed of a central zone of necrotic neutrophils without true caseation. Special stains are not needed to visualize the single or budding globes which are, on average, 8 to 15 μm in diameter, sometimes reaching a maximum of 30 μm, and which have thick refractile walls containing either a clear cytoplasmic mass or varying numbers of granules (Fig. 5-13). Shrinkage of the cytoplasmic

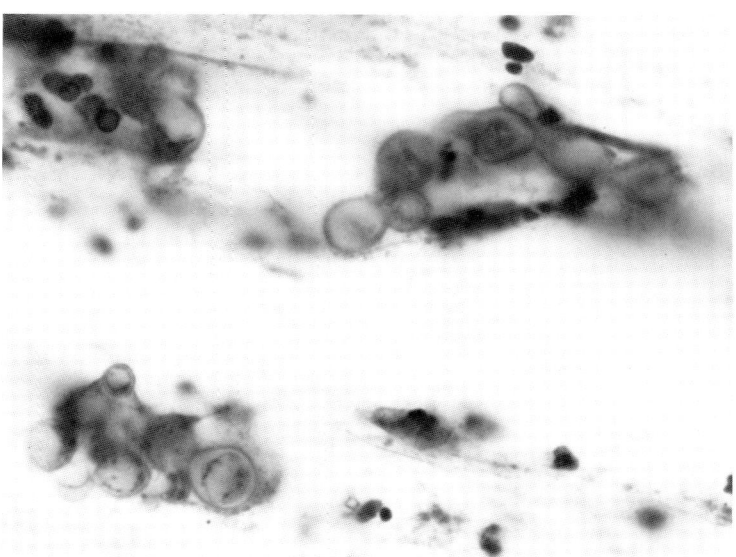

Fig. 5-13 Blastomycosis (sputum). A hallmark of Blastomyces organisms is the broad-based bud that sometimes forms a chain of organisms. (Courtesy of Dr. William W. Johnston, Duke University Medical Center.) (Papanicolaou stain, × 1,000.)

mass may produce a halo effect between the cell wall and the mass. All of these features are characteristic, but the most important feature diagnostically is the broad-based bud[27] of Blastomyces, which distinguishes it from Cryptococcus (with its thin tapering attachment). The organisms may be found either extracellularly within the necrotic granulomas, or within the cytoplasm of macrophages.

The cytologic examination of a bronchopulmonary specimen will reflect the variable inflammatory pattern. Polymorphonuclear leukocytes may accompany, or alternate with, multinucleated giant cells in which the budding yeasts may be found. Organisms have been recovered in pleural effusions. There is nothing specifically diagnostic about the inflammatory pattern; thus, identification of the organism is crucial.[28]

Invasive Fungal Pneumonias

Fungi that cause a pneumonia pattern rather than granulomatous disease are outlined in Table 5-3. In the past, such diagnoses were not targets for cytologic interpretation, as these organisms were not recovered from exfoliated or brushed specimens. Transbronchial biopsy, in some instances, would retrieve diagnostic material. However, with the advent of FNA and enhanced radiologic imaging techniques, needles can be directed to suspicious areas in the lung parenchyma and material can be aspirated, not only for microbiologic identification, but also for cytologic analysis. These organisms do not require special stains for identification, as routine Papanicolaou staining effectively demonstrates them. Their morphology is sufficiently characteristic to allow tentative identification of the organism, so that therapy may be initiated even before definitive culture results are available. This is especially critical in immunocompromised patients with life-threatening infections.

ASPERGILLOSIS

Aspergillus is a saprophytic organism that occurs as an invading pathogen almost exclusively in patients who are in some way immunocompromised. Patients with acute leukemia are particularly prone to this infection. Rare cases of invasive aspergillosis in otherwise normal individuals have been reported.[16] Sputum cultures are frequently negative, making antemortem diagnosis difficult. Even with positive culture results, the identification of Aspergillus as the causative agent is difficult since this organism is so frequently encountered. Open biopsy, transbronchial biopsy, and transbronchial and transthoracic FNA are the most reliable means of identifying the organism as pathogenic. Because of the debilitated condition of most infected patients, the prognosis is poor unless very early diagnosis and aggressive therapy are accomplished.

The tissue pattern is that of a hemorrhagic infarct, with only scattered inflammatory cells. In order to be defined as an invasive process, fungal hyphae should be identified invading blood vessel walls and permeating the alveolar septa. Fungi can behave as arterial thrombi when they occlude the lumina. Another pattern is that of a necrotizing bronchopneumonia. A striking gross pattern, a "target lesion," is formed by a central yellow-grey zone rimmed with a dark periphery. This lesion may be the precursor of a hemor-

Table 5-3 Fungal Pneumonias: Contrasting Histologic Features

	Aspergillosis	Mucormycosis	Candidiasis	Torulopsis Infection
Organism Morphology				
Hyphae	Thin (3 to 5 μm); septate	Wide (10 to 15 μm); nonseptate	—	—
Branching	Dichotomous, 45°	Haphazard, 90°	—	—
Budding yeast	—	—	+	+
Pseudohyphae	—	—	+	—
Tissue Reaction				
Vascular invasion, infarction	+	+	—	—
Acute inflammation, abcesses	—	—	+	+

(From Rosenthal,[6] with permission.)

Fig. 5-14 Aspergillosis (FNA). Aspergillus organisms usually are not obtained in exfoliated material as they grow tenaciously into tissue. FNA is an effective way of obtaining diagnostic material, both for morphology and culture. Note the broad hyphae with 45-degree angle branching. The accompanying inflammation is predominantly acute. Vascular invasion with hemorrhage and infarction is common with this organism. (H&E stain, × 400.)

rhagic infarct, caused by vascular invasion. The fungus probably invades the parenchyma through the bronchial walls.

The morphology of the organism is that of a long, thin, septate mycelium that is approximately 4 µm in diameter and that demonstrates 45-degree branching (Figs. 5-14 and 5-15). Mycelia frequently run parallel to each other, radiating from a central point. Mycelial growth is usually not associated with conidiophores, so mycelia may be misinterpreted as being indicative

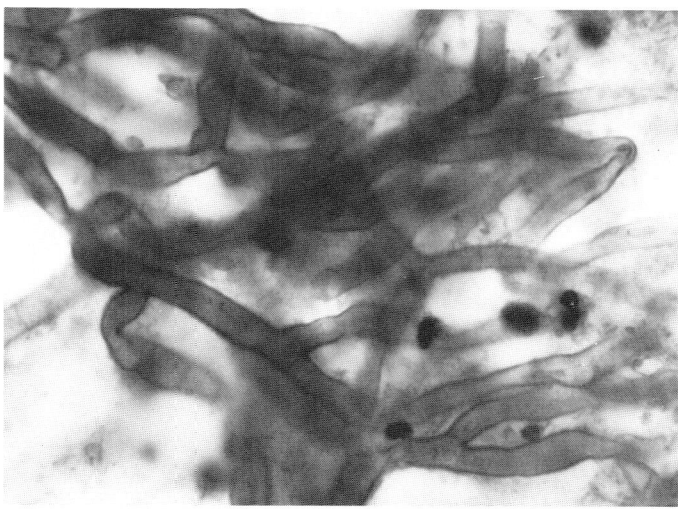

Fig. 5-15 Aspergillosis (FNA). A higher power view of the morphologic features seen in Fig. 5-14 illustrates the acute-angle branching of these remarkably ribbon-like hyphae. (H&E stain, × 1,000.)

of phycomycosis. The distinguishing feature is that in phycomycosis the mycelia are not septate.

Aspergillus and other fungi can produce dysplastic squamous cells that may be misinterpreted as squamous carcinoma. This is particularly true when a cavity develops in a mycetoma (Fig. 5-10). Calcium oxylate crystals in large aggregates can be seen in association with the hyphae,[1,16] and have been retrieved in sputum.[29] These crystals polarize, readily permitting identification. Their presence in a sputum specimen indicates that an Aspergillus infection exists even if the organism is not represented in the sample.[30]

MUCORMYCOSIS (PHYCOMYCOSIS)

The term phycomycosis applies to an acute mycotic infection in which extensive inflammation and vascular thrombi are caused by invasion of vessel walls and lumina by any of a long list of fungi, including Absidia, Mucor, Rhizopus, and Basidiobolus. Underlying debilitating diseases, including diabetes mellitus, the lymphoproliferative diseases, and immunocompromised conditions, predispose patients to these infections. Steroid therapy in otherwise healthy individuals also has been identified as a predisposing factor.

The histologic pattern features extensive parenchymal and vascular invasion by the organism, with subsequent hemorrhagic infarcts and scanty cellular infiltrates. The mycelia of these organisms are ribbon-like and are wider than Aspergillus, measuring 10 to 15 μm in width. Ninety-degree branching differentiates these from the 45-degree branches of Aspergillus.

Fungi Variably Producing Disease

A variety of fungi can be found in respiratory samples; they are usually contaminants, but occasionally are of pathogenic significance. What used to be saprophytes have now become opportunistic infectious organisms. Therefore, the presence of fungi in a respiratory sample can no longer be ignored or minimized. However, the determination of whether or not a fungal organism is responsible for disease in a patient is left to the clinical judgment of the attending physicians. Moreover, definitive confirmation of the type of organism is also not the responsibility of the cytology laboratory, but is the purview of the microbiology staff. However, as reliant on special stains as many pathologists are, experience has shown that the routine Papanicolaou stain is capable of detailing the characteristics of the mycoses sufficiently to obviate the need for other stains. As with any other disease process, if the observer does not consider the possibility of a particular disease, the pathology may not be recognized. Knowledge of infectious diseases endemic to or likely to be brought into an area is important when dealing with probable infectious material.

CANDIDIASIS

Candida species are frequently saprophytic inhabitants of the oral cavity and skin, and occasionally, the respiratory tree. The only way of definitively determining that the organism is pathogenic, rather than merely a contaminant, is to locate the organism within the tissue. Such infections usually occur in immunocompromised patients and present as multisystem diseases. Significant pulmonary involvement, however, is rare.[16] On cytologic examination, Candida species appear as long pseudohyphae with budding yeast, sometimes found in a morular form.

ACTINOMYCOSIS

Actinomyces organisms are usually contaminants of lower respiratory tract specimens, being dragged down by the bronchoscope from the tonsillar area. In order to implicate this organism as a pathogen, tissue sections must be obtained to demonstrate invasion of Actinomyces into the lung tissue.[31] Association of the organism with a pathologic condition cannot be made based solely on the presence of the organism in a cytologic sample from the respiratory tract.

On cytologic examination, Actinomyces species appear in clusters of organisms, with rodlike filaments extending radially from the center. The central structure, the so-called sulfur granule, is not readily recovered in cytologic material.

NOCARDIOSIS

Nocardia, an organism like Actinomyces, produces a disease pattern similar to Actinomyces when the latter is infectious. Dissemination via the bloodstream is common, especially to the central nervous system. In most cases, the diagnosis cannot be made by sputum culture, and lung biopsy or FNA are often required.

A necrotizing acute pneumonia with abscess formation is the common presentation. Poorly formed granulomas, predominantly involving histiocytes, may surround the necrotic areas. A GMS stain allows clear visualization of the organisms. They are also weakly acid-fast and appear as gram-positive with Brown-Hopps or Brown-Brenn techniques. The organisms appear as long, branching, filamentous rods, assuming "Chinese character" configurations and measuring 0.5 to 1.0 μm in diameter. Granules, such as seen in Actinomyces organisms, are not usually present in colonies of Nocardia.

PNEUMOCYSTIS

Pneumocystis carinii has become a major cause of morbidity and mortality among patients with acquired immunodeficiency syndrome (AIDS) and other immunosuppressive conditions, although only a few years ago it was rarely encountered. On pathologic examination, it is characterized by a marked interstitial plasma cell infiltrate and a foamy intraalveolar exudate, hence the archaic name "interstitial plasma cell pneumonia."[16]

Recovery of the organisms in sputa is rare.[32] Brushings and washings occasionally are productive,[27] but the most diagnostic study is bronchoalveolar lavage. Prior to the use of this technique, open lung biopsy was the most highly diagnostic method, with transthoracic percutaneous needle biopsy and transbronchial biopsy being adequate, but less successful than open biopsy. In our institution, bronchoalveolar lavage has essentially replaced the open lung biopsy for diagnosis of pneumocystis.[14] Equally impressive results have been reported by others.[14,33-35]

The frothy honeycomb "exudate" within the alveolar spaces stains pink on H & E sections, and appears rusty brown in cytologic samples stained with Papanicolaou stain (Fig. 5-16). This exudate contains closely packed organisms (Fig. 5-17) that can be revealed clearly by GMS (Fig. 5-18) or Giemsa stain, or by fluorescent emission of Papanicolaou-stained material.[32] These small, cup-shaped organisms mea-

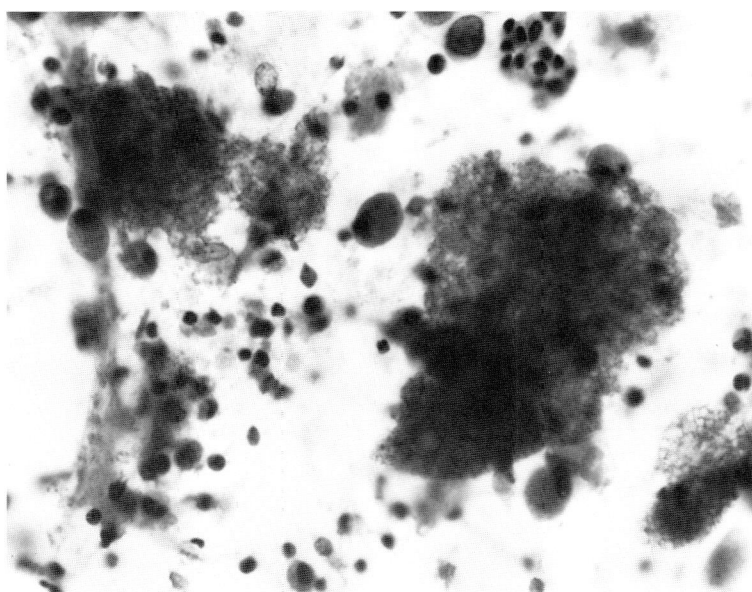

Fig. 5-16 Pneumocystis (bronchoalveolar lavage). Diagnostic material of this opportunistic infection can be obtained readily by lavage. The large groups of tightly packed organisms present as rusty brown sponges. Although silver staining is still considered the standard of practice, Papanicolaou-stained material such as this is considered indisputable. (Papanicolaou stain, × 400.)

198 PRACTICAL CYTOPATHOLOGY

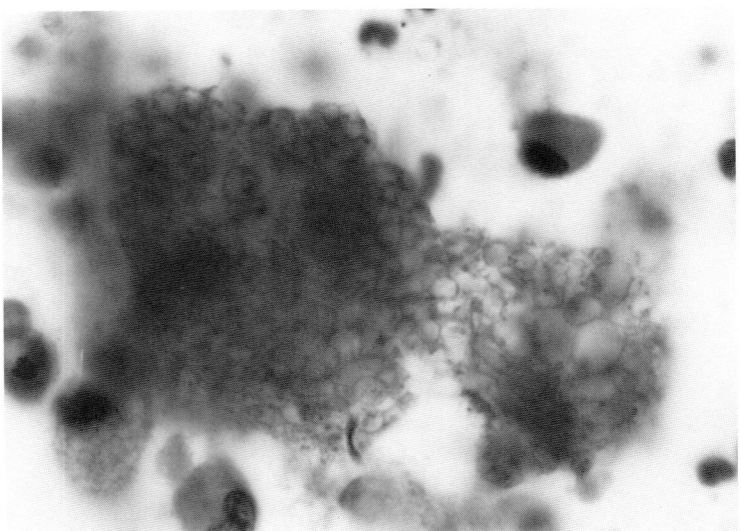

Fig. 5-17 Pneumocystis (bronchoalveolar lavage). A higher power view of Fig. 5-16 shows the outlines of the organisms. This is not truly an "exudate," but a colony of organisms. Compare the size of each "hole" with that of the nearby macrophages. (Papanicolaou stain, × 1,000.)

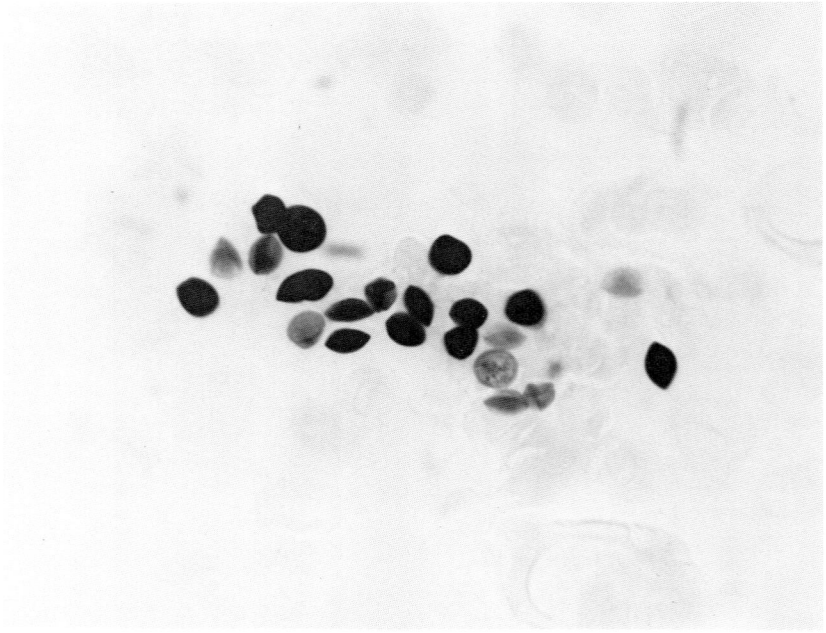

Fig. 5-18 Pneumocystis (FNA). Bipolar organisms stained by traditional silver impregnation. (Silver stain, × 1,000.)

sure 1 to 2 μm and are the intracystic forms of sporozoites.[36] This foamy exudate in cytologic specimens, stained by the Papanicolaou method, is highly diagnostic, and special stains are not required. In immunocompromised patients, an absence of inflammatory reaction is common, attesting to the inability of these patients to respond to infectious organisms.

Viral Infections

The significance of viral infection in the lung has become more critical in recent years as a result of the increasing numbers of immunocompromised patients, and their increased susceptibility to infectious diseases, including viruses. In the well patient, a pulmonary viral infection is usually self-limited, and patients generally return to their previously healthy state. A few patients, especially children, may succumb to an especially virulent strain of virus, or an overwhelming infection of the lung. Until very recently, there has been no definitive antiviral therapy, and supportive measures have been the best that medical science could provide for such patients.[37] As antiviral agents become accepted, effective treatments, diagnosis of the specific infectious agent becomes mandatory in order to match the diagnosis with the appropriate mode of treatment.

The assumption cannot be made that the virus is, indeed, causing the pneumonic process simply because hallmarks of a viral organism may be present (Table 5-4). In a normal population, approximately 80 percent will carry herpes virus, and a lesser but significant percentage will carry cytomegalovirus (CMV) within respiratory cells, without actually experiencing a disease. In order to confirm that an organism is associated with a pneumonia, cultures, immunochemical assays, and DNA probes must be performed on, or cellular morphologic changes must be recognized in, material recovered from the actual pulmonary alveoli. Bronchoalveolar lavage permits the recovery of diagnostic material from the functional airways; cytologic changes in such specimens can indicate infection before culture results are known, and therapy can be initiated on a presumptive basis within a matter of hours.

Whatever the method of sampling, the specimens must be handled rapidly and the changes within the cells quickly fixed. This ensures that any changes that are seen accurately represent viral changes, and not simply degenerative changes secondary to a delay in processing. Stains must be fresh and reveal crisp nuclear detail for the same reasons.

Before the specific cytologic changes of a variety of viruses commonly affecting the respiratory tract are described, nonspecific changes must be addressed. Cilia with attached cytoplasm—ciliocytophthoria—has long been a recognized consequence of viral attack on a cell. This change is quite nonspecific, but can be especially pronounced in adenovirus infections. It was first described by Papanicolaou in 1956.[38] In addition, small, round, eosinophilic masses in the cytoplasm, presumably of degenerative origin, may be observed,[1,3] much like those seen in urothelial cells.

The nonspecific changes that present the greatest diagnostic difficulties are those that accompany re-

Table 5-4 Viral Pneumonias: Light and Electron Microscopic Features

Virus	Ultrastructure	Inclusions		Cellular Alteration	Pathologic Features
		Nuclear	Cytoplasmic		
Cytomegalovirus	100–200 nm; round core; double membrane	+	+	Cytomegaly	Interstitial pneumonia; diffuse alveolar damage
Herpes simplex; varicella-zoster	150–200 nm; round core; double membrane	+	−	−	Necrosis; diffuse alveolar damage
Measles	15–20 nm; tubular filaments	+	+	Multinucleation	Interstitial pneumonia; diffuse alveolar damage
Adenovirus	60–90 nm; icosahedral; crystalline array	+	−	Smudge cells	Necrotizing bronchiolitis; diffuse alveolar damage

(From Rosenthal,[6] with permission.)

generation and repair of the respiratory epithelium. Such atypia may mimic adenocarcinoma or squamous carcinoma unless the wary observer considers cytologic criteria very carefully. If cellular changes are definitely secondary to an infection, they will disappear as the infection progresses and then recedes. If instead the changes are secondary to an adenocarcinoma, the atypia will persist, and may even become more markedly anaplastic, thereby verifying the diagnosis of cancer.

Of importance and interest is the altered inflammatory response manifested by many affected patients, some of whom are unable to respond at all. Therefore, little or no inflammatory reaction will be the norm. Diffuse alveolar damage may be the only pattern seen in tissue sections. A careful search for organisms or their hallmarks is, therefore, an important responsibility of the cytologist, even when significant numbers of inflammatory cells are not present.

SPECIFIC VIRAL INFECTIONS

Herpes Virus Type I

The prototype of viral infections affecting cytologic samples is clearly herpes, no doubt because this family of viruses affects the female genital tract, as well as the respiratory tract and numerous other body sites. The clinical presentation of patients with pneumonia caused by herpes simplex virus usually includes a history of a debilitating disease or immunosuppression. Parenchymal involvement is bronchocentric, with patchy, nodular, or confluent foci of necrosis. The alveolar septa are obliterated, with only their "ghosts" remaining. Alveolar spaces contain a proteinaceous suspension of necrotic neutrophils and cellular debris. Hyaline membranes are equally common. Characteristic intranuclear inclusions (Fig. 5-19) will be found in alveolar lining cells (pneumocytes) or alveolar macrophages at the periphery of the necrosis.[37] If necrosis is too extensive, these inclusions will not be identified.

Herpetic tracheobronchitis is a necrotizing lesion seen in most patients with lung lesions, but it may also occur in patients without these lesions. The ulcerated respiratory epithelium is covered by a fibrinopurulent exudate. The intranuclear inclusions can be identified within cells of the intact mucosa or within submucosal gland epithelium.

Since herpetic tracheobronchitis and esophagitis are relatively common, a true herpetic pneumonia cannot be inferred from the presence of infected cells in bronchoscopic or sputum samples. In order to identify herpes as a cause of a pneumonia, the charac-

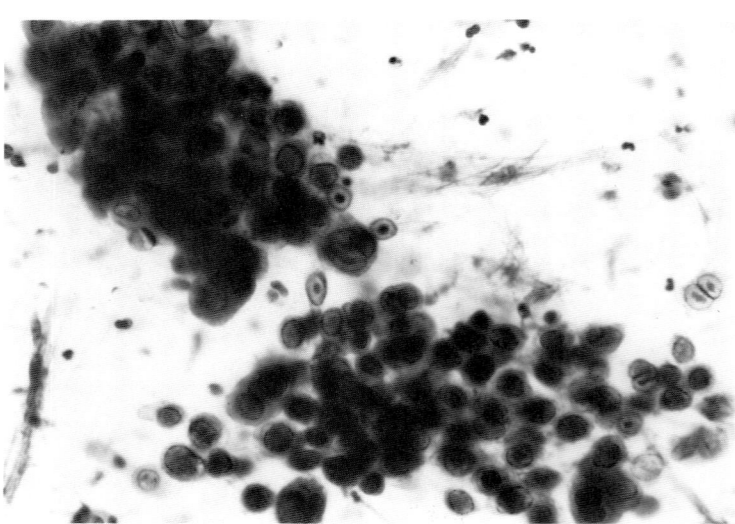

Fig. 5-19 Herpes virus (bronchial brushing). The same criteria that apply to herpes infection of the female genital tract apply to respiratory tract specimens. In this specimen, obtained from a patient with herpetic tracheobronchitis, ground-glass nuclei and intranuclear inclusions are seen. This patient was immunocompromised, suffering from AIDS. (Papanicolaou stain, × 400.)

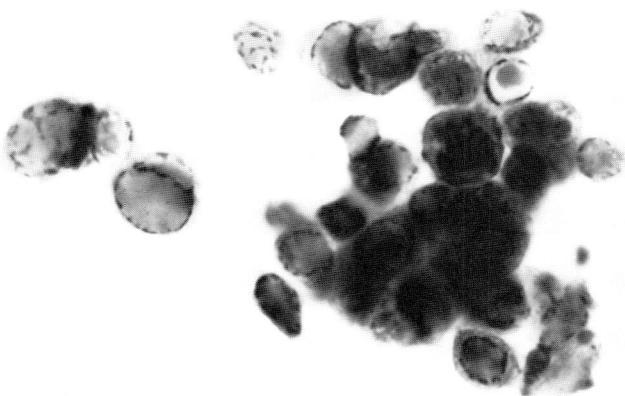

Fig. 5-20 Herpes virus infection (sputum). Note the ground-glass transformation of the nuclei, with margination of the chromatin. Occasional intranuclear inclusions are found in the specimen. The patient was immunocompromised as a result of receiving chemotherapy for oat cell carcinoma. Diagnostic oat cells were found elsewhere in the specimen. (Papanicolaou stain, × 1,000.)

teristic cellular changes must be observed in samples retrieved directly from the pulmonary alveoli, either by transbronchial or transthoracic needle aspiration. Bronchoalveolar lavage can be used to retrieve diagnostic specimens from the pulmonary parenchyma, and in our experience, has provided 100 percent diagnostic yield of infectious material.[14]

Classic herpetic lesions of the lung can be divided into two cytologic types: ground-glass intranuclear inclusions and Cowdry type A inclusions, which are round, eosinophilic, central bodies surrounded by a clear halo and then confined by a thickened, chromatinic membrane[39] (Fig. 5-20). Although multinucleated giant cells may be seen, they are not as common as in herpetic infections elsewhere in the body. The cells are not enlarged; this allows them to be differentiated from those infected with CMV, and herpetic inclusions are bright red or lavender, not the deeply basophilic inclusions that are characteristic of CMV. Cytoplasmic inclusions, often present in CMV-infected cells, are absent in herpetic lesions. Both viruses, however, belong to the same family.

Cytomegalovirus

CMV can be carried by patients who are immunologically intact without any resultant disease. To a large percentage of immunocompromised patients, however, this infectious agent can be lethal. The infection may be opportunistic, but most likely is transferred from patient to patient via blood transfusions. The histologic pattern of CMV infection differs from that of herpes pneumonia in that, in the former, there is an absence of necrosis and a more diffuse pattern. Hyaline membranes, intra-alveolar hemorrhage, and proteinaceous exudates are common findings. Concomitant CMV and *pneumocystis carinii* infections are common.

Rather than wait 7 to 25 days for viral cultures to yield a diagnosis, evidence of the characteristic cellular changes is sought in specimens obtained by open lung biopsy, bronchial brushing,[40] transbronchial and transthoracic needle aspiration, and bronchoalveolar lavage. Diagnostic features include generalized cell enlargement (megalo) and a dramatic, intranuclear, large, basophilic inclusion that is surrounded by a well-defined halo and a very distinct chromatinic rim[41] (Fig. 5-21). In contrast to herpes virus, cells infected with CMV also frequently have single or multiple intracytoplasmic inclusions, which appear as very small spheres (Fig. 5-22). The virus affects respiratory epithelial cells, alveolar lining cells, alveolar macrophages, endothelial cells, and interstitial cells. In addition to the changes appreciated on Papanicolaou-stained material, the inclusions can also be appreciated in PAS-stained specimens.

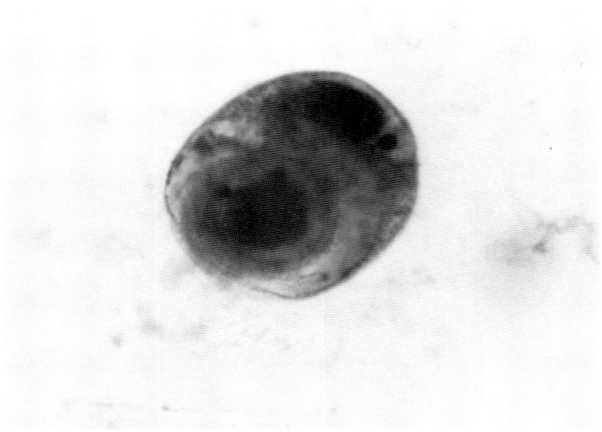

Fig. 5-21 Cytomegalovirus infection (bronchoalveolar lavage). An unusual multinucleated cell, with characteristic intranuclear inclusions and satellite inclusion, is seen. Note the large size of the cell, and the halo rimming the intranuclear inclusion. (Papanicolaou stain, × 1,000.)

Varicella-zoster Virus

Varicella virus, of the same family as herpes simplex and indistinguishable from herpes zoster, causes either chickenpox in children, or shingles in adults who have had previous varicella-zoster infection. This virus causes pneumonia in approximately 15 percent of patients with chickenpox, usually adults. Children who are immunocompromised or otherwise debilitated may develop a varicella pneumonia. Affected adults are not necessarily immunocompromised. If the disease clinically resembles herpes zoster, dissemination will occur in immunocompromised patients, especially in those with underlying malignant diseases, such as Hodgkin's disease. Lung involvement in such patients is very uncommon.

Histologic changes in the lung include those of an acute interstitial pneumonia with hyaline membranes, and proteinaceous exudate within the alveolar spaces. A parabronchial distribution has been described, but focal areas of necrosis are the most common presentation. The intranuclear inclusions are identical to those of herpes simplex, and are most commonly seen within alveolar lining cells. Healing of this pneumonia has been noted to result in diffuse calcification.[16]

Measles Virus

Measles pneumonia is extremely rare, and death as a result of this disease is even more uncommon. However, in immunocompromised children and, rarely in adults, the disease has a significant impact.[42] Although a skin rash is usually present, reports of giant cell pneumonia without skin rash have also been noted;[43] this is because immunocompromised children may not respond to infection in the usual manner.

The histopathology of measles pneumonia is characterized by a dramatic scattering of multinucleated giant cells containing eosinophilic intranuclear and intracytoplasmic inclusions. Such inclusions can also be found within endothelial cells and macrophages. These polykaryocytes may contain up to 50 nuclei with abundant eosinophilic cytoplasm, and are probably the result of the fusion of type 2 pneumocytes (Fig. 5-23). Accompanying the characteristic giant cells is an acute interstitial pneumonia with hyaline membranes and intra-alveolar protein. Although focal necrosis may occur, it is not a consistent or diagnostic finding; it does distinguish measles pneumonia from the giant cell pneumonia caused by respiratory syncytial virus (see the later section on that virus). Bronchial mucosal hyperplasia with focal squamous metaplasia may also be found.[16]

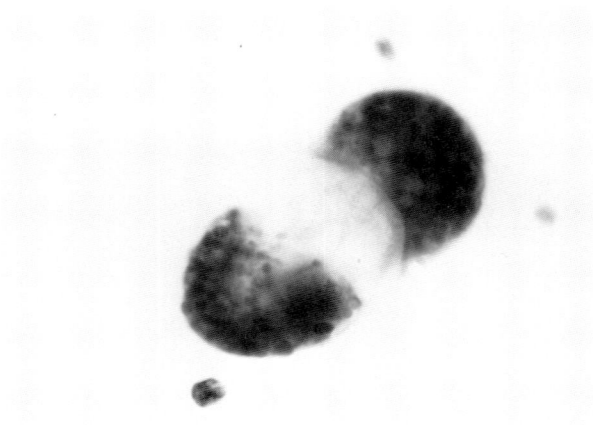

Fig. 5-22 Cytomegalovirus infection (bronchoalveolar lavage). This undivided double cell contains not only intranuclear inclusions (out of the plane of focus), but multiple cytoplasmic inclusions with a buckshot appearance. Note the large size of the cells when compared to that of lymphocytes or red cells. (Papanicolaou stain, × 1,000.)

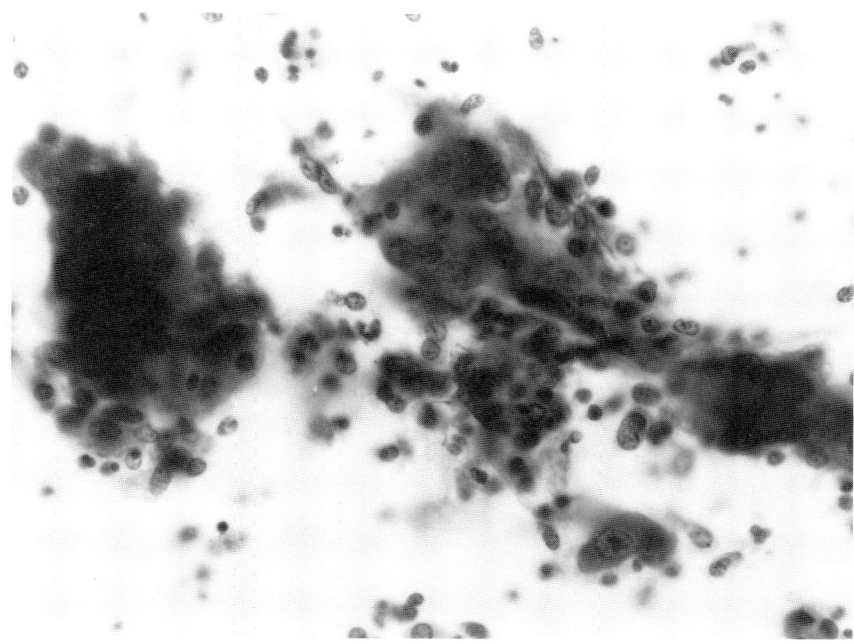

Fig. 5-23 Giant cell pneumonia (touch preparation of lung biopsy material). Material obtained by FNA of a giant cell pneumonia would resemble this material obtained from a touch preparation. Note the multinucleated giant cells and the large epithelioid cells which are consistent with type II pneumocytes. Measles and respiratory syncytial virus are the most common viral diseases producing this picture. (Papanicolaou stain, × 400.)

Adenovirus

Adenovirus usually does not produce severe disease, but simply causes a minor influenza-like syndrome involving the upper respiratory tract and resembling the common cold. Pneumonia, although rare, can be fatal in 40 percent of affected patients. These fatalities usually involve children younger than 1 year of age, but occasionally, deaths have been reported in previously healthy adults and immunocompromised people. Undiagnosed adenovirus infections have been implicated in other forms of chronic lung disease, such as bronchiectasis.[16]

The histologic characteristics of pneumonia secondary to adenovirus include destruction of bronchioles and small bronchi. Multiple, eosinophilic, intranuclear inclusions, each surrounded by a halo, can be seen in respiratory epithelium, which can be recovered in secretions for cytologic examination. As the pneumonia progresses, the epithelia of the bronchi and bronchioles slough, and the lumina become packed with granular, eosinophilic debris, resulting in distal air-trapping. Samples of this debris can be expected to be recovered by bronchoalveolar lavage or bronchial washing. Accompanying this bronchial damage is an acute interstitial pneumonia with intra-alveolar protein exudate and prominent hyaline membranes.

Two types of intranuclear inclusions are found in the bronchiolar epithelium and alveolar lining cells. One is a homogeneous, amphophilic or basophilic mass that almost totally replaces the nucleus. These inclusions are termed "smudge cells" and, owing to their enlargement, are very distinct, even with low-power magnification. The second kind of inclusion is a round, eosinophilic body surrounded by a clear halo that is circumscribed by clumped chromatin. This inclusion is smaller than the Cowdry type A inclusion of herpes virus. Ciliacytophthoria is most pronounced with this infection.

Respiratory Syncytial Virus

Respiratory syncytial virus may cause a severe bronchiolitis that is associated with low mortality, except in immunosuppressed patients.[10] It is a common cause of respiratory infection in the young. The major change in the lung parenchyma is an interstitial pneumonia. Sloughing of the bronchial epithelium and necrotic debris in the lumina are frequent findings.

The cytologic changes include large syncytial cell aggregates that measure 100 μm or more in diameter. Clear halos surround deeply basophilic inclusion bodies within the cytoplasm of these degenerating cells.[3,16] The disease may resemble measles pneumonia, as both viruses result in giant cell formation. However, RSV more consistently and dramatically produces necrosis.

Influenza Virus

Influenza pneumonia is not associated with any specific cytologic changes, but it does produce ciliocytophthoria. Parenchymal changes reflect diffuse alveolar damage characterized by capillary congestion, interstitial and intra-alveolar edema with hyaline membranes, hemorrhage, and inflammation. Necrotizing bronchiolitis and bronchitis can also be complicated by secondary bacterial infections. Bronchiolitis obliterans and interstitial fibrosis may also result.

Bacterial Infections

Because bacteria do not produce specific cytologic changes, our discussion of bacterial lung infections is necessarily limited. Bacteria can be recognized in respiratory tract samples and should be mentioned. However, they are frequently contaminants of the sample during collection,[44] so the presence of bacteria does not necessarily imply infection. Acute inflammation is the usual accompaniment to an acute bacterial infection.

Infectious Rarities

The pathogenic organisms and their disease processes described above can all be considered to be common. Case reports occasionally describe exotic diseases caused by unusual organisms. Lung infections by *Strongyloides stercoralis*[45–48] have been among the most frequently reported. Isolated case reports describe disease caused by Echinococcus,[49] Dirofilaria,[50] *Paracoccidioides brasiliensis*,[51] and *Paragonimus westermanii*.[52]

Organisms not producing disease, but described in the respiratory tract, include trichomonads[53] and *Entamoeba gingivalis*.[54] Seaweed has been reported to mimic fungus in at least one instance.[55]

NEOPLASMS OF THE LUNG

General Considerations

Lung cancer has become a major health problem, and is now the number one cancer killer among both men and women in the United States. The causal link with cigarette smoking is now indisputable,[56,57] but an exact scientific basis for the initiation and promotion of lung cancer by tobacco smoke has yet to be proved.[58] Nonetheless, the general opinion of pulmonologists and most other physicians holds that the best way to prevent lung cancer is for patients to stop smoking tobacco products. The only one of the major primary lung tumors for which this association has not been strongly established is bronchiolo-alveolar carcinoma.

Not only are the incidence, prevalence, and death rate statistics disheartening, but the salvage rate is downright dismal. The overall 5-year survival rate for carcinoma of the lung by latest figures is 9 percent. Squamous carcinoma of the lung still has the most optimistic outlook, with a 25 percent 5-year survival rate. Patients with adenocarcinoma and large cell carcinoma have an expected 12 percent 5-year survival rate. Of those patients with small cell carcinoma, most will die within 1 year, and less than 1 percent of these patients will survive for 5 years. Recent attempts to stage patients with oat cell carcinoma accurately and to evaluate resectability of the tumor, with subsequent surgical resection, have resulted in a few patients surviving for more than 2 years.

The occult nature of most carcinomas of the lung dictates a generally poor outcome. Death usually occurs 1 year after clinical evidence of the disease.[58a] If there were methods for earlier detection during clinically favorable stages of this disease, the salvage rate would most likely improve greatly.[59] Sputum cytology, utilized for mass population screening, was at one time thought to be the answer.[60,61] Several large studies were begun but the results were disappointing, as the cost of detecting an early lesion in an individual patient was exorbitant, making the total survey cost-ineffective.[62] However, screening for squamous carcinoma with sputum samples and chest radiography seems worthwhile; in the Johns Hopkins Lung Project, mortality was reduced by 46.6 percent in patients with squamous carcinoma.[9] Identification and screening of individuals at risk for the development of lung cancer are now being undertaken by most physicians.[63]

The invention of the fiberoptic bronchoscope has made the collection and diagnosis of respiratory cytologic samples highly reliable.[2,64] Not only can brushings, washings, and biopsies be obtained through the flexible bronchoscope, but FNA of both midline and peripheral lung lesions may be performed with precision.[65-74] Accurate staging can be accomplished with the bronchoscope by sampling paratracheal nodes with the fine needle and exploring nonobvious areas of the epithelium with brush and biopsy forceps to determine the presence or absence of in situ lesions. Fluoroscopically controlled transthoracic fine needle aspiration is performed routinely in most major hospitals.[12,75-77] For lesions measuring less than 2 cm, FNA provides hope that early lesions will be detected accurately and that cure will be effected.[78] Now under experimental investigation is the use of hematoporphyrin fluorescence for examination of in situ lesions, directing treatment by laser ablation through the bronchoscope.[2,79] Currently, until cigarette smoking is erradicated, or until an immunologic means of prevention or cure is discovered, an accurate work-up of a patient suspected of having lung cancer is the best that can be done to increase the quality and length of life of these patients.

The diagnosis of lung lesions is necessarily a team approach. Location of the lesion should determine the initial diagnostic tests (Table 5-5). Bronchoscopists and thoracic radiologists have developed techniques to locate and sample lesions, even those of very small dimensions, accurately. Once the samples are obtained, they are routed to the cytopathologist and surgical pathologist, who are responsible for making a definitive diagnosis on the basis of a very small amount of material. This situation dictates extremely careful processing and highly developed diagnostic skills. Intimate collaboration between the cytopathologist and surgical pathologist is a prerequisite for a concordant and accurate diagnosis. Nothing is more confusing to the clinician than an opinion from the surgical pathologist that is in conflict with the cytologic findings. Clinicians should be encouraged to challenge the pathologist if the diagnosis does not mesh with their clinical impression. Only through this interchange, unaffected by ego, will the patient receive the best care.

Table 5-5 Initial Diagnostic Tests for Pulmonary Lesions Based on the Location of the Neoplasm

Central Lesions	Peripheral Lesions
Chest radiography (tomography)	Chest radiography
Fiberoptic bronchoscopy	Tomography
Bronchial washings	CT scan
Bronchial brushings	FNA of mass
Transbronchial FNA	Mediastinoscopy
Primary tumor	Biopsy
Paratracheal nodes	FNA
Mediastinoscopy	
Biopsy	
FNA	

Classification of Lung Tumors

The classification system outlined in Table 5-6 is a modification of the current World Health Organization (WHO) classification of lung tumors,[80] which is quite lengthy and unnecessarily involved for the cytopathologist. The first four categories are the most commonly encountered primary lung tumors, but the microscopist must always anticipate that metastatic disease will be encountered frequently. Most metastatic lesions are carcinomas, especially adenocarcinomas,[81,82] although other entities, such as ma-

Table 5-6 Classification of Cancer of the Lung

Squamous carcinoma
Small cell undifferentiated carcinoma
Adenocarcinoma
Large cell undifferentiated
Carcinoid tumors
Bronchial gland tumors
Carcinosarcoma—blastoma
Sarcoma
Malignant lymphoma
Miscellaneous—including melanoma
Metastatic

lignant melanoma, should be considered. The category of large cell carcinoma is infrequently used at my institution, as we have routinely utilized electron microscopy whenever a cell type has been difficult to categorize. Electron microscopy is especially useful in differentiating between true oat cell carcinomas and other small cell neoplasms.

The need to classify lung lesions accurately according to cell type has been a result of the demands of both the radiologist and chemotherapist, who adjust their treatment based on the presumed cell of origin of the tumor.[83-85] Recently, the inaccuracy of typing lung tumors by light microscopy has been addressed in the literature,[86-89] and now, with the use of immunochemical methods, classification is even more confusing.[90-96] Conceivably, as these increasingly sophisticated diagnostic modalities are tested, their accuracy confirmed, and their significance fully recognized, the next few years will see a major overhaul of the classification of lung tumors. In our experience at UCLA,[6] and also in the experience of others,[88] cellular features in cytologic samples may more accurately categorize a lesion than histologic patterns, the current "gold standard."

SQUAMOUS (EPIDERMOID) CARCINOMA

Pulmonary squamous carcinoma is the primary lethal cancer in males and the third most prevalent cancer killer of females. It accounts for 35 to 50 percent of the lung cancers occurring in males, and 20 percent of those in females. This was the first cell type linked to cigarette smoking. When metastases do occur, they involve nonregional lymph nodes, adrenal glands, liver, kidney, and the contralateral lung. Occasionally, the brain is involved, but the diagnostic yield in spinal fluid is relatively low. Treatment is usually surgical if the patient's tumor is staged as resectable. If not, irradiation is the treatment of choice.

The anatomic location of squamous carcinoma is usually subsegmental or in the segmental bronchial junctions, with growth toward the main stem bronchus. The tumor locally invades bronchial cartilages, regional lymph nodes, and adjoining lung parenchyma. It is a relatively slowly growing lesion, with metastases occurring late in the course of the disease.

Squamous carcinoma of the lung can be subdivided on microscopic examination, into well-differentiated, moderately differentiated, and poorly differentiated forms. The presence of keratin will automatically classify a squamous carcinoma as a well-differentiated lesion, even if only a small number of cells exhibit keratin within the cytoplasm. Moderately differentiated tumors exhibit a squamous cytoplasm and hyperchromatic nuclei, but do not demonstrate keratin. Poorly differentiated tumors, which are difficult to distinguish from poorly differentiated adenocarcinomas, may require electron microscopy for definitive identification.

Cytologic Criteria

Specimens from a patient with classic squamous carcinoma with keratinization will contain cells with large, hyperchromatic nuclei that occasionally are multinucleated, with a variable nucleocytoplasmic ratio (Fig. 5-24). Aberrant cytoplasmic shapes, especially "tadpoles" (Fig. 5-25), are the hallmark of squamous carcinoma of the lung, and keratinized cytoplasm will categorize the lesion as being well-differentiated. Occasionally, the lesion will be so well-differentiated that anucleate keratin will predominate (Fig. 5-26), and no cells displaying truly malignant criteria will be present.

Accompanying the keratinized cells are usually numerous nonkeratinized cells that have similar characteristics; however, the latter have a very opaque green or blue cytoplasm with endoplasmic and ectoplasmic zones (Fig. 5-27). Nucleoli may be a prominent feature, but their presence is not a significant criterion. Accompanying the large tumor cells (both the keratinized and the unkeratinized cells) are hyperchromatic, often pyknotic nuclei mixed with necrotic tumor debris (diathesis) (Fig. 5-28). Such debris may be the first indication of tumor on the initial cytologic examination, and although not diagnostic, should indicate the need for follow-up cytologic specimens.[97]

Careful attention to nuclear chromatin and cytoplasmic boundaries will help distinguish poorly differentiated glandular lesions from squamous lesions (Table 5-7). In the former, shared cell borders, often in a syncytial arrangement, and delicate nuclear chromatin are the norms. Poorly differentiated squamous lesions have a generally coarser chromatin and well-defined, separate cell boundaries. Nucleoli are more

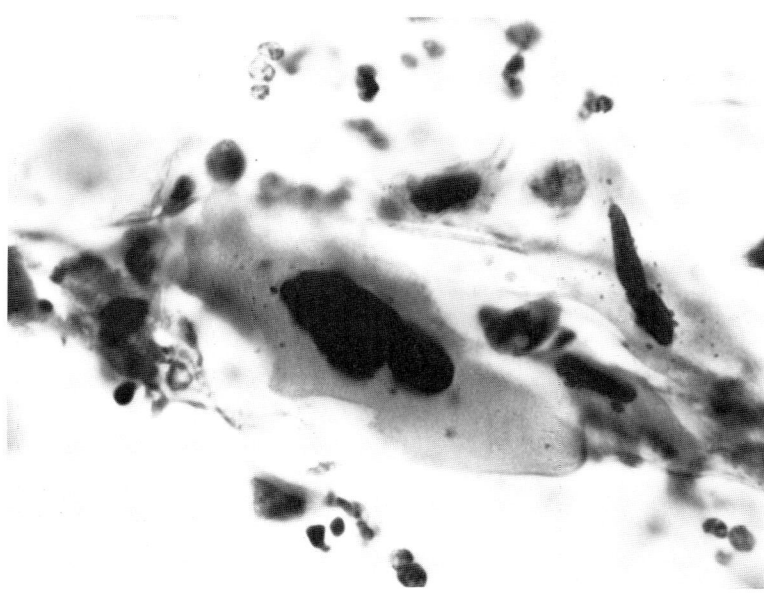

Fig. 5-24 Squamous carcinoma (sputum). The center cell, which is the largest in this field, contains multiple hyperchromatic nuclei of unequal size, surrounded by an aberrantly shaped opaque cytoplasm. If photographed in color, the orange cytoplasm would be apparent. Accompanying cells display less severe, but nonetheless significant, atypia. (Papanicolaou stain, × 1,000.)

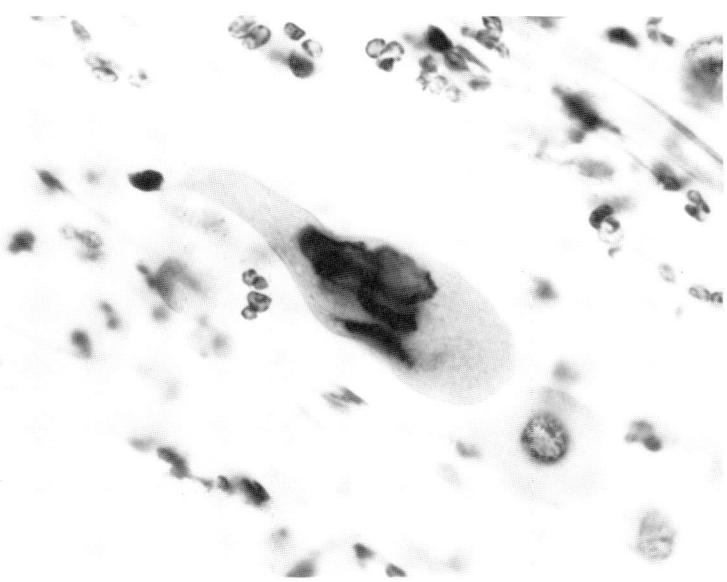

Fig. 5-25 Squamous cell carcinoma (sputum). This "tadpole" is the hallmark of squamous cell carcinoma. The nuclear changes are similar to those seen in the large cell in Fig. 5-24. The aberrantly shaped cytoplasm reinforces the lesion's malignant nature. The accompanying cells possibly reflect an adjacent CIS, as cytoplasmic shapes are less irregular. (Papanicolaou stain, × 1,000.)

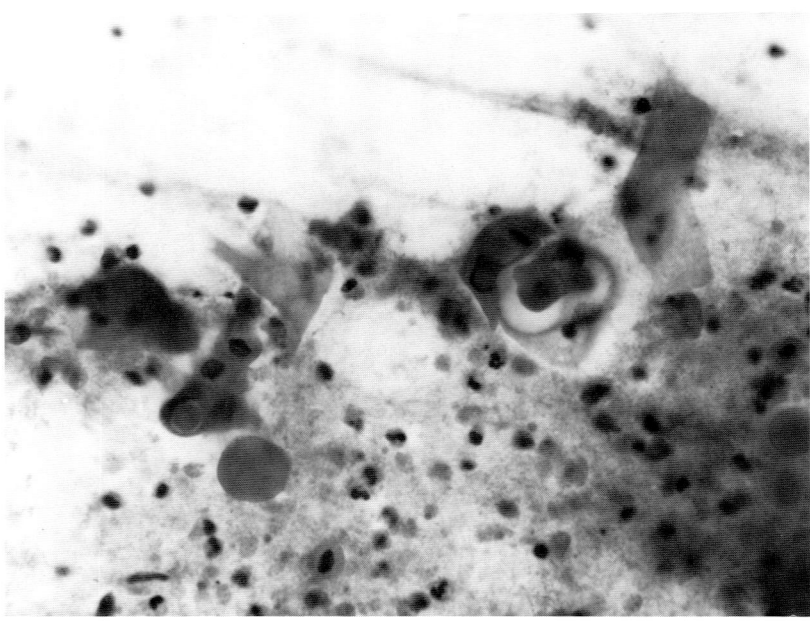

Fig. 5-26 Keratin and necrotic debris (FNA). Opaque cytoplasmic fragments, which stain orange in Papanicolaou preparations, indicate keratin. The nuclear detail is not sufficient to establish a diagnosis of malignant disease. The accompanying necrosis could be from either a cavitary squamous carcinoma or from the keratinized lining of a tuberculoma or mycetoma. This specimen was obtained from a patient with squamous carcinoma. (Papanicolaou stain, × 400.)

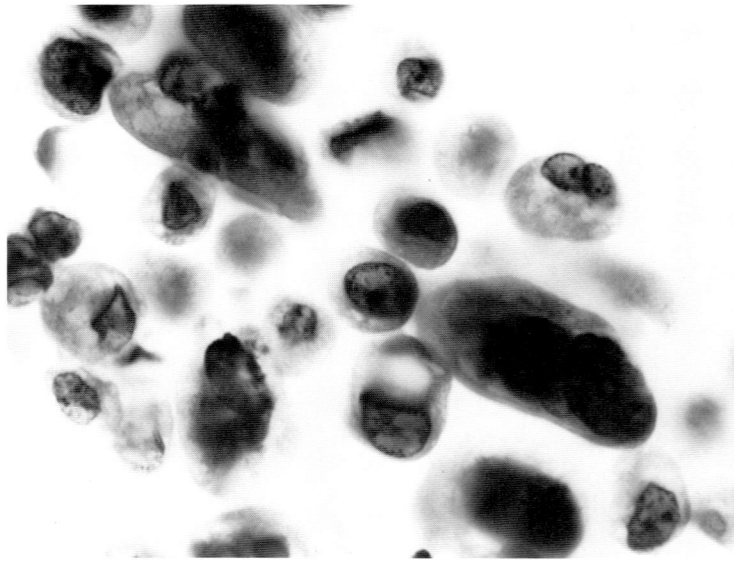

Fig. 5-27 Squamous carcinoma, nonkeratinizing (bronchial wash). Note the multinucleation, the dark, unevenly distributed chromatin, and the irregular nuclear membranes. No two cells appear to be identical, although all are consistent with a nonkeratinizing squamous carcinoma. Occasional vacuoles should not be misconstrued as features of an adenocarcinoma. Such cytoplasmic vacuoles may reflect either persistent mucus production in cells of a transformed respiratory epithelium or simply degenerative vacuoles. (Papanicolaou stain, × 1,000.)

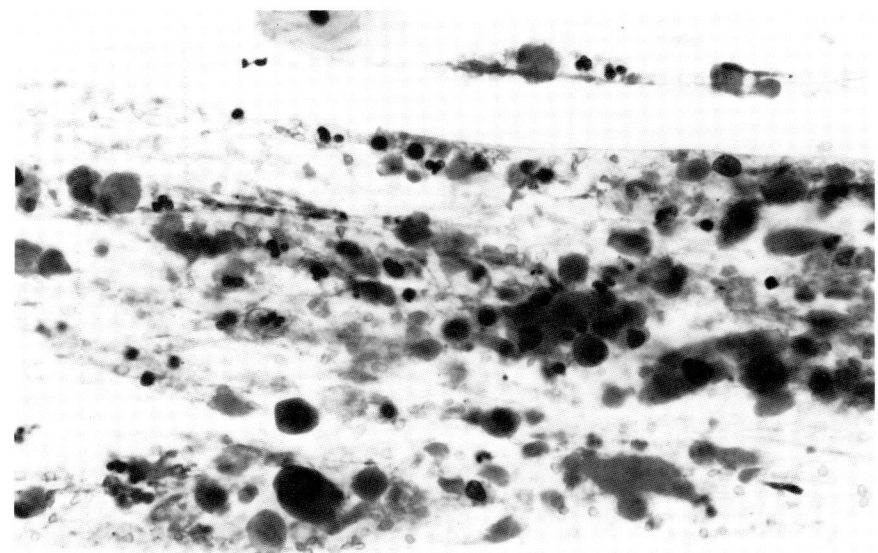

Fig. 5-28 Tumor diathesis (sputum). Fragments of cytoplasmic and nuclear debris can be found in large streams in sputum and other respiratory specimens from patients with cancer. The marked variation in nuclear fragment size is characteristic of squamous cell carcinoma, and should not be interpreted as being indicative of a small cell carcinoma (see Fig. 5-42). Frequently, the cytoplasmic fragments are keratinized, and will suggest the correct diagnosis, which requires the presence of malignant cells. (Papanicolaou stain, × 400.)

Table 5-7 Cellular Features Helpful in Discriminating Between Squamous Carcinoma[a], Adenocarcinoma[a], and Highly Atypical Nonmalignant Lesions

Cellular Features	Squamous Carcinoma	Adenocarcinoma	Benign (Atypical) Lesions
Cytoplasm			
Border	Defined	Poorly defined	Defined
Shape	Variable	Usually oval	Round or oval
Quality	Opaque	Delicate	Delicate
Relation to other cells	Separate	Syncytial	Shared
Nuclear/cytoplasmic ratio	Variable	Moderate	Low
Nucleus			
Border	Irregular	Round to oval	Round or oval
Chromatin	Coarse—variable from cell to cell	Finely granular—monotonous from cell to cell	Delicate
Location in cell	Central	Eccentric/central	Variable
Nucleolus			
Size	Small	Large	Small
Shape	Round	Round/irregular	Round
Prominence	Visible	Prominent	Variable
Number	Single/multiple	Multiple/single	One
Pattern of groups	Multilayered	Balls or papillae	Single or in flat clusters
Single cells	Common	Rare	Rare

[a] Excluding very well-differentiated types.
(from Rosenthal,[6] with permission.)

Table 5-8 Diagnostic Pitfalls Associated With Squamous Carcinoma

Squamous metaplasia: However severe and whether secondary to an underlying malignancy or reparative process, single malignant cells must be present for a diagnosis of carcinoma. In most cases, squamous metaplasia will occur in sheets (i.e., bronchiectasis, pneumonia, etc).

Mycetoma: The cavity lining of a fungal infection may undergo extremely bizarre squamous metaplasia.

Radiation reaction: Special caution must be exercised in evaluating post-irradiation specimens from patients with a previous history of tumor.

Busulfan therapy and other drugs

---

commonly seen and more prominent in adenocarcinoma, but their presence or absence is not diagnostically critical in either type of lesion. In instances in which electron microscopy is not possible, a diagnosis using the term "bronchogenic" with a suspected cell type is all that may be possible. I characterize such cases as "poorly differentiated carcinoma, favor squamous (or adeno) carcinoma."

Diagnostic Pitfalls

Major diagnostic pitfalls arise when differentiating squamous carcinoma from squamous metaplasia, mycetoma, radiation reaction, and chemotherapeutic effect (Tables 5-8 and 5-9). *Squamous metaplasia* is generally considered to be a precursor lesion to squamous carcinoma, just as in the uterine cervix. A spectrum of changes has been identified by several authors.[98-101] *Mycetomas* can be lined by an atypical squamous metaplasia (Fig. 5-10), mimicking squamous carcinoma. *Radiation reaction* causes bizarre cell changes in the lung, identical to those found in the female genital tract and, for that matter, in all other sites of the body (Fig. 5-29). *Chemotherapy* can also produce cytologic changes that mimic carcinoma. The original culprit was busulfan, but numerous other chemotherapeutic agents are now known to

Table 5-9 Squamous Carcinoma—Distinctive Cytologic Features

Cellular Features	Squamous Carcinoma	Metaplasia	Repair	Radiation Drug Reactions
Cytoplasm:				
Border	Sharp	Sharp	Sharp	Delicate
Shape	Aberrant	Uniform	Uniform	Variable
Quality	Opaque	Opaque	Translucent	Often vacuolated
Relation to other cells	Separate	Separate	Separate or syncitial	Separate
Nuclear/cytoplasmic ratio	Variable	Intermediate	Low	Low in large cell forms
Nucleus				
Border	Irregular, variable	Smooth	Smooth	Smooth
Chromatin	Coarse; clumped	Uniform; varies with severity	Fine	Coarse; clumped
Location in cell	Central	Central	Central	Variable
Nucleolus				
Size	Usually small	Small	Large	Large
Shape	Round/irregular	Round	Irregular	Irregular
Prominence	Blends with chromatin	Minimal	Very prominent	Very prominent
Number	Single/multiple	Single	Single/multiple	Single/multiple
Pattern of groups	Haphazard mosaic; thick sheet	Mosaic; flat sheet	Attenuated; flat mosaic	Relatively normal
Single cells	Many	Scattered	Rare	Common
Smear background	Diathesis	Variably inflamed	Variable inflamed	Clean

(From Rosenthal,[6] with permission.)

CYTOLOGIC DIAGNOSIS OF RESPIRATORY DISEASES **211**

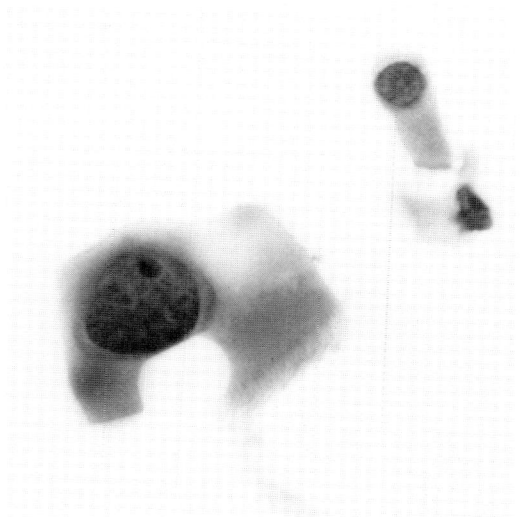

Fig. 5-29 Radiation-induced cellular atypia (bronchial brush). One year following radiation therapy for squamous carcinoma of the lung, these cells were recovered in a brushing. An abortive attempt at cytoplasmic division and a huge nucleus are ominous signs. The presence of cilia places this markedly atypical cell in the benign category. The patient remained disease-free 5 years later. (Papanicolaou stain, × 1,000.)

produce a cytopathic effect[102] (Table 5-1), a reflection of their intended ability to damage the reproductive portion of the cell.

In addition, *head and neck squamous carcinomas* can shed cells that may contaminate pulmonary specimens. The source of these cells is not always apparent. *Esophageal squamous carcinomas* may erode into the bronchus, or such cells may be regurgitated and subsequently picked up in sputa. An accurate history will warn the pathologist of a potentially inaccurate interpretation.

Very well- or very poorly differentiated squamous carcinomas may also present diagnostic difficulties. The former may produce exfoliated cells that are so "differentiated" that they do not look malignant (Fig. 5-26), whereas in the latter, the classic features may not be obvious (Fig. 5-30).

ADENOCARCINOMA

Adenocarcinoma is found both centrally and peripherally, and presents on radiographic examination as a bulky mass. Bronchiolo-alveolar carcinoma is usually peripheral, and grows in either a nodular or

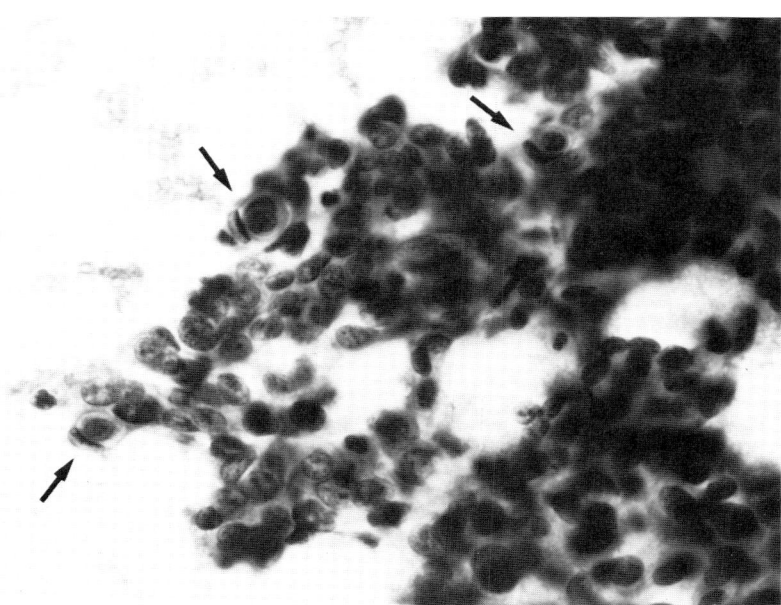

Fig. 5-30 Squamous cell carcinoma, poorly differentiated (FNA). The relationship of the cells in this sheet of poorly differentiated epithelium indicates the squamous origin of the lesion. Note the areas indicated by the arrows; such nuclear-to-cytoplasmic molding and well-defined cytoplasmic borders are characteristic of squamous carcinoma. (Papanicolaou stain, × 400.)

infiltrating pattern. Adenocarcinoma accounts for approximately 30 percent of the lung carcinomas in most series. This represents a definite increase over previous years, probably resulting from the increased incidence of carcinoma of the lung in women, in contrast to the large proportion of squamous carcinomas in men.[103] It is essential that adenocarcinoma be identified as either a primary lesion arising in the lung or a metastatic neoplasm originating elsewhere. Metastases from primary lung tumors can be found in the adrenal glands,[104] brain,[105] vertebrae, regional lymph nodes, and pleura, as well as in the contralateral lung. Treatment is usually surgical if staging indicates a possible cure. The survival rate with surgery is 27 percent at 5 years. If staging indicates metastatic disease, chemotherapy with or without irradiation is the treatment of choice. The overall 5-year survival rate for adenocarcinoma is 12 percent.

Adenocarcinoma may be subdivided into well-differentiated, moderately differentiated, and poorly differentiated types, as well as into the unique subtype of bronchioloalveolar carcinoma. The first three types are subcategorized depending upon the amount of mucin production and recapitulation of glandular structures. The poorly differentiated type is often difficult to distinguish from poorly differentiated squamous carcinoma; electron microscopy and mucin stains are often helpful in such cases. Bronchioloalveolar carcinoma can be divided into type 1 (secretory) and type 2 (nonsecretory) lesions, both of which grow along the existing framework of the alveoli.[106] Type 1 is characteristically mucin-producing, and is clearly an adenocarcinoma. Type 2 has a more hobnailed, individual cell appearance as it lines the framework of the alveoli.

Cytologic Criteria

"Bronchogenic" adenocarcinoma, the most common form of this neoplasm, arises from the bronchial lining or the submucosal glandular epithelium. Cells may occur singly (Fig. 5-31), or they may form a monolayer (Fig. 5-32) or a three-dimensional cluster (Fig. 5-33) in exfoliated material. Cerebroid nuclei

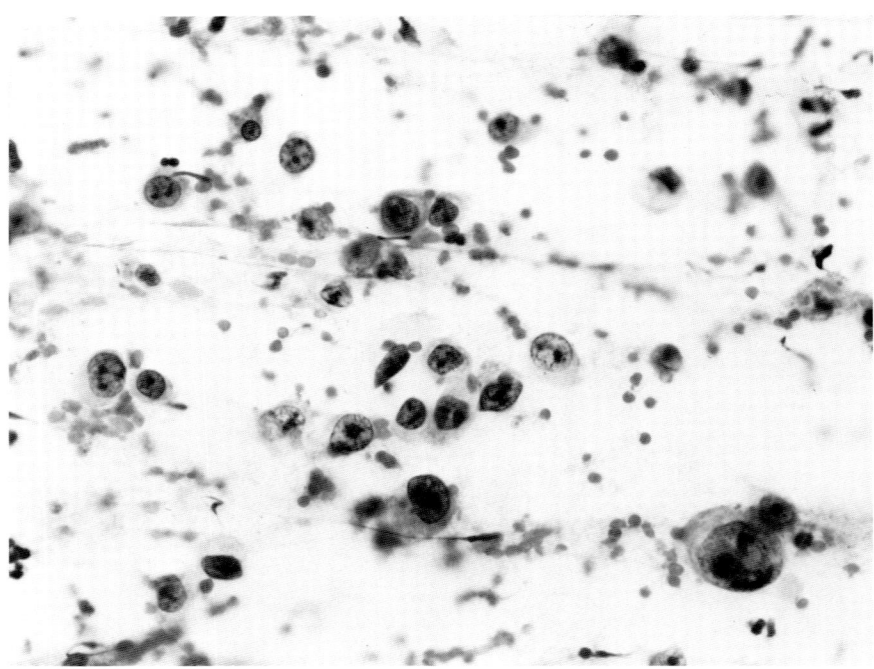

Fig. 5-31 Adenocarcinoma (bronchial washing). Although clusters of malignant glandular cells are common, dispersed single cells from adenocarcinomas are only seen occasionally, and indicate a high-grade lesion. Note the pleomorphism, and remarkably large nuclei, and the prominent nucleoli. Such cells could be mistaken for a lymphoma. Tissue studies verified the diagnosis established by the bronchial washing. Although the pattern is poorly differentiated, a positive mucin stain confirmed the cell type. (Papanicolaou stain, × 400.)

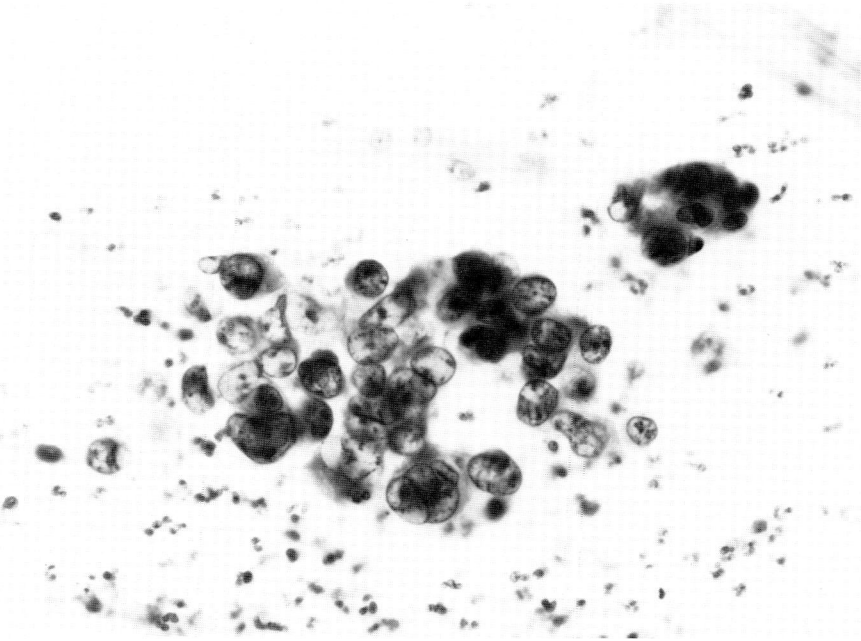

Fig. 5-32 Adenocarcinoma (sputum). Rather than exfoliating in balls of malignant cells, high-grade lesions tend to exhibit cells that appear singly, as in Fig. 5-31, or that occur in somewhat dispersed monolayers, as in this case. Note the marked pleomorphism and anisonucleosis, the unevenly dispersed (although fine) chromatin, and the prominent and irregularly shaped nucleoli. Cell borders are poorly defined, which is characteristic of adenocarcinoma. Although the tissue pattern is moderately differentiated, the individual cells correlate well with those seen in the sputum sample. (Papanicolaou stain, × 400.)

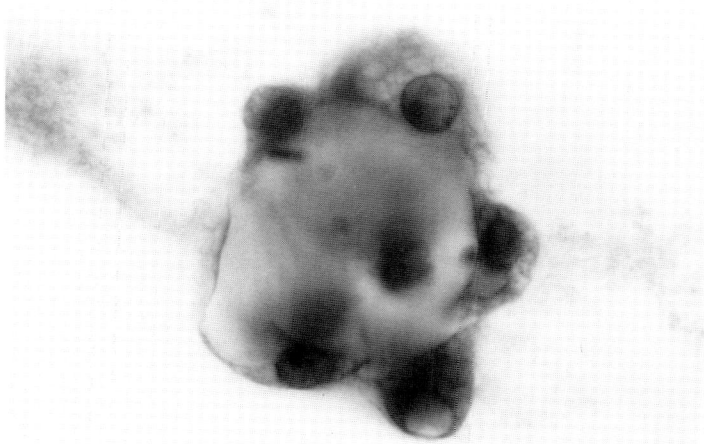

Fig. 5-33 Adenocarcinoma (sputum). The three-dimensionality of cell groups from adenocarcinoma is illustrated by this photograph. The importance of focusing through groups stained by the amazingly transparent Papanicolaou stain cannot be overemphasized. (Papanicolaou stain, × 1,000.)

have a finely granular, nuclear chromatin. Nucleoli are frequently large and irregular. Cytoplasmic borders are characteristically indistinct, with syncytia being quite obvious in brushings or smears of fine needle aspirates. The degree of cytoplasmic vacuolization is variable, and the diagnosis does not depend on its presence.

Papillary adenocarcinoma, a rare form of this lesion, arises from the more proximal bronchial epithelium, and sheds in both clusters and single cells (Fig. 5-34). Cells are uniformly symmetrical, with finely vacuolated cytoplasm, variable nucleoli, and an inconsistent nuclear structure. Clusters are not usually as three-dimensional as those that can be found in bronchiolo-alveolar carcinoma, but both histologic types are difficult to distinguish on cytologic examination. Depending on the degree of differentiation, cells can be quite pleomorphic, and can vary considerably in contrast to the relative uniformity of the bronchiolo-alveolar type (Fig. 5-35). Psammoma bodies and intranuclear cytoplasmic inclusions[107] have been described in this variant of adenocarcinoma.

Bronchiolo-alveolar carcinoma probably arises from the Clara cell, and more rarely, from type II pneumocytes.[108] Two cytologic presentations reflect the two distinct histologic patterns. Cells may occur in three-dimensional clusters (Fig. 5-35), or groups of strikingly uniform cells may be intermixed with abundant histiocytes, which can appear very atypical, making the distinction between histiocytes and tumor cells quite difficult[109] (Fig. 5-36). Single cells may have a hobnailed appearance, with cytoplasm flaring from an eccentric nucleus.[110] The nucleus may be uniformly round and, when seen in clusters, the lack of molding is striking. Nucleoli are conspicuous, but small and uniform. The chromatin pattern is usually powdery, and vacuolization of the cytoplasm

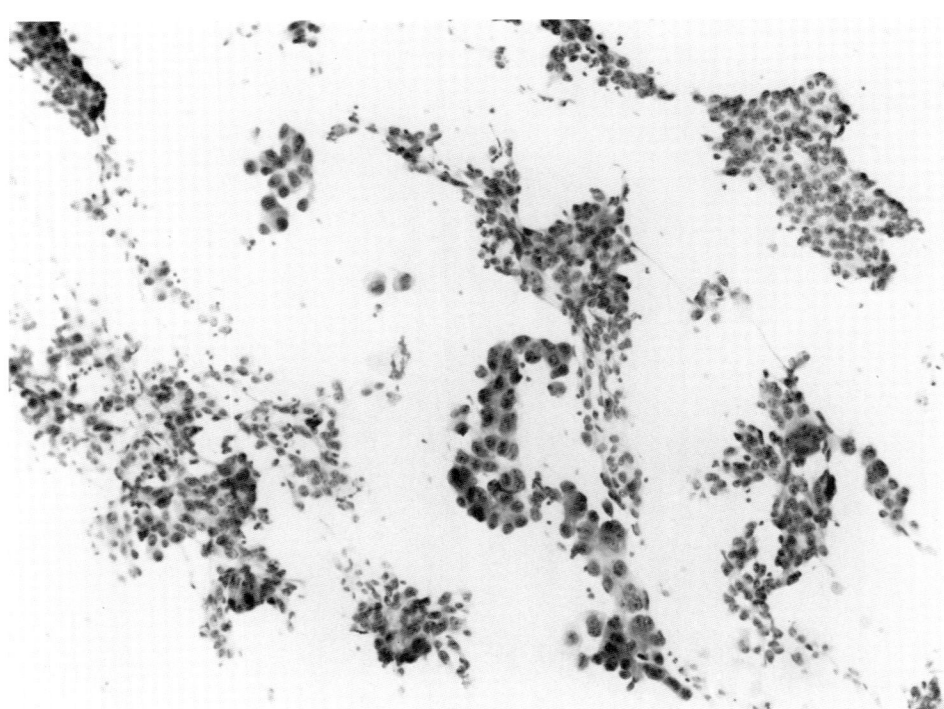

Fig. 5-34 Moderately differentiated adenocarcinoma (transbronchial FNA). The excellent cellular yield is made possible by transmural penetration of the bronchial mucosa by the thin needle guided through the bronchoscope. Pale nuclei, prominent nucleoli, and indistinct cytoplasmic borders are all characteristic of adenocarcinoma. The papillary configuration of the fragments provides a tissue pattern equivalent to that found on histologic section. (Papanicolaou stain, × 100.)

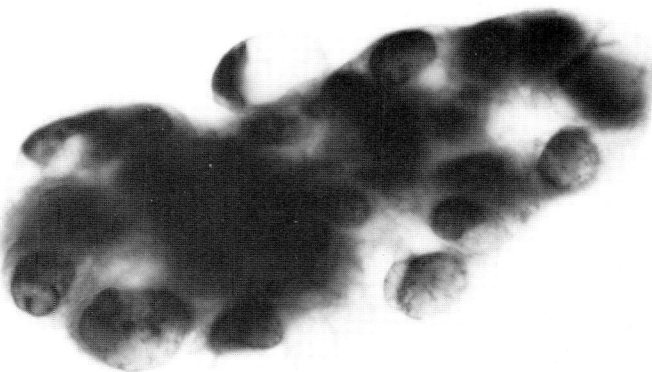

Fig. 5-35 Bronchiolo-alveolar carcinoma (sputum). This lesion is extremely difficult to diagnose because of the variability of its cytologic presentation. The group of cells—a glandular cluster complete with cytoplasmic vacuoles—should be contrasted with the dispersed monolayer of cells seen in Fig. 5-36. (Papanicolaou stain, × 1,000.)

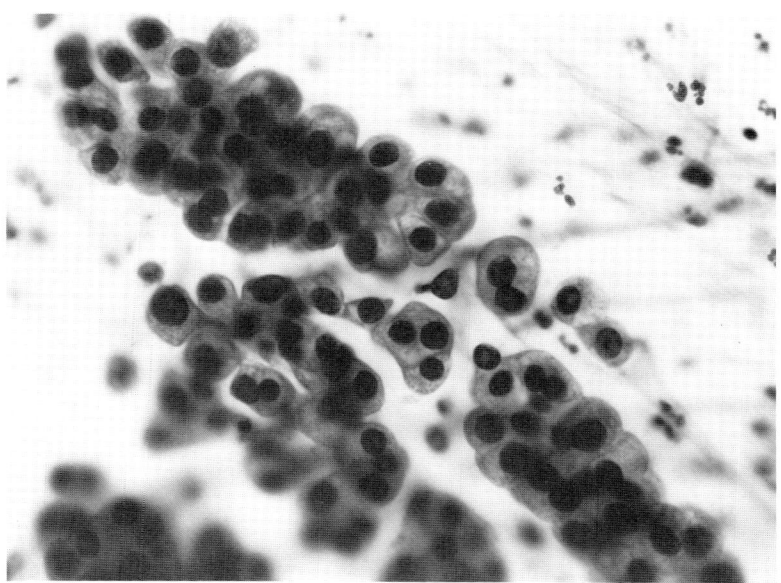

Fig. 5-36 Bronchiolo-alveolar carcinoma (sputum). Monolayers of uniform cells could be mistaken for streams of alveolar macrophages. Such streams are often mixtures of tumor cells and alveolar macrophages. The distinction between the two cell populations is often difficult, a characteristic feature of bronchiolo-alveolar carcinoma. Excess mucus usually completes the picture. (Papanicolaou stain, × 400.)

varies. Abundant mucus is usually evident in the smear background, and reflects the excessive mucus production[111] that often accompanies this tumor.

Diagnostic Pitfalls

Reactive and pneumonic processes can mimic adenocarcinoma[112,113] (Fig. 5-37) (Tables 5-10 and 5-11). In order to avoid such pitfalls, radiologic evidence of a tumor should exist, and the cytologic features should be continuous from one specimen to the other, if not becoming more atypical. Treatment of the lesion with antibiotics will clear the cytologic atypia if the process is inflammatory, but if a neoplasm is present, even in association with a pneumonia, the atypical cells will persist after the pneumonia has resolved. "Creola bodies" are glandular structures that exfoliate after stimulation of the epithelium in such diseases as asthma or chronic bronchitis.[114,115]

Misinterpretation of adenocarcinoma as a *squamous "bronchogenic" carcinoma* may occur when vacuoles are present in the cytoplasm of some squamous tumor cells (Fig. 5-38). Careful search of the sample for other criteria indicative of cell type (e.g., keratin) will usually clarify the issue. If not, a diagnosis of "bronchogenic, non-oat cell carcinoma" is usually sufficient for the clinician to initiate treatment.

Distinguishing between a *metastatic adenocarcinoma* and a primary adenocarcinoma of the lung is often difficult. Consultation with clinicians in an effort to elicit a history of a possible distant primary is essential for avoiding a misdiagnosis. The most common adenocarcinomas to travel to the lung are those originating in the breast and colon.[82] Certain metastatic

Table 5-10 Diagnostic Pitfalls Associated With Adenocarcinoma

Any reactive or pneumonic process

In order to avoid pitfalls, one must be certain of radiologic evidence for tumor, and there must be continuity of the cytologic picture from one specimen to another. If it varies, that process is benign and reactive.

Differentiation from metastatic adenocarcinoma may be impossible. A conference with clinicians may clarify the issue.

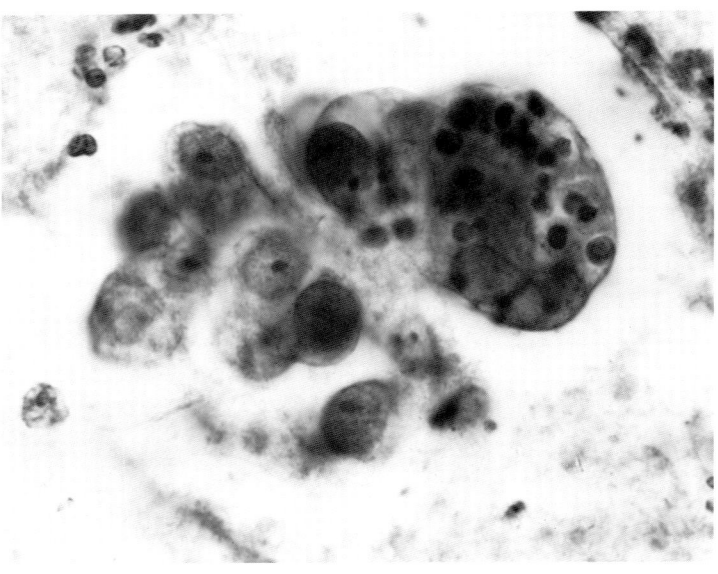

Fig. 5-37 Diffuse alveolar damage with severe atypia (sputum). Cells in sputa from this patient were repeatedly diagnosed as adenocarcinoma. In this group, the intracytoplasmic neutrophils provide a clue that this lesion is, instead, inflammatory. However, the lesion proved lethal after several years of recurrences. Etiology was never established. The severe atypia seen in multiple sputum samples was confirmed in the respiratory epithelium obtained at the time of segmental resection and autopsy. (Papanicolaou stain, × 1,000.)

Table 5-11 Adenocarcinoma—Distinctive Cytologic Features

Cellular Features	Adenocarcinoma	Pneumonia	BAC
Cytoplasm			
Border	Distinct	Indistinct	Distinct
Shape	Round to oval	Round to oval	Round
Quality	Delicate/vacuolated	Vacuolated, with neutrophils	Delicate
Relation to other cells	Shared borders	Shared borders	Distinct/separate
Cilia	Absent	Usually present	Absent
Nuclear/cytoplasmic ratio	Variable	Variable	Uniform
Nucleus			
Border	Slightly irregular	Thin; uniform	Smooth
Chromatin	Finely/coarsely granular	Fine; somewhat granular	Usually fine
Location in cell	Eccentric	Eccentric	Central
Nucleolus			
Size	Large	Small	Small
Shape	Round/irregular	Round	Round
Prominence	Very prominent	Visible	Very prominent
Number	Usually single	Single	Single
Pattern of groups	Round; three-dimensional	Irregular; flat	Variable; papillary—single cells
Single cells	Rare	Rare	Common, with histiocytes
Smear background	Dirty	Inflamed	Clean; much mucus

BAC, bronchioloalveolar carcinoma

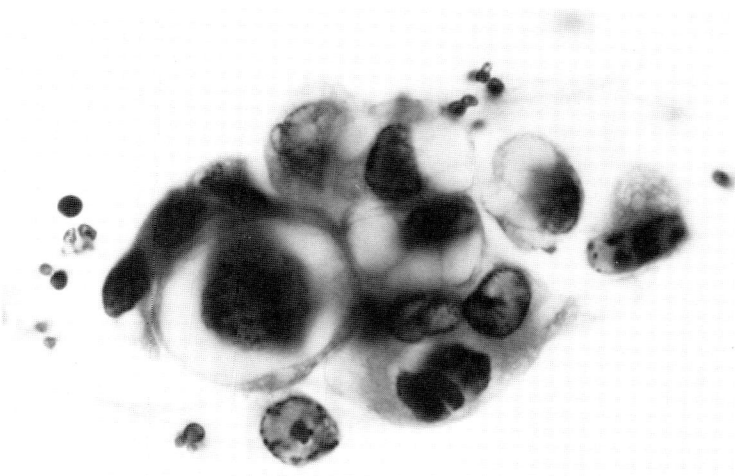

Fig. 5-38 Squamous carcinoma (sputum). The cytoplasmic vacuoles might persuade the observer that the lesion is of glandular origin. Further inspection of the specimen, however, reveals keratinized cytoplasmic fragments indicative of squamous carcinoma. Tissue studies confirmed the diagnosis of squamous carcinoma by virtue of the intraluminal keratin, but also revealed the source of the vacuolated cells. This case is a good example of the validity of the term "bronchogenic." (Papanicolaou stain, × 1,000.)

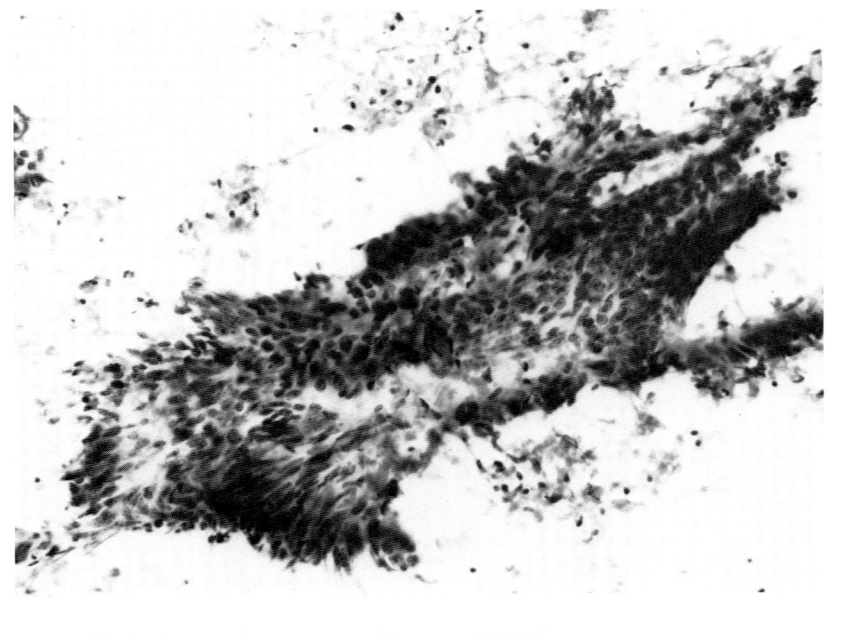

Fig. 5-39 Adenocarcinoma of the colon, metastatic to the lung (FNA). A large tumor fragment was aspirated from a lung nodule. The elongated, slender epithelial cells, aligned along the edges of the fragment, recapitulate the histologic findings, which are so characteristic of colonic carcinoma. Note the debris in the background, indicating necrosis and possible cavitation. (Papanicolaou stain, × 200.)

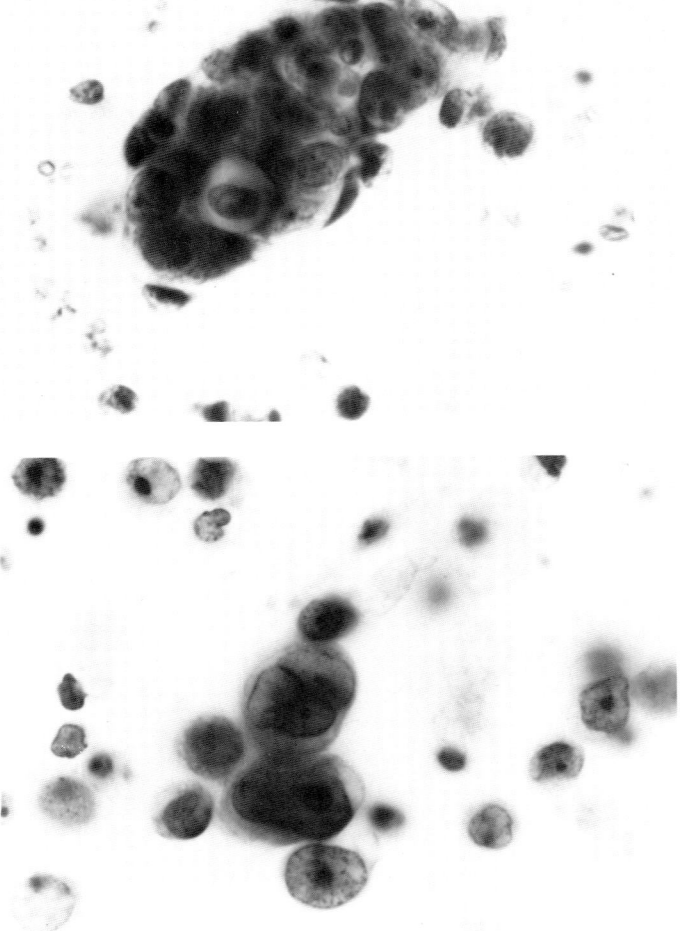

Fig. 5-40 Adenocarcinoma of the breast, metastatic to the lung (sputum). Carcinoma of the breast usually metastasizes to the lung in solid tumor aggregates. When it exfoliates into sputum, clusters of neoplastic glandular cells are the rule. Note the smoothness of the outer edge of the group and the suggestion of cytoplasmic vacuolization and cell separation, which could be mistaken for "windows." This is the classic diagnostic pitfall in differentiating between mesothelial cells and breast carcinoma cells. (Papanicolaou stain, × 1,000.)

Fig. 5-41 Adenocarcinoma of the breast, metastatic to the lung (sputum). Compared with the cells pictured in Fig. 5-40, these cells have exfoliated individually. There is no question as to the malignant nature of these cells, but they are not classically those seen in carcinoma of the breast; in fact, they could be mistaken for a large cell lymphoma (see Fig. 5-47). (Papanicolaou stain, × 1,000.)

carcinomas will mimic the normal histology of the primary site, especially colonic carcinoma, which has elongated cells with carrot-shaped nuclei[3,116] (Fig. 5-39). Breast cancer cells sometimes will appear in morulae or balls (Fig. 5-40), but will also assume a tandem or "Indian-file" arrangement (Fig. 5-41). Highly specific immunochemical assays, such as prostate-specific antigen, can also be of help. The primary tumor should be stained in concert with the metastatic sample to ensure that the parent tumor has the same immunologic character as the metastatic lesion. A problem arises when metastases lose their membrane antigens and the primary tumor still tests positive for membrane antigen. Microscopic comparison with tissue or cytologic samples from the suspected primary site is still the method of choice for resolving diagnostic uncertainties.

SMALL CELL UNDIFFERENTIATED CARCINOMA

Small cell undifferentiated ("oat cell") carcinoma is located centrally, with a tendency toward early spread to and invasion of bronchial, hilar, and mediastinal lymph nodes, as well as soft tissue. This lesion represents approximately 25 percent of all lung cancers, and has a strong association with cigarette smoking.

This type of carcinoma is a multisystem disease process,[117] with metastatic foci frequently becoming clinically evident before the primary lesion is apparent.[118,119] Metastases can be found in the liver, adrenal glands, brain, kidney, and abdominal lymph nodes. Such biologic behavior accounts for the very poor survival rate, which is currently much less than 1 year. Treatment traditionally involves radiation coupled with adjuvant chemotherapy. However, in rare cases, patients who are staged to be free of metastatic disease have been known to survive surgical resection for more than 2 years; adjuvant chemotherapy is usually employed.

This tumor group is perhaps the most fascinating primary lung tumor. "Undifferentiated" is really a misnomer, as these tumor cells are capable of producing a variety of hormones and are thus considered among the amine precursor uptake decarboxylation (APUD) family of cancers.[119–123] This capability is no doubt responsible for the propensity of oat cell carcinomas to create paraneoplastic syndromes.[124]

The cell of origin is generally accepted to be the Kulchitsky cell.[119,125] Two cell types—"lymphocyte-like" cells and intermediate cells—can be seen in the same lesion in tissue and cytologic samples, and may represent different degrees of maturation of the same cell line.

Cytologic Criteria

In sputum samples, streams of small hyperchromatic cells, which are not tightly adherent but are closely related to each other, can be highly diagnostic, even in a single specimen (Fig. 5-42). The cell size is slightly larger than a lymphocyte in the lymphocyte-like cell type, and considerably larger, with a more open chromatin network, in the intermediate cell type[126] (Fig. 5-43). Very scanty, almost indiscernible cytoplasm surrounds a nucleus that is polygonal. Chromatin is powdery, with very inconspicuous nucleoli, if any are at all noticeable. Molding, onion-skinning, and Indian-file, or tandem, arrangements are diagnostic, and are maintained in pleural fluids. Nuclear fragments accompany these tumor cells, and contribute to the diagnosis. In brushings, these fragile cells are easily attenuated when smeared, and assume the elongated, pointed form that provides the name "oat cell," and that corresponds to the crush artifact seen in tissue samples.

Diagnostic Pitfalls

Although the cytologic certainty of a diagnosis of oat cell carcinoma is the highest of all primary lung cancers, the list of diagnostic pitfalls associated with this lesion is lengthy (Tables 5-12 and 5-13). A discussion of some of the conditions that must be considered in the differential diagnosis follows.

Small cell adenocarcinomas have nucleoli, and exhibit a three-dimensional arrangement of cell clusters (Fig. 5-44). *Small cell breast carcinoma* is the most treacherous diagnostic pitfall, as Indian-filing and molding are prominent features; however, crush artifact is absent and nucleoli are usually conspicuous. In tissue samples, the Indian-filing that is characteristic of metastatic breast carcinoma is more uniform and linear in arrangement than the haphazard Indian-filing seen in oat cell carcinoma.

Tumor diathesis, consisting of necrotic debris from a variety of tumors, should not be confused with oat cell carcinoma (Fig. 5-28). Rigid diagnostic criteria

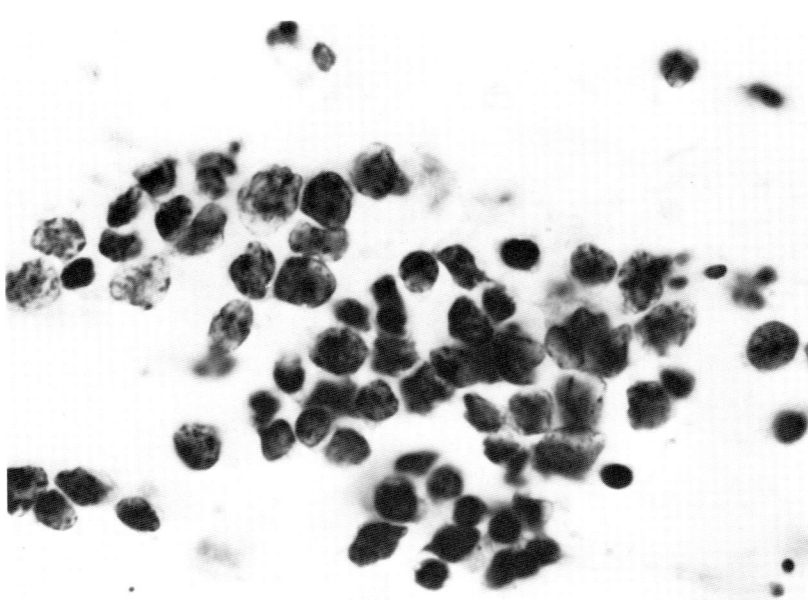

Fig. 5-42 Small cell undifferentiated oat cell carcinoma of the lung (sputum). Streams of associated but disconnected small tumor cells provide a definitive diagnosis of this tumor cell type, even if no more than this amount of material is seen on a single sputum sample. Note the inconspicuous cytoplasm, the absence of nucleoli, and the smudgy nuclear chromatin. Nuclear molding and a tandem arrangement, or Indian-filing, are additional characteristics of oat cell carcinoma. (Papanicolaou stain, × 1,000.)

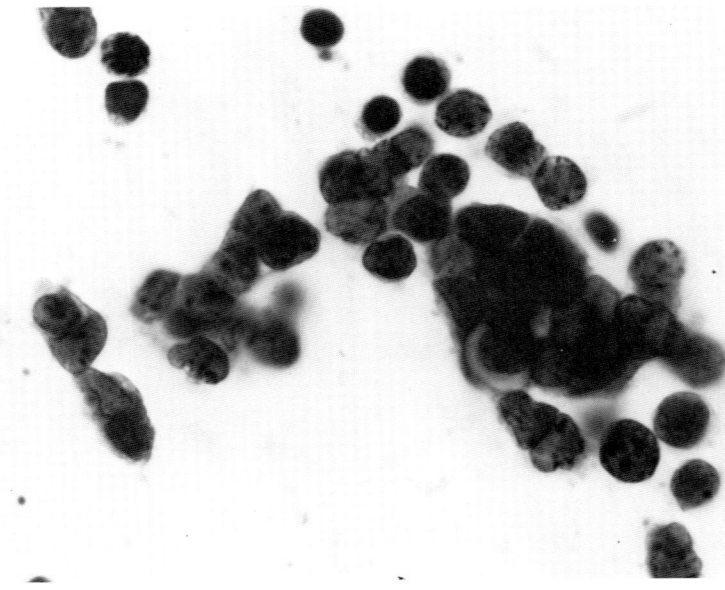

Fig. 5-43 Small cell undifferentiated oat cell carcinoma of the lung (sputum). Compare the size and chromatin distribution of these cells with those in Fig. 5-42. Note the pathognomonic features of Indian-filing, nuclear molding, salt-and-pepper chromatin, absence of nucleoli, and minimal, adherent cytoplasm. Several cells wrap around each other, producing a so-called onion skin effect. (Papanicolaou stain, × 1,000.)

Table 5-12 Diagnostic Pitfalls Associated With Small Cell Undifferentiated Carcinoma

Lymphocytes never mold; although they may occur in streams, they do not interrelate in a shape relationship.

Other small cell tumors (i.e., seminoma) have prominent nucleoli; oat cell carcinoma does not.

Oat cells obtained from a brushing will have a more consistent and open chromatin network than in sputum samples, probably as a result of the freshness of cells. This pattern should be recognized as oat cell carcinoma.

Tumor diathesis of necrotic debris from another type of tumor (i.e., squamous carcinoma or adenocarcinoma).

Debris from a bronchiectasis or other inflammatory process. Molding, onion-skinning or an Indian-file arrangement must be present to make the diagnosis of oat cell carcinoma.

Small cell breast carcinoma can closely mimic oat cell carcinoma, especially with its Indian-file arrangement and molding. A clinical history is essential if the tumor occurs in a female patient.

---

established for oat cell carcinoma must be followed. Debris from bronchiectasis and other inflammatory processes can also mimic oat cell carcinoma.

Squamous aggregates and rosette formations[6] can both be seen within a bonafide oat cell carcinoma. These findings should not prompt the observer to classify the tumor erroneously as a squamous cell carcinoma or adenocarcinoma. However, such double primary combinations have been reported,[127] and should always be considered when confronted with two malignant cell lines.[126]

LARGE CELL UNDIFFERENTIATED CARCINOMA

Large cell undifferentiated carcinoma is usually located peripherally, in a subpleural location. The tumor commonly presents as a large, bulky, demarcated mass that is frequently associated with cavitation. Access to bronchial lumina is usually not possible, so the recovery of diagnostic cells in sputum samples is uncommon.

These tumors constitute approximately 10 percent of primary lung tumors in most series. However, the criteria used to establish whether a carcinoma is of the "large cell" type vary from pathologist to pathologist, so that these figures are unreliable. Many poorly differentiated squamous carcinomas or poorly differentiated adenocarcinomas are included in this category erroneously; most are identified as adenocarcinomas on electron microscopy.[86] Metastases will be found in the liver, adrenal glands, brain, and abdominal lymph nodes, as well as in the contralateral lung. The treatment of choice is resection if the lesion is determined to be technically curable. A 25 percent overall 5-year survival rate can be expected.

Cytologic Criteria

Cellular material indicative of large cell undifferentiated carcinoma is often difficult to distinguish from that of poorly differentiated epidermoid carcinoma or adenocarcinoma, in which case electron microscopy can be helpful. The easiest diagnosis to arrive at is "large cell undifferentiated" if the observer is confronted with a specimen having large undifferentiated cells that happen to exhibit a lack of consistency from one specimen to another, and yet still maintain malignant characteristics. These large, variably shaped cells will have ill-defined cytoplasm marked by inconsistent staining quality. Cells will frequently occur singly, or in cell clusters with or without three-dimensionality (Fig. 5-45). If cavitation is present, and the specimen is a needle aspirate, extensive tumor diathesis will be evident. The giant cell variant is quite rare and dramatic in its cytologic presentation. Huge pleomorphic single cells are the prototypical signs of this malignant disease, but the cells have few characteristics to categorize them other than their epithelial quality.[128] Multinucleation is a consistent feature. Electron microscopy is necessary to appreciate the features that will facilitate cell typing.

Diagnostic Pitfalls

There is usually little chance of a false-positive diagnostic result, as cells of large cell undifferentiated carcinomas present with features that definitely meet the criteria of malignancy. The only usual problem lies in establishing the cell type, an issue that has been addressed earlier. Another possible source of confusion is the large cell lymphoma. A tumor diathesis may not contain definitively malignant cells in the first specimen, and the hyperchromatic nuclear fragments may either mimic an oat cell carcinoma or suggest a bronchiectactic origin.

Table 5-13 Small Cell Undifferentiated (Oat Cell) Carcinoma: Distinctive Cytologic Features

Cellular Features	SCUC	Small Cell Adenocarcinoma	Small Cell Squamous Carcinoma	Lymphocytes	Tumor Debris	Reserve Cell Hyperplasia
Cytoplasm	Appears absent					
Border		Indistinct	Indistinct	Sharp	Fragmentary	Sharp
Shape		Oval	Oval/bipolar	Round to oval	Irregular	"Square"
Quality		Delicate	Delicate	Opaque	Opaque	Opaque
Relation to other cells		Shared borders	Separate	Very separate	Separate	Shared borders
Nuclear/cytoplasmic ratio	1:1	Almost 1:1	Almost 1:1	Almost 1:1	Not applicable	Almost 1:1
Nucleus						
Border	Polygonal	Oval	Oval	Round	Irregular	"Square"
Chromatin	Smudged or stippled	Finely granular	Somewhat coarse	Dark; coarse	Dark; opaque	Dark; opaque
Location in cell	Total	Eccentric	Central	Central	Not applicable	Central
Nucleolus						
Size	Invisible	Small	Small	Invisible	Not applicable	Invisible
Shape		Round	Round			
Prominence		Visible	Indistinct			
Number		Usually one	Usually one			
Pattern of groups	Indian-file; onion-skinning; semi-cohesive	Acinar groups or three-dimensional balls; molding	Thick groups; occasionally, cell-within-cell pearls	Streams, but separate cells	None	Tight clusters
Single cells	Rare	Infrequent	Common	Invariably present	Cell pieces	Rare
Smear background	Dirty	Dirty	Dirty	Inflamed	Dirty	Clean or inflamed

Abbreviation: SCUC, small cell undifferentiated carcinoma.

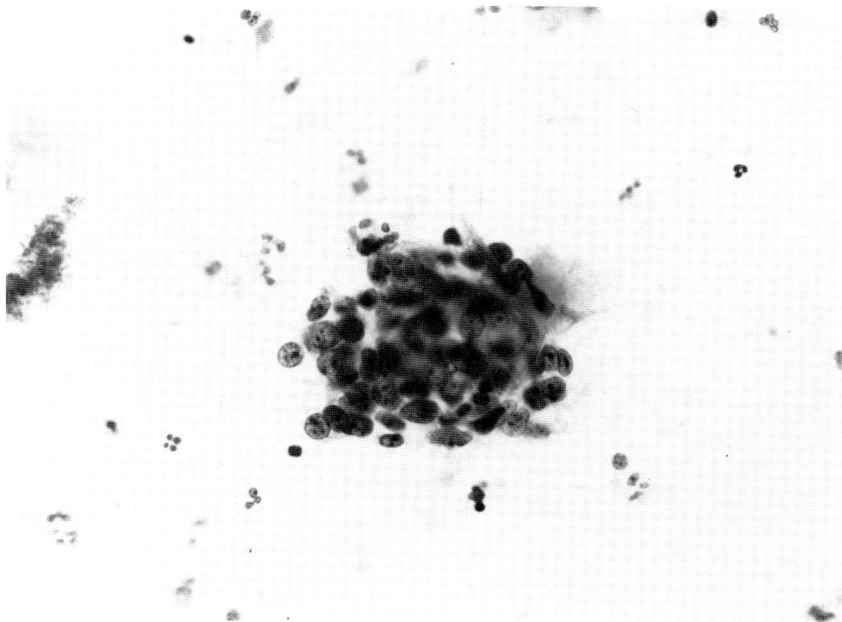

Fig. 5-44 Small cell adenocarcinoma of the lung (bronchial brushing). When small tumor cells are recovered in a respiratory specimen, the differential diagnosis must include lesions other than oat cell carcinoma. If nucleoli are identified, as in this cell group, the diagnosis of oat cell becomes improbable. Adenocarcinoma is the primary diagnosis until proven otherwise. Electron microscopy and other studies are usually needed to define the cell type, a critical distinction for the purposes of proper treatment and determination of prognosis. (Papanicolaou stain, × 400.)

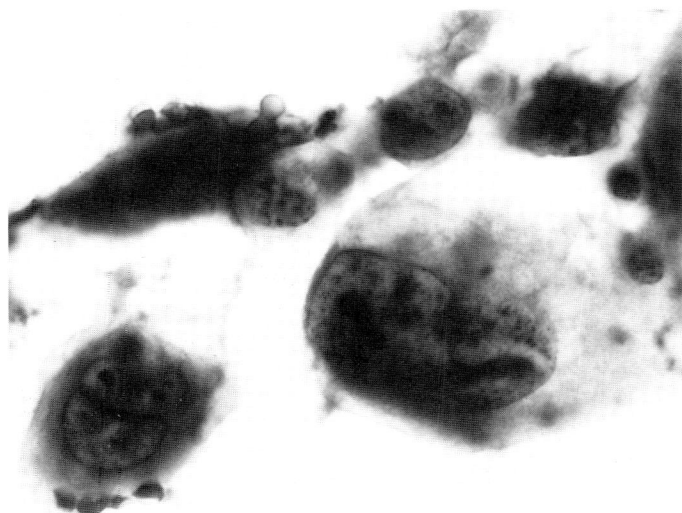

Fig. 5-45 Large cell undifferentiated carcinoma (FNA). Most large cell undifferentiated carcinomas can be cell-typed if careful attention is directed to cytologic criteria. If electron microscopy is performed, most of these lesions are defined as adenocarcinomas. However, sometimes there are no distinguishing criteria by any modality, and the term large cell, especially when cells are this large, is the most appropriate designation. (Papanicolaou stain, × 1,000.)

CARCINOID TUMORS

Carcinoid tumors are rare lesions that usually originate in the large bronchi. They have a so-called iceberg configuration, with the "tip" presenting in the lumen and the bulk of the lesion extending outside of the bronchus. The tumor is thought to originate in Kulchitsky cells of the bronchial epithelium.[125] Rarely, it may give rise to the carcinoid syndrome, or it may manifest a paraneoplastic syndrome, despite its ability to produce a variety of hormones.[129] Carcinoids may also occur peripherally, presenting as solitary nodules.

These lesions account for less than 5 percent of all primary lung neoplasms, and have erroneously been termed bronchial adenomas. The age range of those affected is 9 to 73 years, with a mean age of 45 years, and the tumor occurs with equal frequency in males and females. Metastases occur rarely, but involve regional lymph nodes in 10 percent of the cases; distant metastases or recurrences are unusual events. Survival for 5 years can be expected in 82 percent of the patients. Treatment is most generally surgical.

Cytologic Criteria

Carcinoid tumors are perhaps the most difficult lesions to diagnose by cytologic examination because of the uniformly small cells that appear in cohesive aggregates and have a very benign, almost normal appearance (Fig. 5-46).[130,131] These cell groups often have a three-dimensional configuration. Nucleoli are small and chromatin is very bland. The cells have features that resemble those of reserve cells, but the more atypical tumors can be mistaken for adenocarcinoma[132] or may present as undifferentiated neoplastic cells. Current theory holds that there is a continuous spectrum of neoplastic disease between carcinoid tumor and small cell oat cell undifferentiated carcinoma of the lung, with varying gradations of "atypical carcinoid" in between. These so-called atypical carcinoid cells often are spindle-shaped. Exfoliated

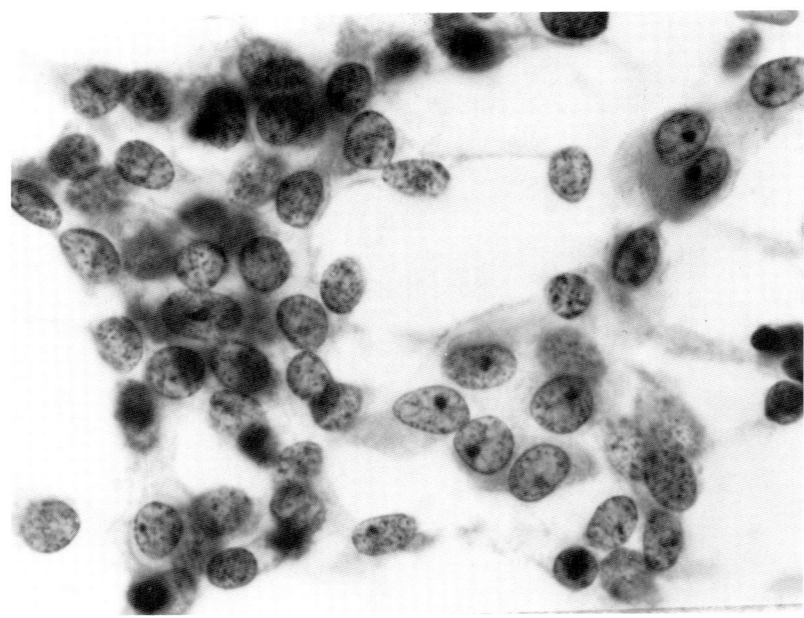

Fig. 5-46 Carcinoid of the lung (FNA). The aspirate from this lesion contains uniform, small tumor cells with diaphanous cytoplasm. Nucleoli are small, but conspicuous. These cells are often so benign-appearing that, in bronchial brushing specimens, they may easily be mistaken for benign, non-neoplastic, respiratory epithelial cells without cilia. Only their large number and monomorphous quality suggest the correct diagnosis. (Papanicolaou stain, × 1,000.)

material in sputum is generally scanty and, therefore, is least reliable for diagnosis; bronchial brush and FNA specimens are most reliable.

Diagnostic Pitfalls

Cells from carcinoids can be mistaken for reactive reserve cells, and the more atypical cells in the atypical carcinoid may be misinterpreted as representing a small cell undifferentiated carcinoma. If nucleoli are prominent, confusion with a seminoma can occur. Because the experience with this tumor is generally minimal and the cytologic findings usually "benign," biopsy is the most frequent means of diagnosing such tumors. Immunochemical stain for chromogranin will differentiate the atypical carcinoid from oat cell carcinoma.[133]

OTHER PRIMARY LUNG TUMORS

The so-called *bronchial adenomas* are unusual tumors that occur in the bronchial submucosal regions, arising from the bronchial glands. Originally thought to be benign, these tumors are now known to metastasize. Adenoid cystic carcinoma,[134] mucoepidermoid carcinoma, pleomorphic adenoma (mixed tumor), and acinic cell tumors have the same histology as their salivary gland counterparts.[135] Rare descriptions of cytologic specimens from these tumors document cellular criteria, most frequently and reliably obtained by FNA.[136] Rarely, metastases to the lung from similar salivary gland tumors may confound the picture, but the peripheral site(s) of the metastases will distinguish them from primary lesions which have a peritracheal location.[137,138]

LYMPHOMAS AND LEUKEMIA

Malignant lymphomas and leukemias may occur de novo or as a result of chemotherapy or another immunosuppressive maneuver in a patient who is threatened by a seemingly unrelated disease.[139] Lymphomas are also common in patients with AIDS. The cytopathologist is, therefore, constantly challenged to recognize malignant lymphoid cells[140–142] as distinct from otherwise mundane chronic inflammatory cells. Consultation with hematologists is strongly recommended.

Although sputa are occasionally diagnostic,[143–145] bronchoalveolar lavage of diffuse infiltrates and FNA of defined masses[146] are the most productive ways to approach these lesions. Fiberoptic bronchoscopy with washings, brushings, and transbronchial biopsy are diagnostic if the lesion is more centrally located. Cytologic criteria (Fig. 5-47) are the same as those for specific lesions in bone marrow, lymph node, or peripheral blood samples. Wright stains are mandatory to allow comparison with hematologic samples for diagnostic confirmation. Sufficient material for a monoclonal antibody panel is helpful in ruling out a polyclonal infiltrate in response to an infectious disease, a common situation in these patients.

MISCELLANEOUS AND RARE TUMORS

The possibility of rare tumors, including carcinosarcomas, pulmonary blastomas, thymomas,[147] metastases from melanomas (Fig. 5-48), primary and secondary sarcomas[148–153] (Figs. 5-49 and 5-50), and unusual metastases to the lungs[138,154,155] must be considered whenever cells in a sputum or other respiratory specimen do not accurately fit any of the cytologic criteria defined earlier. Pulmonary hamartomas and endometriosis are two such examples.[156–158]

METASTATIC CARCINOMA TO THE LUNGS

The distinction between primary and secondary lung cancer is essential to optimal patient management. Most metastatic lesions are adenocarcinoma (see earlier section). In all instances, careful correlation with any tissue available from other tumor sites is mandatory to define the process within the lung.[81] Other epithelial tumors, such as squamous carcinoma from other body sites, can be confused as a primary lung tumor. Such a disastrous assumption can be avoided by careful history-taking. Uncommonly, transitional carcinoma of the bladder can travel to the lung, resembling squamous carcinoma.

As the survival of patients with cancer increases with more effective therapy and earlier diagnosis, a patient's chances of a second primary lesion increase. A lung lesion may be a second primary, should be recognized and managed as such, even in the face of a history of a previous malignancy arising from another site.

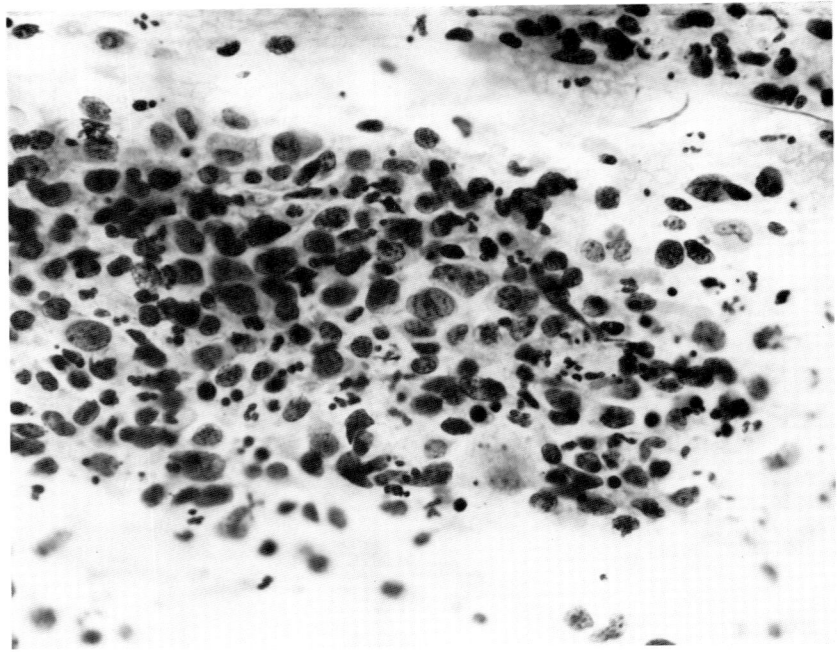

Fig. 5-47 Large cell lymphoma (sputum). Abundant cellular material, consisting of pleomorphic and variably sized primitive cells, indicates an intraluminal lesion of probable nonepithelial origin. Note the mixed character of these cells, ranging in size from that of a small lymphocyte to much larger and often binucleated cells. Chromatin varies considerably, being very fine but unevenly distributed within the largest cells. Nucleoli are often prominent and multiple; nuclear shapes are characteristically cerebroid. (Papanicolaou stain, × 400.)

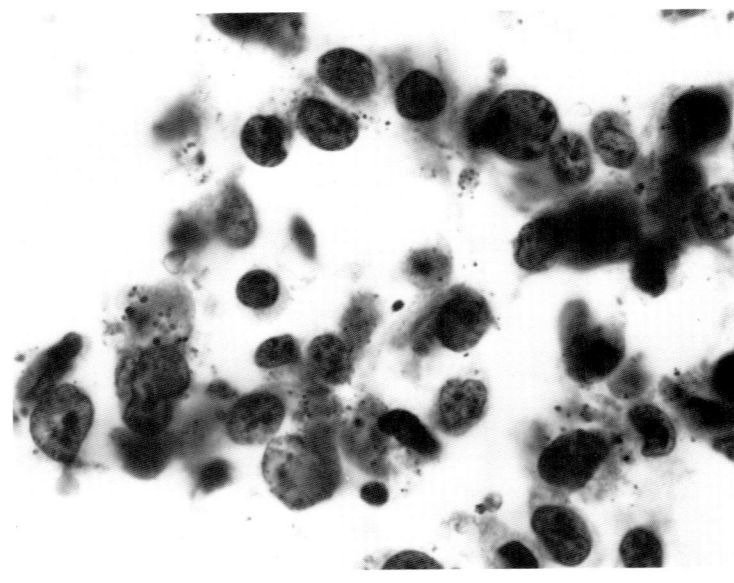

Fig. 5-48 Melanoma metastatic to the lung (bronchial brushing). Large epithelioid cells with obviously malignant nuclei and prominent nucleoli could originate from any epithelial malignant process that is poorly differentiated. The lack of cohesiveness and the presence of melanin pigment, which are fully appreciated with high-power magnification, indicate the correct diagnosis of melanoma. Without the pigment, this could only be considered a poorly differentiated carcinoma; sarcoma must be ruled out. (Papanicolaou stain, × 1,000.)

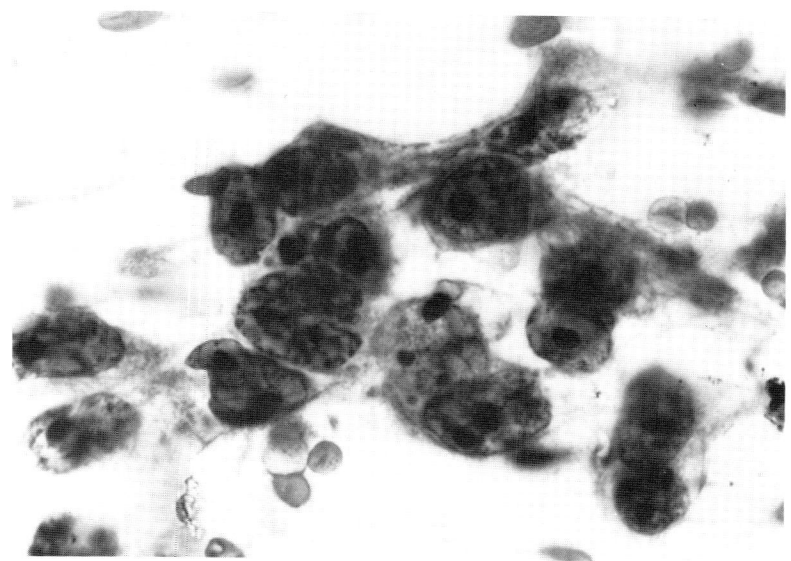

Fig. 5-49 Embryonal carcinoma of the testes, metastatic to the lung (bronchial wash). When large pleomorphic tumor cells with impressively prominent nucleoli are seen, a germ cell tumor should be considered. These cells have scant cytoplasm and dramatic nuclei with a somewhat characteristic "owl eye" clearing around the prominent nucleolus. Other large cell tumors must be considered. The clinical history is most important to verify the diagnosis, as is comparison with any available primary tumor tissue. (Papanicolaou stain, × 1,000.)

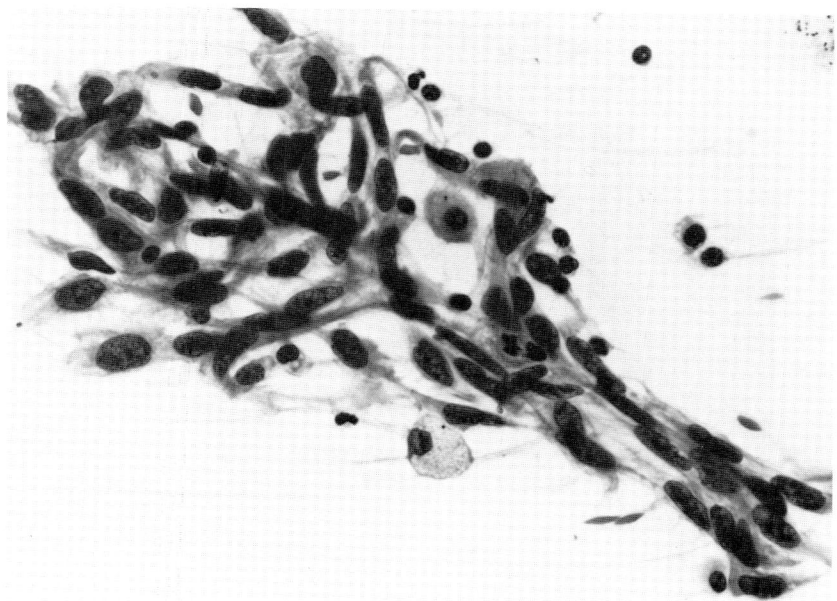

Fig. 5-50 Cystosarcoma phyllodes, metastatic to the lung (FNA of lung). The original breast lesion contains classic components of a cystosarcoma phyllodes (i.e., atypical epithelium and neoplastic fibrous stroma). The FNA specimen contains numerous, neoplastic, spindle-shaped cells, with large, blunt nuclei and irregular nuclear chromatin. The specimen has very few epithelial fragments, so inspection of the original tumor is essential to make an intelligent diagnosis. (Courtesy of McNeil Memorial Hospital, Berwyn, IL and Denise Hidvegi, M.D.) (Papanicolaou stain, × 400.)

SUMMARY

The best ways for the cytologist to refine diagnostic accuracy are as follows:

1. Insist on optimal specimen collection, processing, and staining. Anything less makes consistently reliable diagnoses impossible.
2. Review cytologic and histologic samples from the same or similar cases *before* final sign-out; this provides "instant" reinforcement of criteria.
3. Continually consult with the clinicians. Discussing difficult diagnoses can provide further insight into the most probable choice, and will help direct subsequent work-up.
4. An isolated diagnosis on a single sample can be dangerous. A team approach, using carefully selected diagnostic modalities, is the most efficient and accurate way to achieve the best possible patient care.

REFERENCES

1. Johnston WR, Frable WJ: Diagnostic Respiratory Cytopathology. Masson Publishing, Paris, 1979
2. Kato H, Konaka C, Ono J et al: Cytology of the Lung. Techniques and Interpretation. Igaku-Shoin, Tokyo, 1983
3. Koss LG: Diagnostic Cytology and Its Histopathologic Bases. 3rd Ed. JB Lippincott, Philadelphia, 1979
4. Koss LG: Aspiration Biopsy. Cytologic Interpretation and Histologic Bases. Igaku-Shoin, Tokyo, 1984
5. Linsk JA, Franzen S: Clinical Aspiration Cytology. JB Lippincott, Philadelphia, 1983
6. Rosenthal DL: Cytopathology of pulmonary disease. In Wied GL (ed): Monographs in Clinical Cytology. Vol. 11. S Karger, AG, Basel, 1988
7. Ikeda S: Flexible bronchofiberscope. Ann Otol Rhinol Laryngol 79:916, 1970
8. Carr DT: Lung Cancer. Curr Pulmonol 4:129, 1982
9. National Cancer Institute, National Institutes of Health, U.S. Department of Health and Human Services: Atlas of Early Lung Cancer. Igaku-Shoin, Tokyo, 1983
10. Bedrossian CWM, Accetta PA, Kelly LV: Cytopathology of nonneoplastic pulmonary disease. Lab Med 14:86, 1983
11. Bhatt O, Miller R, Le Riche J et al: Aspiration biopsy in pulmonary opportunistic infections. Acta Cytol 21:206, 1977
12. Bonfiglio T: Cytopathologic Interpretation of Transthoracic Fine-needle Biopsies (Masson Publishing, Paris, 1983
13. Pontiflex AH, Roberts FJ: Fine needle aspiration biopsy cytology in the diagnosis of inflammatory lesions. Acta Cytol 29:979, 1985
14. Nieberg RK, Gong H Jr: Diagnosis of *Pneumocystis carinii* pneumonia by bronchoalveolar lavage in patients with the acquired immunodeficiency syndrome. Am Clin Products Rev 6:23, 1987
15. Blackmon JA, Paris AL: Infectious diseases of the lung. Lab Med 14:77, 1983
16. Katzenstein A, Askin F: Surgical pathology of nonneoplastic lung disease. In Bennington JL (ed): Major Problems in Pathology. No. 13. WB Saunders, Philadelphia, 1982
17. Rosenthal DL: Cytology in the diagnosis of benign lung diseases. Clin Chest Med 8:147, 1987
18. Nasiell M, Roger V, Nasiell K et al: Cytologic findings indicating pulmonary tuberculosis. I. Acta Cytol 16:146, 1972
19. Roger V, Nasiell M, Nasiell K, et al: Cytologic findings indicating pulmonary tuberculosis. II. The occurrence in sputum of epithelioid cells and multinucleated giant cells in pulmonary tuberculosis, chronic non-tuberculous inflammatory lung disease and bronchogenic carcinoma. Acta Cytol 16:538, 1972
20. Baily TM, Akhtar M, Ali MA: Fine needle biopsy in the diagnosis of tuberculosis. Acta Cytol 29:732, 1985
21. Silverman JF, Marrow HG: Fine needle aspiration cytology of granulomatous diseases of the lung, including nontuberculous mycobacterium infection. Acta Cytol 29:535, 1985
22. Silverman JF, Johnsrude IS: Fine needle aspiration cytology of granulomatous cryptococcosis of the lung. Acta Cytol 29:157, 1985
23. Whitaker D, Sterrett G: Cryptococcus neoformans diagnosed by fine needle aspiration cytology of the lung. Acta Cytol 20:105, 1976
24. Gleason TH, Hammar SP, Barthas M et al: Cytological diagnosis of pulmonary cryptococcosis. Arch Pathol Lab Med 104:384, 1980
25. Gupta RK: Diagnosis of unsuspected pulmonary cryptococcosis with sputum cytology. Acta Cytol 29:154, 1985
26. Prolla J, Rosa U, Xavier R: The detection of cryptococcus neoformans in sputum cytology. Report of one case. Acta Cytol 14:87, 1970
27. Johnston W: The cytopathology of opportunistic infection of the lungs and other body sites. p. 282. In Wied GL (ed.) Compendium on Diagnostic Cytology. 5th Ed. Tutorials of Cytology, Chicago, 1983
28. Johnston W, Amatull J: The role of cytology in the primary diagnosis of North American Blastomycosis. Acta Cytol 14:200, 1970

29. Vigorita VJ, Gupta PK, Bargeron CB et al: Occurrence and identification of intracellular calcium crystals in pulmonary specimens. Acta Cytol 23:49, 1979
30. Farley ML, Mabry L, Munoz LA et al: Crystals occurring in pulmonary cytology specimens: Association with Aspergillus infection. Acta Cytol 29:737, 1985
31. Lazzari G, Vineis C, Cugini A: Cytologic diagnosis of primary pulmonary actinomycosis. Acta Cytol 25:299, 1981
32. Markowitz S, Leiman G: Cytologic detection of *Pneumocystis carinii* by ultraviolet light examination of Papanicolaou-stained sputum specimens. Acta Cytol 30:79, 1986
33. Fleury J, Escudier A, Pocholle M-J et al: Cell population obtained by bronchoalveolar lavage in *Pneumocystis carinii* pneumonitis. Acta Cytol 29:721, 1985
34. Greaves TS, Stigle SM: The recognition of *Pneumocystis carinii* in routine Papanicolaou-stained smears. Acta Cytol 29:714, 1985
35. Orenstein M, Weber CA, Heurich AE: Cytologic diagnosis of *Pneumocystis carinii* infection by bronchoalveolar lavage in acquired immune deficiency syndrome. Acta Cytol 29:727, 1985
36. Pintozzi R, Blecka L, Nanos S: The morphologic identification of Pneumocystis carinii. Acta Cytol 23:35, 1979
37. Frable W, Frable M, Seney F Jr: Virus infections of the respiratory tract. Acta Cytol 21:32, 1977
38. Papanicolaou GN: Degenerative changes in ciliated cells exfoliating from the bronchial epithelium as a cytologic criterion in the diagnosis of diseases of the lung. NYSJ Med 56:2647, 1956
39. Frable W, Kay S: Herpesvirus infection of the respiratory tract: Electron microscopic observation of the virus in cells obtained from sputum cytology. Acta Cytol 21:391, 1977
40. An-Foraker S, Haesaert S: Cytomegalic virus inclusion body in bronchial brushing material. Acta Cytol 21:181, 1977
41. Jain U, Mani K, Frable W: Cytomegalic inclusion disease: Cytologic diagnosis from bronchial brushing material. Acta Cytol 17:467, 1973
42. Delage G, Brochu P, Robillard L et al: Giant cell pneumonia due to respiratory syncytial virus: Occurrence in severe combined immunodeficiency syndrome. Arch Pathol Lab Med 108:623, 1984
43. Enders JF, McCarthy K, Mitus A, Cheatham WJ: Isolation of measles virus at autopsy in cases of giant cell pneumonia without rash. N Engl J Med 261:875, 1959
44. Collan Y, Sainio P: Relation of bacteria to exfoliated oral cells. An electron microscopy study. Acta Cytol 14:570, 1970
45. Chaudhuri B, Nanos S: Disseminated Strongyloides stercoralis infestation detected by sputum cytology. Acta Cytol 24:360, 1980
46. Humphreys K, Hieger L: Strongyloides stercoralis in routine Papanicolaou-stained sputum smears. Acta Cytol 236:471, 1979
47. Kenney M, Webber C: Diagnosis of stongyloidiasis on Papanicolaou-stained sputum smears. Acta Cytol 18:270, 1974
48. Wang T, Reyes C, Kathuria S, Strinden C: Diagnosis of Strongyloides stercoralis in sputum cytology. Acta Cytol 24:40, 1980
49. Allen A, Fullmer C: Primary diagnosis of pulmonary echinococcosis by the cytologic technique. Acta Cytol 16:212, 1972
50. Hawkins AG, Hsiu J-G, Smith RM III et al: Pulmonary dirofilariasis diagnosed by fine needle aspiration biopsy. A case report. Acta Cytol 29:19, 1985
51. Tani EM, Franco M: Pulmonary cytology in paracoccidioidomycosis. Acta Cytol 28:571, 1984
52. Willie S, Snyder R: The identification of *Paragonimus westermani* in bronchial washings. Case report. Acta Cytol 21:101, 1977
53. Osborn PT, Giltman LI, Uthman EO: Trichomonads in the respiratory tract: A case report and literature review. Acta Cytol 28:136, 1984
54. Rosenberg M, Rachman R: Entamoeba gingivalis in sputum. Its distinction from entamoeba histolytica. Acta Cytol 14:361, 1970
55. Koizumi J, Hidvegi D: Seaweed (*Undaria pinnatifida*) mimicking fungus. Acta Cytol 25:198, 1981
56. Ayres SM: Cigarette smoking and lung diseases: An update. Respir Care 21:632, 1976
57. Chovil AC: Occupational lung cancer and smoking: A review in the light of current theories of carcinogenesis. Can Med Assoc J 121:548, 1979
58. Ives JC, Buffler PA, Greenberg SD: Environmental associations and histopathologic patterns of carcinoma of the lung: The challenge and dilemma in epidemiologic studies. Am Rev Resp Dis 128:195, 1983
58a. Frost JK, Ball WC, Levin ML et al: Sputum cytopathology: Use and potential in monitoring the workplace environment by screening for biological effects of exposure. J Occup Med 28:692, 1986
59. Fontana RS: Screening for lung cancer. p. 377. In Miller WE (ed): Screening for Cancer. Academic Press, Orlando, FL, 1985
60. Baker RR, Tockman MS, Marsh BR et al: Screening for bronchogenic carcinoma. J Thorac Cardiovasc Surg 78:876, 1979
61. Fontana RS, Sanderson DR, Miller WE et al: The Mayo lung project: Preliminary report of "early cancer detection" phase. Cancer 30:1373, 1972
62. Woolner LB, Fontana RS: Pulmonary cytology in

lung cancer screening. p. 105. In Miller WE (ed): Screening for Cancer. Academic Press, Orlando, FL, 1985
63. Kilburn KH: Medical screening for lung cancer: Perspective and strategy. J Occup Med 28:714, 1986
64. Hayata Y: Lung Cancer Diagnosis. Igaku-Shoin, Tokyo, 1982
65. Kato H, Nishimiya K, Lay J et al: Transbronchial needle aspiration biopsy via fiberoptic bronchoscope. p. 307. In Nakhosteen JA (ed): Proceedings of the Second World Congress for Bronchology, June 2–4, 1980. Bronchology: Research, Diagnostic and Therapeutic aspects. Martinus Nijhoff, The Hague, 1981.
66. Kato H, Ono J, Niizuma M et al: Transbronchofiberscopic aspiration biopsy using a special catheter. Jpn J Thorac Dis 16:774, 1978
67. Lundgren R: A flexible thin needle for transbronchial aspiration biopsy through the flexible fiberoptic bronchoscope. Endoscopy 12:180, 1980
68. Oho K: Transbronchial needle aspiration biopsy (TBAB) (Needle aspiration biopsy via the fiberoptic bronchoscope). p. 118. In Sinner WN (ed): Needle Biopsy and Transbronchial Biopsy. Theime, Stuttgart, 1982
69. Oho K, Kato H, Ogawa I et al: A new needle for transfiberoptic bronchoscopic use. Chest 76:492, 1979
70. Rosenthal DL, Wallace JM: Fine needle aspiration of pulmonary lesions via fiberoptic bronchoscopy. Acta Cytol 28:203, 1984
71. Saccomanno G, Bechtel JJ, Kelley WA: Transbronchial fine needle aspiration cytology of lung tumors. Acta Cytol 27:556, 1983
72. Wang KP, Marsh BR, Summer WR et al: Transbronchial needle aspiration for diagnosis of lung cancer. Chest 80:48, 1981
73. Wang KP, Terry PB: Transbronchial needle aspiration in the diagnosis and staging of bronchogenic carcinoma. Am Rev Respir Dis 127:344, 1983
74. Wang KP, Terry P, Marsh B: Bronchoscopic needle aspiration biopsy of paratracheal tumors. Am Rev Respir Dis 118:17, 1978
75. Lillington GA: The utility of needle aspiration biopsy of the lung. Mayo Clin Proc 55:516, 1980
76. Sinner WN: Needle Biosy and Transbronchial Biopsy. With Special Reference to Carcinoma of the Lung. Thieme, Stuttgart, 1982
77. Zajicek J: Aspiration, Biopsy, Cytology. Part I. Cytology of Supradiaphragmatic Organs. In Wied GL (ed): Monographs in Clinical Cytology. Vol. 4. S Karger, AG, Basel, 1974
78. Hattori S, Matsuda M, Nishihara H et al: Early diagnosis of small peripheral lung cancer—Cytologic diagnosis of very fresh cancer cells obtained by the TV-brushing technique. Acta Cytol 15:460, 1971
79. Hayata Y, Kato H, Konaka C et al: Fiberoptic bronchoscopic laser photoradiation for tumor localization in lung cancer. Chest 82:10, 1982
80. World Health Organization: The World Health Organization histologic typing of lung tumors. 2nd Edition. Am J Clin Pathol 77:123, 1982
81. Johnston W: Percutaneous fine needle aspiration biopsy of the lung: A study of 1,015 patients. Acta Cytol 28:218, 1984
82. Kern WH, Schweizer CW: Sputum cytology of metastatic carcinoma of the lung. Acta Cytol 20:514, 1976
83. Carr DT, Rosenow EC III: Bronchogenic Carcinoma. Basics RD 5:97, 1977
84. Emerson G, Phillips C, Bennett JM, Rubin P: Lung cancer. p. 75. In Rubin P (ed): Clinical Oncology for Medical Students and Physicians: A Multidisciplinary Approach. 5th Ed. American Cancer Society, 1978.
85. Kanhouwa SB, Matthews MJ: Reliability of cytologic typing of lung cancer. Acta Cytol 20:229, 1976
86. Hammar SP, Bolen JW, Bockus D et al: Ultrastructural and immunohistochemical features of common lung tumors: An overview. Ultrastruct Pathol 9:283, 1985
87. Johnston W, Bossen EH: Ten years of respiratory cytology at Duke University Medical Center. II. The cytopathologic diagnosis of lung cancer during the years 1970 to 1974, with a comparison between cytopathology and histopathology in the typing of lung cancer. Acta Cytol 25:499, 1981
88. Mennemeyer R, Hammar SP, Bauermeister DE et al: Cytologic, histologic and electron microscopic correlations in poorly differentiated primary lung carcinoma. A study of 43 cases. Acta Cytol 23:297, 1979
89. Roggli VL, Vollmer RT, Greenberg SD, et al: Lung cancer heterogeneity: A blinded and randomized study of 100 consecutive cases. Hum Pathol 16:569, 1985
90. Battifora H: Recent progress in the immunohistochemistry of solid tumors. Semin Diagn Pathol 1:251, 1984
91. Said JW, Nash G, Banks-Schlegel S, et al: Keratin in human lung tumors. Patterns of localization of different-molecular-weight keratin proteins. Am J Pathol 113:27, 1983
92. Said JW, Nash G, Sassoon AF, et al: Involucrin in lung tumors. A specific marker for squamous differentiation. Lab Invest 49:563, 1983
93. Said JW, Nash G, Tepper G, Banks-Schlegel S: Keratin proteins and carcinoembryonic antigen in lung carcinoma: An immunoperoxidase study of fifty-four

cases, with ultrastructural correlations. Hum Pathol 14:70, 1983
94. Walts AE, Said JW, Banks-Schlegel S: Keratin and carcinoembryonic antigen in exfoliated mesothelial and malignant cells: An immunoperoxidase study. Am J Clin Pathol 80:671, 1983
95. Walts AE, Said JW, Shintaku IP: Epithelial membrane antigen in the cytodiagnosis of effusions and aspirates: Immunocytochemical and ultrastructural localization in benign and malignant cells. Diagn Cytopathol 3:41, 1987
96. Walts AE, Said JW, Shintaku IP et al: Keratins of different molecular weight in exfoliated mesothelial and adenocarcinoma cells—An aid to cell identification. Am J Clin Pathol 81:442, 1984
97. Lavoie RR, McDonald JR, Kling GA: Cavitation in squamous carcinoma of the lung. Acta Cytol 21:210, 1977
98. Johnston WW, Frable WJ: The cytopathology of the respiratory tract: A review. Am J Pathol 84:372, 1976
99. Saccomanno G: Diagnostic Pulmonary Cytology. 2nd Ed. American Society of Clinical Pathologists Press, Chicago, 1986
100. Saccomanno G, Archer VE, Auerbach O et al: Development of carcinoma of the lung as reflected in exfoliated cells. Cancer 33:256, 1974
101. Saccomanno G, Saunders RP, Archer VE, et al: Cancer of the lung: The cytology of sputum prior to the development of carcinoma. Acta Cytol 9:413, 1965
102. Bedrosian CWM, Corey BJ: Abnormal sputum cytopathology during chemotherapy with bleomycin. Acta Cytol 22:202, 1978
103. Smith JH, Frable WJ: Adenocarcinoma of the lung. Cytologic correlation with histologic types. Acta Cytol 18:316, 1974
104. Mitchell ML, Ryan FP Jr, Shermer RW: Pulmonary adenocarcinoma metastatic to the adrenal gland mimicking normal adrenal cortical epithelium on fine needle aspiration. Acta Cytol 29:994, 1985
105. Csako G, Chandra P: Bronchioloalveolar carcinoma presenting with meningeal carcinomatosis. Cytologic diagnosis in cerebrospinal fluid. Acta Cytol 30:653, 1986
106. Donaldson JC, Kaminsky DB, Elliot RC: Bronchiolar carcinoma. Cancer 41:250, 1978
107. Tsumuraya M, Kodama T, Kameya T et al: Light and electron microscopic analysis of intranuclear inclusions in papillary adenocarcinoma of the lung. Acta Cytol 25:523, 1981
108. Clayton F: Bronchioloalveolar carcinomas. Cell types, patterns of growth, and prognostic correlates. Cancer 57:1555, 1986
109. Tao LC, Delarue NC, Sanders D, Weisbrod G: Bronchiolo-alveolar carcinoma. A correlative clinical and cytologic study. Cancer 42:2759, 1978
110. Silverman JF, Finley JL, Park HK et al: Fine needle aspiration cytology of bronchioloalveolar-cell carcinoma of the lung. Acta Cytol 29:887, 1985
111. Ebihara Y, Sagawa H: Mucin-producing bronchioloalveolar-cell carcinoma. With special reference to a characteristic structure revealed by phosphotungstic acid-hematoxylin staining. Acta Cytol 30:643, 1986
112. Jay SJ, Wehr K, Nicholson DP, Smith AL: Diagnostic sensitivity and specificity of pulmonary cytology. Comparison of techniques used in conjunction with flexible fiber optic bronchoscopy. Acta Cytol 24:304, 1980
113. Marchevsky A, Nieburgs HE, Olenko E et al: Pulmonary tumorlets in case of "tuberculoma" of the lung with malignant cells in brush biopsy. Acta Cytol 26:491, 1982
114. Naylor B: The shedding of the mucosa of the bronchial tree in asthma. Thorax 17:69, 1962
115. Naylor B, Railey C: A pitfall in the cytodiagnosis of sputum of asthmatics. J Clin Pathol 17:84, 1964
116. Michel RP, Lushpihan A, Ahmed MN: Pathologic findings of transthoracic needle aspiration in the diagnosis of localized pulmonary lesions. Cancer 51:1663, 1983
117. Aisner J, Aisner SC, Ostrow S et al: Meningeal carcinomatosis from small cell carcinoma of the lung. Acta Cytol 23:292, 1979
118. Bell WR Jr, Johnston WW, Bigner SH: Cytologic diagnosis of occult small-cell undifferentiated carcinoma of the lung. Acta Cytol 26:73, 1982
119. Hoffman PC, Albain KS, Bitran JD, Golomb, HM: Current concepts in small cell carcinoma of the lung. CA 34:269, 1984
120. Baylin SB: Ectopic production of hormones and other proteins by tumors. Hosp Pract 10:117, 1975
121. Pearse AGE: The cytochemistry and ultrastructure of polypeptide hormone-producing cells of the APUD series and the embryologic, physiologic and pathologic implications of the concept. J Histochem Cytochem 17:303, 1969
122. Pearse AGE, Polak JM: Endocrine tumours of neural crest origin: Neurolophomas, apudomas and the APUD concept. Med Biol 52:3, 1974
123. Solcia E, Capella C, Buffa R et al: The contribution of immunohistochemistry to the diagnosis of neuroendocrine tumors. Semin Diagn Pathol 1:285, 1984
124. Nathanson L, Hall TC: Lung tumors: How they produce their syndromes. Ann NY Acad Sci vii:367, 1974

125. Yesner R: Small cell tumors of the lung. Am J Surg Pathol 7:775, 1983
126. Zaharopoulos P, Wong JY, Stewart GD: Cytomorphology of the variants of small-cell carcinoma of the lung. Acta Cytol 26:800, 1982
127. Ebihara Y, Fukushima N, Asakuma Y: Double primary lung cancers. With special reference to their exfoliative cytology and to the rare, malignant "mixed" tumor of the salivary-gland type. Acta Cytol 24:212, 1980
128. Broderick PA, Corvese NL, LaChance T, Allard J: Giant cell carcinoma of lung: A cytologic evaluation. Acta Cytol 19:225, 1975
129. Yang K, Ulich T, Taylor I et al: Pulmonary carcinoids. Immunohistochemical demonstration of brain-gut peptides. Cancer 52:819, 1983
130. Gephardt GN, Belovich DM: Cytology of pulmonary carcinoid tumors. Acta Cytol 26:434, 1982
131. Lozowski W, Hajdu SI, Melamed MR: Cytomorphology of carcinoid tumors. Acta Cytol 23:360, 1979
132. Pilotti S, Rilke F, Lombardi L: Pulmonary carcinoid with glandular features. Report of two cases with positive fine needle aspiration biopsy cytology. Acta Cytol 27:511, 1983
133. Walts AE, Said JW, Shintaku IP, Lloyd RV: Chromogranin as a marker of neuroendocrine cells in cytologic material—An immunocytochemical study. Am J Clin Pathol 84:273, 1985
134. Lozowski MS, Mishriki Y, Solitaire GB: Cytopathologic features of adenoid cystic carcinoma. Case report and literature review. Acta Cytol 27:317, 1983
135. Coulson WF: Surgical Pathology, 2nd Ed. (JB Lippincott, Philadelphia, 1987
136. Tao L-C, Robertson DI: Cytologic diagnosis of bronchial mucoepidermoid carcinoma by fine needle aspiration biopsy. Acta Cytol 22:221, 1978
137. Anderson RJ, Johnston WW, Szpak CA: Fine needle aspiration of adenoid cystic carcinoma metastatic to the lung. Acta Cytol 29:527, 1985
138. Smith RC, Amy RW: Adenoid cystic carcinoma metastatic to the lung. Report of a case diagnosed by fine needle aspiration biopsy cytology. Acta Cytol 29:533, 1985
139. Jenkins PF, Ward MJ, Davies P, Fletcher J: Non-Hodgkin's lymphoma, chronic lymphatic leukaemia and the lung. Br J Dis Chest 75:22, 1981
140. Ludwig RA, Balachandran I: Mycosis fungoides. The importance of pulmonary cytology in the diagnosis of a case with systemic involvement. Acta Cytol 27:198, 1983
141. Rosen SE, Vonderheid EC, Koprowska I: Mycosis fungoides with pulmonary involvement. Cytopathologic findings. Acta Cytol 28:51, 1984
142. Vernon SE: Cytodiagnosis of "signet-ring"-cell lymphoma. Acta Cytol 25:291, 1981
143. Goldstein J, Leslie H: Immunoblastic lymphadenopathy with pulmonary lesions and positive sputum cytology. Acta Cytol 22:165, 1978
144. Reale FR, Variakojis D, Compton J, Bibbo M: Cytodiagnosis of Hodgkin's disease in sputum specimens. Acta Cytol 27:258, 1983
145. Shaheen K, Oertel YC: Mycosis fungoides cells in sputum. A case report. Acta Cytol 28:483, 1984
146. Nguyen G-K, Jeannot A: Cytopathologic aspects of pulmonary metastasis of malignant fibrous histiocytoma, myxoid variant. Fine needle aspiration biopsy of a case. Acta Cytol 26:349, 1982
147. Spahr J, Frable WJ: Pulmonary cytopathology of an invasive thymoma. Acta Cytol 25:163, 1981
148. Kim K, Naylor B, Han IH: Fine needle aspiration cytology of sarcomas metastatic to the lung. Acta Cytol 30:688, 1986
149. Lozowski MS, Mishriki YY, Epstein H: Metastatic malignant fibrous histiocytoma in lung examined by fine needle aspiration. Case report and literature review. Acta Cytol 24:350, 1980
150. Nickels J, Koivuniemi A: Cytology of malignant hemangiopericytoma. Acta Cytol 23:119, 1979
151. Nieberg RK: Fine needle aspiration cytology of alveolar soft-part sarcoma. A case report. Acta Cytol 28:198, 1984
152. Silverman JF, Weaver MD, Gardner N et al: Aspiration biopsy cytology of malignant schwannoma metastatic to the lung. Acta Cytol 29:15, 1985
153. Zaharopoulos P, Wong JY, Lamke CR: Endometrial stromal sarcoma. Cytology of pulmonary metastasis including ultrastructural study. Acta Cytol 26:49, 1982
154. Craig ID, Shum DT, Desrosiers P et al: Choriocarcinoma metastatic to the lung. A cytologic study with identification of human choriogonadotropin with an immunoperoxidase technique. Acta Cytol 27:647, 1983
155. Ehya H: Cytology of mesothelioma of the tunica vaginalis metastatic to the lung. Acta Cytol 29:79, 1985
156. Granberg I, Willems JS: Endometriosis of lung and pleura diagnosed by aspiration biopsy. Acta Cytol 21:295, 1977
157. Ludwig ME, Otis RD, Cole SR, Westcott JL: Fine needle aspiration cytology of pulmonary hamartomas. Acta Cytol 26:671, 1982
158. Ramzy I: Pulmonary hamartomas: Cytologic appearances of fine needle aspiration biopsy. Acta Cytol 20:15, 1976

6

Fine Needle Aspiration of the Thyroid Gland

Theodore R. Miller

Proper management of the patient with a palpable thyroid nodule has been controversial. Although most thyroid nodules are benign, the clinical studies for the diagnosis of these lesions are not specific. Within the last decade, fine needle aspiration (FNA) biopsy has been utilized in this country for the evaluation of the palpable thyroid nodule. Its use has proven to be sensitive, specific, and cost-effective.[1,2] The majority of thyroid nodules have a characteristic cytologic pattern, allowing specific diagnoses to be rendered. When the patterns are not specific, it can usually be determined whether the lesion is benign or malignant. This chapter discusses the diagnosis of the most common carcinomas and benign lesions of the thyroid.

EPIDEMIOLOGY OF THYROID CARCINOMA

The incidence of thyroid carcinoma is increasing in the United States. This may be explained, in part, by the frequent use in the past of irradiation to treat a number of clinical conditions, including large thymus, tonsilitis, external otitis, ringworm, and acne. The incidences of both benign and malignant thyroid neoplasms increase relative to the dose of radiation exposure received. Papillary carcinoma increases in incidence when exposure to radiation ranges from 6.5 to 2000 rad. However, with a dosage greater than 6000 rad, a decreased incidence of carcinoma is observed.[3]

Thyroid carcinoma is more common in women than in men; however, it must be remembered that women also have a significantly greater number of benign nodules than do men. Hence, any palpable nodule in a man is more likely to harbor carcinoma than is one in a woman. The age ranges for thyroid carcinoma vary according to the cell type. The better differentiated and slower growing tumors (follicular and papillary) occur in a relatively younger age group (25 to 55 years of age), whereas undifferentiated carcinoma generally affects patients 60 years of age or older. The most common thyroid carcinoma is the papillary type, which accounts for 60 to 80 percent of all carcinomas. The second most common malignant disease of the thyroid is follicular carcinoma, which may account for up to 25 percent of all malignant thyroid neoplasms. Smaller numbers of medullary carcinomas and undifferentiated carcinomas account for the remaining primary malignant processes that involve the thyroid. The actual number of cases of thyroid carcinoma in the population is not great. It has been estimated that 4 percent of people living in the United States will have a palpable thyroid nodule, whereas less than 0.004 percent of the population will actually harbor a malignant lesion. The majority of thyroid carcinomas are slow-growing, and less than six persons per million die yearly from them in the United States. Undifferentiated carcinomas and medullary carcinomas are aggressive tumors that do not have the indolent course that is characteristic of well-differentiated papillary and follicular carcinomas.[3]

DIAGNOSTIC TESTS FOR THYROID CARCINOMA

Thyroid imaging has been used to determine the malignant potential of thyroid masses. Types of imaging include external scintigraphy, which utilizes iodine-233 (^{233}I) and technetium-99m (^{99m}Tc) pertechnetate. These radioactive substances are taken up by the normal gland, but not by neoplastic processes; thus, potentially malignant lesions will stand out as areas of nonradioactivity (cold areas). This test is not specific, as approximately 80 percent of cold or nonfunctioning nodules are benign. Another type of imaging available for thyroid masses is ultrasonography. This modality allows classification of lesions according to whether they are cystic, solid, or mixed in type. Approximately 20 percent of solid or mixed lesions prove to be malignant.[3]

FNA biopsy has proven to be more sensitive and specific than either of these modalities. A sensitivity and specificity of greater than 90 percent have been achieved with FNA. With FNA, one can not only detect potentially malignant lesions, but specific histologic types can be determined.[4,5] In experienced hands, FNA can establish a definitive benign or malignant diagnosis in 90 percent of cases. "Suspicious" and unsatisfactory rates should be no higher than 5 percent. When compared with core or open biopsy, FNA biopsy has proven to be safe; only rarely have complications been reported.

NORMAL THYROID

Normal thyroid is not usually sampled; however, biopsy of this tissue may be undertaken in patients who have undergone subtotal thyroidectomy and who present with a mass secondary to hyperplasia. FNA biopsy of normal thyroid yields few epithelial cells. Follicular cells occur as bare nuclei or rare tissue fragments with scanty, delicate, granular cytoplasm (Fig. 6-1). Lipofuscin pigment can often be seen within the cytoplasm. The characteristic chromatin pattern of these lymphocyte-sized nuclei is even and

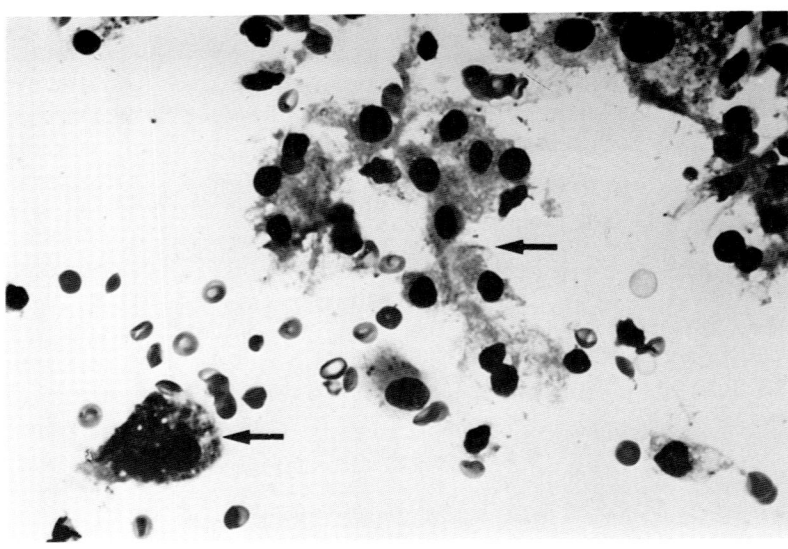

Fig. 6-1 Benign follicular epithelial cells occurring in a small cluster. Note the delicate, slightly granular cytoplasm (long arrow) and the pigment-containing macrophage (short arrow). These epithelial cells are similar to those seen in normal thyroid (MGG stain, × 40.)

finely divided. A small nucleolus may be seen. Colloid from normal glands is not ordinarily of sufficient quantity or quality to be seen.[6]

HYPERFUNCTIONAL THYROID

Hyperfunctional glands, or Grave's disease, has not been studied extensively by FNA; however, these smears have been characterized by a moderately cellular appearance. The cells may appear in small sheets or in aggregates. A feature that has been noted to occur is peripheral vacuolization of the cytoplasm. Upon application of a May-Grünwald-Giemsa (MGG) stain, these vacuoles may become reddish in color and are then referred to as "flame cells." Similar changes may be seen in "hot" adenomas, hyperfunctional areas of multinodular thyroids, and benign macrofollicular adenomas. Another cytoplasmic feature seen in hyperthyroidism is the presence of paravacuolar granulation. Dark, green-black granules may be found in the wall of vacuoles, usually near the nucleus. They have also been noted to occur with a high degree of frequency in patients with resolving subacute thyroiditis. The source of paravacuolar granulation is not known; however, it is possible that it is of lysosomal origin.[6]

MULTINODULAR THYROID

A dominant nodule in a multinodular thyroid is the lesion that is most often sampled in this area. The cytologic presentation of multinodular thyroid is as varied as its histology. Just as the histology may show large colloid lakes, variably micro-sized to macro-sized follicles, and areas of involution, so, too, may the smears. These cytologic features may be equally represented (Fig. 6-2, Plate 6-1), or one pattern may predominate. Colloid stains blue with the Wright stain and blue-green or eosinophilic with Papanicolaou stain. The quality or texture varies from thin and transparent to thick and opaque. Involutional areas show numerous phagocytic cells, which

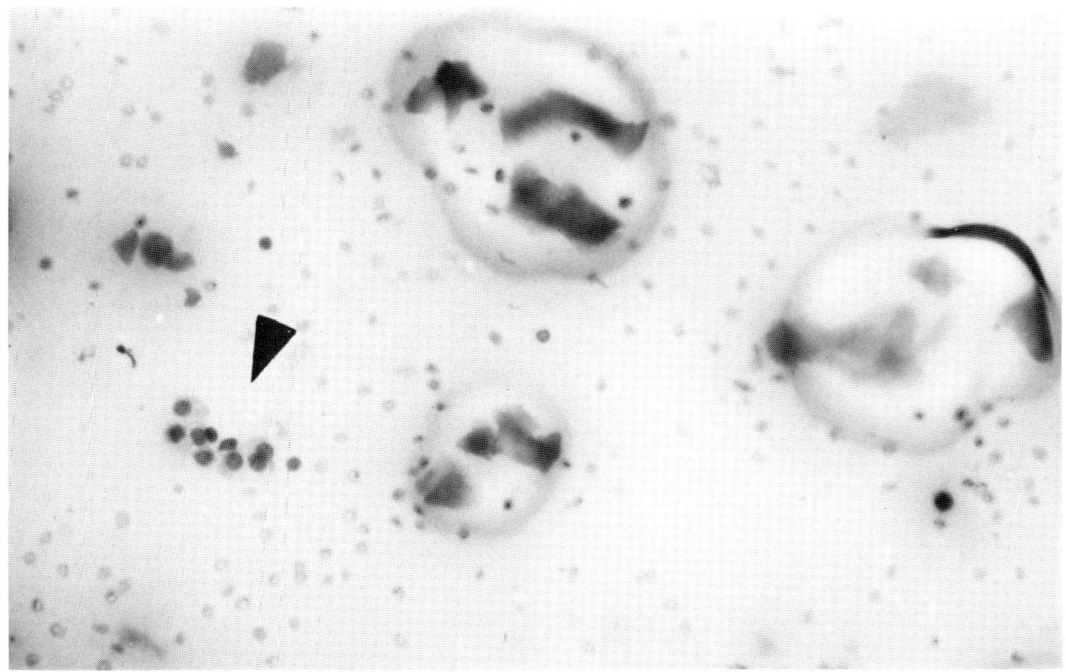

Fig. 6-2 A small cluster of benign follicular cells (arrow) are visible in a field of watery blue colloid. (MGG stain, × 10.) (See Plate 6-1.)

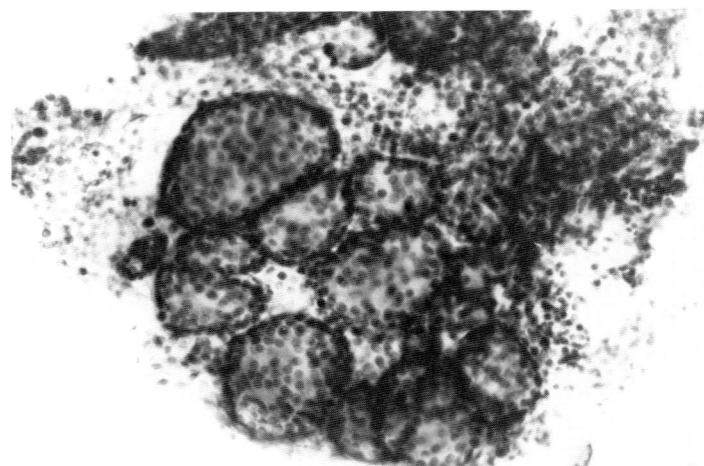

Fig. 6-3 Fragment of intact, benign, follicular structures. This type of moderate-sized, spherical follicular structure is associated with benign thyroid nodules. (Papanicolaou stain, × 10.)

contain ingested colloid as well as hemosiderin (Fig. 6-1). Involutional change is often seen in benign lesions; however, involutional change has also been observed in cystic papillary carcinoma. The risk associated with missing a cystic papillary tumor is not great, as only 1 percent of these cysts are malignant. In order for a cystic lesion to be called benign, epithelial fragments should be evident. Nondisrupted single follicles are represented by intact, three-dimensional structures; with proper focus, glary colloid may be visualized in the center. Occasionally, these follicles may be bound together by fibrous tissue to form microbiopsies (Fig. 6-3). When large follicular structures are ruptured, the epithelium lies flat and the epithelial nuclei are arranged in neat rows and columns. The cytology of the individual cells demonstrates some variability. Cytoplasm is most often scanty and delicate (Fig. 6-1). Occasionally, oxyphilic or Hürthle cell changes may predominate. This change is seen as an increase in nuclear and nucleolar size in conjunction with increased amounts of granular, well-defined cytoplasm. It should be remembered that, in most multinodular thyroids; the pattern is one of abundant colloid or involutional material, or both. Occasionally, however, areas of hyperplasia may have an appearance identical to that of cellular adenomas (see the following section).[3]

THE CLINICAL UNINODULAR THYROID

The clinical uninodular thyroid has three major histologic presentations. In many cases, a clinically solitary palpable thyroid nodule will, upon gross and microscopic examination, be a dominant nodule in a multinodular thyroid. Of greater interest and concern is the solitary nodule that represents a true adenoma. There are two types of adenomas that may be sampled by FNA biopsy: the simple (colloid) type, which is relatively common, and the less common fetal embryonal or trabecular adenoma. This is fortunate because most observers believe that these latter types constitute neoplasms with a propensity for capsular and vascular invasion.

Simple (colloid) adenomas have many of the same histologic and cytologic features as do multinodular thyroids. The aspirate smear of both contains moderate to abundant watery colloid and normal, macrofollicular or, occasionally, microfollicular structures. Pigmented phagocytic cells may also be present. An additional feature of the cytologic specimen is the presence of disrupted follicular elements. The ruptured epithelium lies in a flat sheet with the nuclei evenly dispersed in orderly rows and columns. It is not uncommon to find tissue fragments composed of variably sized, three-dimensional colloid containing follicles and connective tissue. In many cases, only a few epithelial elements can be identified, and the major pattern is that of watery colloid material from a colloid nodule, or proteinaceous material from a "thyroid cyst." The smears from so-called thyroid cysts contain only a few obvious epithelial cells; instead, phagocytic cells predominate. Ingested material includes hemosiderin, colloid, and lipofuscin. In most instances, the epithelium has delicate cytoplasm, with faint or absent cell borders. Although not common, minimal oxyphilic changes may be seen in the cytoplasm, along with increased cytoplasmic density and visible cell borders. Benign cytologic features in follicular epithelium include flame cell changes (as seen in Grave's disease), cytoplasmic lipofuscin, and paravacuolar granulation.[3,6]

Microfollicular and trabecular adenomas have a distinctive presentation in that the smears are cellular and lack the abundant watery colloid of a benign thyroid nodule. A distinctive pattern of microfollicular adenoma is the presence of microfollicles; these follicles are characterized by monolayered structures with nuclei arranged in a circular fashion around a syncytial mass of delicate cytoplasm. Occasionally, small, dense, hyaline-like colloid may be seen in the center of such a mass. A variant of the microfollicle is a small, intact follicle which, when viewed, appears to have a top and bottom but lacks colloid material at its center. The trabecular pattern can be identified as a solid, serpiginous arrangement of disorderly nuclei. Microfollicular and trabecular patterns may occur in tissue fragments composed of both epithelial and connective tissue (Figs. 6-4 and 6-5).[3,6] The cytologic features of simple adenomas or microfollicular or trabecular adenomas include normal to slightly enlarged nuclei. These nuclei rarely, if ever, exceed 90 μ^2 in area, in comparison to the larger nuclei of follicular carcinoma.

A diagnosis of follicular neoplasm is made when microfollicular or trabecular patterns are dominant. The term benign thyroid nodule is applied to these solitary or dominant nodules that have a predominant pattern that is macrofollicular, involutional, or colloid in nature. I believe this designation is justified even though the term benign thyroid nodule may be applied to adenomas of the macrofollicular or normofollicular type. One diagnostic difficulty is that the microfollicular pattern can be present in disorders other than microfollicular adenoma, including mixed microfollicular and macrofollicular adenomas, well-differentiated follicular carcinoma, follicular variant of papillary carcinoma, chronic thyroiditis, and hyperplastic, adenomatous areas of multinodular thy-

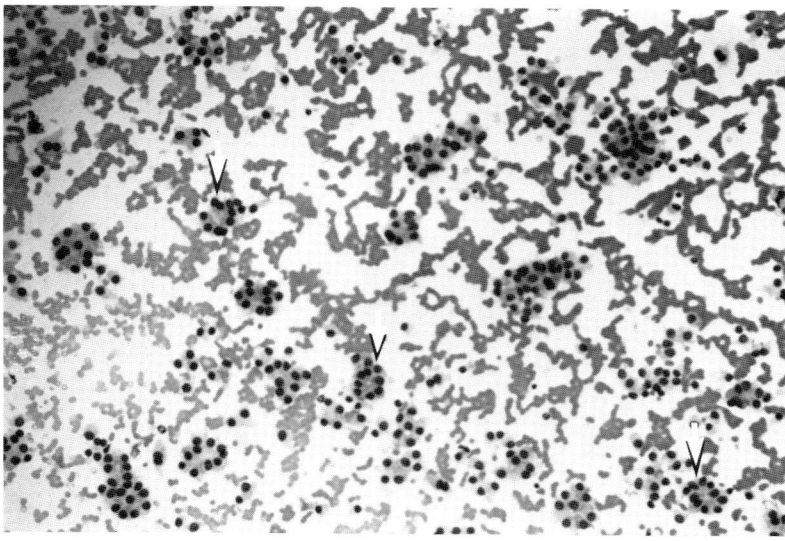

Fig. 6-4 Smear from a follicular neoplasm. Note the absence of colloid in the background and the microfollicular structures (arrowheads) that are evident. (MGG stain, × 10.)

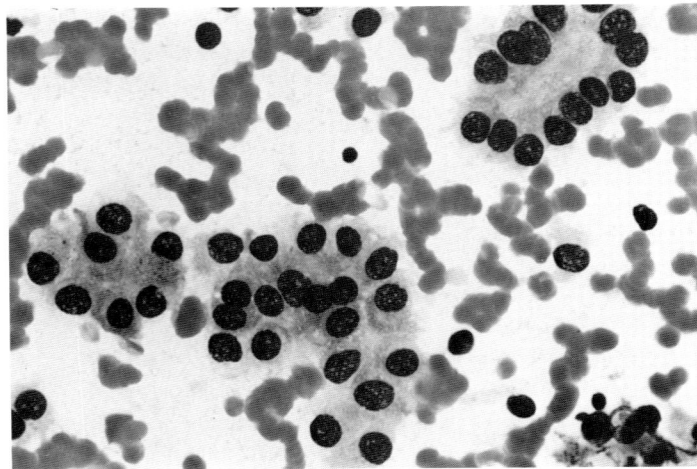

Fig. 6-5 A microfollicular structure is demonstrated (upper right), as is a trabecular structure with some nuclear overlapping (lower left). These findings are characteristic of follicular neoplasms. (MGG stain, × 40.)

roid. Removal of any mass that has a smear dominated by a microfollicular/trabecular pattern is advised.[3] The risk of malignant disease in lesions exhibiting this pattern is about 15 percent.[7]

FOLLICULAR CARCINOMA

It is evident from the literature that well-differentiated follicular carcinoma may resemble benign microfollicular adenoma, and that FNA may not always be able to distinguish between these two entities. There are, however, follicular carcinomas that are not so well differentiated and that will contain features that point to a correct diagnosis. Well-differentiated follicular carcinomas and microfollicular adenomas contain microfollicles and disorderly groups of epithelial cells, but lack the marked nuclear abnormalities of less-than-well-differentiated, overt follicular carcinomas. In the latter, nuclear size is increased in excess of 90 μ^2, nucleoli and chromocenters appear, and considerable variation in shape occurs. The low-power picture is similar to that indicating a follicular neoplasm; trabecular and microfollicular structures predominate, and there is an absence of colloid.[6]

PAPILLARY CARCINOMA

Fortunately, papillary carcinoma, the most common malignant disease affecting the thyroid, has a distinctive cytologic presentation. A number of cytologic features have been proposed as prerequisites for establishing a diagnosis of papillary carcinoma. By use of a stepwise, logistic regression analysis, the most helpful features include: (1) papillary structures without vessels, (2) intranuclear inclusions, and (3) metaplastic cytoplasm. Intranuclear inclusions are invaginations of cytoplasm into the nucleus; they can be differentiated from artifacts by the accentuation of chromatin material on the edge of the inclusion, nuclear chromatin material visible at the depth of the invagination, and a homogeneous center that is similar in texture and chromatically to the surrounding cytoplasm (Fig. 6-6). Papillary structures without vessels consist of thick disorderly groups of tumor cells with a blunt-ended configuration. Upon focusing into these groups, no vessels are visualized (Fig. 6-7). Papillary structures with obvious vessels are found in more than 50 percent of papillary carcinomas; however, they may also be seen in other diseases, such as multinodular goiter and chronic thyroiditis.[8] In papillary carcinoma, the cytoplasm of

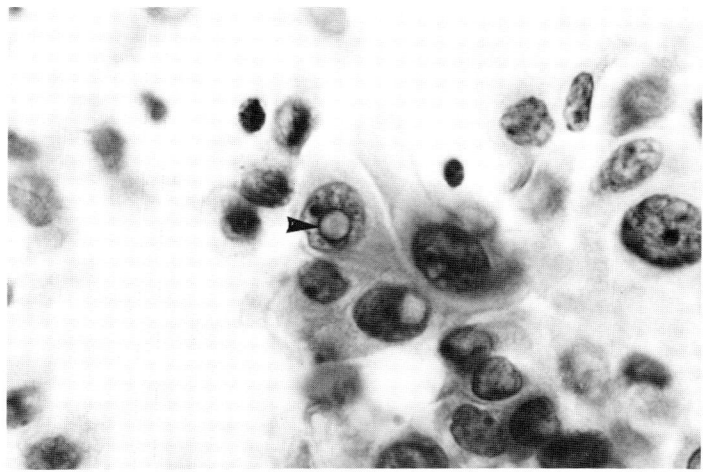

Fig. 6-6 A cluster of cells with metaplastic-type cytoplasm and nuclei with nuclear inclusions. Note the accentuation of chromatin material around the outside of the inclusion (arrowhead). (Papanicolaou stain, × 63.)

tumor cells is denser than that of normal epithelial cells or follicular lesions (Fig. 6-8). The cytoplasm becomes so dense in some cells that they resemble squamous cells. Cells with metaplastic cytoplasm are encountered in about 65 percent of the cases of papillary carcinoma. These cells bear a striking resemblance to immature squamous metaplasia, as seen in the cervix. The individual cells have a dense, waxy cytoplasm with sharply demarcated borders (Figs. 6-9 and 6-10, Plate 6-2).[8]

Other features that may be helpful, but are not necessarily diagnostic, include the presence of psam-

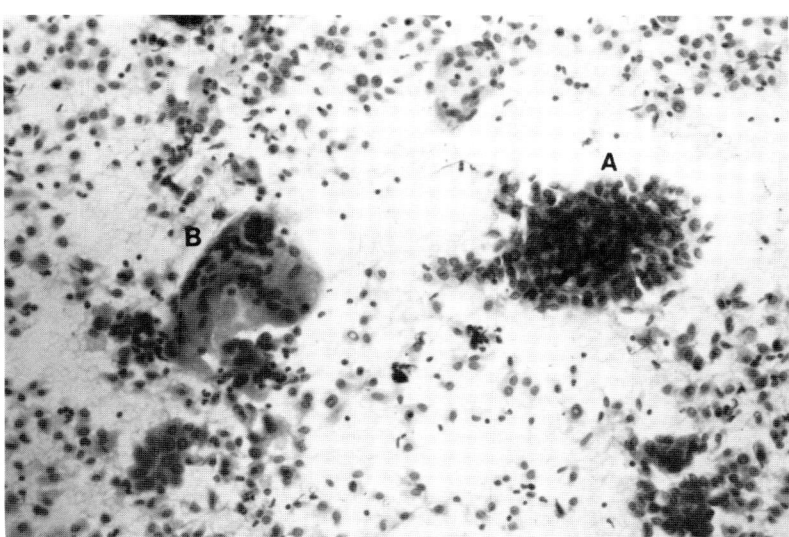

Fig. 6-7 (A) An example of a papillary structure without a discernible vessel. Note the rounded tip. **(B)** An epithelial giant cell. (Papanicolaou stain, × 10.)

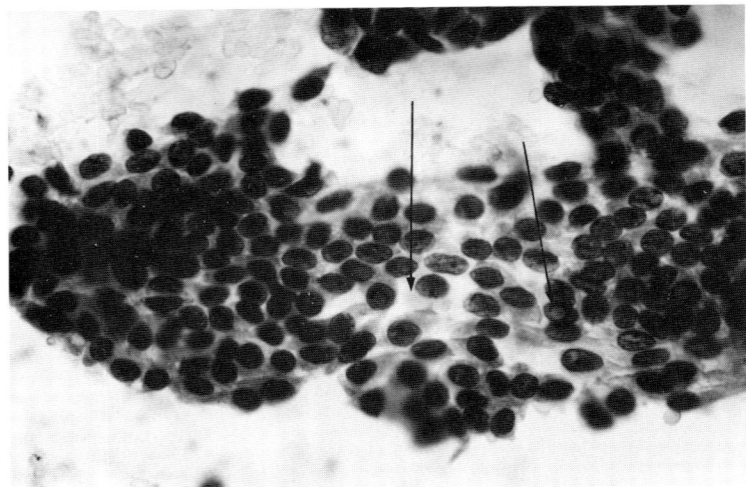

Fig. 6-8 In the central portion of this picture, papillary carcinoma cells are seen in a flat sheet. These cells have denser, more well-defined cytoplasms than do those of follicular lesions. The left edge of this group is thicker and has the appearance of a papillary frond without a discernible vessel. In addition, nuclear inclusions are present (arrows). (Papanicolaou stain, × 40.)

moma bodies and papillary structures with vessels. Psammoma bodies are laminated, calcified structures that, with the Wright stain, are transparent in their center with a condensation of bluish material around their edges (Fig. 6-11). With the Papanicolaou stain, psammoma bodies have a reddish-blue hue. Although psammoma bodies are useful in the diagnosis of papillary carcinoma, they are found in less than 50 percent of all papillary carcinomas, and occur in 1 percent of benign diseases.

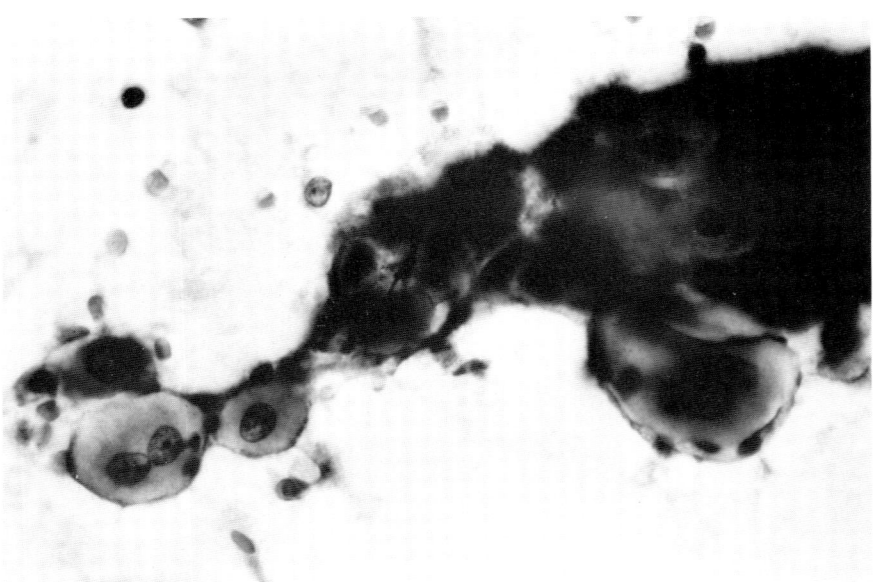

Fig. 6-9 A cluster of cohesive cells from a patient with papillary carcinoma demonstrating metaplastic cytoplasm. (Papanicolaou stain, × 40.) (See Plate 6-2.)

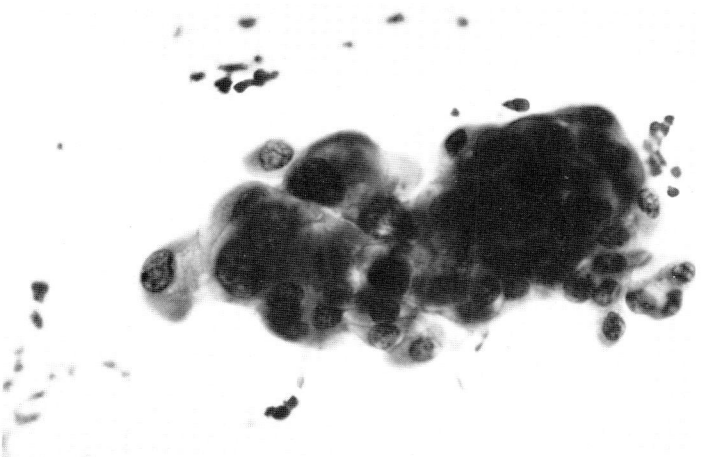

Fig. 6-10 A cohesive group of papillary carcinoma cells demonstrating cytoplasm similar to that of immature metaplastic cells of the cervix. (Papanicolaou stain, × 40.)

Additional features that have been described in papillary carcinomas include septate cytoplasmic vacuoles, epithelial giant cells (Figs. 6-10 and 6-12, Plate 6-3), and "sticky" colloid (Fig. 6-13, Plate 6-4). These features are either nonspecific or occur in a very low percentage of cases, and thus are not of great diagnostic value.[8]

MEDULLARY CARCINOMA

FNA of medullary carcinoma yields a cellular aspirate that demonstrates one of several patterns. The most common pattern is that of individual tumor cells and small cell groups. These individual cells have nuclei that vary in size and shape and have

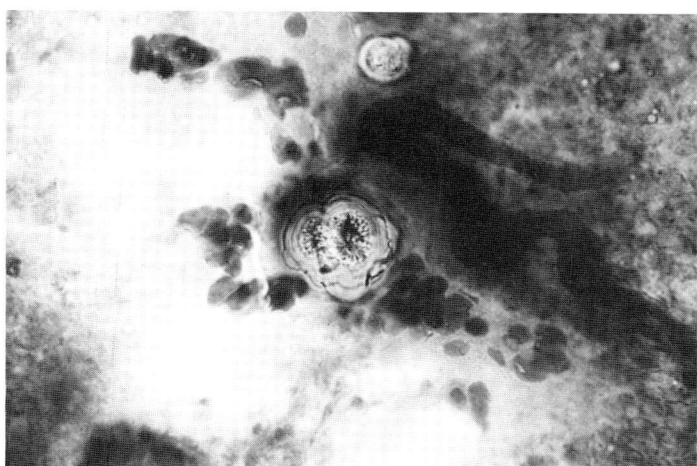

Fig. 6-11 An air-dried smear showing psammoma bodies with discrete laminations. (MGG stain, × 20.)

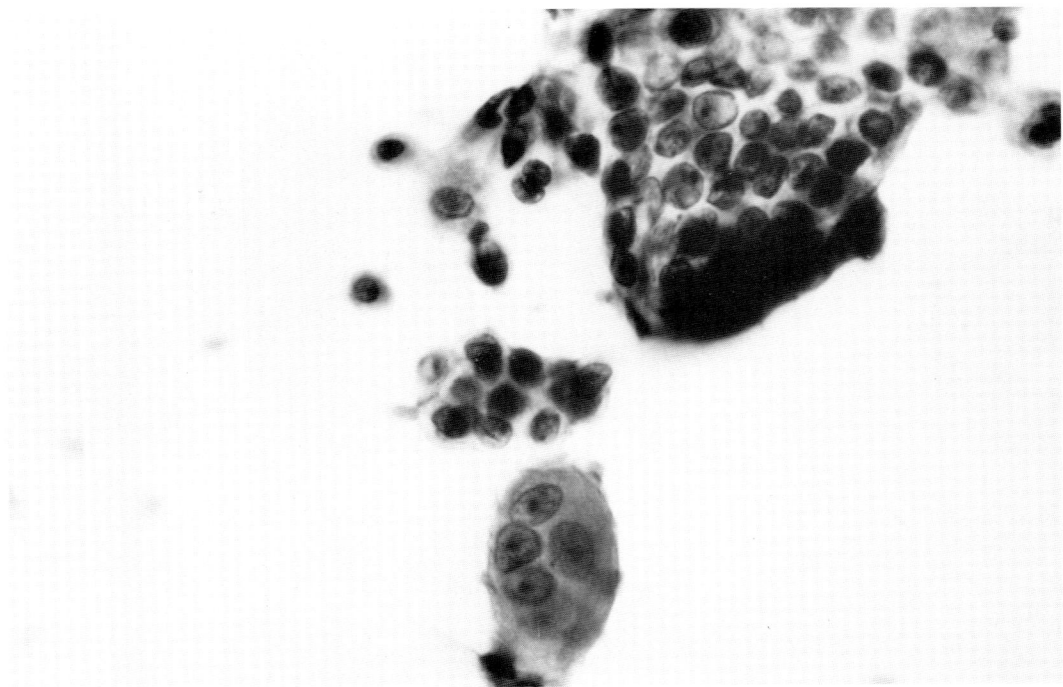

Fig. 6-12 Three features of papillary carcinoma are demonstrated. The upper portion of the figure shows a papillary structure without a demonstrable vessel. In the midportion (arrow), there are epithelial cells with well-defined cytoplasms, and in the lower portion of the field is an epithelial giant cell. (Papanicolaou stain, × 40.) (See Plate 6-3.)

coarse, granular, nuclear chromatin. A second pattern is that of dispersed, uniform, small, single cells that have a monotonous quality, with either a spindle or an epitheloid shape (Fig. 6-14). The cytoplasm in either case is blue-gray on Wright stain and cyanophilic on Papanicolaou stain. A third pattern demonstrates small, bland cells that are mixed with large, multinucleated, giant cells; the latter may exhibit red granulation (Fig. 6-15, Plate 6-5). These cells with red granulations have been noted in all three patterns; however, they are not diagnostic as they have been described in follicular adenomas, carcinomas, and large cell anaplastic tumors of the thyroid. Nucleoli, although not present in all cells, may be prominent.[9]

Occasionally, medullary carcinoma may be associated with nuclear inclusions and be misdiagnosed as papillary carcinoma. A second lesion that medullary carcinoma has been confused with is a Hürthle cell tumor. This misdiagnosis can occur when the medullary carcinoma is associated with abundant granular cytoplasm.

Immunoperoxidase stains for calcitonin may be performed directly on slides stained by the Papanicolaou technique.[10] Amyloid stains may be attempted, but the slides should first be destained.

ANAPLASTIC CARCINOMA

Large cell anaplastic carcinoma of the thyroid is difficult to diagnose by FNA biopsy, not because of a lack of high-grade malignant features within the tumor cells, but rather because of the difficulty in obtaining the cells. These lesions often have large areas of necrosis and inflammation with only a few viable tumor cells per unit area. From this, it is evident that aspiration from several areas is required to ensure that viable tumor material is sampled. The malignant cells, when present, are easily distinguishable, as they have large nuclei, prominent nucleoli, and mitotic figures.[6]

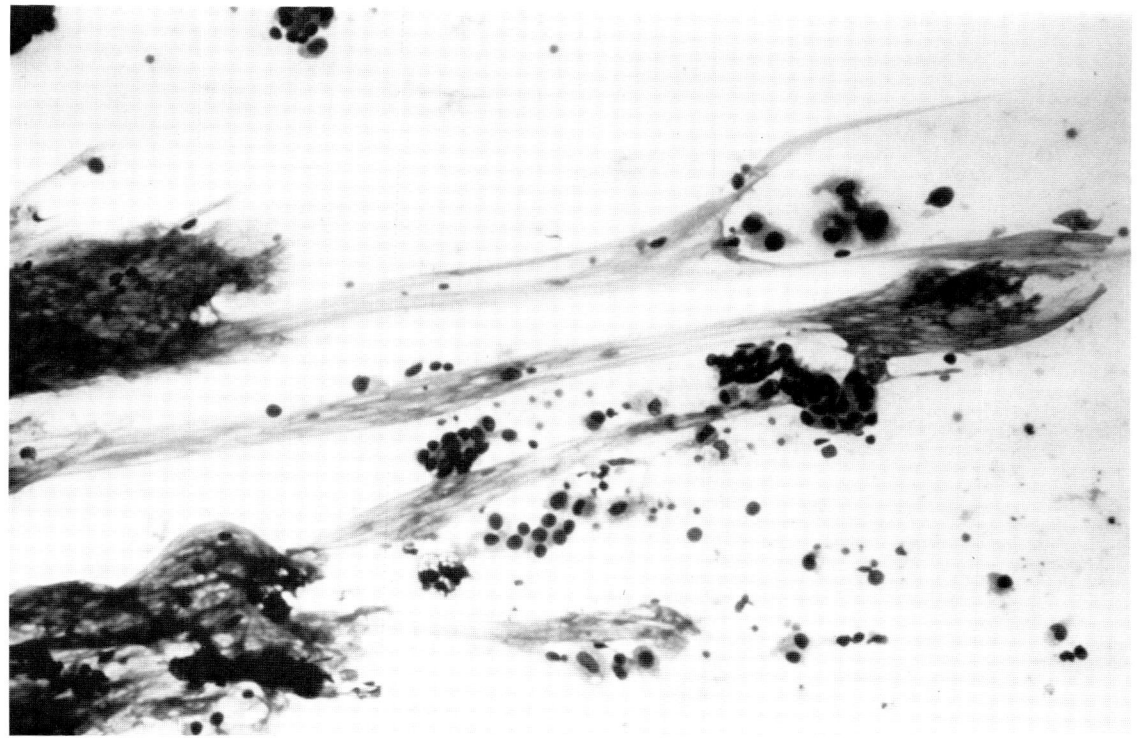

Fig. 6-13 This air-dried smear demonstrates the streaking and smearing effects of "bubble-gum" colloid. (MGG stain, × 10.) (See Plate 6-4.)

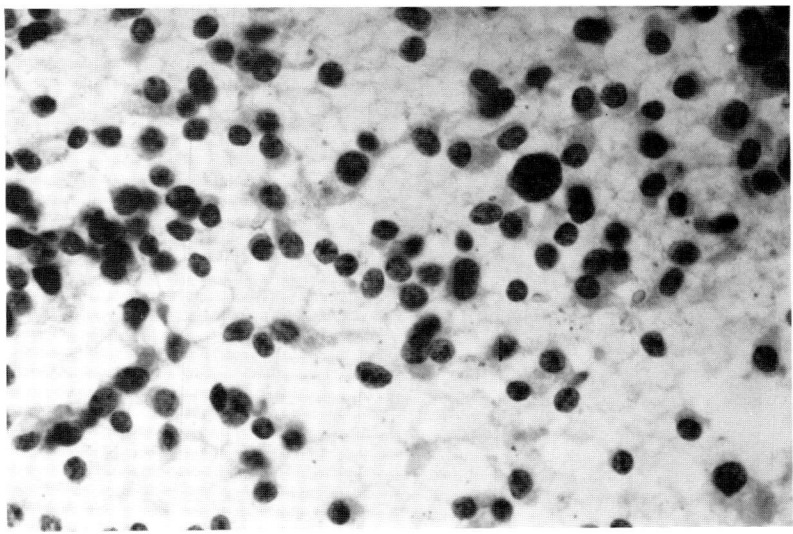

Fig. 6-14 An example of the dispersed cell pattern of medullary carcinoma. Note the presence of both spindle and round nuclei. (Papanicolaou stain, × 40.)

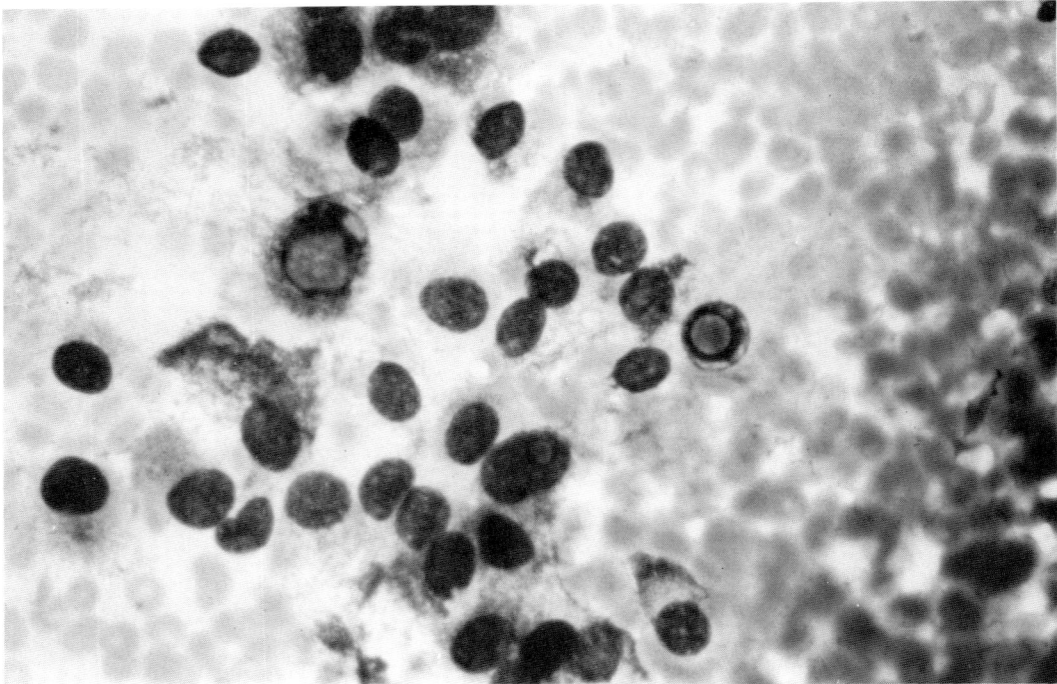

Fig. 6-15 This smear from a medullary carcinoma shows red cytoplasmic granulation as well as nuclear inclusions. (MGG stain, × 40.) (See Plate 6-5.)

Small cell anaplastic tumors are rare. These neoplasms resemble poorly differentiated lymphocytic lymphomas, both histologically and cytologically. Although the potential for finding a true, small cell, anaplastic carcinoma exists, it is uncommon and may be difficult to differentiate from lymphoma.[6] The absence of "blue blobs" (see the following section) in small cell carcinoma facilitates the differential diagnosis.

CHRONIC THYROIDITIS

Chronic thyroiditis is diagnosed without difficulty when its two histologic components—lymphoid cells and Hürthle cells—are evident on FNA biopsy. One feature of these smears is a heterogeneous population of dispersed lymphoid cells similar to those seen in reactive lymph nodes. Additional features of the aspirated lymphoid tissue may include the presence of "blue blobs" and so-called lymphoid stroma. Blue blobs are small, bluish structures, demonstrated on MGG stain, which are similar in size and shape to platelets, but which lack cytoplasm with purple granules. "Lymphoid stroma" consists of mechanically distorted clumps of fragile lymphoid elements. The second component that is characteristic of chronic thyroiditis is the follicular epithelium, which undergoes oxyphilic or Hürthle cell change. This change may be identified on cytologic examination by the presence of cohesive groups of cells with moderate to abundant granular cytoplasm (Figs. 6-16 to 6-18, Plates 6-6 to 6-8). The nucleus tends to be eccentric, and nucleoli may be present.[6]

There are several differential diagnoses to be considered before a definitive diagnosis of chronic thyroiditis is made on the basis of FNA biopsy. If only lymphoid elements are observed, two other possibilities have to be considered. One is that the sample was taken, not from the thyroid, but from a lymph node adjacent to it. A second possibility is that a small cell lymphoma was aspirated. When only the epithelial element is sampled, differential consideration must

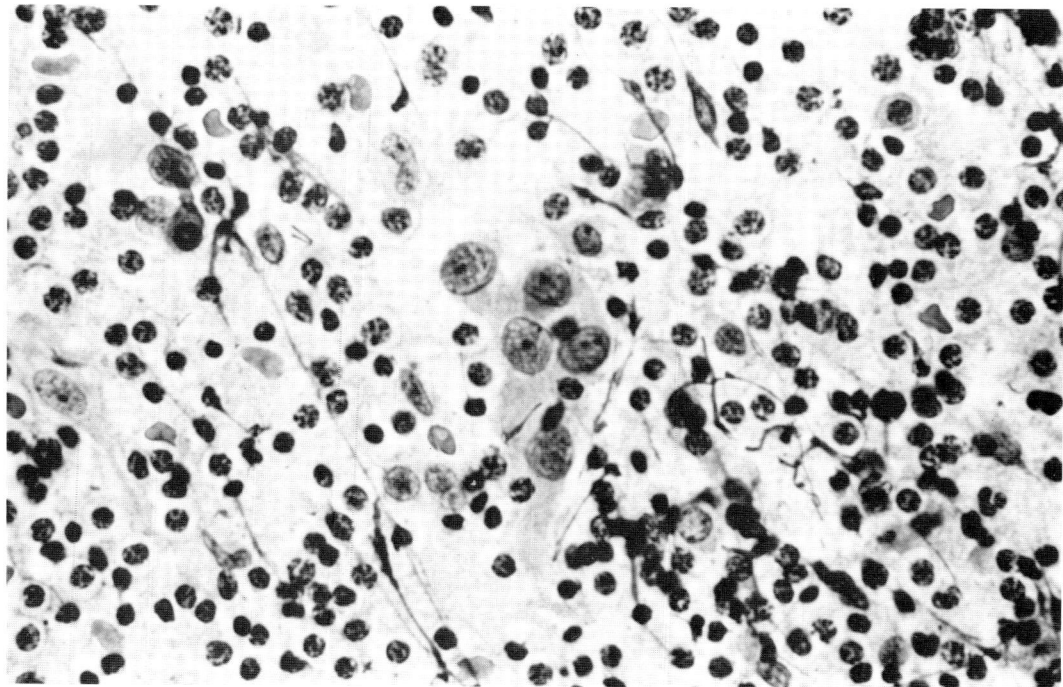

Fig. 6-16 In this example of chronic thyroiditis, a small group of Hürthle cells with abundant granular cytoplasm is seen. They are surrounded by small, mature lymphocytes. (Papanicolaou stain, × 20.) (See Plate 6-6.)

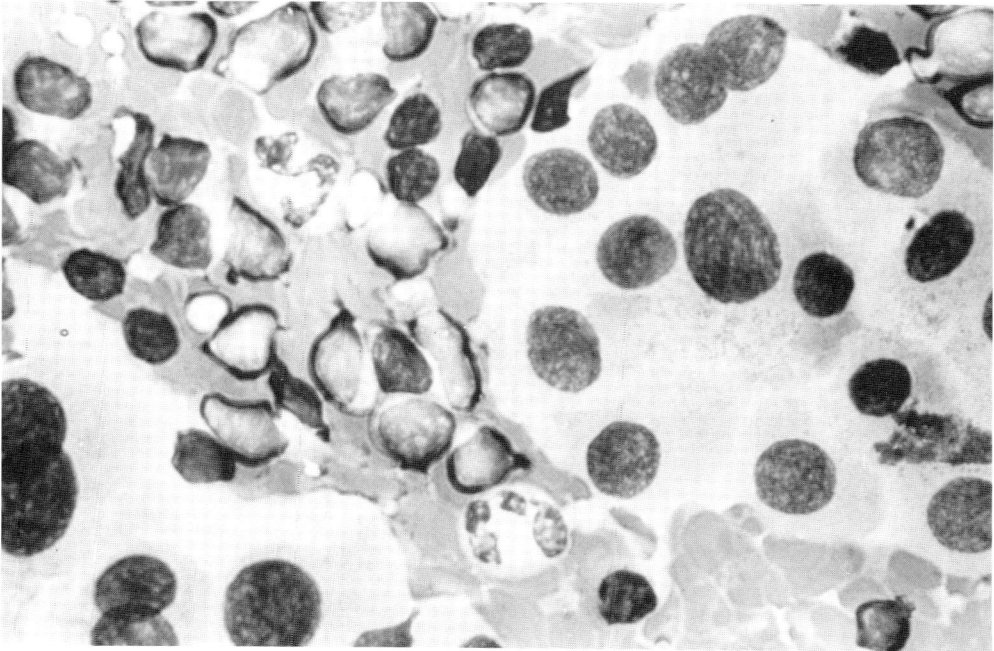

Fig. 6-17 This air-dried smear from a patient with chronic thyroiditis reveals Hürthle cells with abundant, slate-gray cytoplasm. The lymphoid elements are well demonstrated. (Wright-Giemsa stain, × 40.) (See Plate 6-7.)

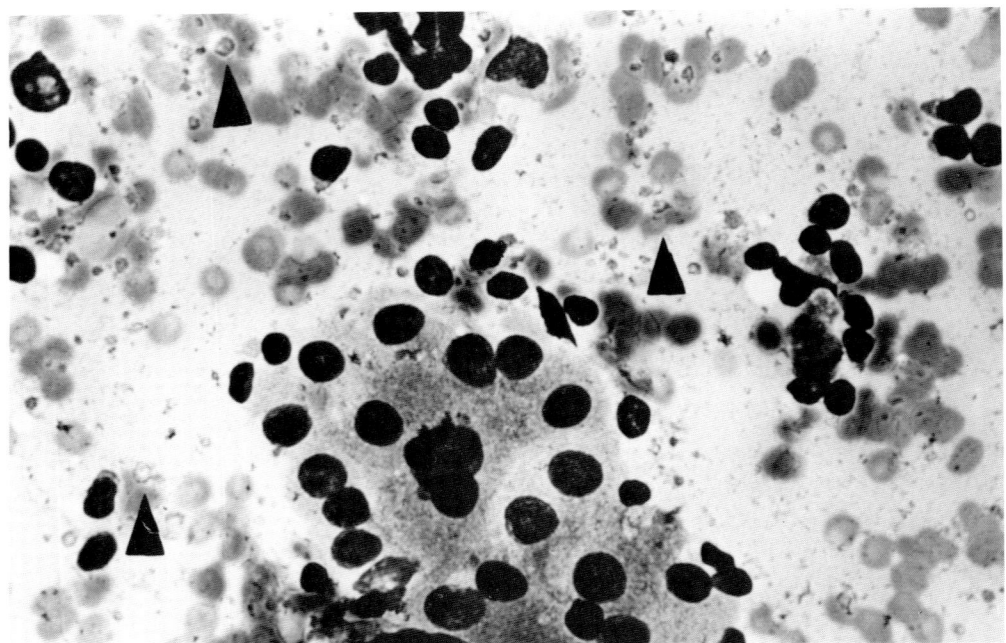

Fig. 6-18 In this example of chronic thyroiditis, air-dried smears reveal "blue blobs" (arrows), as well as Hürthle cells and lymphoid elements. (MGG stain, × 40.) (See Plate 6-8.)

be given to a Hürthle cell tumor or a Hürthle cell nodule in a multinodular thyroid. The cellular elements in the latter two entities are less cohesive when compared to those of chronic thyroiditis (also refer to the section on Hürthle Cell Tumors). Papillary carcinoma may also be a differential consideration. Both Hürthle cells and papillary carcinoma cells have moderate amounts of dense, well-defined cytoplasm. However, Hürthle cell nodules and tumors lack the major features seen in papillary carcinoma.[11]

SUBACUTE THYROIDITIS

Subacute thyroiditis has a characteristic clinical course and history that are useful in understanding its cytologic interpretation. During the early stage of this disease, a biopsy by FNA is quite painful and yields a small amount of material. This scanty specimen consists of a few follicular elements, monocytic cells, and lymphocytes. After a few weeks, when the disease is fully developed, giant cells appear in addition to the lymphocytes and macrophages. Epithelioid cells are usually not abundant; however, when present, they have a moderate amount of delicate cytoplasm, as well as nuclei that vary in shape from round to elongated. Follicular cells, when present, may demonstrate prominent paravacuolar granulation. An aspirate of a subacute thyroiditis that has run its course contains only a few mononucleated cells.[6]

HÜRTHLE CELL TUMORS

Most observers consider the Hürthle cell tumors to be a variety of follicular adenoma, but because of its striking cytologic features, it is considered as a separate entity in this chapter. Aspirate smears from patients with Hürthle cell tumors yield findings similar to those derived from histologic sections. That is, one can tell that the lesion is a Hürthle cell tumor; however, the malignant potential remains uncertain if only the cytologic pattern is considered. Hürthle cells dominate the smear pattern. The cells are an exaggeration of the oxyphilic cells seen in chronic thyroiditis. They have large amounts of dense, granular, well-defined cytoplasm (Fig. 6-19, Plate 6-9). Cytoplasm prepared with the Wright stain is blue-gray, whereas the Papanicolaou-stained cell has a cyanophilic to eosinophilic hue. One difference between Hürthle cell tumors and Hürthle cell nodules in chronic thyroiditis and multinodular thyroid is a loss of cell-to-cell cohesion. The cellular pattern for Hürthle cell tumors is one of single cells with occasional clusters and groups. In aspirates from patients with multinodular thyroid, there is a tendency toward increased cell-to-cell cohesion and aspiration of large tissue fragments. At the cellular level, Hürthle cells from patients with multinodular thyroid and chronic thyroiditis lack large nucleoli, and the general cell and nuclear size is smaller than that seen in neoplastic lesions. Another finding in multinodular thyroid is a spectrum of follicular cell cytology ranging from no Hürthle cell change to marked change.[12]

EPITHELIAL REPAIR

Epithelial repair may cause cytologic changes that can pose some diagnostic difficulties. Diagnostic problems arose early in my experience with so-called thyroid cyst, as sheets of cells containing alarming nuclear detail were evident. The nuclei were enlarged with conspicuous nucleoli. The benign character of the lesion was evident, however, by the orderly arrangement of the nucleus, the abundant cytoplasm, and the hypochromasia. The changes, when compared to the tissue, were those of epithelial repair, similar to those seen in the cervix. The remainder of the cytologic material had features resembling a benign thyroid nodule from a multinodular thyroid.

THYROGLOSSAL DUCT CYSTS

Thyroglossal duct cysts are midline structures that may occasionally be studied by FNA. Upon aspiration, these cysts yield a small amount of fluid which,

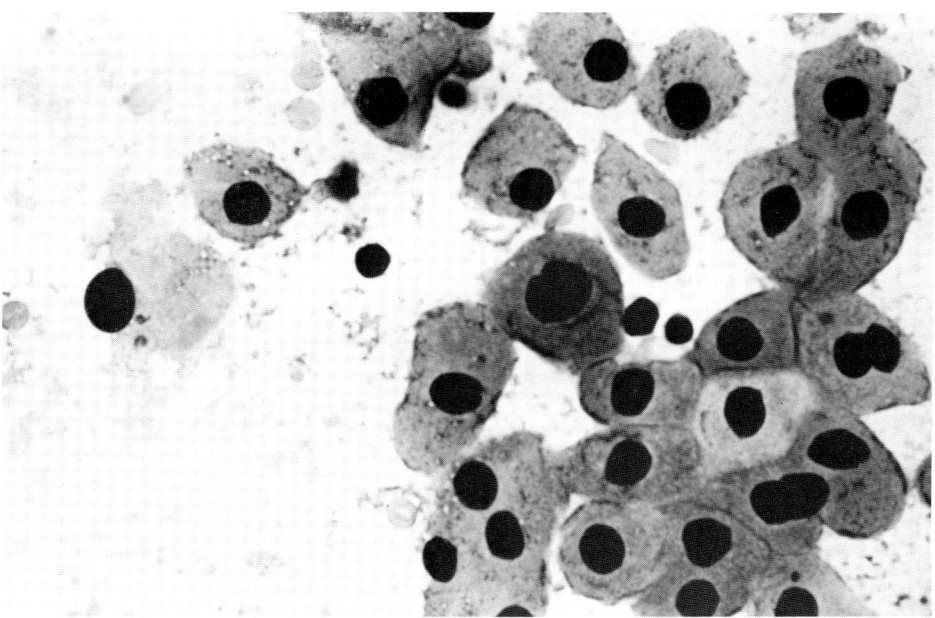

Fig. 6-19 Cells with abundant granular cytoplasm in a very discohesive pattern are seen in this example of a Hürthle cell tumor. In addition to a loss of cohesion, these cells also exhibit prominent nucleoli. (MGG stain, × 20.) (See Plate 6-9.)

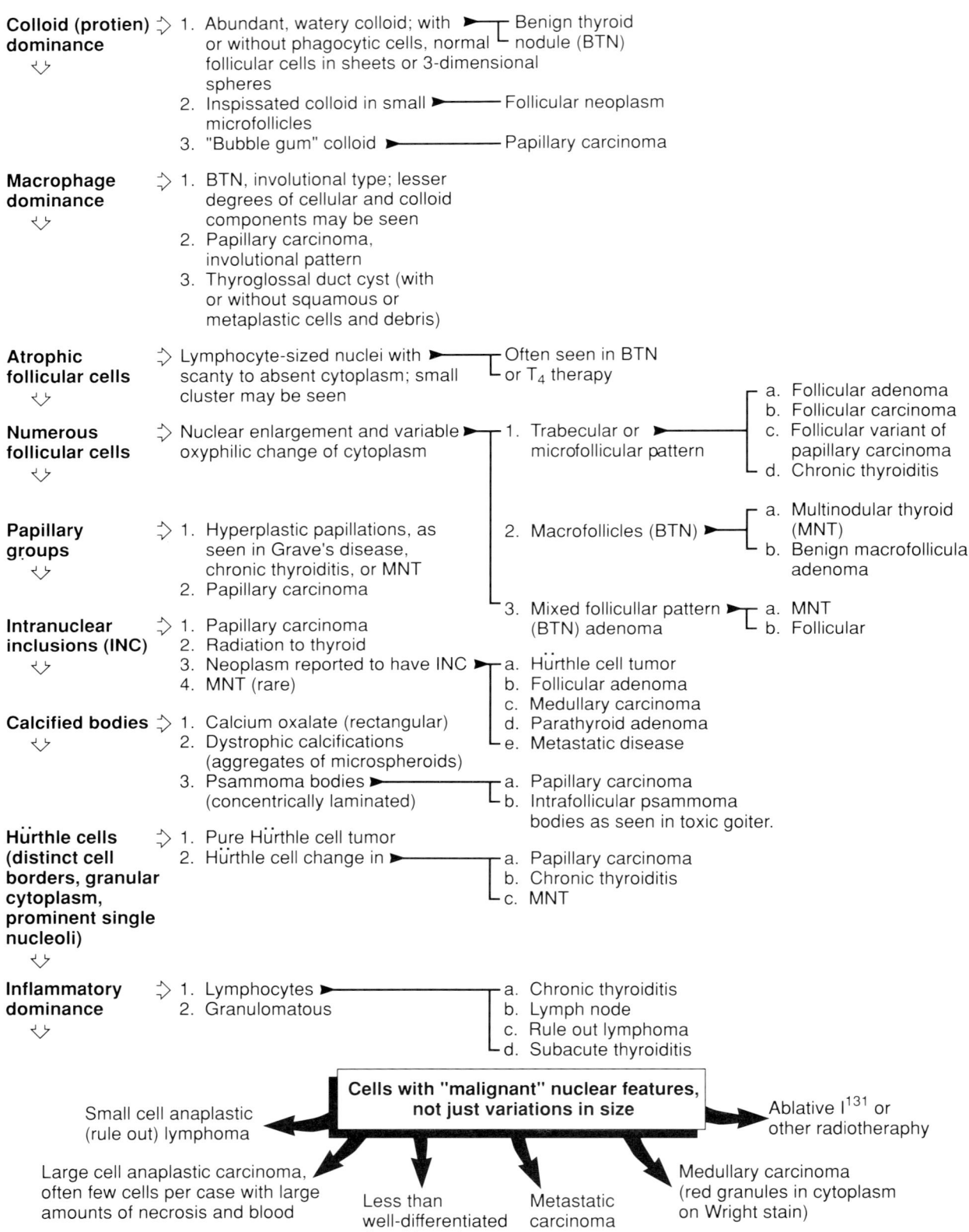

Fig. 6-20 Diagnostic flow chart for FNA of the thyroid. T_4 = thyroxin.

in many cases, is acellular or contains only inflammatory cells. When epithelial elements are present, they are represented mainly by squamous cells, both with and without nuclei. Although extremely rare, columnar epithelial cells may be seen. A diagnostic problem may arise with metastatic cystic squamous carcinoma. In studying this rare disease by FNA, one may obtain bland squamous elements without appreciating the malignant nature of the lesion. In cystic squamous carcinomas, a biopsy of the viable edge is indicated.[6]

Figure 6-20 indicates helpful diagnostic points and consideration, as well as points of overlap.

REFERENCES

1. Ashcraft M, Van Herle AJ: Management of thyroid nodules. II. Scanning techniques, thyroid suppressive therapy, and fine needle aspiration. Head Neck Surg 3:297, 1981
2. Hamburger B, Gharib H, Melton LJ, et al: Fine-needle aspiration biopsy of thyroid nodules. Impact on thyroid practice and cost of care. Am J Med 73:381, 1982
3. Abele JS, Miller TR: Fine needle aspiration of the thyroid nodule: Clinical applications. p. 2983. In Clark O (ed): Endocrine Surgery of the Thyroid and Parathyroid. CV Mosby, St. Louis, 1985
4. Hoffman WH: Diagnostic accuracy of fine needle aspiration biopsy in the diagnosis of thyroid malignancy. Pathologist 40:9, 1986
5. Van Herle AJ, Rich P, Ljung B-ME, et al: The thyroid nodule. Ann Intern Med 96:221, 1982
6. Zajicek J: Aspiration biopsy cytology. Part 1. Cytology of supradiaphragmatic organs. p. 67. In Wied GL, von Haam E, Koss LG, Reagan JW (eds): Monographs in Clinical Cytology. Vol. 4. S Karger AG, Basel, 1974
7. Gharib H, Goellner JR, Zinsmeister AR, et al: Fine-needle aspiration biopsy of the thyroid. The problem of suspicious cytologic findings. Ann Intern Med 101:25, 1984
8. Miller TR, Bottles K, Holly EA, et al: A step-wise logistic regression analysis of papillary carcinoma of the thyroid. Acta Cytol 30:285, 1986
9. Kini SR, Miller M, Hamburger JI, Smith MJ: Cytopathologic features of medullary carcinoma of the thyroid. Arch Pathol Lab Med 108:156, 1984
10. Geddie WR, Bedard YC, Strawbridge HTG: Medullary carcinoma of the thyroid in fine-needle aspiration biopsies. Am J Clin Pathol 82:552, 1984
11. Kini SR, Miller JM, Hamburger JI: Problems in the cytologic diagnosis of the "cold" thyroid nodule in patients with lymphocytic thyroiditis. Acta Cytol 23:506, 1981
12. Kini SR, Miller JM, Hamburger JI: Cytopathology of Hürthle cell lesions of the thyroid gland by fine needle aspiration. Acta Cytol 25:647, 1981

7
Cytology of the Gastrointestinal Tract

Kent Bottles
Para Chandrasoma

Salivary Glands
Kent Bottles

There is not complete agreement about the proper management of the patient with a palpable salivary gland mass. Although open surgical biopsy of salivary gland masses allows histologic characterization of the lesion, head and neck surgeons have not universally advocated this approach. Major problems with such an approach include incisional contamination with tumor, facial nerve damage, fistula formation, and technical problems necessitating subsequent radical neck dissection flaps as a result of the placement of the initial biopsy incision.[1-4] Some have advocated determining the type of surgical excision by gross inspection of the relationship of the mass to the facial nerve,[5] whereas others have advocated surgical exploration with frozen section diagnosis.[6] Consensus rates for intraoperative frozen section diagnosis compared with permanent section histology have been reported to be 89 to 93 percent for benign salivary gland lesions and 36 to 77 percent for malignant salivary gland lesions.[6-8] Obviously, none of these approaches is ideal.

Fine needle aspiration (FNA) biopsy can solve some but not all of the problems of preoperative evaluation of the patient with a salivary gland mass. The procedure is well tolerated by patients, safe, inexpensive, and suitable for outpatient clinical settings. Fears of implanting tumor cells along the needle tract and of decreasing survival rates by hematogenous spread of tumor cells are not valid based on the results of hundreds of thousands of procedures performed worldwide with 22-gauge or smaller needles.[9] Although FNA biopsy cannot classify salivary gland lesions as well as permanent histology, its accuracy rates compare favorably with those of frozen section diagnosis. In a recent salivary gland tumor study, FNA biopsy had an overall accuracy rate of 88 percent, and frozen section diagnosis had an overall accuracy rate of 71 percent.[2] In another salivary gland study, the false-negative rate for FNA biopsy was 4.7 percent, whereas the false-negative rate for frozen section was 11 percent.[4] FNA sensitivity rates for salivary gland tumors range from 56.5 to 87.5 percent; specificity rates range from 88 to 100 percent.[10]

Most salivary gland masses have a characteristic cytologic pattern, permitting a specific FNA diagnosis to be rendered. However, there are some salivary gland masses that are difficult, if not impossible, to classify by this procedure. Luckily, the easily classified lesions are much more common than the problematic cases. In a California outpatient clinic series of 308 consecutive salivary gland lesions, the breakdown of FNA biopsy diagnoses was as follows: benign salivary gland tissue, 27 percent; inflammation, 24 percent; pleomorphic adenoma, 19 percent; Warthin's tumor, 11 percent; lymphoid hyperplasia, 9 percent; suspicious, 5 percent; carcinoma, 3 percent; and lymphoma, 2 percent.[11] The problem cases are usually cellular pleomorphic adenomas with no stroma, mucoepidermoid carcinomas, some cystic lesions, some lymphoid lesions, and rare tumor types.[2–4,11,12] These cases should be signed out descriptively with a differential diagnosis, and frozen or permanent sections, or both, performed to arrive at a definitive diagnosis. The relatively small number of problem cases should not prevent the use of FNA in the preoperative evaluation of the majority of patients with easily classifiable lesions. For FNA biopsy to be successful in the diagnosis of salivary gland masses, close communication between the clinician and a pathologist who is experienced in performing, smearing, and interpreting the aspiration biopsies is required.

APPEARANCE OF NORMAL SALIVARY GLANDS ON FNA BIOPSY

Histologic sections reveal that salivary gland tissue is composed of multiple lobular acinar units that are suspended within a fatty matrix and joined by a network of ductular structures.[11] FNA smears contain each of these three components: acinar units, fat, and ducts. The acinar cells form tightly packed, ball-like structures with considerable nuclear overlap; this can be misinterpreted as architectural evidence of well-differentiated adenocarcinoma. However, the small size of the nuclei (1.5 times that of red cells), the uniform chromatin pattern, the single small nucleolus, and the characteristically small, ill-defined cytoplasmic vacuoles allow the cytopathologist to recognize them as benign acinar cells. Adipose tissue is often seen at the periphery of these lobular acinar units (Fig. 7-1), and ductular structures lined by small cuboidal nuclei are frequently seen emerging from the acinar units. Ductular cells are also sometimes seen as flat sheets of cells with a typical honeycomb appearance.[11]

BENIGN LESIONS

Lipomas

The needle moves within a lipoma with minimal resistance and the aspirate has a characteristic yellow gross appearance on the slide. Microscopic examination reveals normal adipose cells.[11,12]

Sialosis

Sialosis presents as painless nodules in the salivary gland, and the needle moves within the mass with some resistance, but not a gritty sensation. On gross examination, the aspirate consists of clear fluid and particles. Microscopic examination reveals acinar units, bare nuclei, and a blue granular background on May-Grünwald-Giemsa (MGG) stain. Inflammatory cells and ductular cells are not seen.[11]

Sialadenitis

Acute sialadenitis presents as a painful, hot swelling of the salivary gland. Puncture usually releases copious purulent material that should be drained as thoroughly as possible. Smears should be prepared, and material sent for microbacterial cultures. After drainage, any hard nodular areas should be reaspirated. Microscopic examination reveals neutrophils,

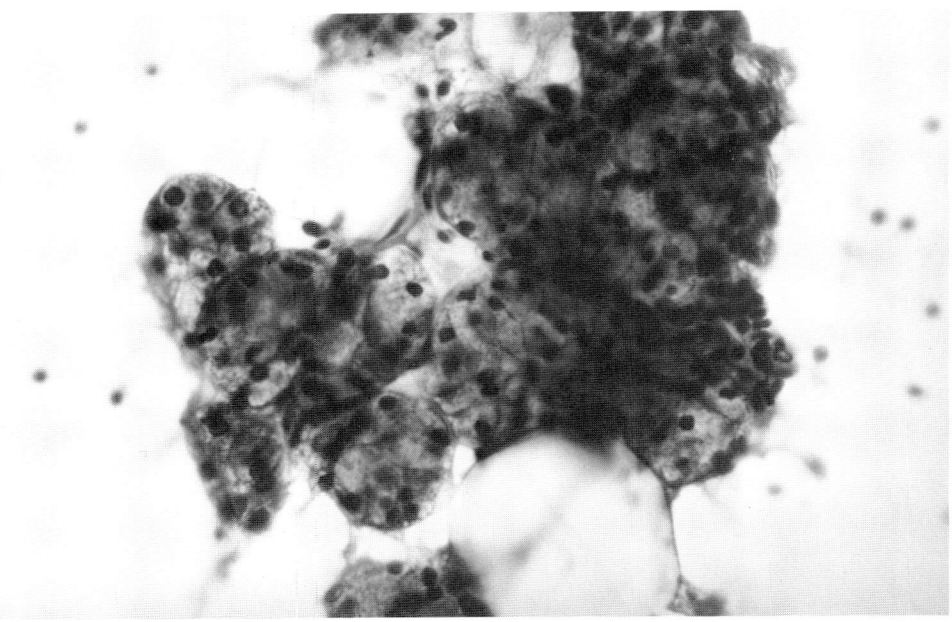

Fig. 7-1 Smear from a benign salivary gland nodule. The cluster of bland cells arranged in ball-like structures is surrounded by fat cells. (Papanicolaou stain, × 200.)

necrotic debris, and delicate interconnecting vessels that represent areas of granulation tissue. Aspirates from patients with chronic sialadenitis may yield normal salivary gland tissue, lymphocytes, plasma cells, or fibroblasts.[12]

Sarcoidosis

Sarcoidosis can involve the salivary glands. Aspirates from this lesion reveal discrete, well-formed granulomas composed of epithelioid histiocytes.[12]

Cysts

Non-neoplastic and neoplastic cysts occur in the salivary gland. Non-neoplastic cysts can yield abundant cyst fluid which may or may not contain epithelial and inflammatory cells. Cysts should be drained, and it is imperative that any residual mass be sampled by repeat FNA biopsy.[13] Cysts may occur with some frequency in some neoplasms, including mucoepidermoid carcinomas, pleomorphic adenoma, and Warthin's tumor.[2,3,11,12]

Lymphocyte-containing Entities

Lesions having abundant lymphocytes include benign lymphoepithelial lesions, Sjögren's syndrome, intraparotid lymphoid hyperplasia, and malignant non-Hodgkin's lymphomas.[14] The first three benign lesions are characterized by a polymorphic infiltrate consisting of lymphocytes, plasma cells, immunoblasts, and histiocytes. The non-Hodgkin's lymphomas are, for the most part, associated with a monomorphic infiltrate consisting of one type of malignant lymphoid cell. Although some non-Hodgkin's lymphomas can be diagnosed accurately by FNA, confirmatory surgical biopsy is usually suggested before definitive treatment is begun.[14]

TUMORS

Pleomorphic Adenoma

The key criteria for making the cytologic diagnosis of benign pleomorphic adenoma are stromal characteristics and the bland nature of the epithelial cells with eccentric nuclei.[11,12,14–16] The stroma appears intensely purple on MGG stain, and gray to pink on Papanicolaou-stained smears. The stroma is usually arranged in fern-like, fibrillar bundles, and bland epithelial cells are embedded within the stroma (Fig. 7-2, Plate 7-1). Reactive stroma can be seen with both neoplastic and inflammatory conditions, and is not diagnostic of pleomorphic adenoma. In contradistinction to the pleomorphic adenoma stroma, reactive stroma often contains inflammatory cells, fat, hyperplastic blood vessels, and necrotic debris. Pleomorphic adenoma stroma is "clean" stroma; reactive stroma is "dirty" stroma.

The bland epithelial cells that are characteristic of pleomorphic adenoma can be found in groups and as single cells. The nuclei are small, with a diameter about 1.5 times that of a red cell. The nuclear chromatin is evenly distributed, and a single small nucleolus can be identified. Single cells often have well-defined cytoplasm and eccentric nuclei (Fig. 7-3).[11,12,14–16]

Although the diagnosis of pleomorphic adenoma is usually straightforward, some of these tumors may present problems in attempting diagnosis by FNA. These problematic cases have included tumors without the typical biphasic pattern (smears with only stroma or smears with only epithelial cells), tumors with cystic changes, tumors with epithelial atypia, tumor cells with intracellular mucin, and tumors with squamous cells.[12] Often, careful search of all the smears, or reaspiration, will reveal typical stroma and epithelial cells that confirm the diagnosis of pleomorphic adenoma.

Monomorphic Adenoma

The cytologic criteria for benign monomorphic adenoma are bland epithelial cells arranged mostly in groups and a lack of abundant pleomorphic adenomatous stroma. The epithelial cells are similar to those seen in pleomorphic adenoma, but single cells are uncommon. The differential diagnosis of this lesion includes pleomorphic adenoma with prominent epithelial cell components and scant stroma. In some

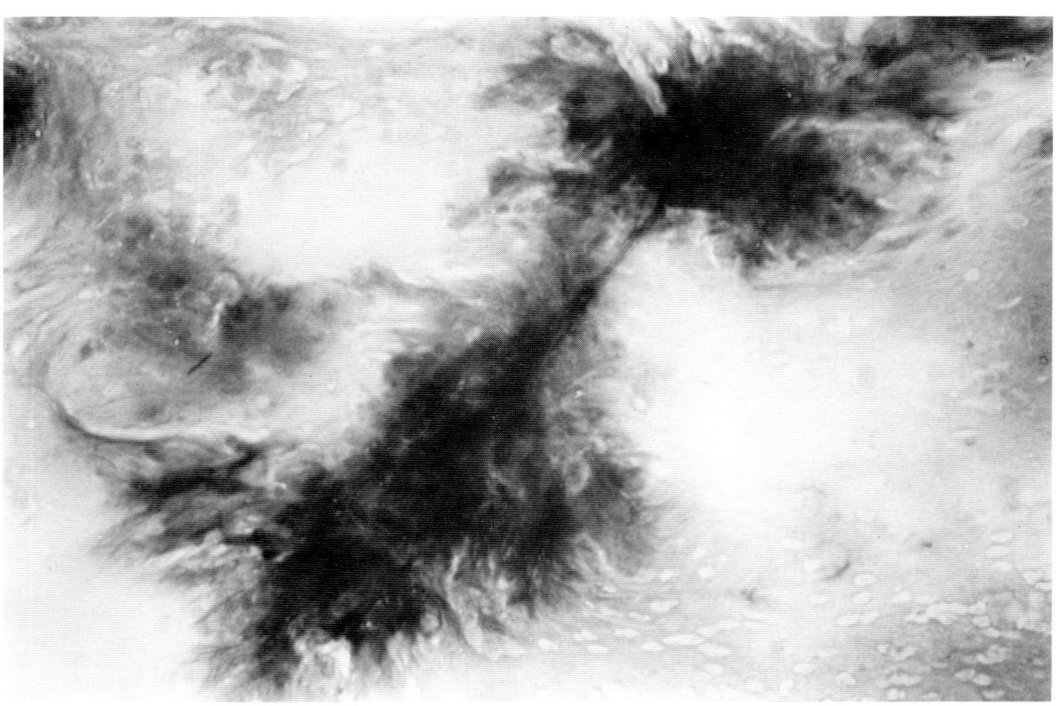

Fig. 7-2 Smear from a pleomorphic adenoma. The stroma of a pleomorphic adenoma stains intensely purple and has a fernlike arrangement. (MGG stain, × 200.) (See Plate 7-1.)

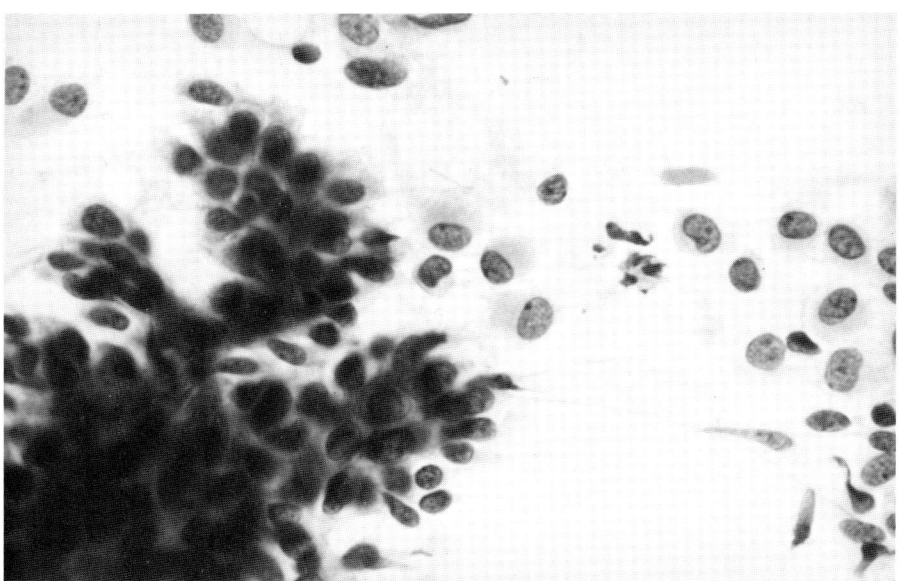

Fig. 7-3 Smear of a pleomorphic adenoma showing the characteristic bland epithelial cells with eccentric nuclei. (Papanicolaou stain, × 400.)

cases, it is difficult to distinguish between these two benign tumors by FNA biopsy.[11,12]

Warthin's Tumor

The three key cytologic criteria for this benign tumor are oncocytes, lymphocytes, and mast cells.[16,17] The oncocytes are typically arranged in flat sheets. The oncocytic nuclei can vary tremendously in size, but all have a single, centrally placed nucleolus and abundant granular cytoplasm (Fig. 7-4). Lymphocytes are easily identified in the background by their scant cytoplasm and fragility. The mast cells are seen best in the MGG stain, and appear as cells with red cytoplasmic granules. These mast cells are superimposed both on the sheets of oncocytes and in the background with the lymphocytes (Fig. 7-5, Plate 7-2).

Using these three criteria, one can easily identify most Warthin's tumors. Problems usually arise when cystic or mucoid material obscures the characteristic microscopic features.[12] Also, inexperienced cytopathologists sometimes may misinterpret the variable sizes and shapes of benign oncocytes as a feature of malignant disease.

Oncocytoma

Oncocytoma, an uncommon benign neoplasm, presents on FNA biopsy as clusters of overlapping oncocytes unassociated with lymphocytes, mast cells, or mucoid material (Fig. 7-6, Plate 7-3). The oncocytes with their single nucleolus and granular cytoplasm are similar to those seen in Warthin's tumor, but the architectural arrangement is more complex than the flat sheets seen in Warthin's tumor. Diagnostic problems can occur when oncocytic metaplastic cells predominate in a smear from a patient with sialadenitis, but oncocytomas, with their clean background and lack of significant inflammation, can usually be differentiated from such benign inflammatory conditions.[12,14–16]

Acinic Cell Carcinoma

The key cytologic features of acinic cell carcinoma are a cellular smear with cells that resemble normal salivary gland cells, a clean background, an absence of fat surrounding the clusters of epithelial cells, an absence of ductular structures, and occasional psammoma bodies[12,14–16,18] (Fig. 7-7). Although the indi-

256 PRACTICAL CYTOPATHOLOGY

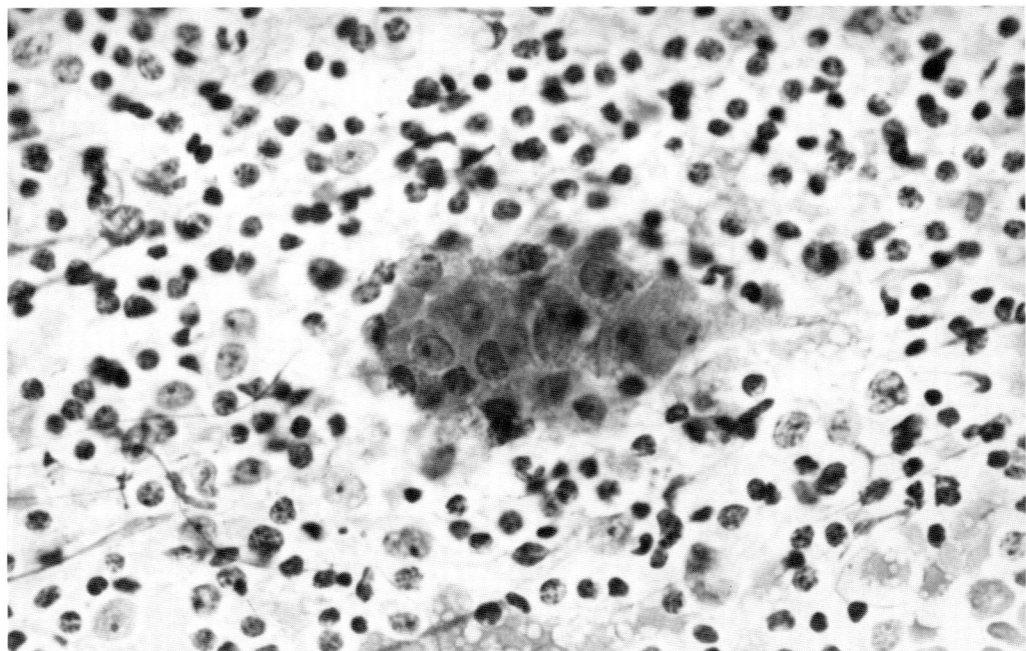

Fig. 7-4 Smear from a Warthin's tumor which shows a group of oncocytes with nucleoli and granular cytoplasm. The background is dominated by lymphocytes. (Papanicolaou stain, × 400.)

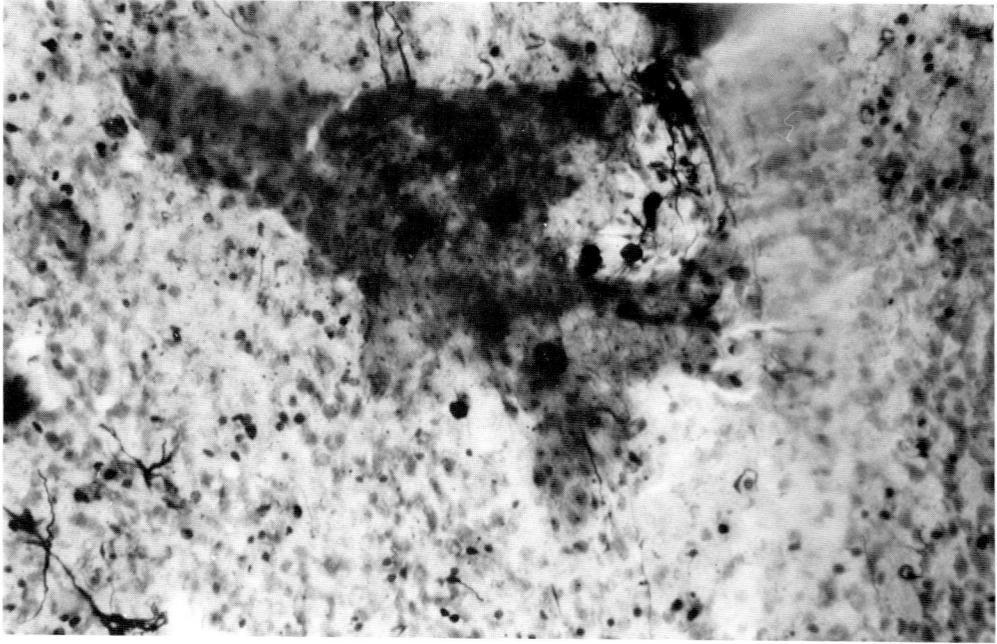

Fig. 7-5 Smear from a Warthin's tumor showing numerous mast cells with their characteristic red cytoplasmic granules. The mast cells are superimposed on a sheet of oncocytes. (MGG stain, × 300.) (See Plate 7-2.)

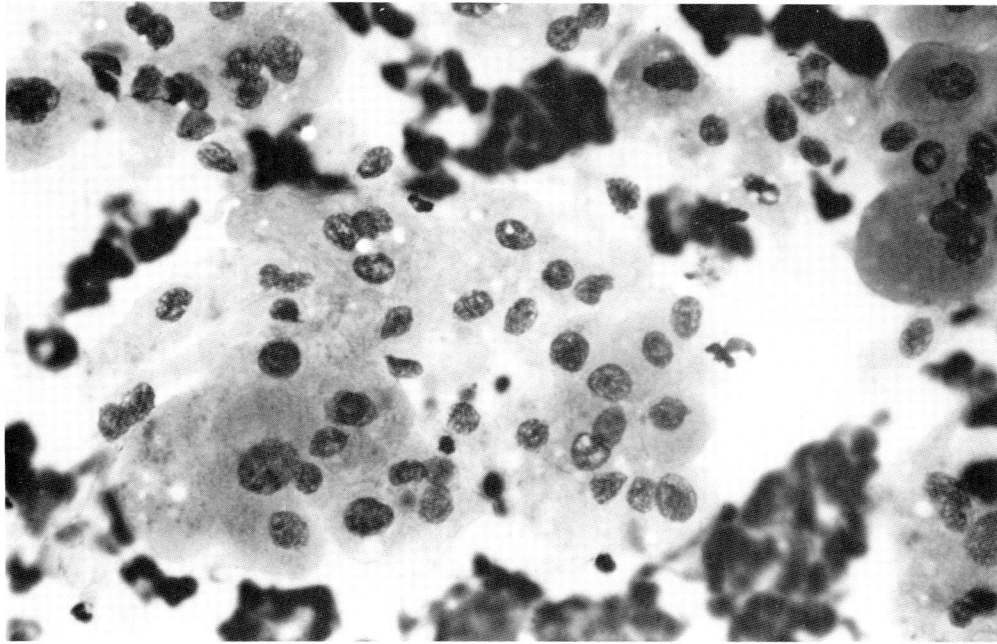

Fig. 7-6 Smear from an oncocytoma. The oncocytes show considerable variation in nuclear size, as well as an intensely granular cytoplasm. (MGG stain, × 400.) (See Plate 7-3.)

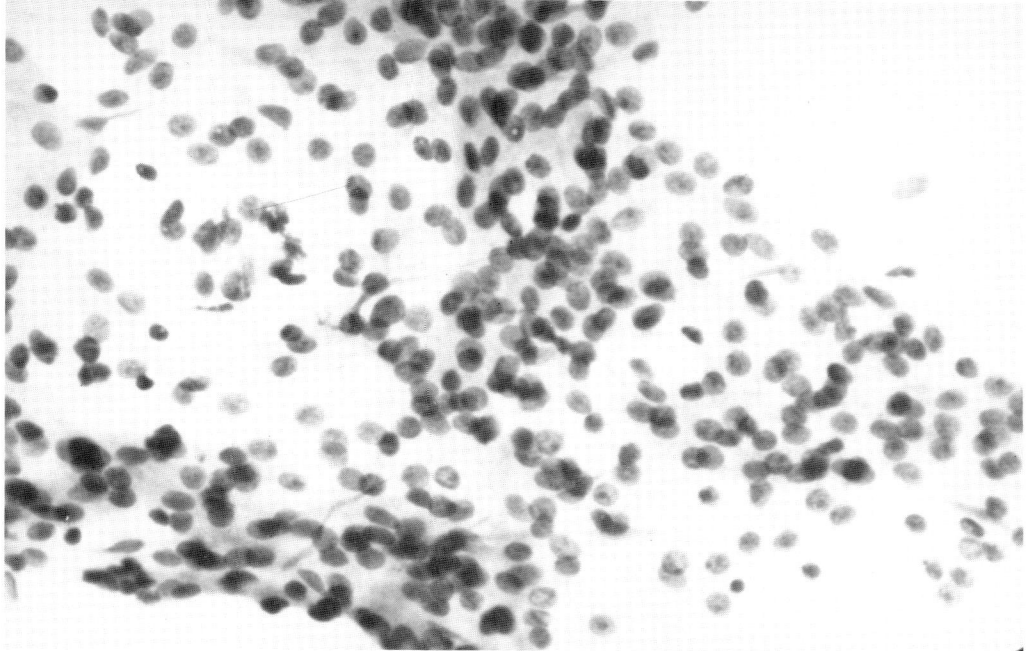

Fig. 7-7 Smear from an acinic cell carcinoma. The cells resemble normal salivary gland cells, but the architectural arrangement and lack of fat and ducts around the periphery of the clusters are important clues to the correct diagnosis. (Papanicolaou stain, × 300.)

vidual cells in acinic cell carcinoma smears resemble normal salivary gland cells, their architectural arrangement belies their innocent appearance. These bland cells are arranged in cohesive clusters, not in the well-developed, lobular, acinar structures with associated fat or ducts of a benign lesion. Psammoma bodies are a rare but useful feature of FNA biopsies of acinic cell carcinomas.[18]

Some cases of acinic cell carcinoma can be confused with normal salivary gland, oncocytomas, Warthin's tumor, and mucoepidermoid carcinomas. Differentiation between acinic cell carcinoma smears and normal smears is based on the different architectural arrangements described earlier. Tumors containing oncocytes (oncocytomas and Warthin's tumors) can usually be distinguished from acinic cell carcinomas by careful examination of the cytoplasm by both MGG and Papanicolaou stains. Acinic cell cytoplasm is finely vacuolated, whereas oncocyte cytoplasm is intensely granular. Although more poorly differentiated, acinic cell carcinomas can also be confused with mucoepidermoid carcinoma. The absence of intracytoplasmic mucin in acinic cell carcinoma can facilitate differentiation between these two tumors.[12]

Adenoid Cystic Carcinoma

The two most well known cytologic features of adenoid cystic carcinoma are rigidly spherical stromal balls and bland, uniform nuclei.[11,12,14–16] These stromal balls stain intensely red on MGG stain (Fig. 7-8, Plate 7-4). On Papanicolaou-stained material, round collections of the bland nuclei can be appreciated (Fig. 7-9). The nuclei are small (less than 1.5 times the diameter of a red cell) and have a bland chromatin pattern.

When numerous, rigidly spherical stromal balls are present, the diagnosis is straightforward. When a few apparent stromal balls and the fern-like stroma that is characteristic of pleomorphic adenoma are seen on the same slide, the correct diagnosis is probably pleo-

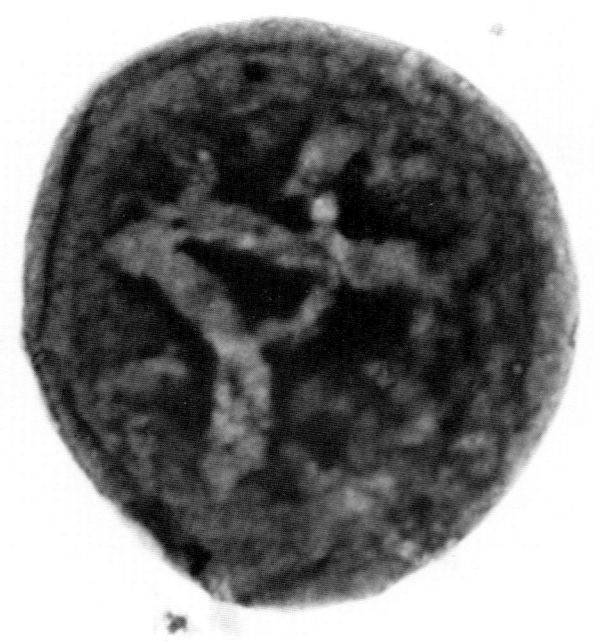

Fig. 7-8 Smear of a rigidly spherical stromal ball that is characteristic of adenoid cystic carcinoma. (MGG stain, × 400.) (See Plate 7-4.)

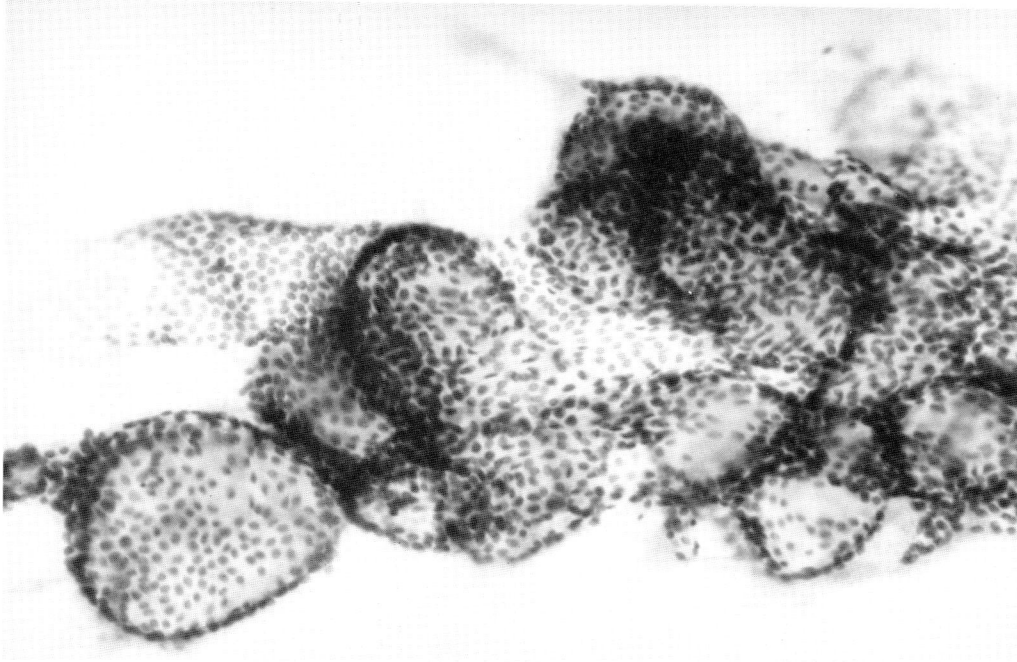

Fig. 7-9 Smear of an adenoid cystic carcinoma with characteristic bland nuclei. (Papanicolaou stain, × 200.)

morphic adenoma. Poorly differentiated adenoid cystic cancers do not always have numerous stromal balls; in such cases, it is easy to arrive at a diagnosis of malignant disease, but difficult to subclassify the tumor correctly.[12]

Mucoepidermoid Cancer

Key criteria for the diagnosis of mucoepidermoid carcinoma by FNA biopsy include malignant squamous cells, intermediate cells, clusters with overlapping epithelial cell nuclei, cells with intracytoplasmic mucin, extracellular mucin, and necrotic debris (Figs. 7-10 and 7-11, Plate 7-5).[11,12,14,16] When malignant squamous cells and cells with intracytoplasmic mucin are both abundant, the cytologic diagnosis can be made easily. Unfortunately, many tumors do not present with such clear-cut microscopic findings.

Some mucoepidermoid carcinomas pose as great a diagnostic challenge as the cytopathologist will face in all of aspiration cytology. Well-differentiated lesions can look deceptively bland, and one must correctly identify the squamous, intermediate, and adenocarcinomatous components. Poorly differentiated mucoepidermoid lesions are easily identified as malignant, but are difficult to subclassify as mucoepidermoid cancers.[19] Benign cysts can present with extracellular mucin, necrotic debris, and reparative benign epithelial cells that mimic the malignant epithelial cells of mucoepidermoid cancer.[12] The fact that mucoepidermoid cancers often undergo cystic change makes differentiating between atypical benign cysts and cystic mucoepidermoid cancer even more difficult.

Adenocarcinoma

The key cytologic features of adenocarcinoma are hyperchromatic nuclei with large nucleoli, intracellular mucin, and three-dimensional tumor glands.[14] Obviously, one must search carefully to exclude the presence of squamous cells and intermediate cells which would point to a mucoepidermoid carcinoma rather than a primary adenocarcinoma.

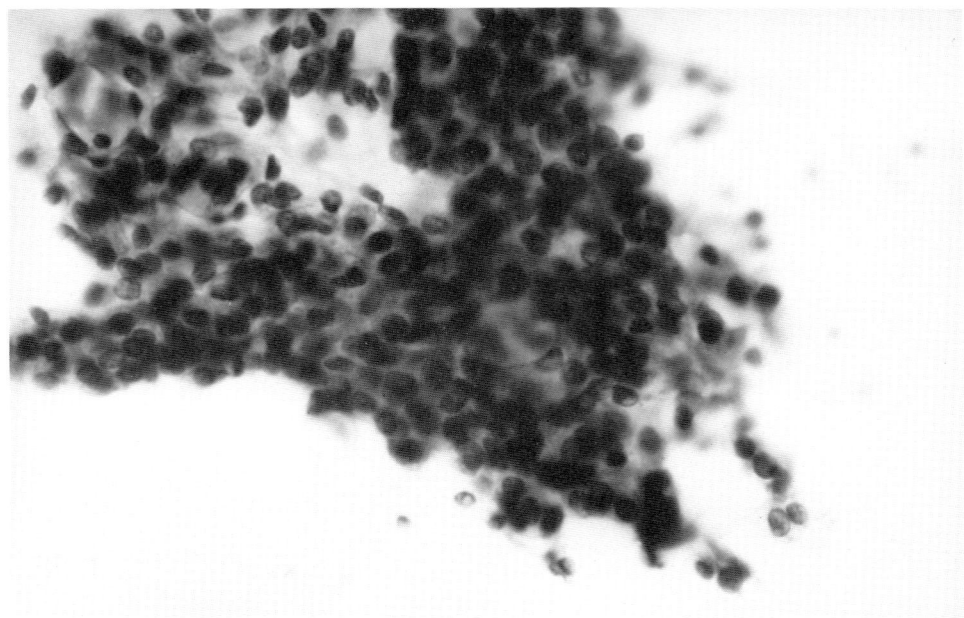

Fig. 7-10 Smear exhibiting the nuclear overlap that is characteristic of a mucoepidermoid carcinoma. (Papanicolaou stain, × 200.)

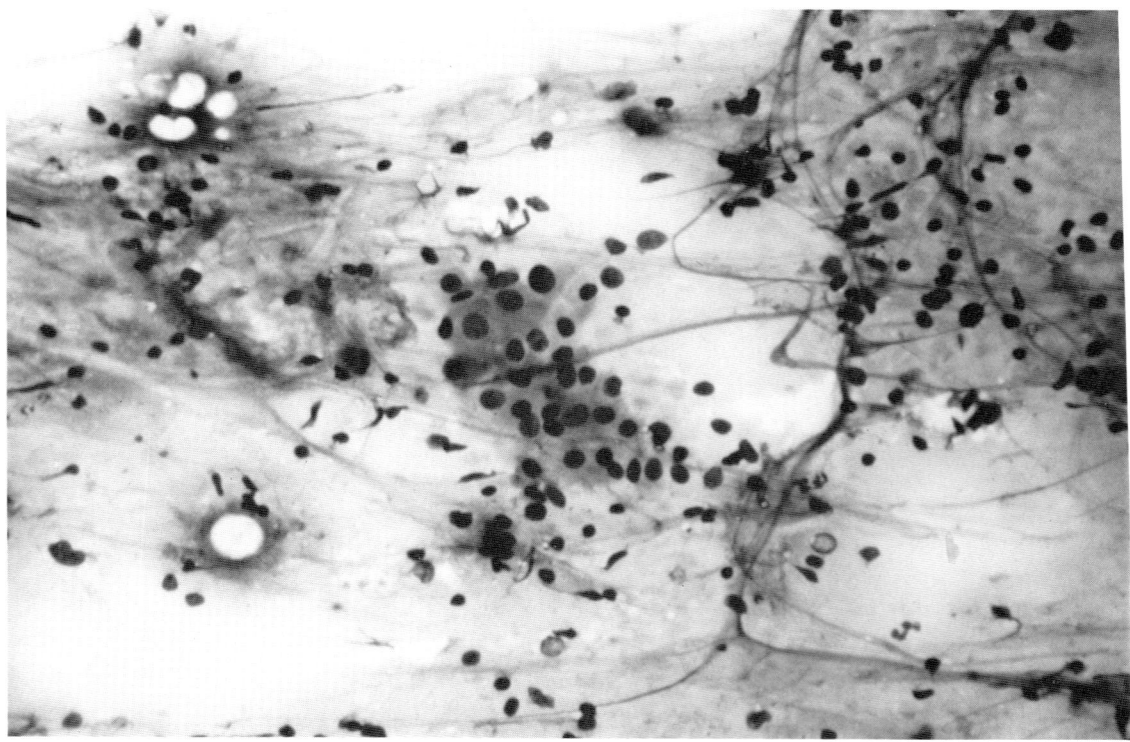

Fig. 7-11 Smear from a patient with mucoepidermoid carcinoma. Note the extracellular mucin. (MGG stain, × 300.) (See Plate 7-5.)

SUMMARY

FNA biopsy can diagnose many, but not all, salivary gland masses preoperatively. For it to be successful, the cytopathologist must recognize the relatively few problematic cases for which a description of the findings with a differential diagnosis is more appropriate than a definitive diagnosis. Close communication between the clinician and the cytopathologist is essential so that a patient's nodule can be assigned to either the large group of lesions that can be diagnosed definitively or to the smaller group of lesions requiring further diagnostic work-up.

Esophagus, Stomach, Duodenum, and Colon
Para Chandrasoma

The greatly increased availability of fiberoptic endoscopy has made much of the gastrointestinal tract accessible to direct visualization and specimen collection. Upper gastrointestinal endoscopy permits sampling of the esophagus, stomach, and duodenum. The second part of the duodenum, which contains the ampulla of Vater, is easily accessible, and via this the bile duct and pancreatic duct can be cannulated for specimen collection. Colonoscopy permits examination of the entire colon and, in some cases, the terminal ileum. The remainder of the small intestine from the duodenojejunal junction to the terminal ileum is not accessible to endoscopy, and it is a fortunate coincidence that epithelial neoplasms are rare in this part of the gastrointestinal tract.

ESOPHAGUS

Normal Cytology

The esophagus is lined by nonkeratinizing, stratified, squamous epithelium up to the gastroesophageal junction, where there is a transition to cardiac-type gastric mucosa. The submucosa of the esophagus contains numerous mucous glands resembling those in the gastric cardia. All methods of specimen collection involve approaching the esophagus from the lumen, and a normal esophageal specimen is composed predominantly of superficial squamous epithelial cells. A few intermediate cells may be present, but basal cells and glandular cells are not usually seen.

Specimen Collection

By far the most common method of obtaining cytologic specimens from the esophagus is by direct brushing of the surface of a lesion visualized at endoscopy.[20] The brush is retrieved from the endoscope and smeared, with force, on slides that are fixed in 95-percent ethanol. After making two to four slides in this manner, the brush is washed in saline where the specimen is processed through a millipore filter. Because of its greater accuracy, direct brush cytology has replaced the blind saline lavage technique of obtaining specimens from the esophagus.[21]

In China, where the incidence of carcinoma is high, mass screening utilizing a balloon catheter has proved successful.[22] After the catheter is swallowed, a balloon at the tip is inflated and the catheter is pulled up. The entire mucosa of the esophagus is scraped. The surface of the balloon is smeared on a slide, fixed with 95-percent ethanol, and stained. The advantage of balloon catheter cytology is that it permits detection of dysplasia and carcinoma in situ (CIS) at a time when a lesion may not be visible on endoscopy. Its use in countries where the incidence of esophageal carcinoma is too low to justify mass population screening is limited.[23]

Cytology of Non-Neoplastic Lesions

INFECTIONS

Infections are uncommon except in immunocompromised patients, particularly those with acquired immune deficiency syndrome (AIDS). In this population, *Candida albicans* esophagitis is common, and is used as a criterion for the diagnosis of AIDS. *Candida albicans* is a normal commensal in the pharynx, and may be seen in small numbers in gastroesophageal specimens. The diagnosis of Candida esophagitis should be made only when the specimen has been obtained from a lesion that was clinically consistent with that diagnosis, and when there are more than a few organisms on the smear. *Candida albicans* appears in smears as characteristic budding yeasts and pseudohyphae which may be associated with numerous, anucleate squames and inflammatory cells. The finding of yeasts growing within anucleate squames is highly suggestive of Candida infection.

Viral esophagitis is uncommon. Rarely, the esophagus is affected in patients with chickenpox. Herpes simplex esophagitis may occur in immunocompromised patients. Brush cytology specimens from ulcerated herpetic lesions show squamous epithelial cells exhibiting multinucleation, ground glass nuclei, and eosinophilic intranuclear inclusion bodies surrounded by a halo.[24] Although the cells appear to be atypical, their features are so distinctive that there is little risk of false-positive diagnosis of malignant disease. Cytomegalovirus esophagitis occurs mainly in patients with AIDS. Unlike Herpes simplex and Herpes varicella-zoster, which infect squamous epithelial cells, cytomegalovirus infects submucosal endothelial cells. As a result, it is rare to find cytomegalovirus-infected cells in cytologic specimens, and biopsy is much more sensitive as a method of diagnosis. In ulcerated lesions, one may rarely find infected cells scattered among numerous inflammatory cells. Cytomegalovirus-infected cells are greatly enlarged, have a very large eosinophilic intranuclear inclusion surrounded by a halo, and have granular basophilic cytoplasmic inclusions.

REFLUX ESOPHAGITIS

Reflux esophagitis is an extremely common lesion. The early stages are associated with a reactive hyperplasia of the basal layers of the epithelium. Brush specimens from such an early lesion may show increased numbers of parabasal cells. In the later stages of reflux esophagitis, ulceration and inflammation are dominant. In these cases, brush cytology shows numerous squamous epithelial cells in a background of necrotic debris and inflammatory cells. The squamous epithelial cells show regenerative (repair) changes with large nuclei and prominent nucleoli that have a superficial resemblance to squamous carcinoma (Fig. 7-12). The regenerative cells show excellent cell-to-cell cohesiveness with very few single cells, and have a finely distributed, very uniform, chromatin distribution, features that permit differentiation from malignant cells.

BARRETT'S ESOPHAGUS

Barrett's esophagus refers to the occurrence of gastric metaplasia of the esophagus. The cause is uncertain, although current evidence suggests that it is related to acid reflux.[25] Islands of Barrett's esophagus are most common in the lower one third of the esophagus, but may be found in the upper two thirds as well. Barrett's esophagus, which is being recognized increasingly at endoscopy, is characterized by an island of reddened, slightly elevated mucosa that contrasts with the white squamous epithelium. On histologic examination, Barrett's mucosa is characterized by three types of glandular epithelium. The most distinctive is the specialized columnar epithelium that has a villous surface and contains intestinal-type epithelium with goblet cells. The second type resembles gastric cardia, whereas the third type resembles gastric fundus. It is not uncommon to find

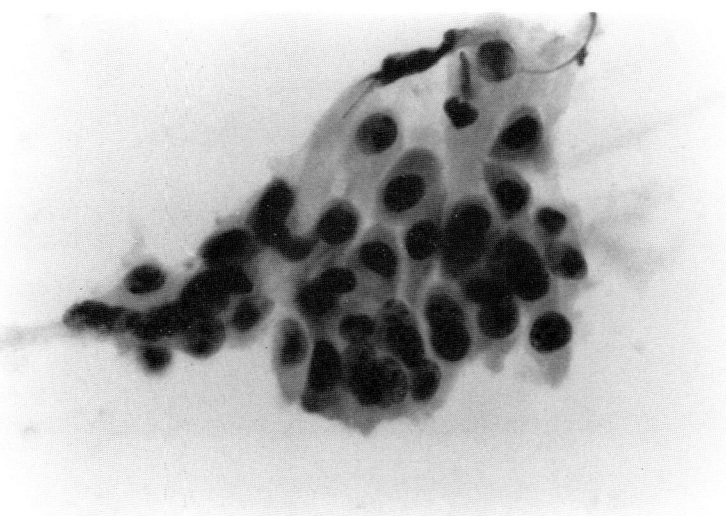

Fig. 7-12 Esophageal brush cytology. Repair showing a flat, cohesive group of squamous epithelial cells with enlarged nuclei. The nuclei are round and show hyperchromasia and moderate pleomorphism. (Papanicolaou stain, × 158.)

all three types of epithelium in one case. Cytologic specimens from patients with Barrett's esophagus exhibit groups of columnar epithelial cells (Fig. 7-13). The specialized epithelium is characterized by goblet cells with basal nuclei, as well as cytoplasm that is distended with mucus and that shows a brush border. The gastric-type epithelia have basal nuclei with uniformly distributed apical mucin. Barrett's esophagus is a premalignant lesion that progresses through increasing degrees of dysplasia to adenocarcinoma (see the later section on adenocarcinoma).

PEMPHIGUS VULGARIS

Pemphigus vulgaris rarely involves the esophagus,[26] and usually affects patients who have coexistent cutaneous and oral lesions. Very rarely, the esophagus represents the first site involved. Pemphigus vulgaris is characterized by acantholysis involving the suprabasal cells of the squamous epithelium as a result of immunologic destruction of the intercellular attachments. The acantholysis results in vesicle formation and ulceration. Smears from lesions of pemphigus vulgaris show large numbers of basal and parabasal cells that are extremely discohesive and that appear as small groups and single cells. These cells have a high nucleocytoplasmic ratio and large nuclei with very prominent nucleoli that have a characteristic oval shape. The chromatin distribution is very uniform and delicate. The cytologic features resemble those of repair, but are more likely to be mistaken for carcinoma because of the discohesive nature of the cells.

RADIATION CHANGE

Radiation-induced changes may involve the esophagus in patients undergoing irradiation for pulmonary and mediastinal disease. Radiation changes in the squamous epithelium include enlargement of the cells, which have abundant, vacuolated cytoplasm. The nuclei are pale and smudgy with irregular clumping.

Cytology of Neoplastic Lesions

SQUAMOUS CARCINOMA

Squamous carcinoma of the esophagus is uncommon; it is responsible for about 6 percent of cancers occurring in the United States. It is a disease that usually affects those older than 50 years of age and that is more prevalent in men than in women. There

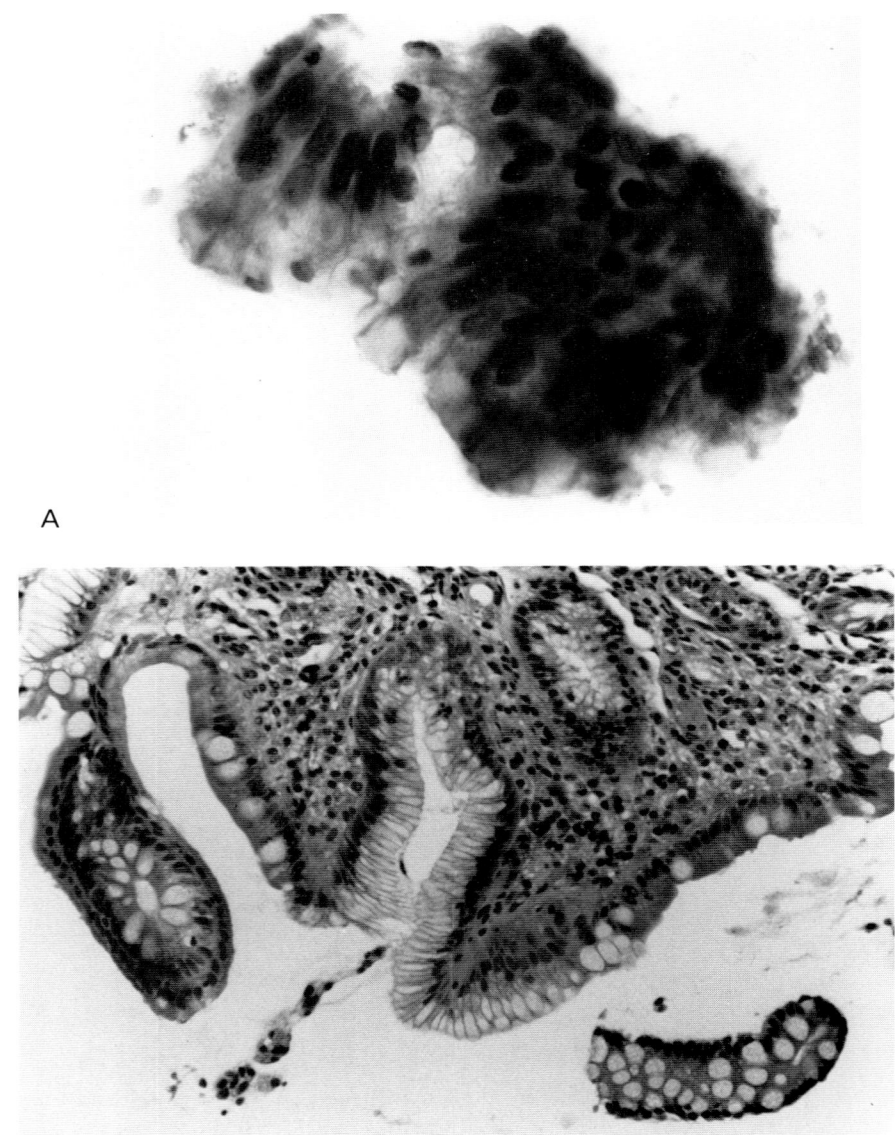

Fig. 7-13 (A) Esophageal brush cytology. Barrett's esophagus showing a group of columnar epithelial cells. Note the columnar cells with basal nuclei and apical, mucin-filled cytoplasm. This represents gastric-type epithelium; no goblet cells are present. (Papanicolaou stain, × 158.) **(B)** Esophageal biopsy showing Barrett's esophagus with specialized epithelium composed of a mixture of gastric and intestinal epithelial cells.

is a high incidence of carcinoma of the esophagus in the Honan Province of China. Known premalignant lesions that predispose one to the development of squamous carcinoma are lye ingestion and Plummer-Vinson syndrome. The latter predisposes one to carcinoma of the upper third of the esophagus.

It is very likely that squamous carcinoma of the esophagus is preceded by increasing dysplasia.[27] Because dysplasia is asymptomatic, the incidence and relationship of dysplasia to carcinoma cannot be evaluated without mass screening of the normal population. Limited data from China, where such studies

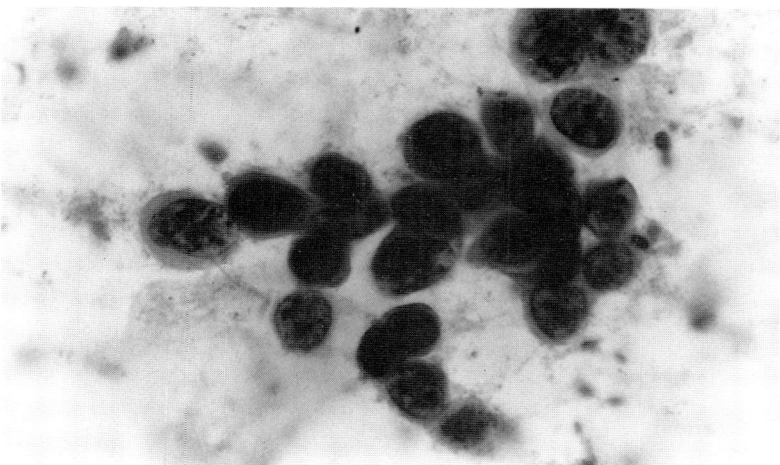

Fig. 7-14 Esophageal brush cytology in a patient with squamous carcinoma. The cells are markedly enlarged and have scant, glassy cytoplasm and round, somewhat pleomorphic nuclei with coarse chromatin but without prominent nucleoli (Papanicolaou stain, × 158.)

have been done, indicate that squamous dysplasia occurs, and probably progresses to carcinoma, at a variable rate.

Squamous carcinoma of the esophagus may occur at any level of the esophagus. Most of these lesions are well-differentiated, keratinizing, squamous carcinomas. On cytologic examination, they appear as groups of abnormal squamous cells with orangeophilic cytoplasm, which is often abundant, and with irregular, highly pleomorphic nuclei (Fig. 7-14). Bizarre cells with markedly hyperchromatic nuclei are common (Fig. 7-15), as are spindle-shaped parakeratotic cells containing hyperchromatic pyknotic nuclei.

Squamous carcinomas that are less well differentiated show discohesive cell groups and single cells that

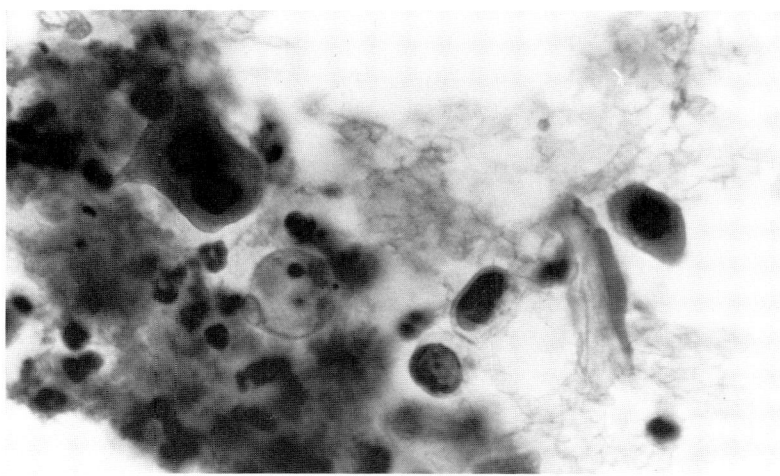

Fig. 7-15 Esophageal brush cytology. Squamous carcinoma showing bizarre single cells with abundant keratinized cytoplasm and markedly enlarged, irregular, hyperchromatic nuclei. (Papanicolaou stain, × 158.)

are characterized by a high nucleocytoplasmic ratio, scant cytoplasm without orangeophilia, and nuclei with irregular nuclear membranes, hyperchromasia, and irregularly clumped chromatin. Rare squamous carcinomas have basaloid features, and others are composed predominantly of spindle cells (spindle cell carcinoma, carcinosarcoma).

The accuracy of diagnosis of squamous carcinoma by brush cytology is excellent.[28,29] The method has a diagnostic rate of 80 to 90 percent, with few false-positives or false-negatives.

SMALL CELL UNDIFFERENTIATED (NEUROENDOCRINE) CARCINOMA

Small cell undifferentiated (neuroendocrine) carcinoma is an uncommon neoplasm in the esophagus.[30] It resembles oat cell carcinoma of the lung, as it is characterized by small to intermediate-sized cells with hyperchromatic nuclei, absent nucleoli, and nuclear molding in the cohesive cell clusters. The diagnosis of neuroendocrine carcinoma should be confirmed by immunohistochemical means (positive neuron-specific enolase and synaptophysin) and by the demonstration of neurosecretory granules on electron microscopy.

ADENOCARCINOMA

Adenocarcinoma accounts for about 10 percent of all cases of esophageal carcinoma. Most cases are believed to arise in Barrett's epithelium,[31] and it is believed that patients with the specialized columnar epithelium associated with intestinal metaplasia have the highest risk of cancer. Adenocarcinoma of the esophagus is usually well-differentiated. Cytologic examination reveals rounded groups of columnar epithelium in which the cells have an increased nuclear/cytoplasmic ratio, hyperchromasia, abnormal chromatin distribution, and large nucleoli. The cytoplasm is granular, and frequently has the foamy vacuolated appearance that is typical of adenocarcinoma (Fig. 7-16). Acinar groupings with central lumina may be seen.

The presence of atypical columnar cells in an esophageal specimen should raise the possibility of dysplasia in Barrett's esophagus.[32] Differentiating between adenocarcinoma in situ and a well-differentiated invasive carcinoma on the basis of cytologic examination can be difficult. Clinical correlation often helps.

Spread of gastric adenocarcinoma to the lower esophagus is more common than primary adenocarcinoma of the esophagus. When the carcinomatous cells are poorly differentiated, and particularly when they are signet ring cells, the possibility of gastric adenocarcinoma must be considered. Again, clinical correlation is essential.

OTHER NEOPLASMS

Other neoplasms affecting the esophagus include leiomyosarcoma and primary malignant melanoma, but are very rare.

THE STOMACH

Normal Cytology

The stomach is lined by columnar epithelium that has a characteristically uniform appearance and that is composed of tall cells with basal nuclei and apical mucin. Goblet cells are not present. The different parts of the stomach contain different kinds of mucosal glands. The cardia and pyloric antrum contain mucous glands. Acid- and enzyme-secreting glands with parietal and chief cells are found in the body and fundus. The most actively proliferative cells in the mucosa are found in the gastric pit, where the glands open onto the surface epithelium.

Specimens from normal stomach usually contain only surface epithelium. These cells appear as sheets and groups with the typical honeycomb appearance. The cells are columnar, with ovoid nuclei that contain fine chromatin and uniformly distributed mucin in the apical part of the cell (Fig. 7-17). Rarely, cells from deeper gastric glands may be seen. These contain parietal cells, which are round with abundant eosinophilic granular cytoplasm, and interspersed chief cells, which are cuboidal and have a basophilic granular cytoplasm.

Specimen Collection

Most gastric cytologic specimens are obtained by brushing a lesion that is visualized at endoscopy. The smears are prepared in a manner similar to that de-

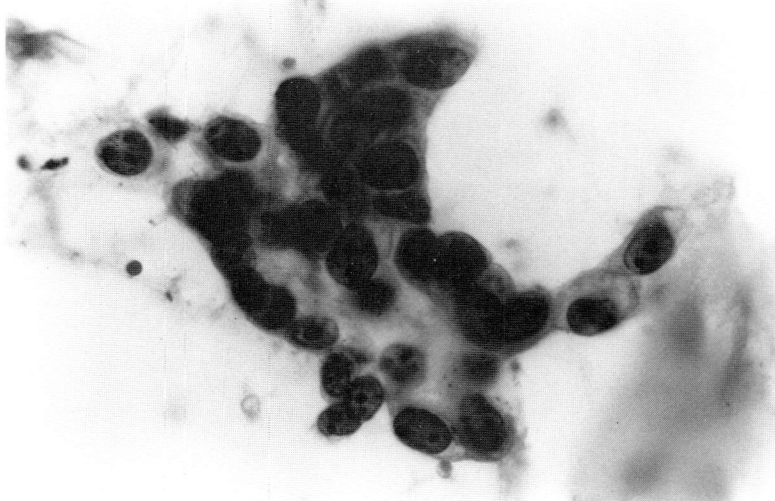

Fig. 7-16 Esophageal brush cytology in a patient with adenocarcinoma. Note the cluster of enlarged cells with abundant, vacuolated cytoplasm and nuclei with prominent nucleoli. (Papanicolaou stain, × 158.)

scribed for the esophagus. Imprint smears of biopsy specimens are used in Japan, but are rarely utilized in the United States. Studies indicate that a touch imprint improves the diagnostic accuracy of endoscopic biopsy.[33] Lavage techniques for obtaining specimens from the stomach for cytologic examination have become obsolete.

Cytology of Non-Neoplastic Lesions

The aim of gastric cytology is to diagnose malignant neoplasms. Although numerous non-neoplastic lesions occur in the stomach, they do not produce features that are sufficiently characteristic on cyto-

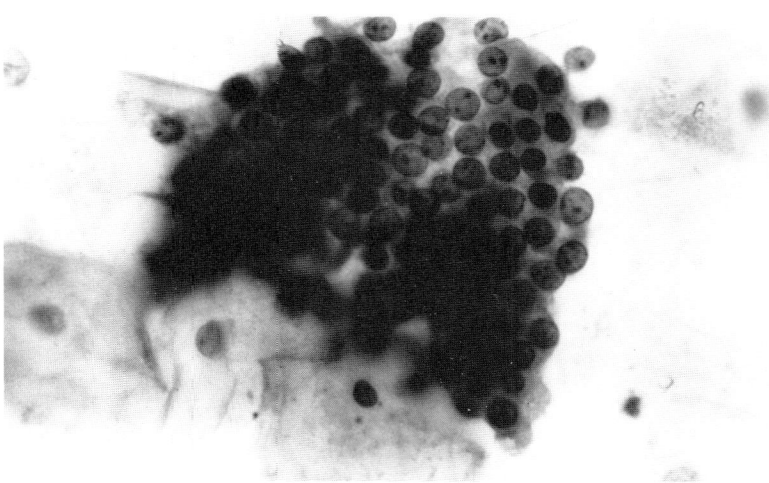

Fig. 7-17 Gastric brush cytology. Normal gastric epithelium. (Papanicolaou stain, × 158.)

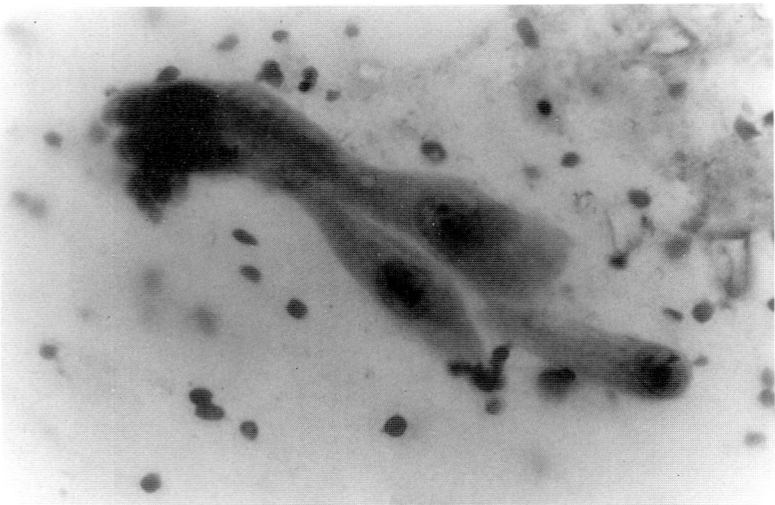

Fig. 7-18 Gastric brush cytology. Reparative epithelial cells showing enlargement, abundant cytoplasm and large, round nuclei with fine chromatin pattern and prominent nucleolus. (Papanicolaou stain, × 158.)

logic examination for specific diagnosis. The main purpose of studying non-neoplastic conditions is, therefore, to familiarize the pathologist with the range of epithelial atypia that occurs in inflammatory and reparative processes. The atypia associated with gastric ulcers and gastritis may be so severe as to mimic carcinoma, leading to a false-positive diagnosis.[34] Atypical cells usually occur in groups without single cells, and are composed of cells with high nucleocytoplasmic ratios, large round nuclei with prominent nucleoli, and a fine chromatin distribution (Fig. 7-18). Intestinal metaplastic cells are also com-

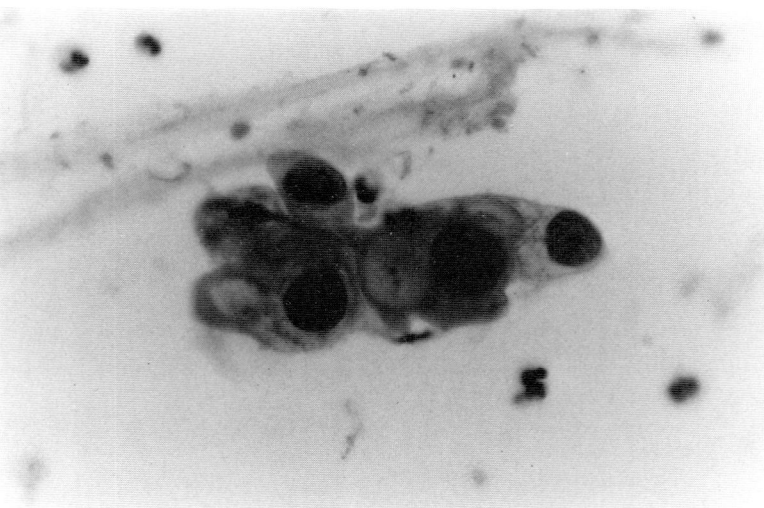

Fig. 7-19 Gastric brush cytology in a patient with atypical intestinal metaplasia. The cells have enlarged, hyperchromatic nuclei and the cytoplasm appears to be distended with a vacuole of mucin (goblet cell). (Papanicolaou stain, × 158.)

mon in chronic gastritis and gastric ulcer (Fig. 7-19). Reactive lymphoid cells are frequently present on smears from patients with ulcers.

PERNICIOUS ANEMIA

Pernicious anemia represents a specific disease in which gastric cytology plays a role in management. Patients with pernicious anemia have an atrophic gastritis that predisposes them to carcinoma. Carcinoma in these patients is preceded by increasing dysplasia, the detection of which is an indication for prophylactic gastrectomy. In patients who have not been treated with vitamin B12, the epithelial cells may show enlargement with nuclear abnormalities similar to those seen in folate deficiency. These changes disappear with vitamin B12 treatment. Epithelial dysplasia in treated patients is characterized by an increase in nuclear/cytoplasmic ratio with nuclear hyperchromasia and abnormal chromatin clumping.

INFECTION

Infection with *Campylobacter pylori* is common. Its significance is currently highly controversial. *Campylobacter pylori* appears on smears as very small, curved bacilli that are usually found entrapped in mucus. Other infections are uncommon. *Candida albicans* is frequently present on the surface of gastric ulcers, but its presence is of little significance. We have observed cytomegalovirus-infected gastric epithelial cells in patients with AIDS.

Cytology of Neoplastic Lesions

GASTRIC ADENOCARCINOMA

The most common gastric malignant disease is gastric adenocarcinoma. In the United States, its incidence has declined in the past two decades; however, it has an extremely high prevalence in Japan and South America. Adenocarcinomas may occur in all parts of the stomach.

The recognition of early gastric carcinoma (defined as a tumor that is restricted to the mucosa and submucosa) has improved the outlook for survival of this disease.[35] Compared to late cancers (those that have invaded the muscle wall), which have a 5-year survival rate of about 10 percent, early gastric cancer has a 5-year survival of about 85 percent. Unfortunately, detection of early gastric cancer has been successful only in those countries where mass population screening is undertaken. In Japan, for example, approximately 40 percent of the gastric cancers are in the early stages, compared to less than 5 percent in the United States. Most early gastric cancers are asymptomatic; rarely, they may cause symptoms resembling those of peptic ulcer disease.

On histologic examination, two types of gastric carcinoma are recognized:[36] (1) the well-differentiated or intestinal type, which is believed to arise in intestinal metaplasia;[37] and (2) the poorly differentiated, diffuse, or gastric type, which is believed to arise in gastric epithelium. The latter type is frequently composed of signet ring cells. Some studies suggest that the intestinal type has a slightly better prognosis than does the gastric form.[38]

Cytologic specimens from intestinal-type carcinomas reveal groups of malignant cells that either have an acinar arrangement or that appear as sheets (Fig. 7-20). The cells are columnar and have round nuclei. The nucleocytoplasmic ratio is increased, there is nuclear hyperchromasia and irregular chromatin clumping. Nucleoli are usually prominent. In carcinomas that are not as well differentiated, the cells have less cytoplasm and are arranged in smaller groups and singly. The nuclear features appear more obviously malignant, and scattered bizarre cells are seen. Well-differentiated, intestinal-type gastric carcinoma is difficult to differentiate from dysplasia such as occurs in adenomatous polyps of the stomach and pernicious anemia. Careful clinical correlation is very helpful.

Smears of the gastric- or diffuse-type of gastric carcinoma usually reveal numerous single cells with scattered cell groupings. The cells are round and commonly appear as signet ring cells with vacuolation of the cytoplasm by intracytoplasmic mucin, which pushes the hyperchromatic nucleus to a side of the cell and ultimately flattens it (Fig. 7-21). The cells are very pleomorphic, with some cells having small, dense nuclei and others having larger nuclei with coarse chromatin clumping and prominent nucleoli. In some patients with extremely infiltrative tumors, the neoplastic cells may be restricted to the wall without mucosal ulceration; in such cases, a false-negative cytologic result is likely.

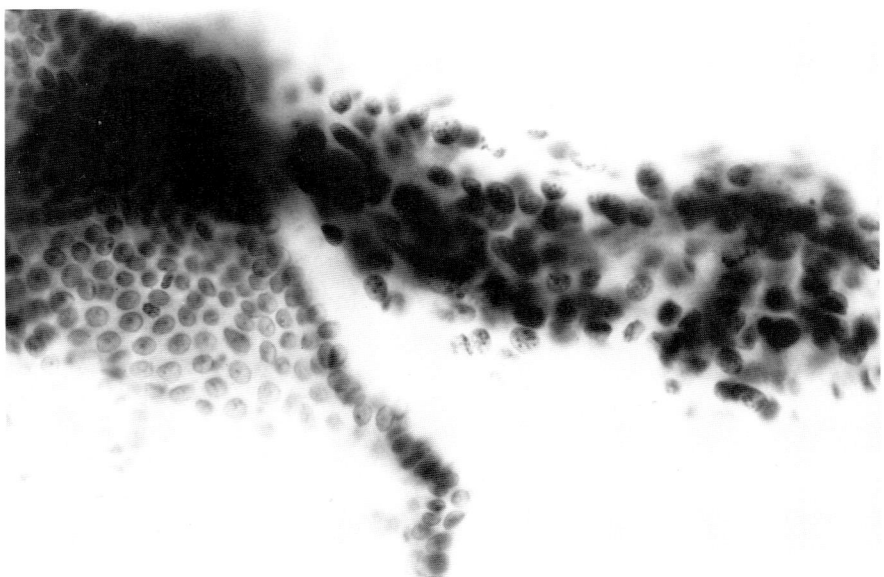

Fig. 7-20 Gastric brush cytology in a patient with well-differentiated (intestinal) adenocarcinoma. The malignant cells appear as a disorganized sheet of cells and exhibit mild enlargement, pleomorphism, and abnormal chromatin distribution. This contrasts with the group of benign gastric epithelial cells adjacent to them (Papanicolaou stain, × 158.)

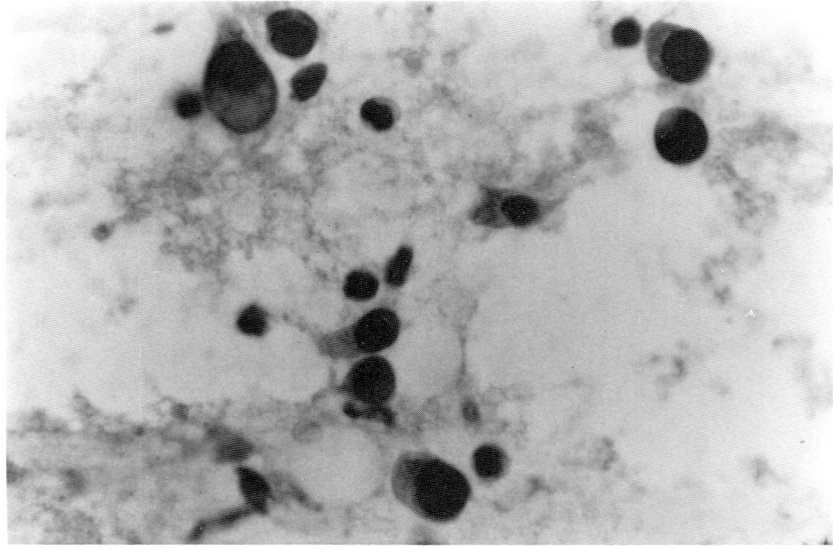

Fig. 7-21 Gastric brush cytology in a patient with a poorly differentiated adenocarcinoma. The cells appear as discohesive single cells with hyperchromatic nuclei pushed to the side by intracytoplasmic mucin. (Papanicolaou stain, × 158.)

The cytologic appearance of both early and late gastric cancer is identical.[39] Differentiation between early and late cancers is only possible on examination of the resection specimen, as diagnosis depends on determining the depth of invasion of the gastric wall by the neoplasm.

MALIGNANT LYMPHOMA

The stomach is a common extranodal site for the occurrence of malignant lymphoma. Most gastric lymphomas are high-grade B-cell lymphomas, including Burkitt's lymphoma and immunoblastic lymphoma. These lesions present with thickened rugal folds, which are often associated with large submucosal masses and ulceration. Smears usually reveal no diagnostic material, and are composed predominantly of necrotic debris from the ulcer base. When diagnostic cells are present, they appear as a dense, monomorphous population of transformed lymphocytes (Fig. 7-22).[40] In most cases, it is difficult to differentiate between a reactive lymphoid proliferation (so-called pseudolymphoma) and a malignant lymphoma on the basis of cytologic preparations, and biopsy material is necessary to confirm the presence of a monoclonal lymphocytic population.

LEIOMYOSARCOMA

Leiomyosarcoma accounts for about 5 percent of all gastric malignant diseases. It usually presents as a bulky intramural mass with crater-like mucosal ulceration. Failure to obtain diagnostic material at endoscopy is common in patients with this predominantly submucosal neoplasm, and false-negative results frequently occur. When neoplastic cells are present on smears, they appear as spindle cells that resemble smooth muscle cells (Fig. 7-23).[41] They frequently show nuclear enlargement and hyperchromasia. In most cases the biologic behavior of smooth muscle neoplasms cannot be predicted on cytologic grounds alone; however, the presence of mitoses and/or necrosis reinforces the diagnosis of malignancy. Some smooth muscle tumors are characterized by epithelioid cells which are round and have central, round nuclei surrounded by vacuolated cytoplasm (epithelioid leiomyosarcoma). The cells are discohesive and appear mainly as single cells, although they may occur in larger groups. Rarely, the cytoplasmic vacuole pushes the nucleus to the side in the same manner as a signet ring cell, thereby mimicking carcinoma.

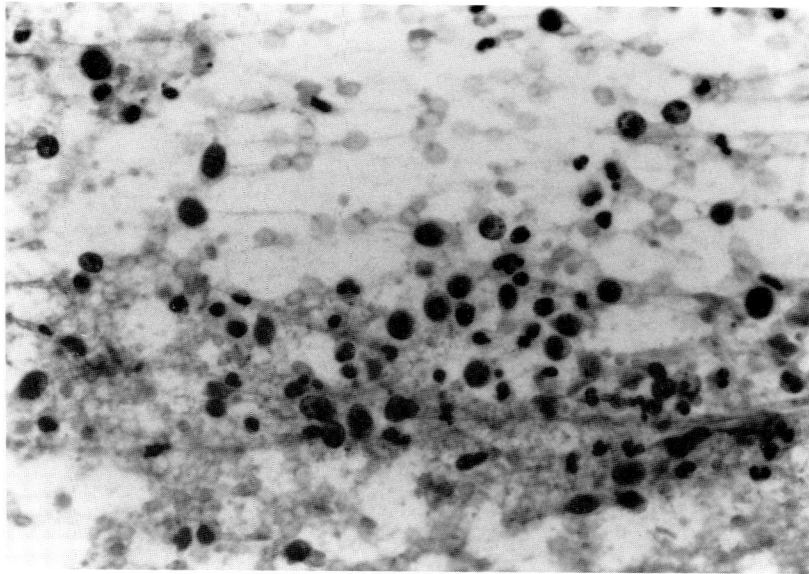

Fig. 7-22 Gastric brush cytology in a patient with malignant lymphoma. The cells are discohesive and have round nuclei and scant cytoplasm. The chromatin distribution resembles that seen in transformed lymphocytes. (Papanicolaou stain, × 158.)

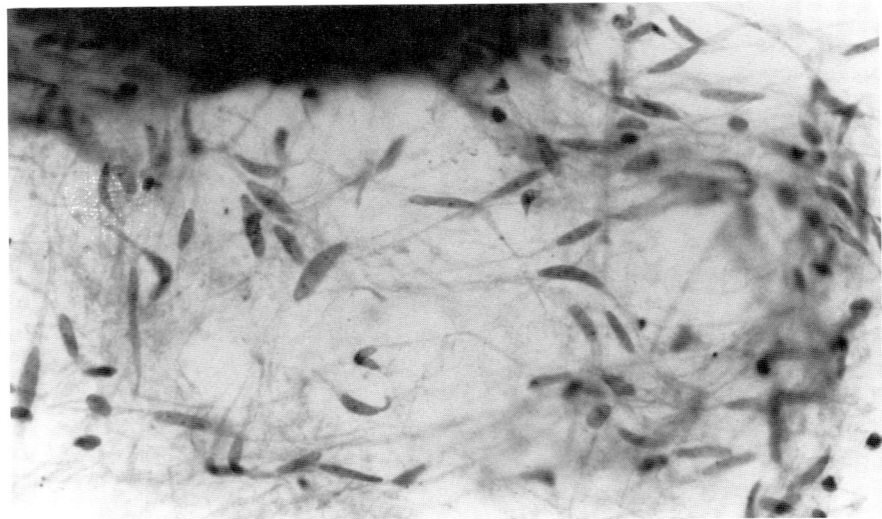

Fig. 7-23 Gastric brush cytology from smooth muscle neoplasm composed of dispersed single cells and loose clusters of cells with enlarged spindle and cigar-shaped nuclei. (Papanicolaou stain, × 100.)

THE DUODENUM

Normal Cytology

Normal duodenal and ampullary aspirates may include duodenal epithelium, which is columnar, with numerous interspersed goblet cells that appear as spaces or windows (Fig. 7-24), and cells from the larger pancreatic and bile ducts. The latter appear as uniform, cohesive groups of columnar epithelial cells with small, regular nuclei and abundant, pale cytoplasm, typically appearing as honeycomb-like clusters. Pancreatic and bile duct epithelium does not contain goblet cells.

Specimen Collection

Endoscopy of the upper gastrointestinal tract now has the ability to reach the second part of the duodenum, cannulating the pancreatic and bile ducts through the ampulla of Vater (endoscopic retrograde cholangiopancreatography, [ERCP]). Brush cytology specimens may now be obtained from grossly visible tumors in the periampullary region, which include carcinomas arising in the duodenal mucosa, carcinomas of the ampullary part of the bile duct, and carcinomas of the head of pancreas. In addition, specimens of bile and pancreatic juice may be aspirated directly from the cannulated ducts.

Cytology of Pathologic Conditions

INFECTION WITH *GIARDIA LAMBLIA*

Doudenal aspiration is the best method for diagnosing infection with the protozoan parasite *Giardia lamblia*. Superficially, Giardia trophozoites appear on smears as pale-staining, naked nuclei. On closer examination, each trophozoite is pear-shaped, with two nuclei containing prominent chromocenters, and each has a terminal flagellum (Fig. 7-25).

CHRONIC CHOLECYSTITIS, CHOLELITHIASIS, AND PANCREATITIS

The range of epithelial changes in non-neoplastic diseases of the pancreas and biliary system is considerable. Patients with chronic cholecystitis and cholelithiasis frequently demonstrate inflammatory and re-

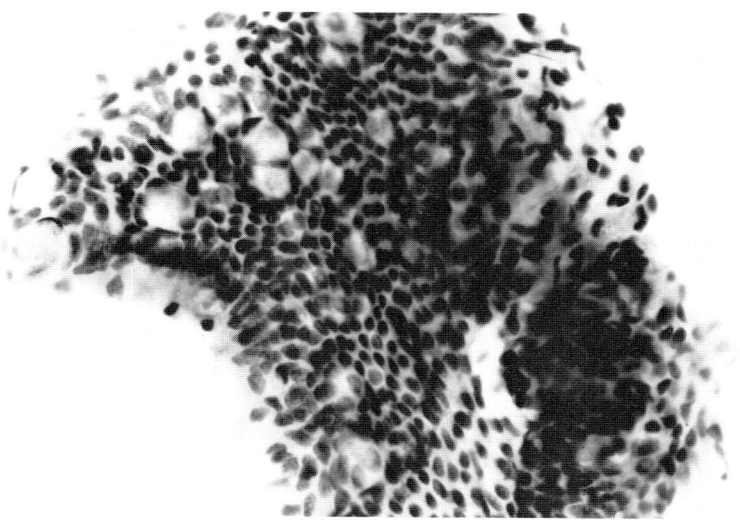

Fig. 7-24 Duodenal brush cytology. Normal duodenal mucosa showing numerous goblet cells that appear as "windows" in the cell cluster. (Papanicolaou stain, × 158.)

generative atypia of the epithelium. These findings are difficult to distinguish from dysplastic changes, which also occur frequently in patients with cholelithiasis. Chronic pancreatitis is also associated with marked atypia of the pancreatic duct epithelium.

PERIAMPULLARY ADENOCARCINOMAS

Periampullary adenocarcinomas are usually very well differentiated. The distinction between adenocarcinoma and reactive atypia must be made with a

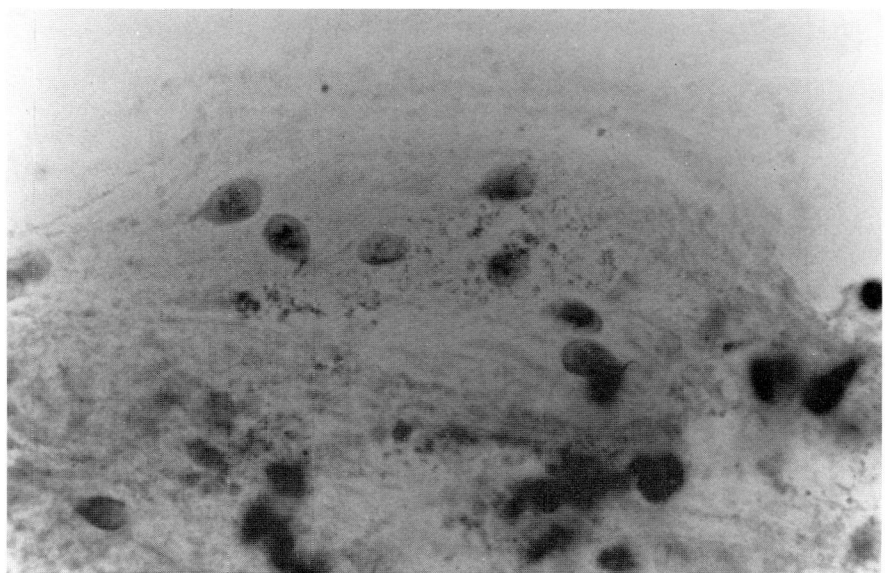

Fig. 7-25 Duodenal aspirate. *Giardia lamblia* trophozoites. (Papanicolaou stain, × 158.)

great deal of caution, particularly in aspirated specimens from the bile and pancreatic ducts. Strict criteria for diagnosing malignant disease must be satisfied, including a high degree of cellularity, the presence of discohesive cell clusters with many single cells, cell enlargement, increased nuclear/cytoplasmic ratio, nuclear pleomorphism, prominent nucleoli, hyperchromasia, and irregular chromatin clumping (Fig. 7-26). The carcinomas of this region that are less differentiated show marked cytologic abnormalities, including malignant spindle cells and giant cells (pleomorphic and sarcomatoid carcinoma of the pancreas).

The accuracy of cytologic diagnosis depends on whether a tumor is visualized in the duodenum, permitting brush cytology. In this setting, the diagnostic accuracy is greater than 90 percent. When a tumor is not visualized, the diagnostic accuracy depends on the location of the neoplasm. In carcinoma of the head of the pancreas or terminal bile duct, a definitive positive diagnosis is possible upon examination of an aspirated specimen from the cannulated ampulla in about 50 to 65 percent of cases; in carcinoma of the tail and body and more proximal biliary system, the true positive rate drops to less than 25 percent.[42] Differentiation between adenocarcinoma of the bile duct, pancreas, and duodenum is not possible on cytologic examination.

When a sample is composed predominantly of malignant spindle cells, the possibility of a leiomyosarcoma of the duodenal wall should also be considered. Other neoplasms of the duodenum and pancreas are extremely uncommon. Granular cell tumors of the bile duct may cause strictures resembling carcinoma. They are characterized by large, discohesive cells with small, central nuclei and abundant, pale, granular cytoplasm. Carcinoid tumors, islet cell tumors, gangliocytic paragangliomas, and Brunner's gland neoplasms rarely occur in the duodenum, but cannot be expected to be diagnosed on cytologic examination because of their submucosal location.

THE COLON

Colonic cytology as a diagnostic method has not experienced the same increase in popularity as cytology in other sites. In my institution, colonic specimens are rarely submitted for cytology, despite a very active gastroenterology service performing numerous colonoscopies and colonic biopsies.

Specimen Collection

Direct brush cytology from a lesion visualized at colonoscopy is the most common method for obtaining a specimen for cytologic examination.[43] It is performed in a manner similar to that for the upper intestinal tract. The accuracy of brush cytology in the diagnosis of carcinoma is around 80 percent when

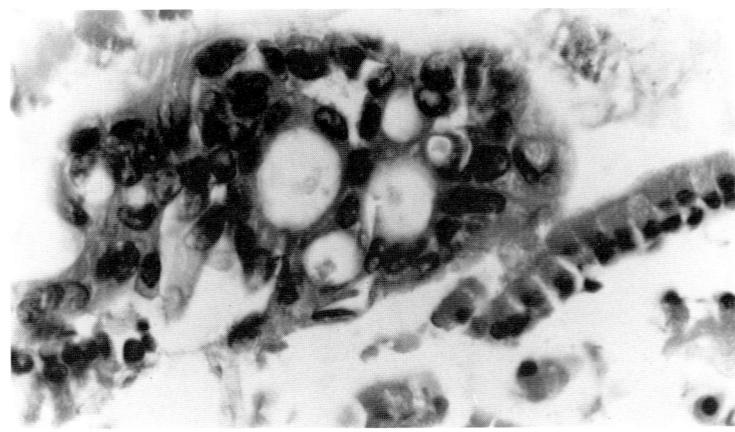

Fig. 7-26 Duodenal brush cytology. Periampullary adenocarcinoma showing increased cellularity, increased nuclear/cytoplasmic ratios, nuclear pleomorphism, and hyperchromasia. (Papanicolaou stain, × 158.)

compared with biopsy, and in almost all studies, cytologic examination does not add significantly to the accuracy rate of biopsy.

In diseases in which there is no visible lesion, specimens may be obtained by saline lavage of the colon. This method is particularly useful in evaluating epithelial dysplasia in patients with chronic ulcerative colitis, as it has the advantage of sampling the entire mucosa and may theoretically be superior to random biopsies. Saline lavage has not proved to be a popular method of specimen collection because it is time-consuming and difficult for the patient to tolerate.

Cytology of Pathologic Conditions

DIARRHEA

The identification of neutrophils in a smear obtained either from feces or from the gloved finger after rectal examination is very useful in the differential diagnosis of an inflammatory versus secretory cause of diarrhea. Rarely, a specific infectious agent, such as *Entamoeba histolytica,* can be identified in a stool sample. Cysts and ova of parasites may also be present.

IDIOPATHIC INFLAMMATORY BOWEL DISEASE

Idiopathic inflammatory bowel diseases, which include ulcerative colitis and Crohn's disease, are characterized by the presence of neutrophils in smears of either stool or specimens obtained for cytologic examination. The epithelium may exhibit changes of inflammatory atypia caused by inflammation and regeneration. Regenerative colonic epithelium is characterized by large, cohesive groups of uniformly columnar cells with abundant granular cytoplasm; enlarged nuclei with a uniform and delicate chromatin distribution; thin, regular nuclear membranes; and prominent nucleoli. Ulcerative colitis is a premalignant disorder, and may exhibit the epithelial changes of dysplasia.[44] High-grade dysplasia in ulcerative colitis is characterized by groups of columnar cells exhibiting marked pleomorphism, increased nuclear/cytoplasmic ratio, hyperchromasia, and coarse chromatin clumping. Some cell discohesiveness may be seen.

ADENOMAS OF THE COLON

Adenomas of the colon are extremely common neoplasms. They are most commonly polypoid lesions, but they may be sessile and they may enlarge greatly. They have an architecture that commonly contains tubular and villous structures in varying proportions. Adenomas are premalignant lesions, with the greatest risk of carcinoma being associated with a purely villous, sessile adenoma. Adenomas are characterized by adenomatous change in the epithelium, which is equivalent cytologically to mild dysplasia. Adenomatous epithelium is characterized by nuclear enlargement and hyperchromasia, and frequently shows stratification of the nuclei within the gland. The nuclei have a typical oval shape and retain their normal polarity with the longitudinal axis of the nucleus being perpendicular to the basement membrane. The amount of cytoplasmic mucus in the cell is reduced. An increasing degree of dysplasia in adenomas is reflected by increasing nuclear size and hyperchromasia, with loss of polarity of the nuclei. Differentiation between adenocarcinoma and adenoma is based on the presence of invasion, not on cytologic findings. On the basis of cytologic preparations, it is very difficult, if not impossible, to distinguish between an adenoma with high-grade dysplasia and well-differentiated adenocarcinoma.

ADENOCARCINOMA OF THE COLON

The second most common cause of cancer death in the United States, when both sexes are considered together, is adenocarcinoma of the colon. This disease has an incidence of 120,000 cases per year, with 55,000 deaths annually. Most colonic carcinomas arise from premalignant lesions, the most common of which are adenomas. Less commonly, ulcerative colitis and familial polyposis syndromes may be the precursors of colonic carcinoma. In cytologic preparations (most commonly brush specimens from a lesion visualized at colonoscopy), well-differentiated carcinoma appears as sheets of columnar cells.[43] The cells have crowded nuclei arranged haphazardly and without polarity. The nuclei are large, with hyperchromasia, a coarse chromatin pattern, and prominent nucleoli. The cytoplasm is granular (Fig. 7-27). Carcinomas that are less differentiated show discohesion with numerous single cells and greater degrees of cytologic abnormality.

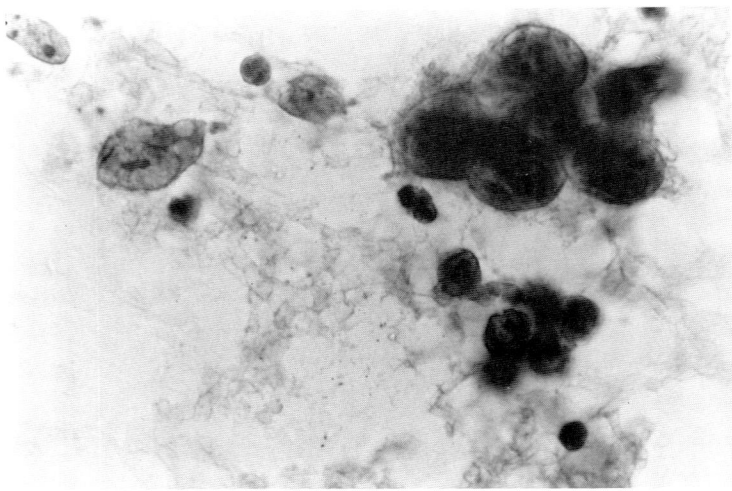

Fig. 7-27 Colonic brush cytology. Adenocarcinoma. (Papanicolaou stain, × 158.)

REFERENCES

1. Webb AJ: Cytologic diagnosis of salivary gland lesions in adult and pediatric surgical patients. Acta Cytol 17:51, 1973
2. Cohen MB, Ljung BME, Boles R: Salivary gland tumors: Fine needle aspiration vs. frozen-section diagnosis. Arch Otolaryngol Head Neck Surg 112:867, 1986
3. Young JEM, Archibald SD, Shier KJ: Needle aspiration cytologic biopsy in head and neck masses. Am J Surg 142:484, 1981
4. Layfield LJ, Tan P, Glasgow BJ: Fine needle aspiration of salivary gland lesions: Comparison with frozen sections and histologic findings. Arch Pathol Lab Med 111:346, 1987
5. Patey DH: The treatment of tumors of the parotid gland. Proc R Soc Med 59:431, 1965
6. Wheelis RF, Yarington CT: Tumors of the salivary glands. Arch Otolaryngol 110:76, 1984
7. Miller RM, Calcaterra TC, Paglia DE: Accuracy of frozen section diagnosis of parotid lesions. Ann Otol Rhinol Laryngol 88:573, 1979
8. Hillel AD, Willard FE: Evaluation of frozen section in protid gland surgery. Arch Otolaryngol Head Neck Surg 109:230, 1983
9. Bottles K, Miller TR, Cohen MB, et al: Fine needle aspiration biopsy: Has its time come? Am J Med 81:525, 1986
10. O'Dwyer P, Farrar WB, James AG et al: Needle aspiration biopsy of major salivary glands: Its value. Cancer 57:554, 1986
11. Abele JS, Miller TR, Knoll R: Fine needle aspiration diagnosis of salivary glands. p. 283. In Abele JS, Miller TR (eds): Seventh Annual Symposium on Fine Needle Aspiration. University of California, San Francisco, San Francisco, 1987
12. Orell SR, Sterrett GF, Walters MN-I et al: Manual and Atlas of Fine Needle Aspiration Cytology. Churchill Livingstone, New York, 1986
13. Matsuyama T, Fuji Y, Takeichi N et al: Aspiration biopsy cytology: A highly diagnostic procedure for assessing neck masses, excluding thyroid tumors. Jpn J Surg 16:239, 1986
14. Koss LG, Woyke S, Olszewski W: Aspiration Biopsy: Cytologic Interpretation and Histologic Bases. Igaku-Shoin, New York, 1984
15. Kline TS, Merriam JM, Shapshay SM: Aspiration biopsy cytology of the salivary gland. Am J Clin Pathol 76:263, 1981
16. Linsk JA, Franzen S, Perrone-Donnorso R: Aspiration biopsy cytology of the salivary glands. p. 85. In Linsk JA, Franzen S (eds): Clinical Aspiration Cytology. JB Lippincott, Philadelphia, 1983
17. Bottles K, Lowhagen T, Miller TR: Mast cells in the aspiration cytology differential diagnosis of adenolymphoma. Acta Cytol 29:513, 1985
18. Bottles K, Lowhagen T: Psamomma bodies in the aspiration cytology diagnosis of acinic cell tumors. Acta Cytol 29:191, 1985
19. Qizilbash AH, Sianos J, Young JEM et al: Fine needle aspiration biopsy cytology of major salivary glands. Acta Cytol 29:503, 1985

20. Qizilbash AH, Castelli M, Kowalski MA et al: Endoscopic brush cytology and biopsy in the diagnosis of cancer of the upper gastrointestinal tract. Acta Cytol 24:313, 1980
21. Graham DY, Spjut HJ, Estrada RG: Comparisons of three methods of collecting cytology specimens with the Olympus fiberscope. Front Gastrointest Res 5:21, 1979
22. Shu YJ: Esophageal cytopathology in China. Abstracts of the Scientific Sessions of 28th Annual Scientific Meeting of the American Society of Cytology. Acta Cytol 25:454, 1981
23. Cooper WA, Papanicolaou GN: Balloon technique in the cytological diagnosis of gastric cancer. JAMA 151:10, 1953
24. Lightdale CJ, Wolf DJ, Marcucci RA et al: Herpetic esophagitis in patients with cancer: Ante-mortem diagnosis by brush cytology. Cancer 39:223, 1977
25. Messian RA, Hermos JH, Robbins AH et al: Barrett's esophagus. Clinical review of 26 cases. Am J Gastroenterol 69:458, 1978
26. Raque CJ, Stein KM, Samitz MH: Pemphigus vulgaris involving the esophagus. Arch Dermatol 102:371, 1970
27. Ushigome S, Spjut HJ, Noon GP: Extensive dysplasia and carcinoma in situ of esophageal epithelium. Cancer 20:1023, 1967
28. Hishon S, Lovell D, Gummer JW et al: Cytology in the diagnosis of esophageal cancer. Lancet 1:296, 1976
29. Young JA, Hughes HE, Lee FD: Evaluation of endoscopic brush and biopsy touch smear cytology and biopsy histology in the diagnosis of carcinoma of the lower esophagus and cardia. J Clin Pathol 33:811, 1980
30. Rosen Y, Moon S, Kim B: Small cell epidermoid carcinoma of the esophagus. An oat-cell-like carcinoma. Cancer 36:1042, 1975
31. Hawe A, Payne WS, Weiland LH et al: Adenocarcinoma in the columnar epithelial lined lower (Barrett) esophagus. Thorax 28:511, 1973
32. Belladonna JA, Hajdu SI, Bains MS et al: Adenocarcinoma in situ of Barrett's esophagus diagnosed by endoscopic cytology. N Engl J Med 291:895, 1974
33. Tamura K, Masuzawa M, Akiyama T et al: Touch smear cytology for endoscopic diagnosis of gastric carcinoma. Am J Gastroenterol 67:463, 1977
34. Prolla JC, Xavier RG, Kirsner JB et al: Morphology of exfoliated cells in benign gastric ulcer. Acta Cytol 15:128, 1971
35. Kasugai T: Prognosis of early gastric cancer. Gastroenterology 58:429, 1970
36. Lauren P: The two histological main types of gastric carcinoma: Diffuse and so-called intestinal type carcinoma. Acta Pathol Microbiol Immunol Scand 64:31, 1965
37. Morson BC: Carcinoma arising from areas of intestinal metaplasia in the gastric mucosa. Br J Cancer 9:377, 1955
38. Stemmermann GN, Brown C: A survival study of intestinal and diffuse type of gastric carcinoma. Cancer 33:1190, 1974
39. Pilotti S, Rilke F, Clemente C et al: The cytologic diagnosis of gastric carcinoma related to the histologic type. Acta Cytol 21:48, 1977
40. Kline TS, Goldstein F: The role of cytology in the diagnosis of gastric lymphoma. Am J Gastroenterol 62:193, 1974
41. Cabre-Fiol V, Vilardell F, Sala-Cladera E et al: Preoperative cytological diagnosis of gastric leiomyosarcoma. A report of three cases. Gastroenterology 68:563, 1975
42. Takeda M: Duodenum and pancreas. In Takeda M (ed): Atlas of Diagnostic Gastrointestinal Cytology. Igaku-Shoin, New York, 1983
43. Bemvenuti GA, Prolla JC, Kirsner JB et al: Direct vision brushing cytology in the diagnosis of colorectal malignancy. Acta Cytol 18:477, 1974
44. Cook MG, Goligher JC: Carcinoma and epithelial dysplasia complicating ulcerative colitis. Gastroenterology 68:1127, 1975

8
Fine Needle Aspiration of the Pancreas

Para Chandrasoma

Located in the upper retroperitoneum, the pancreas is one of the most difficult organs from which to obtain tissue. As recently as five years ago, before fine needle aspiration (FNA) gained acceptance, a histologic diagnosis was made only in those patients in whom surgery was indicated. In most patients for whom surgery was not indicated, either because the pancreatic lesion was not thought to be neoplastic or because the neoplasm was deemed to be inoperable, only a clinical diagnosis was established. In those patients who underwent surgery, either in an attempt to resect the tumor or as a palliative procedure, no preoperative diagnosis was determined. Diagnosis in these patients was made by core needle biopsies performed during surgery. The error and deferment rate for frozen sections of core needle biopsy specimens obtained from patients with pancreatic neoplasms was very high, and the frequent failure of intraoperative diagnosis led to difficulties in patient management.[1] Clearly, when radical surgery is performed based on a surgeon's impression after palpation of the gland, a significant error rate is inevitable. In Lee's series, 4 of 48 patients who underwent radical surgery at our institution based on clinical impression alone had no carcinoma.[2]

Given this background, it is probably true that FNA has had a greater positive impact on the management of patients with mass lesions of the pancreas than in most other sites. In a general review of thoracic and abdominal FNA procedures performed at the Toronto General Hospital, pancreatic aspirations accounted for 344 of 1,952 abdominal aspirates, being second only to liver aspirations in number.[3]

In our hospital, most patients with pancreatic masses that are visualized by radiographic means, including ultrasonography and computed tomography (CT), are subject to an image-directed FNA biopsy as almost the first diagnostic maneuver. This provides a positive, reliable diagnosis in about 50 percent of the cases of pancreatic carcinoma, with a near 100 percent specificity and a 100 percent predictive value of a positive test. False-negative diagnoses are common, making the predictive value of a negative test approximately 60 percent.[4]

For those patients who go on to surgery without a positive diagnosis of neoplasia but in whom that possibility still remains on the basis of clinical evaluation, the most appropriate intraoperative diagnostic test has changed from a frozen section evaluation of a core needle biopsy specimen to intraoperative FNA.

The latter has yielded far superior results with fewer complications and an accuracy rate approaching 100 percent.[1]

OVERVIEW OF PANCREATIC PATHOLOGY

From the point of view of the cytopathologist, there are only two disease processes affecting the pancreas that are commonly encountered. These are pancreatic neoplasms and chronic pancreatitis.

Pancreatic Neoplasms

Pancreatic neoplasms are classified according to the cell of origin in the pancreas (Table 8-1). A more useful classification in the context of aspiration cytology when there is fairly close communication between pathologist and radiologist is the division of pancreatic neoplasms into solid and cystic masses. The differential diagnosis of a solid mass includes ductal and acinar cell carcinoma and islet cell neo-

Table 8-1 Classification of Pancreatic Neoplasms

Neoplasms of pancreatic ducts
    Ductal adenocarcinoma (80–90%)
        Well-differentiated
        Poorly differentiated
            Sarcomatoid carcinoma
            Pleomorphic giant cell carcinoma
            Carcinoma with osteoclast-like giant cells
    Mucinous cystic neoplasms (5%)
        Mucinous cystadenoma
        Mucinous cystadenocarcinoma
    Neuroendocrine neoplasms (very rare)
        Carcinoid tumor
        Neuroendocrine carcinoma
Neoplasms of pancreatic acinar cells
    Acinar cell carcinoma (1–2%)
    Serous cystadenoma (1%)
Neoplasms of pancreatic islets[a] (5–10%)
    Islet cell adenoma
    Islet cell carcinoma
Other neoplasms
    Infantile pancreatic carcinoma (very rare)
    Papillary low-grade carcinoma (also called solid and papillary epithelial neoplasm of the pancreas)

[a] Also classified according to type of hormones secreted.

plasms. Cystic mucinous tumors and serous cystadenoma must be considered in the differential diagnosis when the mass is cystic.

DUCTAL ADENOCARCINOMA

By far the most commonly encountered pancreatic neoplasm is ductal adenocarcinoma (implied when the unqualified term, pancreatic carcinoma, is used). This lesion accounts for 80 to 90 percent of all pancreatic neoplasms. Its frequency is increasing in the United States, and it represents the fourth leading cause of cancer deaths in males. The lesions, which occur in the head of the pancreas in about 60 percent of affected patients, often cause biliary obstruction which is their most common presentation. Carcinomas in the body and tail of the pancreas present at an advanced stage of disease, and commonly are associated with liver metastases at the time of presentation. Ductal adenocarcinoma varies histologically in terms of its degree of differentiation. The well-differentiated carcinomas may exhibit few cytologic abnormalities, even when they are located around nerves or in lymph nodes. Carcinomas that are less well differentiated may exhibit giant cells, and may resemble sarcomas. The prognosis for patients with any type of ductal carcinoma is very poor. Only a small percentage of these lesions are surgically resectable at presentation, and even with radical surgery, the prospect of a cure is not good.

ACINAR CELL CARCINOMA

Acinar cell carcinoma is very rare and differs from ductal carcinoma in that it is composed of solid cellular masses that resemble pancreatic acinar cells. These cells are relatively more uniform, have prominent nucleoli, and abundant granular cytoplasm. Ultrastructural examination reveals zymogen granules, a finding which permits the most definitive differentiation from ductal carcinoma. Immunohistochemical studies are necessary to differentiate acinar cell carcinoma from islet cell neoplasms, the latter of which will exhibit positive neuroendocrine markers, such as neuron-specific enolase and chromogranin. Very rarely, acinar cell carcinoma secretes lipase into the blood, leading to elevated serum lipase levels and disseminated fat necrosis. The latter change frequently involves the skin and bone marrow, producing multiple, lytic, skeletal lesions, as well as polyarthritis and skin lesions. Acinar cell carcinoma has a prognosis similar to that of ductal carcinoma.

ISLET CELL NEOPLASMS

Islet cell neoplasms commonly secrete hormones and are named accordingly (insulinoma, gastrinoma, etc). About 40 percent of these lesions secrete more than one hormone, as demonstrated by positive reactivity of cells for multiple hormones on immunohistochemical studies. Differentiation between islet cell adenoma and carcinoma can be accomplished reliably only when there are metastases; cytologic features are of little value in predicting biologic behavior.

CYSTIC NEOPLASMS

Cystic neoplasms of the pancreas, although rare, are an important group of lesions. Cystic mucinous neoplasms are classified into cystadenoma and cystadenocarcinoma, based on the presence of invasion and the greater cytologic abnormality of the latter. Some controversy persists regarding the existence of a benign mucinous cystadenoma, and thorough sampling is necessary before this benign diagnosis can be made. Mucinous cystadenocarcinoma of the pancreas is a far more responsive malignant neoplasm than the usual pancreatic carcinoma, and should be treated aggressively. With complete surgical removal, the 5-year survival rate is around 70 percent. Serous and mucinous cystadenomas are benign lesions.

Chronic Pancreatitis

Chronic pancreatitis is a common disease, and in most cases, it involves the pancreas diffusely and is easy to distinguish clinically from pancreatic carcinoma. Chronic pancreatitis is characterized by atrophy of the acinar structures, ductal dilatation, fibrosis, chronic inflammation, and focal calcification. The dilated ducts contain inspissated secretions and may have a hyperplastic epithelial lining that may show considerable amounts of cytologic atypia.

In certain situations, however, the distinction between cancer and chronic pancreatitis can be very difficult, if not impossible on the basis of radiologic and clinical evaluation. The most difficult diagnostic situation arises when the chronic pancreatitis appears as a focal process, producing a mass lesion that may cause biliary obstruction. Such lesions resemble pancreatic carcinoma even when palpated grossly at surgery. Another difficult situation is created when chronic pancreatitis complicates a carcinoma that has obstructed the pancreatic ductal system. Unless sampling is very precise, such cases may be associated with a false-negative biopsy result. Finally, there may be diffuse involvement of the pancreas by carcinoma, in which case the absence of a focal lesion may argue against a clinical diagnosis of carcinoma.

TYPES OF CYTOLOGIC SAMPLES IN PANCREATIC DISEASES

Two distinct types of samples from the pancreas may be encountered by the cytopathologist. First, an aspirate of pancreatic juice may be obtained directly from the cannulated pancreatic duct at the time of endoscopic retrograde cholangiopancreatography (ERCP). This method yields a sample that generally affords reliable results.[5] Second, FNA of the pancreas using a 20- to 22-gauge needle may be performed, employing the same technique used for all FNA procedures. This procedure may be performed percutaneously with radiologic guidance, or at surgery, guided by palpation. The actual placement of the needle in the appropriate location is done by the radiologist (in percutaneous aspirations) or the surgeon (in intraoperative aspirations). The actual aspiration may also be performed by these individuals if they have been trained in the technique of aspiration; otherwise, the aspiration is performed by the pathologist in attendance. The availability of FNA of the pancreas has increased greatly with the realization that ultrasonography, which is a relatively inexpensive and more readily available means of guidance, is comparable in effectiveness to CT scanning.[6]

Immediately upon collection, the aspirate is smeared on slides which are stained at the bedside to determine specimen adequacy. We use a rapid hematoxylin and eosin (H&E) stain for this purpose after fixing the smear with 95% ethanol. The use of air-dried May-Grünwald-Giemsa (MGG) stains is also popular at many centers. Once adequacy of the specimen is established, other smears are fixed for Papanicolaou staining and immunohistochemical evaluation, and the remainder of the tissue is processed for routine histologic examination (cell block preparation). When indicated, tissue can also be processed for electron microscopy.

It is important to evaluate these two specimen types differently. When the specimen is an aspirate obtained from within the duct by ERCP, all of the cells are necessarily ductal epithelial cells. When there is chronic pancreatitis, the hyperplasia and cytologic atypia associated with the ductal epithelium may be a potential source of error. On the other hand, an FNA specimen is characterized by the presence of more than one cell type, and the presence of a single cell population has some meaning. It must be stressed, however, that patients with chronic pancreatitis frequently exhibit replacement of the entire area by fibrosis and dilated ducts, and only ductal cells may be present in an aspirated sample.

CYTOLOGY OF THE NORMAL PANCREAS

On FNA, the normal pancreas is characterized on smear and cell block by the presence of large numbers of acinar cells that form cohesive glandular structures (Fig. 8-1). These structures are composed of cells that have small, round, regular nuclei and abundant, somewhat basophilic, granular cytoplasm. Scattered ductal epithelial cells can be recognized in the smear as flat sheets of columnar epithelial cells with a honeycomb arrangement. The constituent cells have central, round, regular nuclei that are larger than those of the acinar cells, as well as abundant eosinophilic cytoplasm. The nuclei have a delicate, finely stippled, chromatin pattern and pinpoint nucleoli. Strips of columnar cells may also be seen, particularly at the periphery of the cell clusters. Islet cells are very difficult to identify as specific cell types in the smear of a fine needle aspirate, as they closely resemble acinar cells.

When an aspirate of the main pancreatic duct is examined, the smear is made up exclusively of ductal epithelial cells in cohesive groups. Mild variation in cell and nuclear size and shape is normally present. It is important to study and become aware of the degree of cytologic abnormality present in pancreatic ductal cells in the normal pancreas, as well as in patients with chronic pancreatitis.

CYTOLOGY OF PANCREATIC DISEASE

Chronic Pancreatitis

In chronic pancreatitis, an FNA specimen from a "mass" is often characterized by an admixture of acinar cells, ductal epithelial cells, and inflammatory cells. The cell block may reveal fibrosis. The poly-

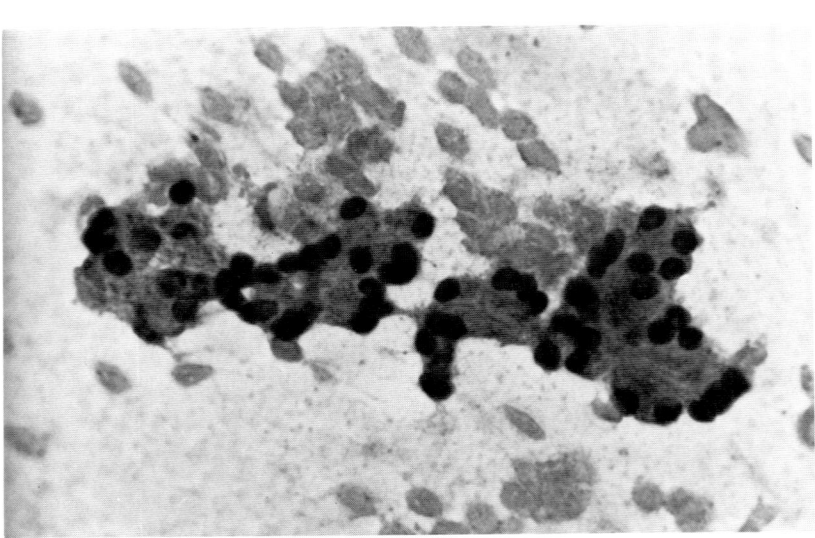

Fig. 8-1 Pancreas, FNA smear revealing normal acini. (Papanicolaou stain, × 158.)

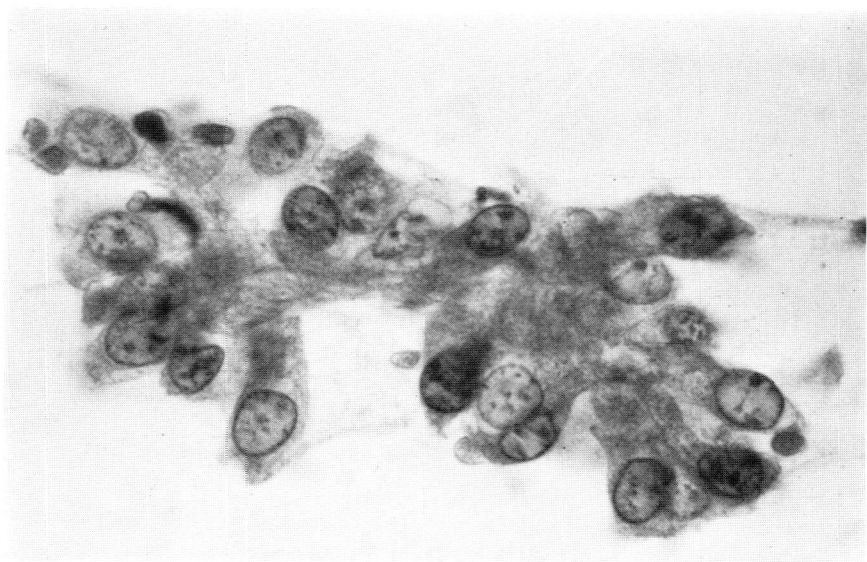

Fig. 8-2 ERCP aspirate, smear. Atypical pancreatic ductal epithelial cells are evident in this example of chronic pancreatitis. The cells are enlarged, with only a slight increase in the nuclear/cytoplasmic ratio. The nuclei are round, have a fine distribution of chromatin, and the nucleoli are not prominent. (H&E stain, × 100.) (See Plate 8-1.)

morphous nature of the smear permits recognition of the process in these cases.

Frequently, chronic pancreatitis is characterized by complete atrophy of the acinar component. This occurs most commonly in those cases in which the pancreas appears to be most dense and indurated because of replacement fibrosis. Aspirates from such areas reveal a predominance of large epithelial cells from the dilated ducts, and may resemble the smears obtained from a well-differentiated ductal carcinoma (Fig. 8-2, Plate 8-1). The differentiation of chronic pancreatitis from carcinoma in this setting must be made purely on cytologic grounds. The hyperplasia and cytologic atypia that occur in chronic pancreatitis overlap, to some extent, with the appearance of ductal cells in well-differentiated carcinoma; this overlap is responsible for the fairly high (approximately 50 percent) false-negative rate in most series of pancreatic carcinoma. This same cytologic overlap is also the reason that there is a high false-negative rate in the diagnosis of pancreatic carcinoma on the basis of an aspirate of pancreatic juice obtained by ERCP.

Chronic sclerosing pancreatitis may also be associated with hyperplastic foci of endocrine cells that may be seen in aspirates, leading to a diagnosis of islet cell neoplasm. This topic is considered more fully in the section on Cytology of Islet Cell Neoplasms.

Ductal Carcinoma of the Pancreas

The cytologic diagnosis of ductal carcinoma is made when ductal epithelial cells show unquestionable features of a malignant process (Fig. 8-3). Three criteria are basic to such a diagnosis. First, cell enlargement is an important feature in all cases of ductal carcinoma. The cells frequently exhibit considerable pleomorphism, and appear on smears both as cohesive cell groups and as scattered single cells. Second, nuclear changes, including nuclear enlargement, pleomorphism, and hyperchromatism, are usually prominent. The chromatin pattern may vary from uniform, coarse stippling to considerable irregularity. Nuclear membrane irregularity is common. Third, the cytoplasm is usually abundant, although the nucleocytoplasmic ratio is increased considerably. The cytoplasm is eosinophilic and has no specific features.

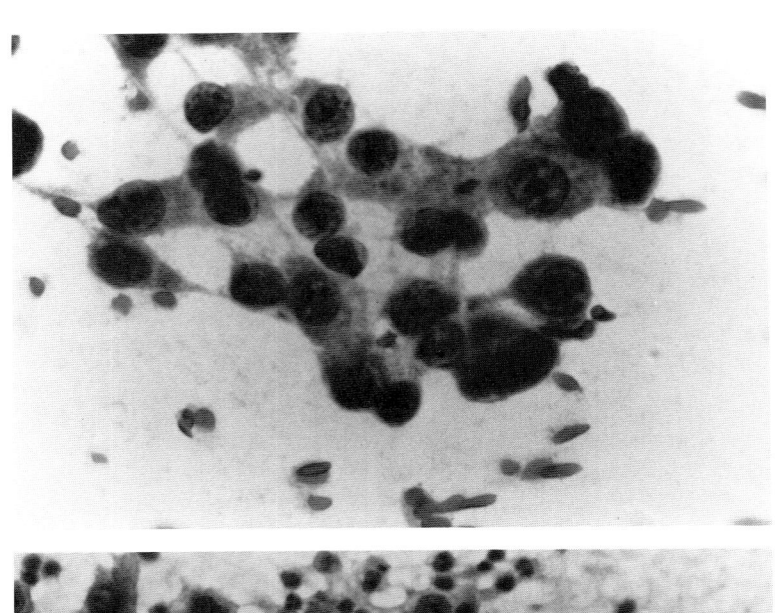
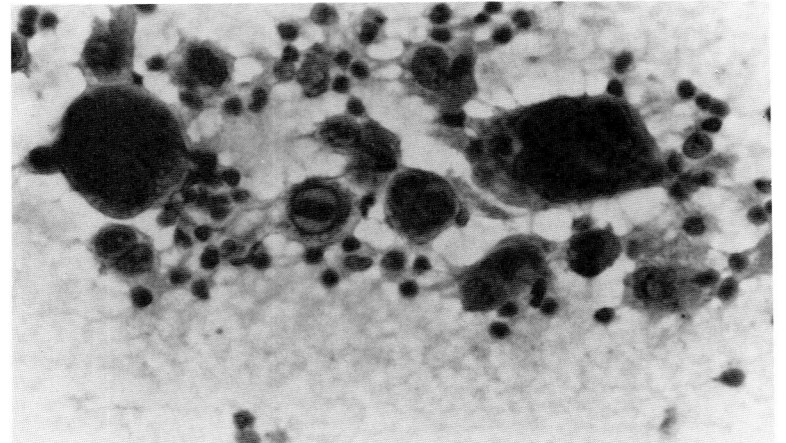
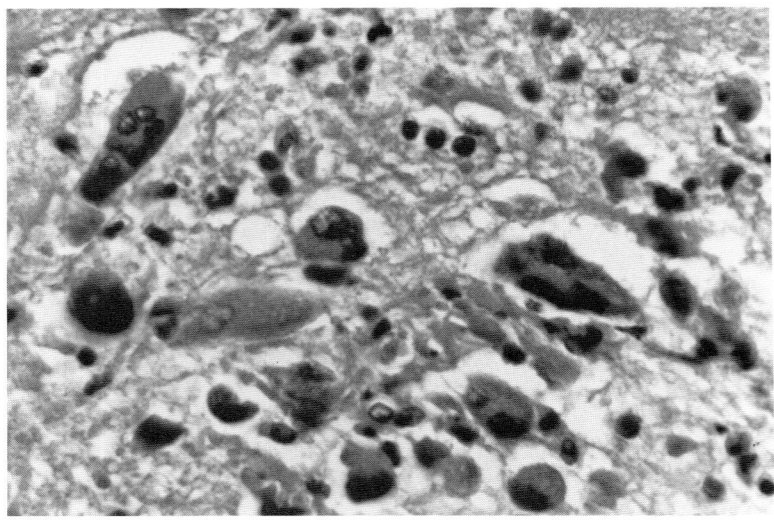

Fig. 8-3 (A) Pancreas, FNA. A smear reveals well-differentiated adenocarcinoma. (Papanicolaou stain, × 158.) **(B)** Pancreas, FNA, smear. A poorly differentiated adenocarcinoma with pleomorphic giant cells is demonstrated. (Papanicolaou stain, × 158.) **(C)** Pancreas, FNA. A cell block demonstrates a pleomorphic giant cell carcinoma. (H&E stain, × 100.)

The variants of ductal carcinoma that are less well-differentiated appear to be unquestionably malignant cytologically, but progressively lose their epithelial characteristics. The presence of malignant spindle cells in sarcomatoid carcinomas and pleomorphic giant cells in giant cell carcinomas may necessitate the use of immunoperoxidase studies to demonstrate keratin positivity before a diagnosis of carcinoma can be established. Rarely, squamous differentiation may be identified.[7]

The diagnosis of ductal carcinoma of the pancreas is the main objective of most cytologic evaluations of pancreas, whether it be examination of pancreatic juice removed at ERCP or an FNA specimen. Most studies indicate that the specificity of a positive diagnosis of carcinoma is close to 100 percent, indicating that most pathologists require that the most stringent criteria for carcinoma be satisfied before the diagnosis is made. The sensitivity and false-negative rates are less than 100 percent in most series, and range from between 50 and 100 percent (Table 8-2). These are appropriate rates that indicate recognition of the potential impact of a positive diagnosis of ductal carcinoma. A positive diagnosis may lead to total pancreaticoduodenectomy if the tumor is deemed resectable. If the lesion is not considered resectable, the patient may be advised of a prognosis with a drastically shortened life expectancy. In this setting, it is imperative that no false-positive diagnoses be made.

The reasons for false-negative diagnoses are many. Probably the most common reason in my experience is the technical failure of the aspirate, meaning that the material obtained is not representative of the neoplasm. This is especially true in patients in whom the carcinoma is associated with chronic pancreatitis, making selection of the target point difficult. In some cases, the material obtained may consist only of inflammatory cells and fibrous tissue, and there may be no epithelial cells to evaluate. Such a specimen is clearly inadequate.

The most significant false-negative results are obtained from examination of aspirates in which epithelial cells are present on the smear but are regarded as nondiagnostic for carcinoma. In my experience, at least some of these cases represent technical failures, with the aspirate being derived from areas of chronic pancreatitis adjacent to the carcinoma. In such instances, and indeed in all instances in which there is a firm suspicion of carcinoma based on clinical and radiologic evaluation, a second aspirate may provide diagnostic material.

In other false-negative cases, ductal epithelial cells are present on the smear that do not satisfy the criteria for diagnosis of carcinoma. The main differential diagnosis is between well-differentiated carcinoma and the atypical, hyperplastic epithelium that is characteristic of chronic pancreatitis. For an individual pathologist, the incidence of false-negative diagnoses decreases with increasing experience with pancreatic FNA. It is clear, however, that even for most experienced pathologists, there will almost always be a small percentage of false-negative results. Attempting to eliminate false-negative diagnoses completely has the potential of increasing the risk of false-positive diagnoses, and is not recommended.

Table 8-2 Results of Percutaneous FNA of the Pancreas

Study	No. of Patients	Sensitivity (%)	False-negative rate	Inconclusive
Hancke et al.[6] (1975)	21	84	3	—
Goldstein et al. (1978)	21	73	NR	NR
Evander et al. (1978)	52	64	14	7
Yamanaka et al. (1979)	22	86	NR	NR
Mitty et al. (1981)	43	86	6	—
Bret et al. (1982)	66	77	2	12
Grant et al. (1983)	15	100	—	—
Mitchell et al. (1985)		79		
Fekete et al.[4] (1986)	42	50	16	5

Abbreviation: NR, not reported.

Acinar Cell Carcinoma

Acinar cell carcinoma is rare. It has a clinical and radiologic presentation that is identical to ductal carcinoma except in those very rare functional cases in which it causes lipase secretion and disseminated fat necrosis.

Acinar cell carcinoma is characterized cytologically by a much more uniform population of cells than is seen with ductal carcinoma (Fig. 8-4). The cells appear as discohesive single cells, as well as in glandlike clusters. The cells in the glandlike clusters retain their cytoplasm, which has a distinctive, finely granular, somewhat basophilic appearance. The nuclei are round, central, have a finely stippled chromatin distribution, and commonly contain a single, prominent nucleolus. The single cells commonly appear as naked nuclei without cytoplasm. The cells resemble pancreatic acinar cells, but are much larger and show a greater degree of discohesion than do those in the normal pancreas. The cytologic appearance is very similar to that seen in islet cell neoplasms of the pancreas, which is the main differential diagnosis. The diagnosis of acinar cell carcinoma is best established by (1) demonstrating zymogen granules on electron microscopy, and (2) performing immunohistochemical studies that show positive staining for keratin intermediate filaments and negative staining for neuroendocrine markers and islet cell hormones.

Islet Cell Neoplasms

It is uncommon for pancreatic islet cell neoplasms to warrant FNA. Most of these neoplasms present with clinical evidence of excess hormone secretion, and the specific diagnosis of the radiologically delineated pancreatic mass is rarely in doubt.

FNA is performed only in those rare cases in which the islet cell neoplasm does not produce hormones that are clinically evident, and the patient presents with a solid pancreatic mass. Many of these patients will have evidence of liver metastases at the time of presentation, and it is as common to obtain a liver aspirate as it is a pancreatic aspirate.[8]

Aspiration smears from islet cell neoplasms are hypercellular and consist of monomorphic, medium-

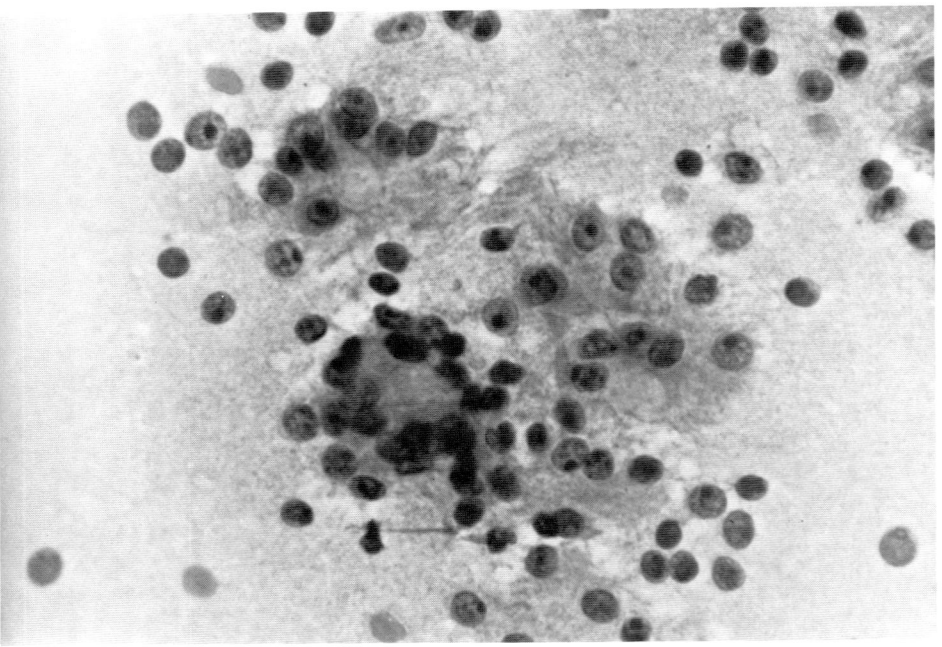

Fig. 8-4 Pancreas, FNA, smear. In this example of acinar cell carcinoma, the cells have formed loosely cohesive acinar structures. Many single naked nuclei are present. The nuclei are moderately enlarged, round, and have a fine chromatin distribution and large nucleoli. (H&E stain, × 158.)

sized cells that are arranged singly and in loose clusters (Fig. 8-5). A tendency toward trabecular and acinar formation may be detected, particularly in cell block preparations. The tumor cells may also have a tendency to cluster around capillary blood vessels in the smear. The cells are very regular, with round, central, or slightly eccentric nuclei and abundant, finely granular cytoplasm. The nuclear membrane is regular and the chromatin pattern is finely granular and evenly dispersed. One or two small nucleoli are commonly present. In my experience, as well as in most reported cases, the degree of pleomorphism observed in smears of islet cell neoplasms is minimal. A few scattered large cells with hyperchromatic nuclei may be seen, and should not be taken as evidence of malignant disease. In the absence of liver metastases, the differentiation of islet cell adenoma from carcinoma is probably impossible on cytologic grounds. These cases should, therefore, be reported simply as islet cell neoplasms.

When the initial smear suggests a diagnosis of islet cell neoplasm, it is imperative to process tissue for immunohistochemical examination and, if possible, electron microscopy. Immunohistochemistry is best done on the cell block preparation, and it is important to ensure that adequate material be available for this purpose. Islet cell neoplasms stain variably with keratin and positively with neuroendocrine markers, such as neuron-specific enolase, chromogranin, and synaptophysin. Demonstration of specific hormones in the tumor, such as insulin, glucagon, gastrin, and vasoactive intestinal polypeptide, is also feasible, and may be possible even when the neoplasm has not shown clinical evidence of satisfactory function. Electron microscopy reveals neurosecretory granules in all cases.

Hyperplastic islets are commonly found in sclerosing chronic pancreatitis, and may reach a diameter of 0.3 cm. The cytologic features of such hyperplastic islets are indistinguishable from those of islet cell neoplasms, and careful clinical and radiologic correlation is essential.[9]

It should be emphasized that pancreatic carcinoid tumors cannot be differentiated from islet cell neoplasms unless an islet cell hormone, such as insulin, glucagon, gastrin, or vasoactive intestinal polypeptide, can be demonstrated. Carcinoid tumors are believed to arise in neuroendocrine cells of the large

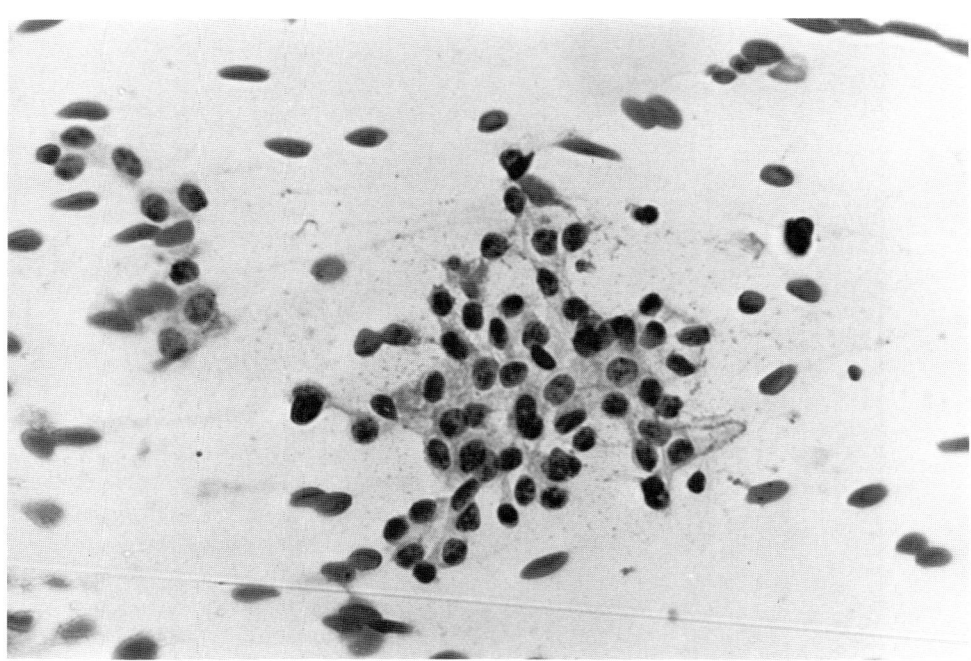

Fig. 8-5 Pancreas, FNA, smear. Islet cell neoplasm. (Papanicolaou stain, × 158.)

pancreatic ducts and have features that are very similar to islet cell neoplasms on cytologic, electron microscopic, and immunohistologic examination.

Cystic Pancreatic Masses

PANCREATIC PSEUDOCYST

By far the most common cystic pancreatic mass is a pancreatic pseudocyst. A pseudocyst usually follows an episode of acute pancreatitis by several months, or occurs in a patient with a history of chronic, relapsing, alcoholic pancreatitis. In such cases, the diagnosis of pseudocyst is made clinically, and the patient is taken directly to surgery. In a small percentage of patients with pseudocysts, however, there is no clinical history of pancreatitis and the patient presents with a cystic mass in the pancreas. When the lesion is in the head of the pancreas, it may cause obstructive jaundice. In such cases, FNA may be performed.

Pancreatic pseudocysts are inflammatory fluid collections that are filled with serosanguinous fluid and are lined with granulation tissue that undergoes progressive fibrous thickening. These pseudocysts commonly communicate with the pancreatic duct system, as evidenced by the high amylase content of the cyst fluid and the fact that they can be filled with dye by injecting contrast material into the main pancreatic duct.

Aspiration of a pseudocyst results in the withdrawal of a large volume of brownish fluid. Satisfactory smears are difficult to make at the time of aspiration. Although the diagnosis of pseudocyst becomes apparent when the fluid is withdrawn, it is probably worthwhile to send some of the fluid for amylase estimation. Smears and cell block preparations show scanty cellular material composed mainly of inflammatory cells. Ductal epithelial cells are usually absent, but the communication of the cyst with the duct system may result in the presence of a few benign epithelial cells.

PANCREATIC ABSCESS

Pancreatic abscesses may rarely be encountered at the time of FNA. These are characterized by purulent fluid in which large numbers of neutrophilic leukocytes are demonstrated. Fluid culture is necessary in such cases.

PANCREATIC ADENOCARCINOMAS

Pancreatic adenocarcinomas may also exhibit necrosis and cystic degeneration, and may result in the withdrawal of fluid during FNA. In most such cases, malignant epithelial cells can be demonstrated in the cytologic preparation. Elevated levels of carcinoembryonic antigen (CEA) in the fluid have been reported in cystic pancreatic carcinomas, so it is of value to send some of the aspirated fluid for this study.

MUCINOUS CYSTIC NEOPLASMS

Mucinous cystic neoplasms of the pancreas represent an uncommon but important lesion to diagnose accurately. Mucinous cystic neoplasms are usually unilocular or have several large locules with mucinous contents and a mucinous epithelium. In mucinous cystadenoma, the entire epithelial lining is composed of a uniform, single-layered, columnar epithelium with small basal nuclei and abundant, mucinous cytoplasm. By comparison, the lining in mucinous cystadenocarcinoma becomes grossly thicker and microscopically more complex, with stratification of cells and increased cytologic abnormalities (Fig. 8-6).

There is only one reported case of a mucinous cystadenocarcinoma being diagnosed by FNA.[10] At my institution, there has been a case involving traumatic rupture of a mucinous cystadenocarcinoma from which fluid was obtained intraoperatively for diagnosis. The diagnosis of this neoplasm depends on the finding of tall columnar cells arranged in sheets and papillary formations. The nuclei show enlargement with hyperchromatism, coarse chromatin, and prominent nucleoli. The cytoplasm contains vacuoles composed of mucinous material. In cases in which there is any significant degree of cytologic atypia, the diagnosis of mucinous cystadenocarcinoma should be made. In mucinous cystadenoma, the epithelial cells resemble benign endocervical cells. Cases in which all of the epithelial cells in the sample have a benign appearance should be reported as "cystic mu-

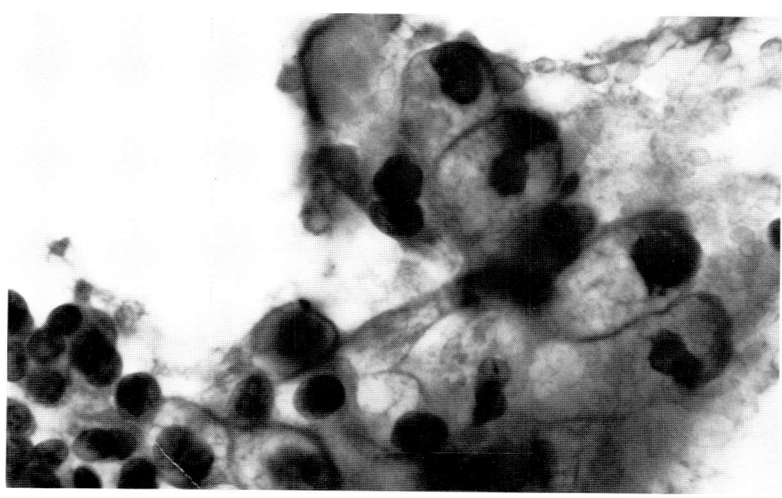

Fig. 8-6 Pancreas, FNA. A smear reveals mucinous cystadenocarcinoma. (H&E stain, × 158.)

cinous neoplasm" with the comment that complete evaluation of the lesion is necessary to exclude mucinous cystadenocarcinoma. Mucinous cystic neoplasms should be resected surgically as they are associated with an excellent 5-year survival rate following surgery.

SEROUS (MICROCYSTIC OR GLYCOGEN-RICH) CYSTADENOMA

Serous (microcystic or glycogen-rich) cystadenoma is a benign cystic neoplasm of the pancreas. It is typically microcystic and resembles a honeycomb on gross examination. The radiologic appearance of serous cystadenoma is very distinctive, and an accurate diagnosis can be made by most experienced radiologists. The microcysts are lined by cuboidal epithelial cells with round nuclei that frequently exhibit hyperchromatism and pleomorphism. The cytoplasm is moderate in amount and clear, staining positively with periodic acid-Schiff (PAS) reagent for glycogen. I have encountered two cases of serous cystadenoma, both of which were associated with inadequate samples at FNA biopsy. In one of these cases, an attempt was made to obtain an imprint preparation following surgical resection, but a cellular smear could not be obtained. This indicates that the cells lining the microcysts are tightly cohesive to the cell wall, and are difficult to dislodge.

REFERENCES

1. Beazley RM: Needle biopsy diagnosis of pancreatic cancer. Cancer 47:1685, 1981
2. Lee Y-TN: Tissue diagnosis for carcinoma of the pancreas and periampullary structures. Cancer 49:1035, 1982
3. Tao LC, Sanders DE, Weisbrod GL, et al: Value and limitations of transthoracic and transabdominal fine-needle aspiration cytology in clinical practice. Diagn Cytopathol 2:271, 1986
4. Fekete PS, Nunez C, Pitlik DA: Fine needle aspiration biopsy of the pancreas. A study of 61 cases. Diagn Cytopathol 2:310, 1986
5. Kameya S, Kuno N, Kasugai T: The diagnosis of pancreatic cancer by pancreatic juice cytology. Acta Cytol 25:354, 1981
6. Hancke S, Holm HH, Koch F: Ultrasonically guided percutaneous fine needle biopsy of the pancreas. Surg Gynecol Obstet 140:361, 1975
7. Leiman G, Markowitz S, Svensson LG: Intraoperative cytodiagnosis of pancreatic adenosquamous carcinoma. A case report. Diagn Cytopathol 2:72, 1986
8. Sneige N, Ordonez NG, Veanattukalathil MS, Samaan NA: Fine-needle aspiration cytology in pancreatic endocrine tumors. Diagn Cytopathol 3:35, 1987
9. Nguyen G-K, Rayani NA: Hyperplastic and neoplastic endocrine cells of the pancreas in aspiration biopsy. Diagn Cytopathol 2:204, 1986
10. Emmert GM, Bewtra C: Fine needle aspiration biopsy of mucinous cystic neoplasm of the pancreas: A case study. Diagn Cytopathol 2:69, 1986

9
Fine Needle Aspiration of the Liver

Para Chandrasoma

The liver, situated in a fixed position under the right lower costal margin, is one of the most accessible intra-abdominal organs. Core needle biopsy of the liver has been used successfully and with very little risk for many years. It is not surprising, then, that fine needle aspiration (FNA) of the liver has also proven to be very successful, as it is associated with an even smaller risk and complication rate than core needle biopsy.

It is important to understand the advantages and disadvantages of FNA as compared with those of core needle biopsy. Core needle biopsy has the advantage of providing a core of liver tissue for histologic examination, thereby permitting an accurate evaluation of the architecture of the liver. This is of considerable importance in the diagnosis of diffuse, non-neoplastic diseases of the liver for which core needle biopsy is preferred over FNA. However, core needle biopsy also has several disadvantages. First, it is a blind procedure that is performed without radiologic guidance. This is because the risk of complications using a large needle is directly related to the transit time of the needle in the liver, and the time taken to guide the needle radiologically would make the procedure unsafe. Second, the area of liver that can be studied by biopsy is restricted to a relatively small area under the capsule. Because of these disadvantages, core needle biopsy is inadequate in the evaluation of many localized mass lesions of the liver.

By contrast, FNA is the method of choice for mass lesions because it can be guided radiologically into the lesion, however deep inside the liver the mass is located. The risk of complications with FNA is minimal, even when the needle remains deep in the liver for a significant length of time. The amount of material obtained from correctly performed FNA is much greater in volume than that obtained by core biopsy, and with a well-prepared cell block preparation, considerable information can be gleaned regarding hepatic architecture. Ho et al. achieved an 87 percent detection rate of hepatic malignant disease with FNA, compared to a 25 percent detection rate with core biopsies performed on the same patients.[1]

At my institution, core needle biopsy is performed for the evaluation of diffuse, non-neoplastic lesions of the liver, in which case tissue samples are processed for histologic examination without ever reaching the cytopathology department. In some institutions, the needle used for the core biopsy is processed separately for cytologic study. Although we do not routinely do this, there is evidence that it may slightly increase the diagnostic yield from the liver biopsy. FNA is the primary diagnostic method for hepatic mass lesions. Aspiration is performed in the radiology department with ultrasonographic or computed tomography (CT) guidance and with the pathologist in attendance.

NORMAL CYTOLOGY OF THE LIVER

Aspiration of normal liver produces a highly cellular smear composed of cohesive hepatocytes. These appear as large, polygonal cells with small, round, central nuclei and abundant cytoplasm (Fig. 9-1). The cytoplasm is finely granular and eosinophilic on smears stained with hematoxylin and eosin (H&E). In Papanicolaou-stained smears, hepatocytes have fine red cytoplasmic granules. The nuclei have a very delicate chromatin distribution, and usually contain a prominent nucleolus. In the large groups of liver cells, it is often possible to make out a sinusoidal pattern and to identify nuclei between the hepatocytes that represent Kupffer cell nuclei and endothelial cells. These are smaller and more irregular than hepatocyte nuclei, and are oval- to spindle-shaped.

Normal liver smears contain rare groupings of biliary epithelial cells. It is usual to find only a very small number of biliary epithelial groups in a smear. Biliary epithelial cells appear as cohesive, small, columnar cells arranged in sheets with a typical honeycomb pattern (Fig. 9-1).

Incidental abnormalities are very common in liver aspirates that are performed to diagnose a mass lesion, and these must be identified. Cytoplasmic vacuoles representing fatty change are very common (Fig. 9-2). Frequently, the fat pushes the hepatocyte nucleus to one side, giving the appearance of a signet ring cell. A variety of pigments may be seen in the liver cell, including bilirubin, which is globular and has a greenish-yellow color; hemosiderin, which is golden brown and finely granular; and lipofuscin, which is golden yellow and finely granular. Another common finding in normal liver are intranuclear vacuoles, which correspond to glycogenosis of hepatocyte nuclei. They resemble intranuclear inclusions.

OVERVIEW OF LIVER PATHOLOGY

The cytopathologist must have a great deal of experience in the diagnosis of hepatic lesions in order to

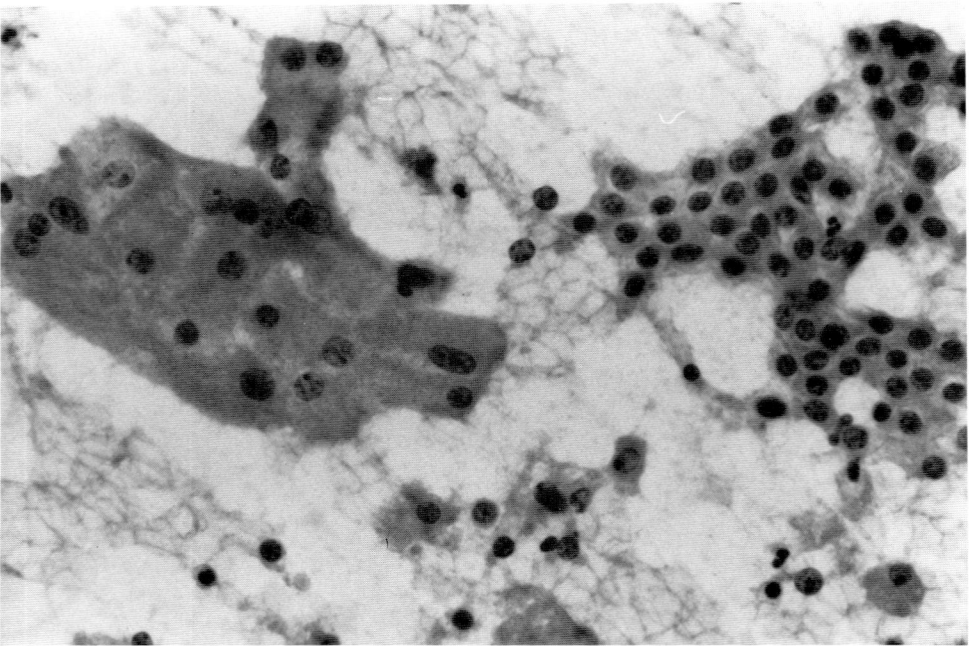

Fig. 9-1 Liver aspiration. Normal liver showing a group of normal hepatocytes (*left*) and biliary epithelium (*right*). (Papanicolaou stain, × 100.)

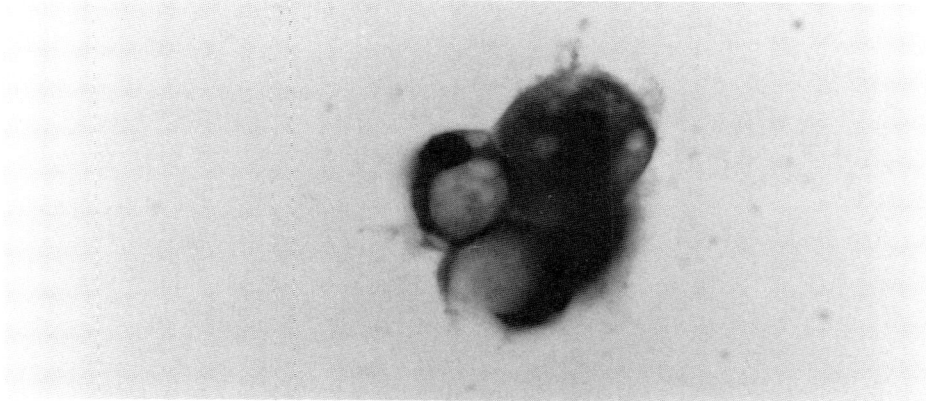

Fig. 9-2 Liver aspiration. Fatty change is evident from the appearance of the liver cells, which show nuclei that have become flattened and pushed to the side of the cell by a macrovacuole of lipid. (Papanicolaou stain, × 158.)

interpret FNA specimens. Liver diseases may be classified into two categories. The first includes diffuse, non-neoplastic diseases, among which are the various types of acute and chronic hepatitis, fatty change, alcoholic liver disease, biliary obstruction, cirrhosis, and others. These diseases are characterized by changes involving the entire liver, as well as the absence of radiologic mass lesions. Exceptions to this rule may be seen in a few cases. A large regenerative nodule in a cirrhotic liver may rarely be interpreted as a mass; likewise, obstruction of a large hepatic duct may produce changes restricted to one lobe of the liver. The second category is composed of localized, mass lesions of the liver, which are usually neoplastic, although they can include inflammatory mass lesions, such as abscesses and granulomas. These mass lesions are usually identified by radiologic studies, primarily ultrasonography or CT scan. Although the radiologic studies are very efficient at delineating the mass, the actual diagnosis of the type of mass can be made only by pathologic examination.

DIAGNOSIS OF DIFFUSE LIVER DISEASE

FNA is not commonly used for the diagnosis of diffuse liver diseases, such as acute hepatitis, fatty change, biliary obstruction, chronic hepatitis, and cirrhosis. However, it is important for cytopathologists to be familiar with these diseases, as they may appear in specimens obtained by FNA. It is also possible to routinely process core needle biopsies to provide cytologic material. This is done by washing the needle used for the core biopsy and processing this by membrane filtration. This procedure is then followed by Papanicolaou staining.[2] In general, the diagnosis of diffuse liver lesions by cytologic means is less popular in the United States than it is in Europe.[3]

Acute hepatitis is characterized by a pleomorphic hepatocyte population with multinucleated hepatocytes and many degenerating forms. Numerous lymphoid cells are also present.[4] Chronic liver disease—including both chronic hepatitis and cirrhosis—is characterized by increased numbers of biliary epithelial cell groupings that correspond to the bile duct hyperplasia that is commonly associated with these conditions. Perry and Johnston found this feature in only 15 percent of the cases of chronic hepatitis and cirrhosis they studied.[2] The presence of fibrous tissue in a smear is of little diagnostic specificity; in Perry and Johnston's series, only 21 percent of patients with fibrosis had evidence of cirrhosis on biopsy examination.[2]

The presence of pleomorphic and cytologically abnormal hepatocytes in cirrhosis is of great importance in the cytologic evaluation of the liver. Brits described the occurrence of such severe nuclear abnormalities in cirrhotic livers that a diagnosis of hepatocellular carcinoma could be entertained (Fig. 9-3).[4] In Perry and Johnston's series, high-grade nuclear abnormalities were uncommon in cirrhosis.[2] Cirrhosis of the liver is a premalignant disease, and there is a

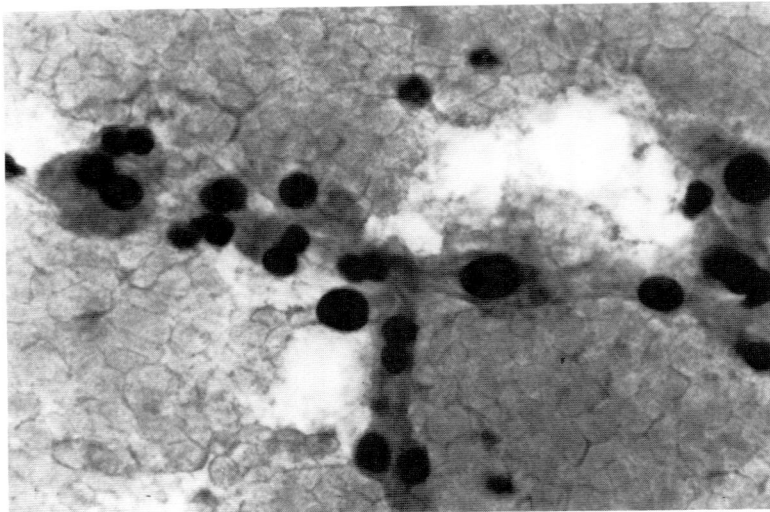

Fig. 9-3 Liver aspiration. Atypical hepatocytes in a patient with cirrhosis. The cells have enlarged, hyperchromatic nuclei. (Papanicolaou stain, × 158.)

suggestion that hepatocytes progress through increasing degrees of dysplasia before they transform into carcinoma. There is no method currently available to identify these premalignant changes in hepatocytes.

FNA has been used at my institution to evaluate iron storage in hepatocytes in patients suspected of having hemochromatosis. In this setting, smears are prepared for routine H&E stains, as well as for a Prussian Blue stain. Hemosiderin pigment appears as a platelike, refractile, golden brown pigment that stains strongly with the Prussian Blue technique. There is good correlation between the amount of iron in the liver and that estimated in aspirated material.[5] However, the reliability of diagnosis by smears has been questioned; Perry and Johnston made the correct diagnosis in only four of nine cases diagnosed by biopsy.[2]

Smears can be used reliably to quantitate fatty change in the liver. Aspiration has also been used in the diagnosis of hepatic storage disease.[6]

DIAGNOSIS OF MASS LESIONS OF THE LIVER

FNA of the liver accounts for about 30 percent of abdominal aspiration procedures, and the liver is the largest single site aspirated in the abdomen.[7] Both the frequency of aspirations and the accuracy of diagnosis of mass lesions of the liver (Table 9-1) have increased dramatically in the past decade.

Hepatocellular carcinoma constitutes more than 80 percent of the primary malignant hepatic neoplasms at my institution.[8] However, the incidence of hepatocellular carcinoma varies in different institutions because of the marked geographic variation in its incidence. The incidence of hepatic adenomas related to the use of oral contraceptives may be increasing.[9] Hepatic adenomas have also been described in athletes taking anabolic steroids. Cholangiocarcinoma accounts for about 10 percent of all primary malignant diseases of the liver, and is radiologically indistinguishable from hepatocellular carcinoma. Epithelioid hemangioendothelioma is an uncommon primary neoplasm that is important to recognize because of its slow but relentless progression. Cavernous hemangioma is a common liver neoplasm that is usually found at autopsy as an incidental finding. Although it does not produce clinical symptoms, its finding at radiologic examination may warrant an aspiration biopsy.

The frequency with which metastatic carcinoma is encountered also varies among different institutions. In many patients, FNA is performed merely to confirm that a given liver lesion in a patient with cancer

Table 9-1 Mass Lesions of the Liver

Lesion	Clinical Presentation
Hepatocytic	
Focal nodular hyperplasia	Solitary mass; associated with oral contraceptive use
Liver cell adenoma	Solitary mass; associated with steroid use, including oral contraceptives
Hepatocellular carcinoma	Solitary or multiple masses; associated with marked elevation of AFP levels; common in Far East Asia and Africa
Biliary epithelial	
Cholangiocarcinoma	Solitary or multiple masses
Biliary cystadenoma and cystadenocarcinoma	Large unilocular cystic mass; rare
Bile duct "adenoma"	Small (less than 2 cm in diameter), subcapsular, sclerotic lesion
Mesenchymal	
Hemangioma	Very common, usually cavernous
Epithelioid hemangioendothelioma	Large, infiltrative mass
Sarcoma	Rare
Metastatic neoplasms	Very common lesion, with adenocarcinoma being the most common; squamous carcinoma, melanoma, and sarcoma also are seen
Malignant lymphoma	Rare as a presenting feature
Inflammatory masses	
Abscess	Bacterial, amebic
Granuloma	

is metastatic. Such information is vital to the proper staging of lesions that is required in many oncologic treatment protocols. In a few patients, a liver metastasis will represent the chief manifestation of malignant disease; the primary lesion may remain occult, even with an extensive work-up.

The importance of the clinical history cannot be overemphasized in the interpretation of FNA biopsies of hepatic mass lesions. A history of a previous cancer at another site makes the likelihood of metastasis very high, although primary hepatocellular carcinoma has occurred in such patients. Review of the radiographs with the radiologist at the time of the FNA may also provide information regarding extrahepatic lesions. A history of steroid use—either oral contraceptives or anabolic steroids—is of critical importance in the diagnosis of a hepatocytic lesion like focal nodular hyperplasia or liver cell adenoma. A knowledge of serum alpha-fetoprotein (AFP) levels is very helpful when an unknown liver mass is being evaluated. The patient's race is also of great importance, as is the knowledge of a positive hepatitis B antigen test. Individuals from Far East Asia and certain parts of Africa have a high incidence of hepatocellular carcinoma, which is probably related to the high incidence of hepatitis B in these areas.

Like aspiration biopsy elsewhere in the body, liver aspirations must be viewed as a clinicopathologic problem. When viewed in this manner, liver aspirations fall into several problem categories (Table 9-2).

Table 9-2 Problem Categories Encountered at FNA

1. Diagnostic for hepatocellular carcinoma
2. Hepatocytes with cytologic abnormalities—benign? carcinoma? Same finding in a patient with a history of steroid use—adenoma? focal nodular hyperplasia? carcinoma?
3. Poorly differentiated carcinoma—hepatocellular? metastatic?
4. Adenocarcinoma—metastatic? cholangiocarcinoma?
5. Diagnostic for specific types of metastatic disease (islet cell/carcinoid tumors, small cell carcinoma, melanoma, sarcoma, renal adenocarcinoma, malignant lymphoma)
6. Malignant cells present—type?

In many cases, the clinical history (e.g., a previous or coexisting primary neoplasm) and laboratory findings (e.g., a marked elevation of AFP or other tumor markers, or a positive serum hepatitis B surface antigen [HBSAg] test) provide critical information. Hypercalcemia is associated with many cancers; in the liver, it has been associated with primary sclerosing hepatocellular carcinoma.

Hepatocellular Carcinoma

Most hepatocellular carcinomas are well-differentiated, with the neoplastic cells closely resembling normal hepatocytes (Fig. 9-4, Plate 9-1). The cells usually appear as moderate-sized groupings exhibiting discohesion at the periphery where single cells separate. The nuclei are round with mild hyperchromasia and minimal alteration in chromatin distribution in many cases. A central, prominent nucleolus is characteristic. Nipplelike protrusions of the nucleus are common. Intranuclear inclusions are common, but do not invariably indicate malignant disease, as they also occur frequently in benign hepatocytes. The cytoplasm is abundant and retains its finely granular appearance. The cytoplasm is commonly found to contain large amounts of glycogen on periodic acid-Schiff (PAS) stain. Fat vacuoles are present in about 20 percent of hepatocellular carcinomas. Bile pigment may be seen in about 30 percent of cases, but even when present, it is found in a small number of cells, and a careful search is necessary. Bile is useful in confirming the hepatocytic origin of the cell, but is not of value in distinguishing benign from malignant lesions. The cells differ from benign hepatocytes in their higher nucleocytoplasmic ratio (which is a con-

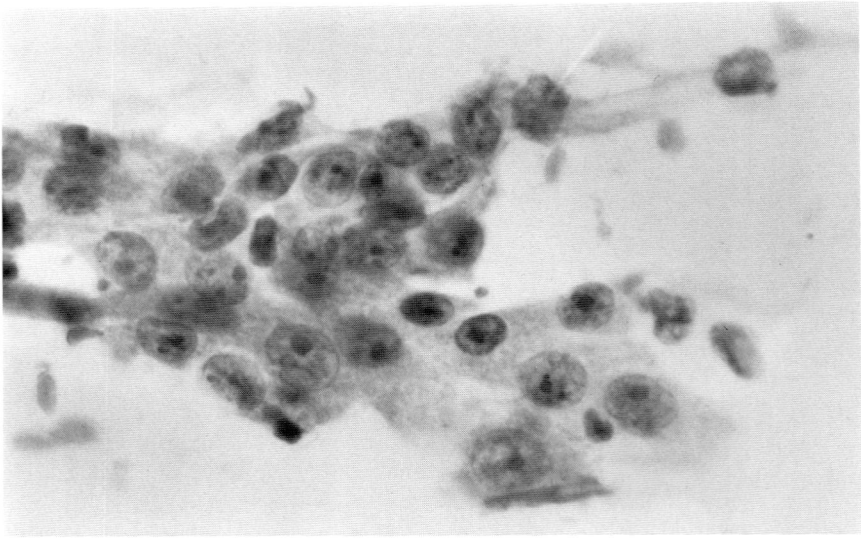

Fig. 9-4 Liver aspiration. A smear reveals well-differentiated hepatocellular carcinoma. The cells are enlarged slightly, have an increased nuclear/cytoplasmic ratio, and exhibit moderate nuclear abnormalities. (Papanicolaou stain, × 158.) (See Plate 9-1.)

stant finding), nuclear enlargement, and abnormal chromatin distribution.

In most well-differentiated hepatocellular carcinomas, there is no question on the smear appearance that the process involves hepatocytes. In many cases, however, differentiation between the benign, atypical liver cells seen in chronic liver disease, liver cell adenoma, and hepatocellular carcinoma is difficult. The cytologic changes associated with cirrhosis include nuclear enlargement and hyperchromasia, but these usually are not associated with the pronounced increase in nuclear/cytoplasmic ratio that is seen in carcinoma. The diagnosis of liver cell adenoma should be considered in patients with a history of steroid therapy, including young women taking oral contraceptives and athletes receiving anabolic steroids. Differentiation of liver cell adenoma from carcinoma is difficult, if not impossible, on the basis of aspiration cytology. Even in resected specimens, the differential diagnosis can be difficult, and depends on the identification of vascular invasion in carcinomas.

The cell block preparation is invaluable in the positive diagnosis of hepatocellular carcinoma. The appearance of cohesive, rounded cell groupings that are surrounded by a layer of endothelial cells is pathognomonic for hepatocellular carcinoma (Fig. 9-5). Similarly, the finding of a trabecular pattern of abnormal liver cells in which trabeculae that are 4 to 8 cells thick are separated by endothelium-lined sinusoids is also characteristic. The formation of "glandular" structures is not uncommon in hepatocellular carcinoma, and may lead to confusion with cholangiocarcinoma. Note that the cell block should be used only for identifying architectural features, not cytologic features; in alcohol-fixed material, groups of hepatocellular carcinoma resemble squamous carcinoma, a potential source of error.

Variants of hepatocellular carcinoma sometimes can be diagnosed by FNA. The most important of these is fibrolamellar carcinoma,[10] which occurs mainly in young females without cirrhosis of the liver in whom AFP levels are usually not elevated. Fibrolamellar carcinoma is characterized histologically by broad bands of collagen separating liver cells that are very large and polygonal and that have abundant eosinophilic cytoplasm. The cytologic features are distinctive enough to permit specific diagnosis on smears.[11] The importance of fibrolamellar carcinoma is that it is the type of hepatocellular carcinoma that is most amenable to surgical resection because of its lack of association with cirrhosis; it is also the type of hepatocellular carcinoma that has the best prognosis.

Another variant of hepatocellular carcinoma that has clinical significance is sclerosing hepatocellular carcinoma, which is associated with hypercalcemia. It is characterized histologically by extensive fibrosis. The diagnosis cannot be made on the basis of smears, as they do not permit differentiation from regular hepatocellular carcinoma. However, this disease should be suspected if the patient has hypercalcemia. Note that the presence of collagen in FNA biopsies is not used as a criterion for diagnosis because it is seen in many benign, as well as malignant, diseases.

In hepatocellular carcinomas that are less well-differentiated, the cytologic features deviate progressively from those of normal hepatocytes. As this happens, the cytologic features of malignant disease increase, so that the question to be answered at the time of biopsy changes from "Are these benign or malignant hepatocytes?" to "Are these malignant cells derived from hepatocellular carcinoma or some other carcinoma, or even some other malignant neoplasm?" In many of these cases, the diagnosis of hepatocellular carcinoma rests on the identification of diagnostic features in the better-differentiated cells in the smear. Note that normal liver cells may be present in aspirates from metastatic lesions, and may show cytologic atypia, necessitating caution. The cell block preparation is very helpful because the trabecular pattern is frequently maintained, even in poorly differentiated hepatocellular carcinoma.

The value of serum AFP levels in the diagnosis cannot be overemphasized. Serum AFP is elevated in 80 to 90 percent of hepatocellular carcinomas. Elevated AFP levels also occur in several other liver diseases, but the elevation is usually mild. When the level exceeds 3,000 IU/L, the diagnosis of hepatocellular carcinoma is almost certain. It must be remembered that testicular germ cell neoplasms also are associated with a marked elevation of serum AFP, and that metastatic germ cell neoplasm must be considered in the diagnosis when high AFP levels are present. In my institution, the results of serum AFP assays are usually not available at the time of FNA, but serve mainly to confirm the cytologic diagnosis. When differentiation between hepatocellular carcinoma and metastatic carcinoma is difficult, serum AFP levels provide a useful adjunct to FNA diagnosis.

298 PRACTICAL CYTOPATHOLOGY

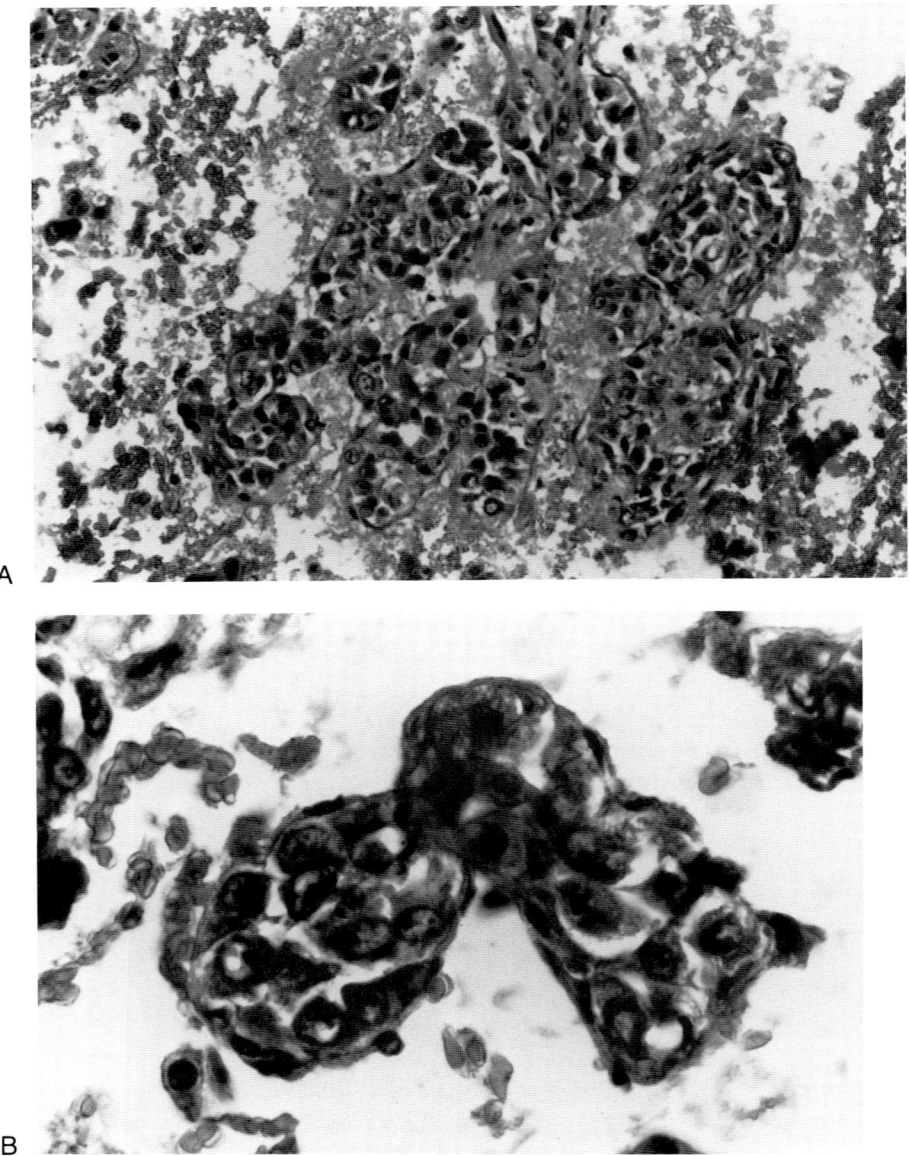

Fig. 9-5 (A) Liver aspiration, cell block. Well-differentiated hepatocellular carcinoma showing "balls" of malignant hepatocytes that are lined on the outside by endothelial cells. (H&E stain × 50.) **(B)** A higher power magnification. (H&E stain, × 158.)

Immunohistochemical evaluation is of limited usefulness in differentiating between hepatocellular and metastatic carcinoma. I routinely process our FNA biopsy specimens for immunohistochemical examination. Both hepatocellular carcinoma and metastatic carcinoma are positive for keratin, although the intensity of staining is often not as great in hepatocellular carcinoma as it is in the latter. Positive staining for AFP on the cell block section is less sensitive than serum AFP determinations; indeed, I have seen several cases in which the tissue tested negative in the presence of a markedly elevated serum AFP level.

Staining for chymotrypsin has been reported to occur in cells from patients with hepatocellular carcinoma; this may be somewhat more helpful than AFP levels in establishing a diagnosis.

Adenocarcinoma of the Liver

Adenocarcinoma of the liver is a common diagnosis made by FNA, and it is one that is encountered fairly uniformly in all institutions. At my institution, the diagnosis of adenocarcinoma of the liver is used because we do not believe it is possible to distinguish primary cholangiocarcinoma from metastatic adenocarcinoma.

Cholangiocarcinoma is an uncommon neoplasm, but it has a clinical and radiologic appearance that is very similar to that of hepatocellular carcinoma. It occurs predominantly in an older age group, and usually has no predisposing factors; in the Far East, there is an association between cholangiocarcinoma and *Clonorchis sinensis* infection. Cholangiocarcinoma is not characterized by increased serum levels of AFP, and there are no tumors markers associated with it. On histologic examination, it is usually a well-differentiated adenocarcinoma that can be distinguished from certain hepatocellular carcinomas in which glandular formations are present by the fact that, unlike hepatocellular carcinoma, it is commonly mucin-positive. The cells of cholangiocarcinoma do not contain bile.

Well-differentiated adenocarcinoma—both metastatic carcinoma and cholangiocarcinoma—exhibit on smears the usual features of adenocarcinoma (Fig. 9-6). It is important to estimate the number of glandular structures on a smear. Normal liver contains relatively rare groups of biliary epithelium, whereas chronic liver disease is characterized by increased numbers of biliary epithelial cells. When the smear is composed predominantly of glandular groupings, however, the diagnosis of adenocarcinoma must be considered even when the cytologic features are bland. Adenocarcinomatous cells usually appear as small, sometimes alveolar groups, and as discohesive single cells. The cells are large, with a central, round nucleus and a prominent nucleolus. The cytoplasm frequently contains vacuoles, and cell block preparations may demonstrate intracytoplasmic mucin. Many of the cytologic features of adenocarcinoma, including glandlike formations, prominent nucleoli, and vacuolation of cytoplasm, may be seen in hepatocellular carcinoma, and differentiating between the two may be difficult. Important in the differentiation

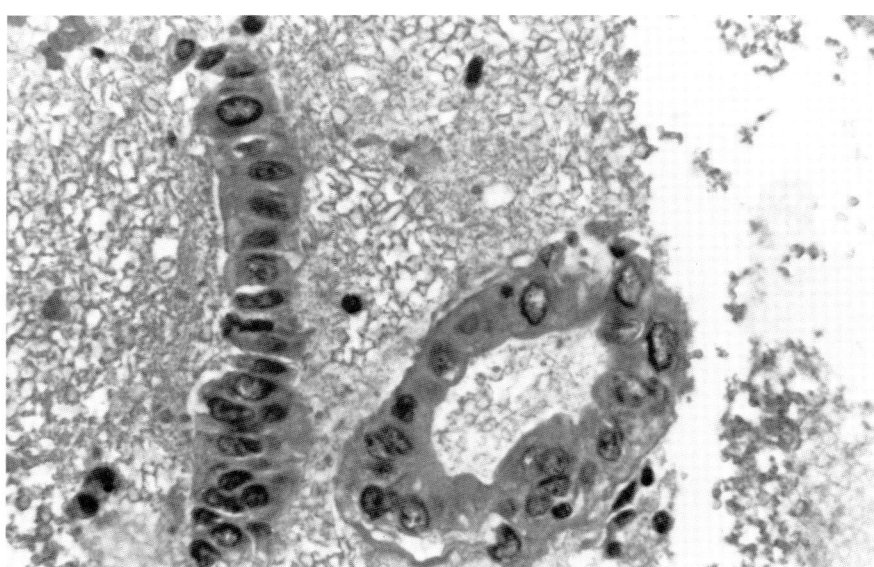

Fig. 9-6 Liver aspiration, cell block. Adenocarcinoma showing duct-like and glandular groupings of large neoplastic columnar cells containing round nuclei and prominent nucleoli. (Papanicolaou stain, × 158.)

is a positive mucin stain. The presence of bile in the cells, an elevated serum AFP level, and positive immunoperoxidase staining for AFP or chymotrypsin in the cells makes adenocarcinoma unlikely. In general, it is not advisable to attempt to identify the primary site of a metastatic adenocarcinoma on the basis of cytologic examination. Although there are specific cytologic features that suggest breast, gastric, colonic, and pancreaticobiliary carcinoma, the overlap between these entities prevents an accurate prediction of the origin of the primary lesion.

Adenocarcinomas that are less well differentiated have increased degrees of cytologic atypia, and although easily recognizable as malignant neoplasms, they are more difficult to characterize. Of greatest difficulty are sarcomatoid carcinomas and pleomorphic giant cell carcinomas, which may masquerade as sarcoma.

Specific Types of Metastatic Neoplasms

Certain types of malignant neoplasms are readily recognized by their cytologic features. They are discussed in the following sections.

MALIGNANT MELANOMA

Malignant melanoma is characterized by malignant cells that contain melanin pigment. In amelanotic melanomas, the cytologic features, which include large, round cells with abundant, granular cytoplasm and large nuclei containing prominent nucleoli, may mimic those of hepatocellular carcinoma. When a diagnosis of melanoma is suspected, confirmation is relatively easy because these lesions stain negatively for keratin and positively for vimentin, S100 protein, neuron-specific enolase, and melanosome-specific antigen (HMB45).

CARCINOID AND ISLET CELL TUMORS

Carcinoid and islet cell tumors present as a uniform population of small, round cells on smears. The cells are predominantly discohesive, but may form small groupings. The diagnosis can be confirmed by immunoperoxidase studies that show positive staining for keratin and neuroendocrine markers, such as neuron-specific enolase, chromogranin, and synaptophysin. Markers for hormones such as gastrin, insulin, and pancreatic polypeptide may be positive in islet cell tumors.

SMALL CELL UNDIFFERENTIATED CARCINOMA

Small cell undifferentiated carcinoma is characterized by hyperchromatic small cells with a very high nuclear/cytoplasmic ratio and nuclear moulding. Most small cell carcinomas have as their primary site the lung, although they may originate in a variety of other sites.

RENAL ADENOCARCINOMA

Typically, renal adenocarcinoma appears on smears as very large cells with abundant, granular cytoplasm and an eccentric nucleus that contains a prominent nucleolus. These cytologic features bear some resemblance to those of hepatocellular carcinoma, a similarity that is enhanced by frequent negative testing for keratin on immunoperoxidase staining. The cell block may show a typical clear cell appearance. In most cases of renal adenocarcinoma, the presence of a renal mass has been detected by the time of the biopsy. This is because the kidney is included in the radiologic field of the liver, and it is unusual to have a renal metastasis without an obvious primary lesion.

SQUAMOUS CARCINOMA

Squamous carcinoma can be readily identified by cytologic means when it is well-differentiated. Most squamous carcinomas of the liver are metastatic, and are usually derived from esophagus, lung, and cervix, although rarely hepatocellular carcinoma may show squamous differentiation.

SARCOMA

Sarcomas are characterized by a malignant spindle cell population. Without a history of a primary lesion elsewhere, diagnosis of this entity presents a rare but difficult problem. The differential diagnosis includes primary sarcoma of the liver, which is extremely rare; metastatic sarcoma originating in an occult primary lesion, such as a leiomyosarcoma of the uterus or gastrointestinal tract; and sarcomatoid carcinoma. Immunoperoxidase studies are not very helpful in this setting. Many sarcomatoid carcinomas are vimentin-positive and may stain either weakly or negatively for keratin, a staining pattern that is similar to that of both primary and metastatic sarcoma. In many such cases, the appropriate final diagnosis is simply malignant spindle cell neoplasm.

Epithelioid sclerosing hemangioendothelioma of the liver is an uncommon primary sarcoma of the liver. It is characterized by an extensively infiltrative neoplasm that commonly presents with hepatomegaly and a large liver mass, identified by CT. The growth rate of this neoplasm is very slow but relentless. Because it remains localized to the liver for a long period, liver transplantation is a feasible mode of treatment for these tumors. On histologic examination epithelioid hemangioendothelioma is characterized by small, irregular spaces lined by malignant, epithelioid, endothelial cells that infiltrate the liver diffusely. Extensive sclerosis is the rule. On aspiration, the malignant cells appear as small cell groups resembling glandular spaces. The cells forming these groups have large, irregular, often lobulated nuclei with hyperchromasia and rare nucleoi. They stain negative for keratin and positive for factor VIII.

MALIGNANT LYMPHOMA

Rarely, malignant lymphoma presents as a liver mass. The correct diagnosis, which is suggested on the smear by the presence of a monomorphous population of round, discohesive, transformed lymphocytes, must be confirmed by immunologic marker studies.

Inflammatory Mass Lesions

Pyogenic abscesses, amebic abscesses, granulomas, and parasitic cysts may occasionally be identified by FNA. Recognition of the inflammatory nature of such lesions at the time of aspiration biopsy should lead to appropriate microbiologic work-up of the specimen. I have encountered *Clonorchis sinensis* ova in fluid aspirated from a cystic lesion in a patient with oriental cholangiohepatitis (Fig. 9-7).

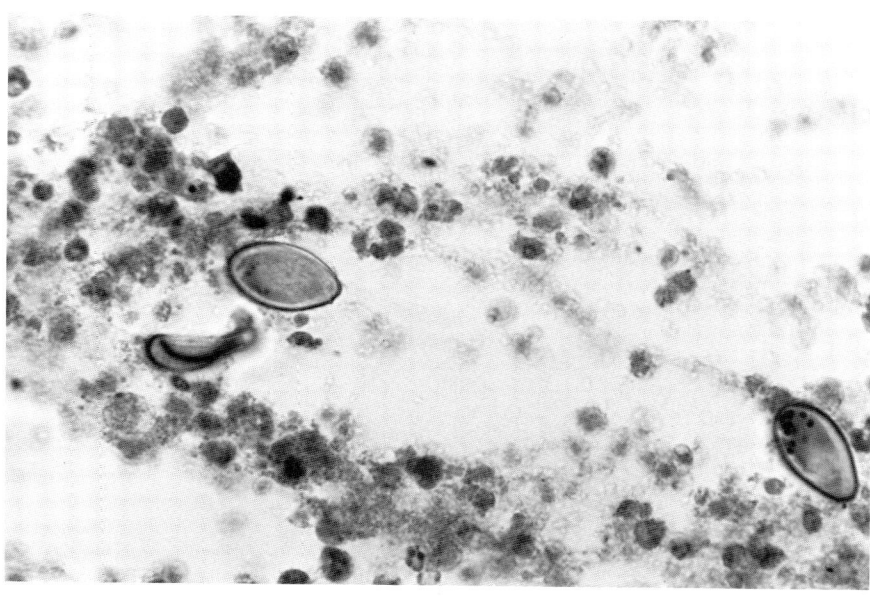

Fig. 9-7 Liver aspiration, smear. Operculated ova of *Clonorchis sinensis* in a patient with a clinical diagnosis of oriental cholangiohepatitis. (Papanicolaou stain, × 100.)

REFERENCES

1. Ho CS, McLoughlin MJ, Tao LC, et al: Guided percutaneous fine needle aspiration biopsy of the liver. Cander 47:1781, 1981
2. Perry MD, Johnston WM: Needle biopsy of the liver for the diagnosis of nonneoplastic liver diseases. Acta Cytol 29:385, 1985
3. Lundquist A: Fine needle aspiration biopsy of the liver: Applications in clinical diagnosis and investigation. Acta Med Scand 520(Suppl.):5, 1971
4. Brits CJ: Liver aspiration cytology. S Afr Med J 48:2207, 1974
5. Lundin P, Lundquist A, Lundvall O: Evaluation of fine needle aspiration biopsy smears in the diagnosis of liver iron overload. Acta Med Scand 186:369, 1969
6. Lundquist A, Ockerman PA: Fine needle aspiration biopsy of human liver for the enzymatic diagnosis of glycogen storage disease and gargoylism. Acta Pediatr Scand 59:293, 1970
7. Tao LC, Sanders DE, Weisbrod GL, et al: Value and limitations of transthoracic and transabdominal fine needle aspiration cytology in clinical practice. Diagn Cytopathol 2:271, 1986
8. Edmondson HA, Peters RL: Neoplasms of the liver. p. 1101. In Schiff L, Schiff ER (eds): Diseases of the Liver. 5th Ed. JB Lippincott, Philadelphia, 1982
9. Klatskin G: Hepatic tumors: Possible relationship to use of oral contraceptives. Gastroenterology 73:386, 1977
10. Craig JR, Peters RL, Edmondson HA et al: Fibrolamellar carcinoma of the liver: A tumor of adolescents and young adults with distinctive clinicopathologic features. Cancer 46:372, 1980
11. Suen KC, Magee JF, Halparin L, et al: Fine needle aspiration cytology of fibrolamellar hepatocellular carcinoma. Acta Cytol 29:867, 1985

10
Urologic Cytology

Dorothy L. Rosenthal

CYTOLOGIC DETECTION OF UROTHELIAL LESIONS

In 1989 an estimated 47,100 new cases of bladder cancer were detected, and approximately 10,200 people died from carcinoma of the bladder. When compared with the incidence and death rates of carcinoma of the breast and lung, these figures may seem insignificant. What is significant, however, is the biologic behavior of most urothelial lesions of the urinary tract, which include those involving the ureters and renal pelves. Generally speaking, 5-year survival rates encompass too short a time to tell the full natural history of these tumors, which can easily span 15 to 20 years. This increased survival rate is not always attributable to the use of recently developed, more effective chemotherapeutic agents, but may simply be the nature of this somewhat unique neoplasm.

The urothelial lining of the urinary tract can give rise to either synchronous or metachronous tumors, which can vary in stage and grade when they occur simultaneously and side by side. Thus, the clinician and patient are faced with a long-term commitment to control a neoplastic process in the urinary tract because obliteration of a low-grade tumor in one site is no guarantee that another tumor, perhaps of a higher grade, will not occur in another area that may be inaccessible to the probing eye of the cystoscope.

Cytology plays an increasingly important role in the management of these patients,[1-8] for although cystoscopy can be used to visualize and locate for biopsy papillary lesions of the urinary bladder, lesions involving the urethra, ureters, and renal pelves are not nearly so accessible.[9] Certainly, radiographic demonstration of so-called filling defects can provide evidence that neoplastic lesions are present, but the incidence of false-positive clues on intravenous pyelograms (IVPs) or retrograde films is too high for this modality to be used for definitive diagnosis. Therefore, urine cytology is relied upon to advise the surgeon whether operative removal of a tumor is indicated. The decision, based on cytologic findings, to remove a kidney or divert the collecting system into an ileal loop because of suspected ureteral tumors places a grave burden of responsibility upon cytologists.

Thus, in order to establish criteria for diagnosing low-grade urothelial lesions in the upper urinary tract (ureters and renal pelves), the cytologist must refine diagnostic criteria[10-13] in order to distinguish low-grade papillary lesions from hyperplasias or benign atypias, and should not relinquish the diagnosis of low-grade tumors to the cystoscopist. The diagnosis of low-grade urothelial lesions is accomplished by comparing cytologic specimens derived from bladders that contain histologically confirmed low-grade neoplasms. At the appropriate time, the cytologist can then utilize these learned criteria and apply them to the diagnosis of upper tract lesions.

Although the discipline of cytology involves all lesions of the urinary tract, both benign and malignant, only the most common diagnostic problems

304 PRACTICAL CYTOPATHOLOGY

are addressed in this chapter. Ambitious students may refer to the list of references to further their education. One of the most important factors in becoming proficient in urinary cytology is to collaborate with the urologists who submit cytologic specimens. A lesion of the upper tract should never be diagnosed unless the radiographic findings are reviewed with the urologist and a discussion of the cytologic findings considered in the light of such evidence. Such close collaboration will not only enhance the cytologic diagnosis, but will also provide the urologist with an understanding of the difficulties and problems involved in rendering a reasonable decision.

Anatomic Considerations

The urinary tract can be divided into three regions: the kidney; the calyces, pelves, and ureters (upper collecting system, or upper tract); and the bladder and urethra (lower collecting system, or lower tract). From a cytologic standpoint, the kidneys are rarely of concern, for the tumors of the renal parenchyma are infrequently recovered in urinary specimens.

The major portion of the collecting system is lined by urothelium (transitional epithelium). Variable areas of the bladder and urethra may be lined by glandular epithelium, especially in the trigone of the bladder and the dome of the bladder (the vestigial urachus). Paraurethral glands, which provide lubrication for the urethra, may also be a source of glandular epithelium from that area. Cystitis cystica, arising in Brunn's nests in the bladder mucosa, may shed groups of atypical glandular cells that should not be confused with similar cells arising from an adenocarcinoma of the bladder or prostate. In addition, the prostate and accessory sex glands are lined by columnar epithelium. Therefore, if glandular cells are seen within a urine sample, any of these sources should be considered, in addition to the tubular epithelium of the kidney.

Squamous epithelium can occur as a result of squamous metaplasia or as a congenital area, especially within the trigone of women. The more distal portions of the penile urethra are lined by squamous epithelium. In women, vaginal contamination can be a source of squamous epithelium.

The transitional epithelium itself is a unique mucosa,[11,14] specialized for the urinary tract in its disten-

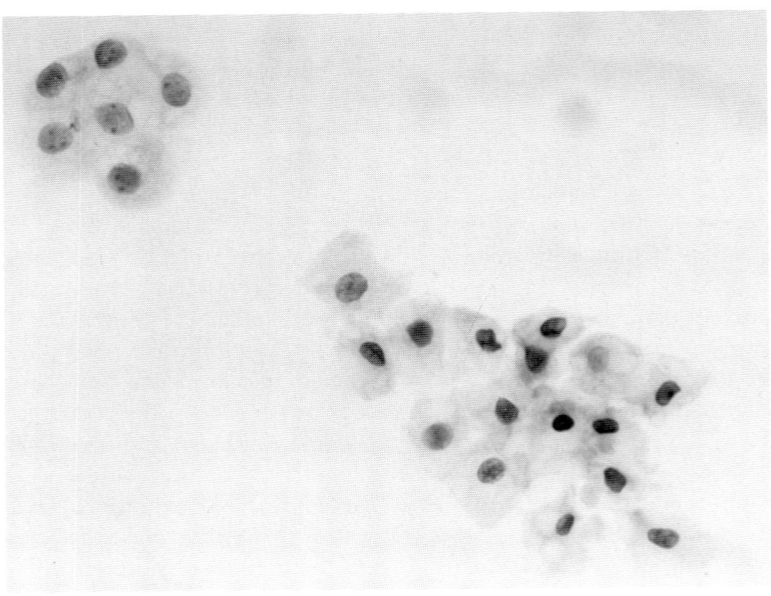

Fig. 10-1 Benign transitional cells (bladder washing). Groups of urothelial cells have abundant delicate cytoplasm and nuclei with fine chromatin and inconspicuous nucleoli. (Papanicolaou stain, × 400.)

sibility and its role as a barrier against toxic urine. This stratified epithelium is intermediate between cuboidal and squamous, hence the name transitional. When collapsed, the bladder is lined by a layer that is 4 to 5 cells thick, with the basal cells acquiring a roughly cuboidal shape, the intermediate cells assuming a polygonal shape, and the surface cells becoming round and large, and often binucleate. When distended, the mucosa may be only 2 to 3 layers thick, and the intermediate and surface cells may appear to be quite flattened.

The surface cells, the most obvious ones found in cytologic samples, have abundant cytoplasm, the luminal surface of which may appear to be thickened (Fig. 10-1). The nuclei of these superficial cells, often called umbrella cells because of their situation over more than one intermediate or basal cell, may have prominent nucleoli, and may be multinucleate.

The physiologic role of the urothelium is fascinating, and is as unique as its histologic appearance. The purpose of the urinary epithelium is to provide a barrier between the blood and the usually hypertonic toxic urine, which contains the majority of wastes from the body. The plasma membranes on the surface of umbrella cells are thicker than most other cell membranes. Interdigitating cell junctions permit great distention of the epithelium without damage to the integrity of the mucosal surface. The epithelium is connected to a basement membrane that is invisible by light microscopy. The basal layer may be deeply indented by strands of underlying connective tissue that contain capillaries.

The histology of the other parts of the urinary tract—the ureters, renal pelves, and calyces—is essentially identical to that of the bladder, except that the cells are smaller. A cross section of a contracted ureter reveals its large mucosal folds, which flatten if the ureter is distended.

Benign Urothelial Atypias

Urothelial cells react to inflammation in a similar way to all epithelial cells—that is, with accentuated nucleoli, slightly coarsened chromatin, and a variably increased nucleo-cytoplasmic ratio (Figs. 10-2 to 10-4). In contrast to cells from low-grade transitional

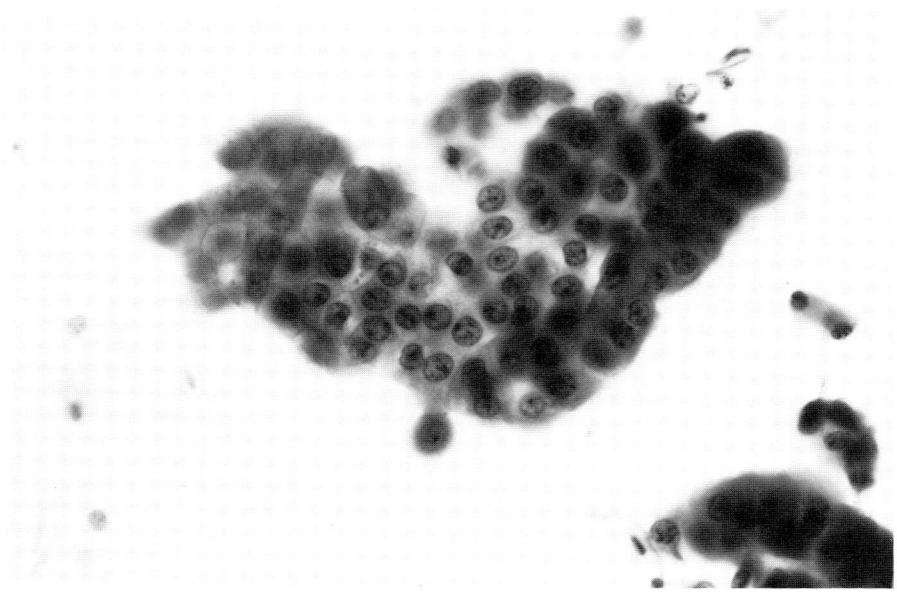

Fig. 10-2 Inflammatory atypia of urothelial cells (catheterized urine). This sheet of urothelium contains large cells that are distinctly separated (honeycomb pattern) and that have nuclei with prominent nucleoli. (Papanicolaou stain, × 400.)

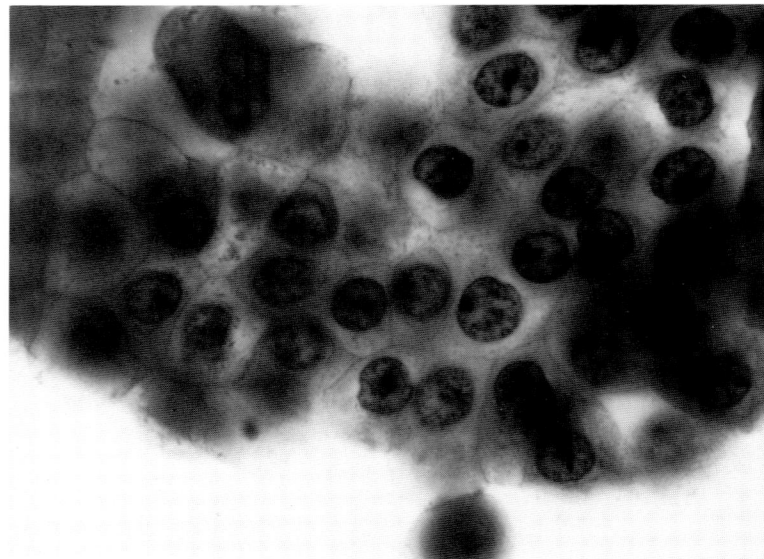

Fig. 10-3 Inflammatory atypia of urothelial cells (catheterized urine). A higher power view of Fig. 10-2 clearly demonstrates the honeycomb separation of cells, prominent nucleoli, and moderate nuclear/cytoplasmic ratio. Compare this chromatin pattern with that in Figs. 10-7, 10-9, 10-10 and 10-12. (Papanicolaou stain, × 1,000.)

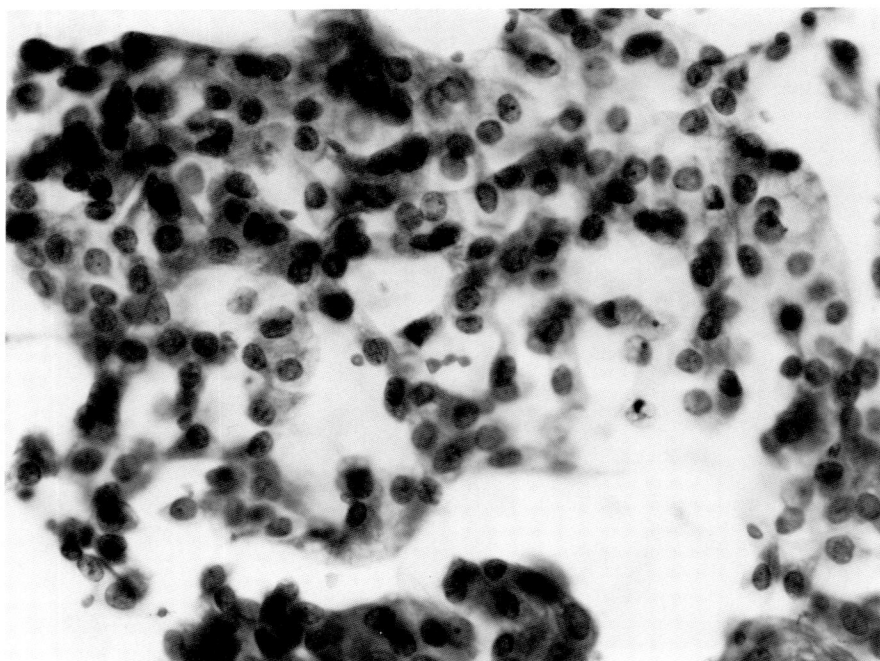

Fig. 10-4 Transitional cell atypia (saline washing). This large sheet of urothelium can be compared with that obtained by catheterization in Figs. 10-2 and 10-3. An increased amount is obtained, and the cell preservation is improved. The large amount of cytoplasm and the fine chromatin place this tissue in a benign category. (Papanicolaou stain, × 400.)

cell carcinoma, reactive urothelial cells are identified by their prominent nucleoli, whereas cells of low-grade transitional cell carcinoma have indiscernible nucleoli.

Most infectious agents are not obvious, but occasionally, trichomonads or evidence of polyomavirus (decoy cells)[15] or human papillomavirus (koilocytes)[11] may be seen. Rarely in our practice, schistosoma ova have been found and have been deemed to be responsible for profound squamous metaplasia.

Grading of Urothelial Neoplasms (Transitional Cell Carcinoma)

The current, generally accepted grading system for transitional cell carcinoma subdivides the lesions into three grades (I to III).[16,17] In those systems that add a fourth grade, equivalence can usually be accomplished by including papillomas in the grade I category. This practice is based on the experience that these benign-appearing papillomas will, in time, progress to become invasive carcinomas in most cases.[18,19] From a patient management standpoint, all papillary lesions of the urinary bladder can be considered cancerous. However, the currently held opinion that the most treacherous lesions are the high-grade sessile (flat) lesions, which are capable of invading quickly, makes the papillary lesions less noteworthy now than they were previously considered.

Table 10-1 outlines the histologic changes to be expected within the three grades, according to Koss.[16] Although the cytologic criteria for the low-grade tumors are only minimally different from those designating normal tissue or benign atypia, I believe that, given a well-preserved sample and sufficient experience with similar lesions, the distinctive features of these lesions can be appreciated.

Cytology of Low-Grade Urothelial Tumors

According to most authors,[20-28] great difficulty is generally experienced in making cytologic diagnoses of low-grade transitional cell carcinoma. One of the obvious reasons is that these lesions do not shed cells as readily as do the higher grade lesions; therefore, the amount of diagnostic material obtained in a given sample will be minimal. The other reason lies in the fact that the DNA content of grade I tumors is diploid or near-diploid,[29] so the nuclei of these cells are essentially identical to those of normal mucosa.

Although the nuclear criteria may not provide evidence of neoplasia, the growth pattern is often a significant clue to the ongoing process.[30,31] In a spontaneously voided urine, a sufficient sample for diagnosis may never be obtained.[32] An irrigation specimen obtained during cystoscopy is the best source of sufficient epithelium[33,34] to appreciate cellular crowding, which is produced by increased nuclear/cytoplasmic ratios, and perhaps a disorderly arrangement of cells. In the lowest-grade lesions and in hyperplastic states (Fig. 10-5), cellular crowding is the first clue that the epithelium is unusual.[35] (Table 10-2). Distinguishing an atypical hyperplasia (Figs. 10-6 and 10-7) from a low-grade papillary tumor (Fig. 10-8) by cytologic means is essentially impossible. Discussion with the cystoscopist will usually clarify the issue.

In the case of upper tract lesions, the problem becomes much more difficult and challenging.[36] Careful consideration of IVPs or retrograde films, as well

Table 10-1 Grading of Papillary Tumors of the Bladder

	Number of Epithelial Cell Layers	Nuclear Abnormalities	
		Enlargement	Hyperchromasia
Papilloma	≤7	Not significant	Absent
Papillary carcinoma, grade I	≤7	Slight to moderate	Slight, in occasional cells
Papillary carcinoma, grade II	>7; usually a marked increase	Moderate to marked	Slight to moderate in 25 to 50% of cells
Papillary carcinoma, grade III	>7; often a marked increase	Marked; extreme variability of sizes	Marked in 50% or more of cells

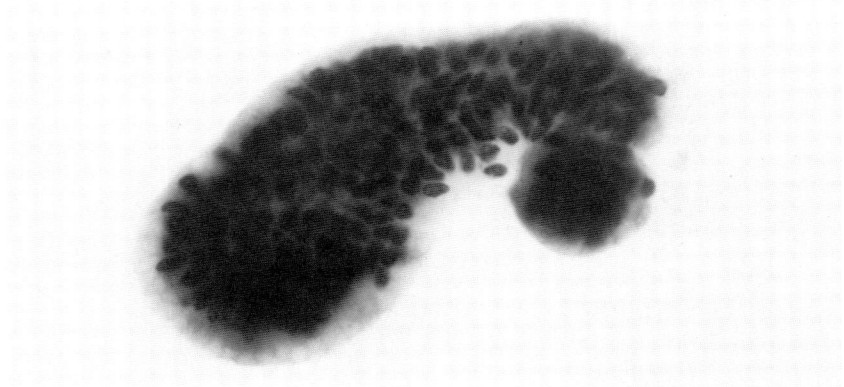

Fig. 10-5 Urothelial hyperplasia (voided urine). A papillary fragment of urothelium can arise in either a hyperplasia or a papillary carcinoma. The size of the nuclei, the chromatin pattern, and the nuclear/cytoplasmic ratio all contribute to the final diagnosis. The small size of the nuclei and the uniform seam of cytoplasm around the papillary fragment are suggestive of a non-neoplastic process. (Papanicolaou stain, × 400.)

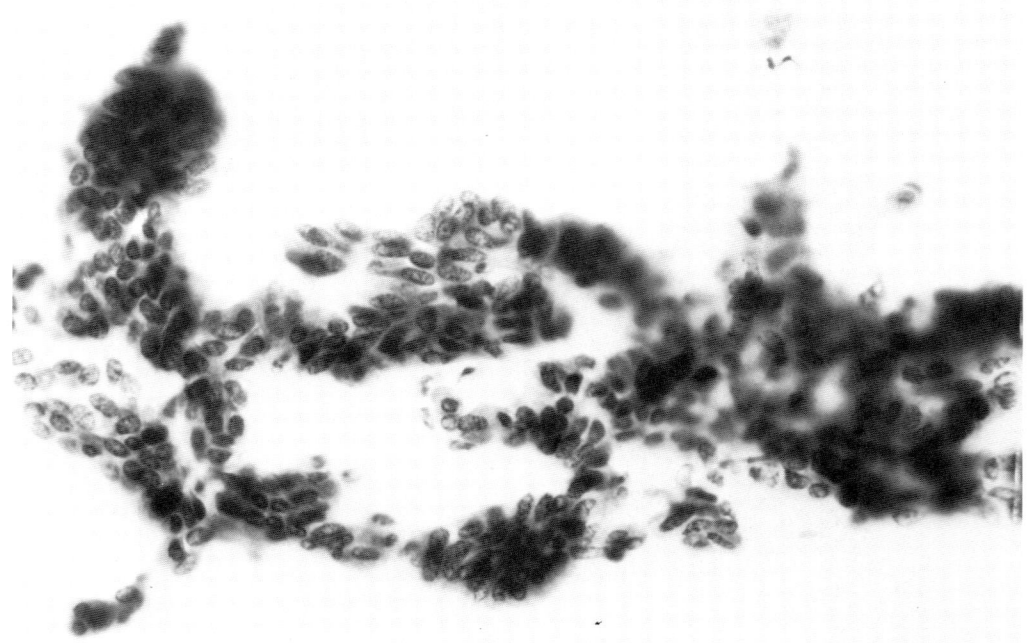

Fig. 10-6 Atypical urothelial hyperplasia (catheterized urine). This elaborate branching fragment of tissue was removed during catheterization. Although some of the fragment could be artifactual, the smooth borders in the more papillaroid areas provide evidence of the actual growth pattern of this tissue. (Papanicolaou stain, × 400.)

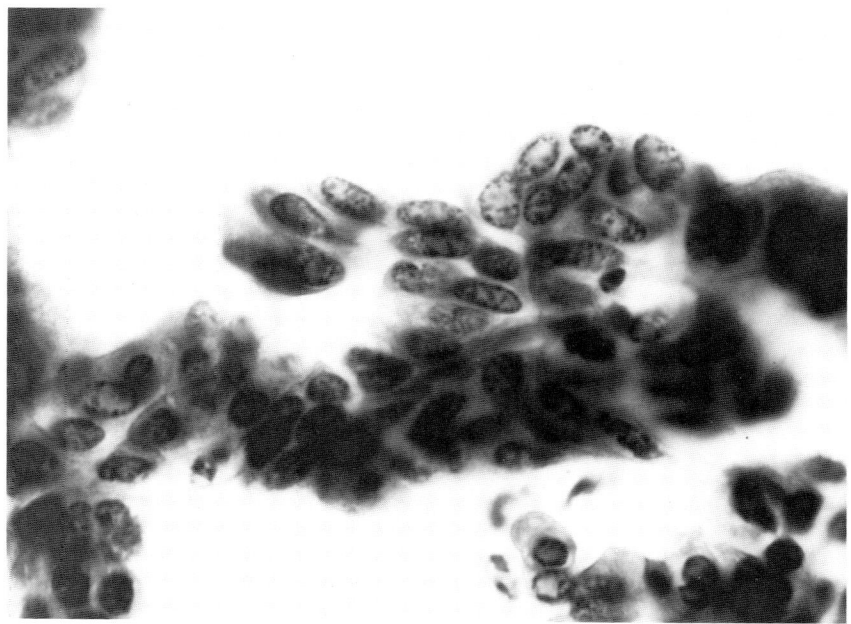

Fig. 10-7 Atypical urothelial hyperplasia (catheterized urine). Note the enlargement of the nuclei, the increased nuclear/cytoplasmic ratio, the coarsened chromatin (partially secondary to degeneration), and the packing of the cells. Cytologic study cannot differentiate between this lesion and a low-grade transitional carcinoma. (Papanicolaou stain, × 1,000.)

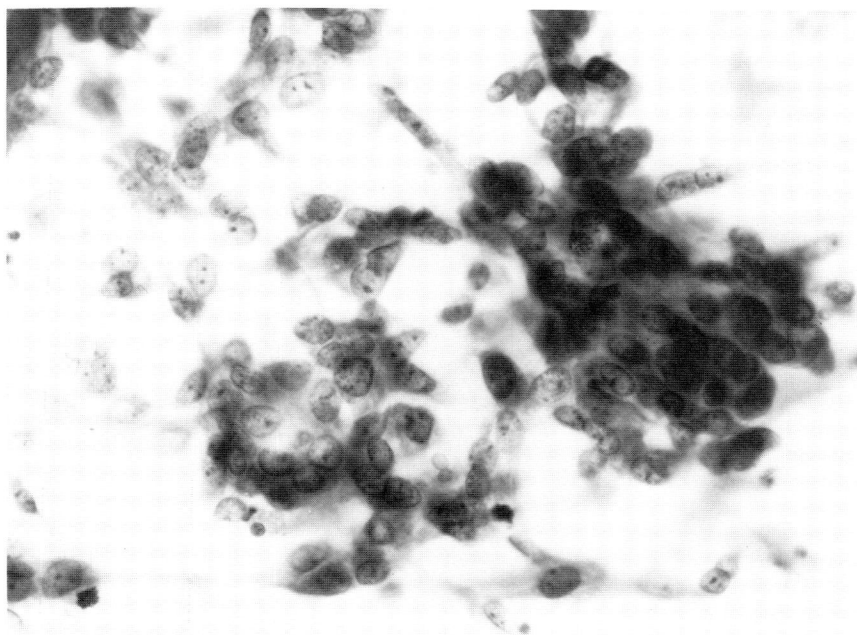

Fig. 10-8 Low-grade transitional cell carcinoma (bladder washing). Compare this tissue with that seen in Fig. 10-4. The cells have obviously larger nuclei, and the nuclear outlines are irregular. The chromatin is fine, which is consistent with a low-grade neoplasm. (Papanicolaou stain, × 400.)

310 PRACTICAL CYTOPATHOLOGY

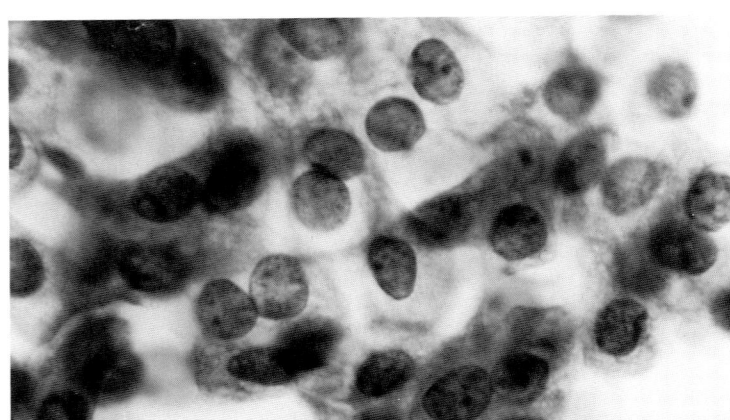

Fig. 10-9 Urothelial atypia (bladder washing). Compare the cytologic features visible at this power (from the same case as in Fig. 10-4) with the nuclear detail in Fig. 10-10 (from the same case as Fig. 10-8). Figs. 10-9 and 10-10 are both taken at the same power; nuclear size is appreciably smaller in Fig. 10-9, and chromatin quality and distribution is different. Nuclear outlines are also more atypical in Fig. 10-10. (Papanicolaou stain, × 1,000.)

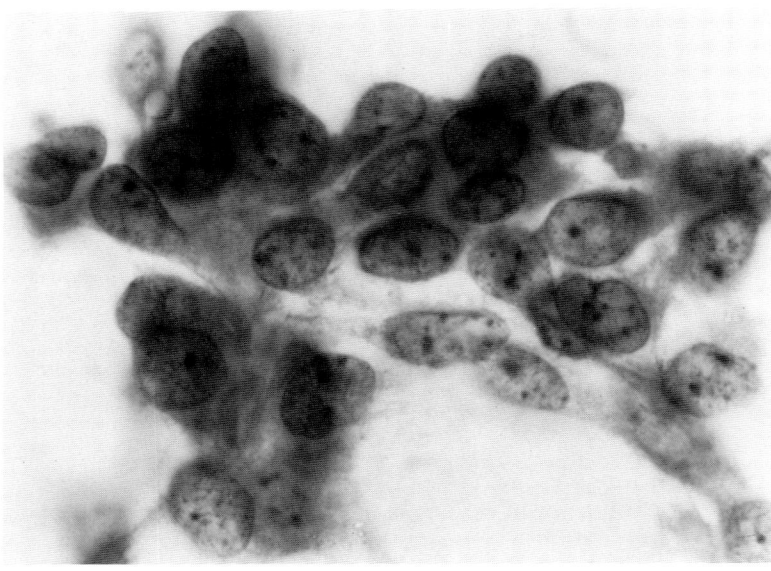

Fig. 10-10 Low-grade transitional cell carcinoma (bladder washing). See legend accompanying Fig. 10-9. (Papanicolaou stain, × 1,000.)

Table 10-2 Progressive Cytologic Changes in the Grading of Urothelial Neoplasms

Diagnosis	Cytologic Criteria
Hyperplasia	Cellular crowding Nuclear enlargement "Honeycomb" present
Grade I	Chromatinic coarseness Loss of honeycomb pattern Irregularities in nuclear shape Cellular enlargement Indistinct nucleoli
Grade II	Definite increase in nuclear/cytoplasmic ratio Haphazard growth pattern Mitoses Generalized gross cell enlargement Distinct chromatinic irregularities Distinct nucleoli
Grade III	Very high nuclear/cytoplasmic ratio Cytoplasmic differentiation (i.e., glandular/squamous) Irregular nuclear outlines Prominent nucleoli

as the urologist's index of suspicion, will play an important role in the final decision. Considerable caution must be incorporated into any diagnosis of a low-grade lesion in the upper tract because of the therapeutic implications. Loss of a kidney because an atypical hyperplasia was originally diagnosed as a neoplasm is a serious false-positive consequence.

If the specimen is of optimal quality, the distinction between atypical urothelial hyperplasia (Fig. 10-9) and a low-grade neoplasm (Fig. 10-10) may be appreciated by noting the size of the nuclei, which are enlarged in carcinoma, as well as any coarsening of the nuclear chromatin.[37] In addition, large papillary fragments lend support to a malignant diagnosis.[38] Admittedly, years of diligent learning are necessary before one feels any degree of confidence in making such a distinction. Biopsy confirmation is clearly indicated before nephrectomy is performed. Careful follow-up is usually employed in the absence of radiographic evidence of a neoplasm in these borderline instances.

High-grade Lesions

Recognition of high-grade lesions is far easier than of the low-grade lesions simply because the well-established criteria for malignancy also apply to urinary tract cytology. When examining these cases, the cytology student (even the more experienced one) should take the opportunity to appreciate the subtle changes in nuclear shape that distinguish true grade I lesions, in which an oval or round configuration is retained, from grade II lesions, in which the first sign of neoplastic advancement is an irregular nuclear outline. Even in the face of bland chromatin, if there is mild anisonucleosis and consistent deviations in nuclear shape from oval or round, then the lesion can be considered a grade II carcinoma. In the slightly higher grade II lesions that approach classification as grade III lesions, the chromatin is obviously coarsened and irregularly distributed (Figs. 10-11 and 10-12). The nuclear size increases in such lesions, as does the overall size of the cell (Fig. 10-13). In tissue fragments (Fig. 10-14), definite disorganization and, often, mitotic figures are evident.

In grade III transitional cell carcinomas, anaplasia will be evident, even to the new student. All of the criteria of malignancy will be present (Fig. 10-15), and once again, the opportunity for comparison should be taken. In these higher grade lesions, differentiation into squamous and glandular cell types (Fig. 10-16) can be seen, but should not change the diagnosis from transitional or urothelial. These "metaplasias" are characteristic of this epithelium, especially when it becomes neoplastic. Even if mucin stains are positive, this finding should be interpreted cautiously, for a grade III papillary carcinoma with glandular features is treated in a considerably different manner from an adenocarcinoma of the bladder. The latter warrants cystectomy, whereas a high-grade papillary carcinoma can be treated conservatively, depending upon staging and clinical considerations.

Carcinoma In Situ

"The past preoccupation with the clinically apparent exophytic papillary neoplasms may prove to be a major error in identifying the enemy, if the aggressive clinical behavior of invasive bladder carcinoma originates in flat carcinoma in situ."[17] Our frame of reference for carcinoma in situ (CIS) unfortunately is

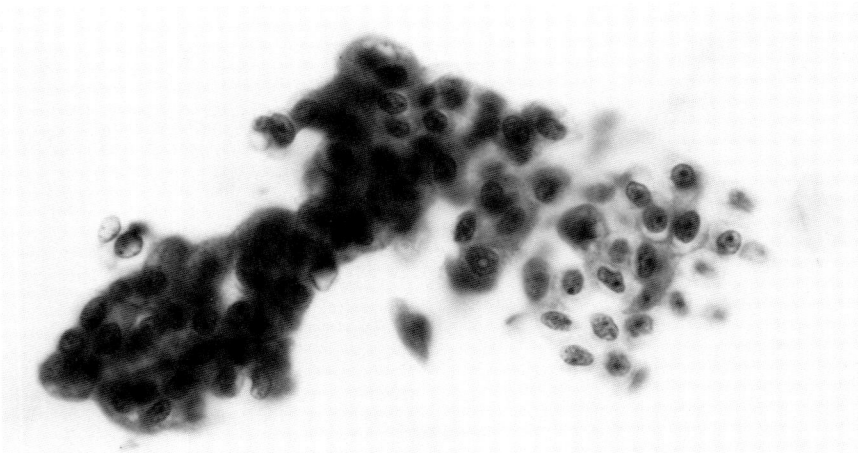

Fig. 10-11 Medium-grade transitional cell carcinoma (right ureteral brushing). This fragment is deceptive because the nucleocytoplasmic ratios are low, but the nuclear outlines are quite irregular, and an intranuclear inclusion can be identified in the middle. (See Fig. 10-12.) (Papanicolaou stain, × 400.)

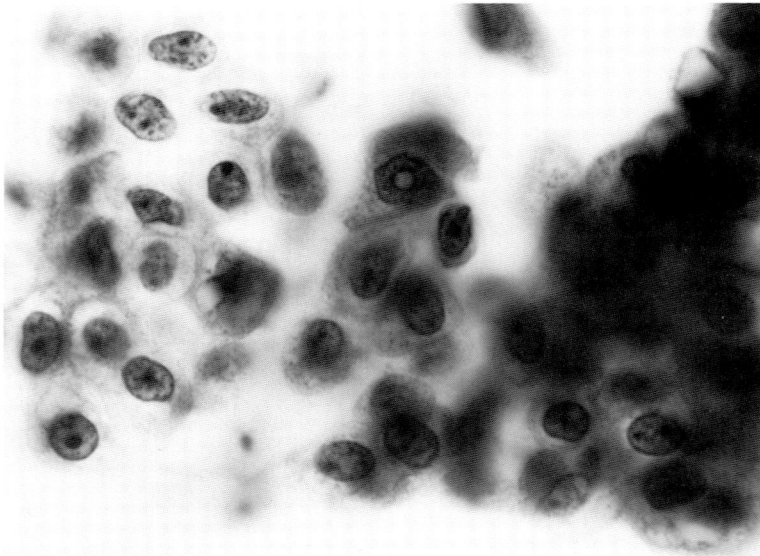

Fig. 10-12 Medium-grade transitional cell carcinoma (right ureteral brushing). Higher power view of Fig. 10-11 demonstrates the irregular nuclear outlines, the uneven chromatin distribution and particle size, and the prominent intranuclear inclusion. The honeycomb is still well preserved, which is the only characteristic that is not consistent with a malignant lesion. (Papanicolaou stain, × 1,000.)

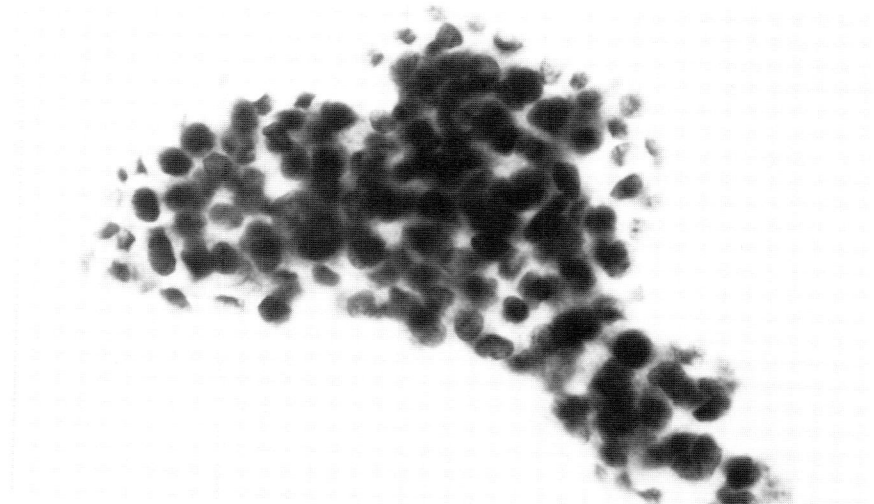

Fig. 10-13 Medium-grade transitional cell carcinoma (bladder washing). This three-dimensional fragment of urothelium is difficult to visualize because of its thickness. The crowding and three-dimensionality indicate neoplasm, whereas the enlarged size of the nuclei indicate the tumor grade. (Papanicolaou stain, × 400.)

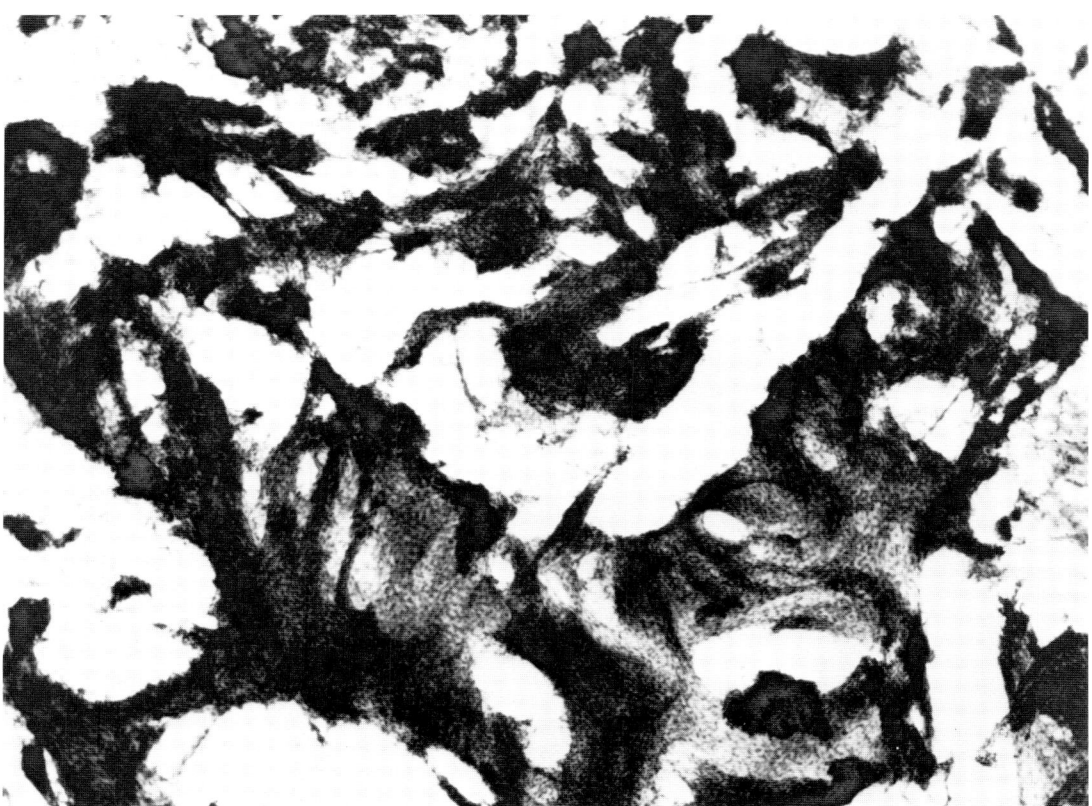

Fig. 10-14 Medium-grade transitional cell carcinoma (right ureteral brushing). A low power view of the case presented in Figs. 10-12 and 10-13 displays the abundant tissue obtainable by a brush inserted into a ureteral orifice. Although this is a somewhat delicate procedure, the yield is great. (Papanicolaou stain, × 40.)

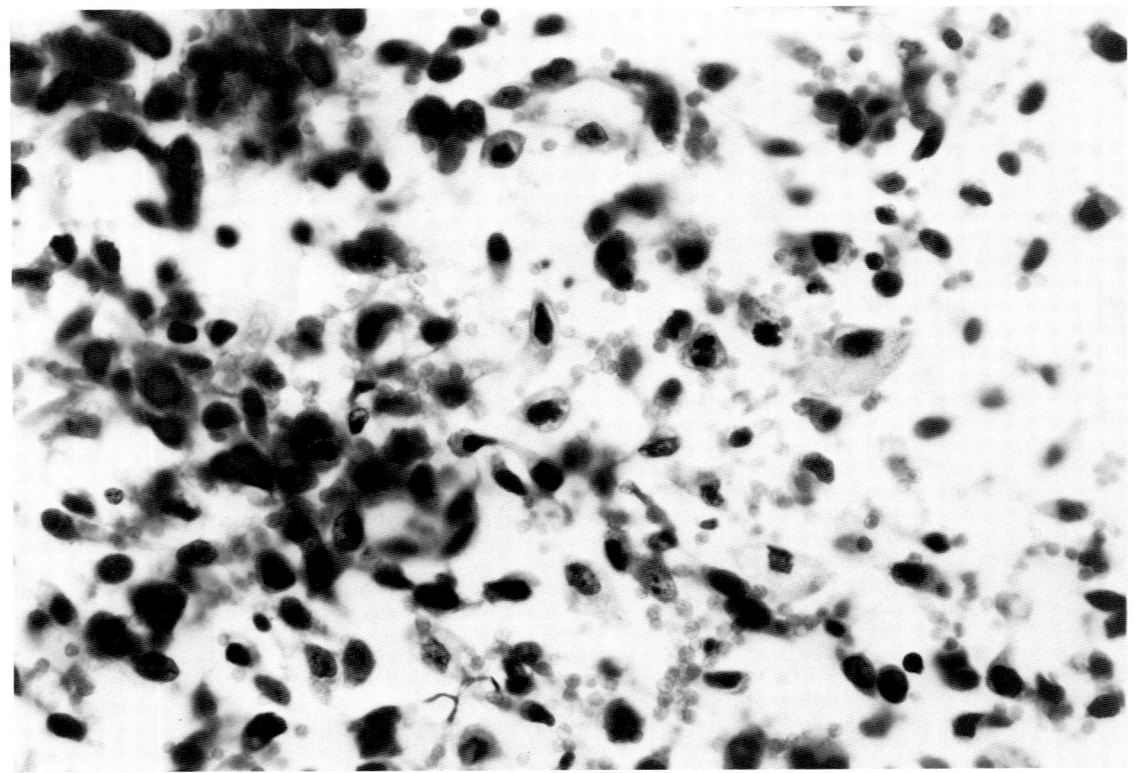

Fig. 10-15 High-grade transitional cell carcinoma, invasive (left kidney washing). These cells, obtained from the renal pelvis by a washing, are hyperchromatic and pleomorphic, and all cells occur singly. These characteristics all indicate a highly malignant disease process. Note the abundant blood in the background. (Papanicolaou stain, × 400.)

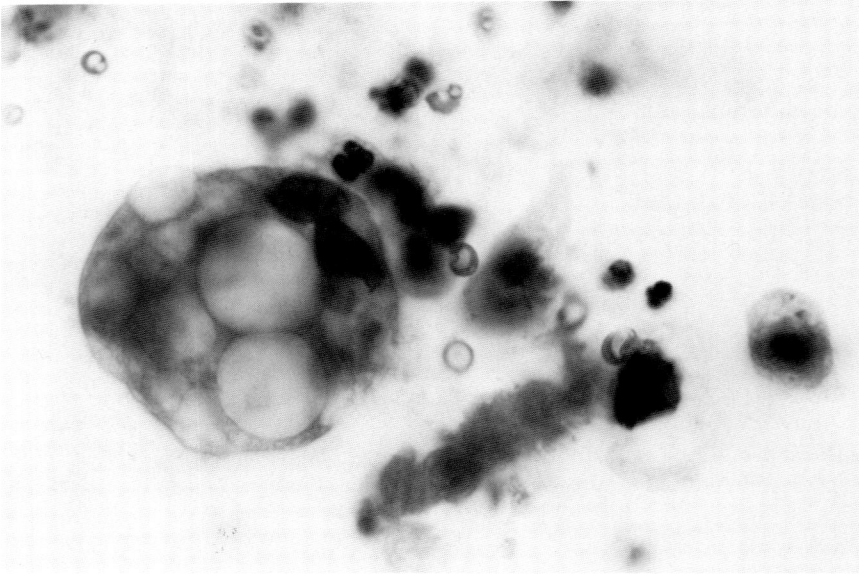

Fig. 10-16 High-grade transitional cell carcinoma with vacuoles (voided urine). Transitional cells can display features of both squamous and glandular cells, hence their name transitional. Vacuoles also can be caused by degeneration or treatment, either with chemical agents or radiation. The ultimate diagnosis is based on the predominant cell type and the pattern in tissue. (Papanicolaou stain, × 1,000.)

learned in the context of the lesion arising in the uterine cervix. Cervical CIS has a very long natural history, and many of the lesions never progress to invasive disease. Such is not the case with CIS of the urinary bladder.[39] This lesion is almost invariably of high grade, is rapidly invasive (generally within 3 years of diagnosis[17]), and is, therefore, ultimately fatal. Moreover, it often accompanies the more obvious low-grade lesions.[40] This combination provides a treacherous setting to the unwary physician. Fortunately, most urologists and cytopathologists are becoming educated about this lesion, its detection, and management. Koss wisely emphasizes that "carcinoma in situ is a primary target for cytologic diagnosis."[11] Although he still considers CIS to be a "precursor lesion," Koss emphasizes the importance of considering the entire urinary tract as being suspect for CIS whenever a lower grade papillary carcinoma is detected. He states that "the status of the peripheral epithelium of the bladder must be determined by cytology of the urinary sediment and by multiple biopsies . . . in all patients with neoplastic diseases of the bladder."[11]

Indeed, perhaps Koss' greatest contribution to pathology has been his emphasis on the variety of grades of urologic neoplasms that can be found in a single individual's bladder. His technique of "bladder mapping"[41] gives testimony to his meticulous scientific approach, and has provided us with a clear understanding of urothelial neoplasia. Therefore, in any patient who either currently has a bladder tumor, or who has a history of one, the cytologic sample must not only be examined to verify the obvious—the grossly visible lesion—but it should be scrutinized carefully for even a few single cells that may indicate a high-grade lesion, the insidious CIS.

HISTOLOGIC CRITERIA

The diagnosis of flat (sessile) lesions is made difficult by the variable and often deceptive thinness of the mucosa, which may be 3 to 20 cells thick. Critical to the diagnosis is the atypia found in individual cells, as this correlates so closely with the cytologic findings. Although some authors have described a dysplastic precursor state[42] that essentially is equivalent to intraepithelial neoplastic lesions of the uterine cervix, the classic CIS lesion of the urinary bladder demonstrates enlarged cells, a high nuclear/cytoplasmic ratio, nuclei that display hyperchromasia, irregular nuclear membranes, and disoriented polarity. The overall impression of the urothelium is one of pleomorphic disorganization.[17]

CYTOLOGIC CRITERIA

As the name implies, CIS is not associated with invasion; therefore, the background of any sample will be without blood and without significant inflammation or cellular debris. The cells of a CIS classically shed singly, are enlarged to a size that is at least four times that of normal basal urothelial cells, and have very high nuclear/cytoplasmic ratios, irregularly clumped chromatin, irregular nuclear outlines, and often, prominent nucleoli (Figs. 10-17 and 10-18).

When the sample is obtained by catheterization or washing, tissue fragments may be present, and these should be carefully examined to appreciate the enlarged nuclear size, the increased nuclear/cytoplasmic ratios, and the other features just mentioned, as well as evidence of disorganized growth. The background will indicate that the lesion is in situ, the cytologic details of the cells will suggest the appropriate high grade, and the combination of these two factors should prompt the observer to diagnose CIS.

In view of Koss' emphasis on the multiplicity of urothelial lesions within a given patient's bladder,[16,41] the microscopist should attempt to sort out the variety of cells and tissue fragments that might be present in a sample, sharing with the clinician as much information as possible.

Special Circumstances

ILEAL LOOP

A common technique following cystectomy or ureteral diversion performed because of obstruction by an inoperable neoplasm is construction of a loop of ileum into a "bladder." The stoma exits through the skin, and an external collecting bag is utilized by the patient. With this approach, patients can expect a longer survival than if the bladder lesion were allowed to invade, or their ureters were allowed to obstruct and destroy the kidneys.

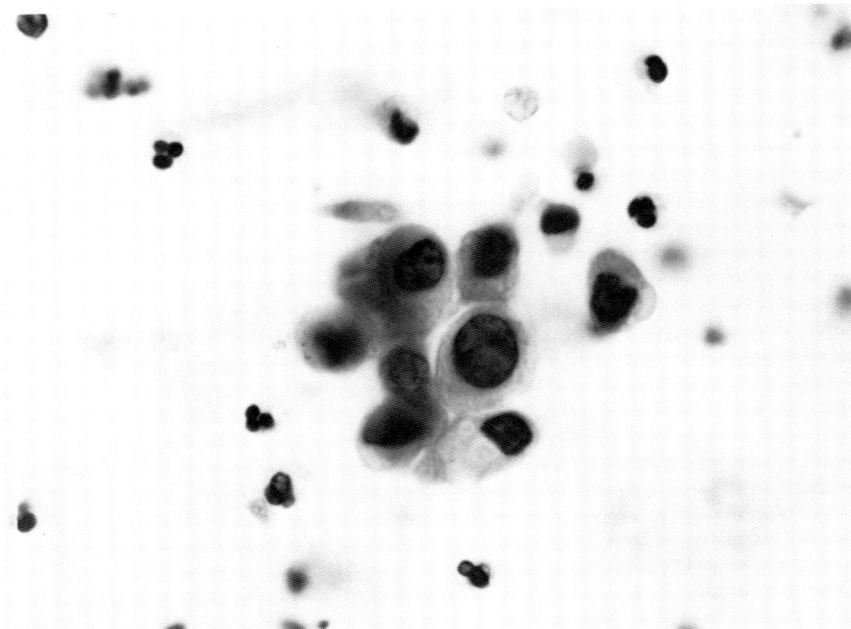

Fig. 10-17 High-grade transitional cell carcinoma (voided urine). The grade of these cells is established by their nuclear/cytoplasmic ratio, their hyperchromasia, and their irregular distribution of nuclear chromatin. If there is no significant inflammation or cellular debris in the background, these cells would qualify as originating in an in situ lesion. (Papanicolaou stain, × 1,000.)

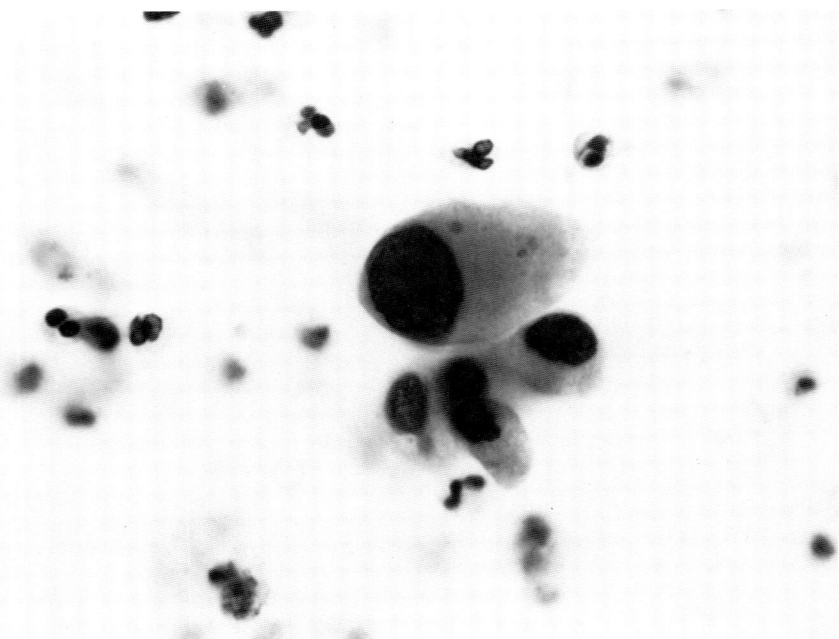

Fig. 10-18 High-grade transitional cell carcinoma (voided urine). Although most high-grade lesions have a very high nuclear/cytoplasmic ratio, occasionally, cells will have abundant cytoplasm, usually with an eccentrically placed nucleus. The size of the cell and the quality of the nucleus indicates the diagnosis of the high-grade lesion. (Papanicolaou stain, × 1,000.)

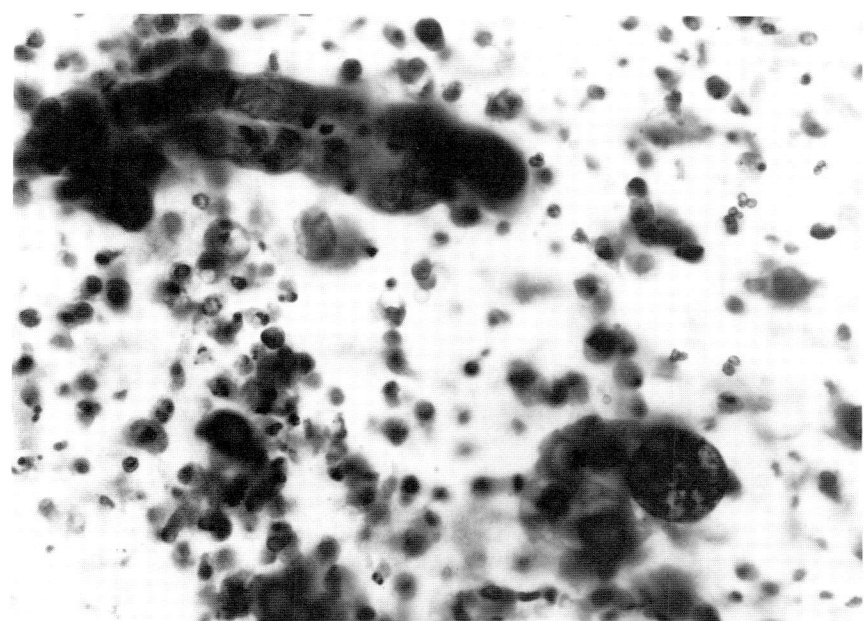

Fig. 10-19 High-grade transitional cell carcinoma (ileal loop urine). In the background of this cellular smear are numerous, small, round cells with features suggestive of a histiocytic origin. Most, however, are ileal columnar cells that have undergone degeneration secondary to toxic urine. In addition, capillary fragments and large malignant cells characteristic of a high-grade lesion are present in this specimen. (Papanicolaou stain, × 400.)

The cytologist must sort through the abundance of ileal mucosal fragments, which often are degenerated and almost unrecognizable as glandular epithelium, to find any recurrent, residual, or new tumor cells[43] (Fig. 10-19). If the specimen is freshly prepared, the stain good, and the smears thin enough, this is not too difficult to accomplish. If there is any suspicion of tumor, a repeat specimen is certainly indicated. The major problem occurs when neoplastic cells are found; the ureters are difficult to cannulate through the ileal mucosa, so that retrograde samples are not so easily obtained as when the ureters empty into the bladder. Therefore, the site of tumor cell origin may not be determined. An IVP may be the only way to localize the lesion.

LITHIASIS

The diagnostic problems posed by urinary calculi are well established.[11,12] Passage of a stone provokes not only blood and inflammatory cells, but nuclear irregularities and hyperchromasia that can mimic carcinoma. Fortunately, the cytologic changes usually subside, virtually disappearing once the calculus is passed. Therefore, if a history of stones is elicited and the cytology is highly atypical, an interval of a few weeks between collection of the questionable specimen and the next collection usually clarifies the issue. If the atypia persists, a neoplasm should be excluded, as there is an increased incidence of renal pelvic neoplasms in patients with a history of renal pelvic calculi.

Drug-Induced Cytologic Atypia

DRUGS USED FOR TREATMENT OF UROTHELIAL NEOPLASMS

Once a diagnosis of CIS is made, the clinician and patient are faced with the decision of cystectomy or conservative treatment. For most patients, cystectomy is a last resort, and three drugs have proven to be variably efficacious for the control of high-grade in situ lesions of the bladder. These drugs,—Bacille Calmette-Guérin (BCG) vaccine, mitomycin, and thiotepa—result in an inflammatory reaction that produces atypia of the urothelium (detailed later) and, in the case of BCG, submucosal granulomas. At UCLA, the most success has been achieved with BCG and mitomycin, with the former being less expensive.

DRUGS USED FOR TREATMENT OF SYSTEMIC ILLNESS, AND NOT SPECIFICALLY FOR UROTHELIAL DISORDERS

The prototype of drug-induced cellular atypia in patients without urothelial disorders is cyclophosphamide (Cytoxan), a drug commonly used in patients with lymphoproliferative neoplasms. The drug can produce an idiosyncratic reaction that is characterized by hemorrhagic cystitis, as the drug is excreted in toxic quantities in the urine. There is no correlation between the cytologic atypia and the drug dosage, and although the changes may regress, a few cases have been reported to progress to invasive carcinoma.

CYTOLOGIC CRITERIA

The cytologic changes secondary to pharmacologic agents resemble those caused by radiation reaction, but are more pronounced[44] (Fig. 10-20). There is variable cell enlargement with some preservation of the nuclear/cytoplasmic ratio, although the nuclear enlargement usually precedes the cytoplasmic changes. The enlarged nucleus may be eccentric and irregularly shaped, with marked hyperchromasia and coarse, evenly distributed chromatin, presenting a "salt and pepper" appearance. The nucleolus may be enlarged and distorted in the very early stages. Later, nuclear pyknosis and karyorrhexis, or a large and hyperchromatic nucleus with glassy chromatin, may result.

As in radiation-induced changes, the cytoplasm is often vacuolated and sometimes contains particles of foreign material or neutrophils. Aberrant cytoplasmic shapes are frequently encountered. The most severe changes may "imitate urothelial carcinoma to perfection."[11]

In addition to cyclophosphamide, busulfan has also been reported to produce severe cytologic atypia. As a practical rule of thumb, whenever a patient has a

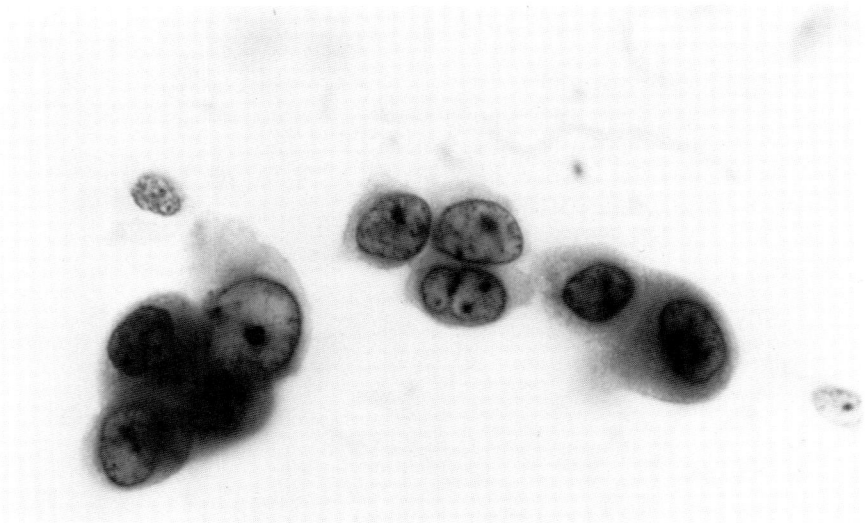

Fig. 10-20 Urothelial atypia secondary to therapy (catheterized urine). These large cells can easily be mistaken for those of a high-grade lesion. However, the chromatin is fine, and the total chromatin complement of the cell nucleus is low. Nucleoli are prominent, further attesting to the reactive stage of the cell. (Papanicolaou stain, × 1,000.)

history of using a cytotoxic agent, the urothelium may be a "target organ," and any cytologic changes must be viewed with skepticism.

Radiation-induced Cytologic Atypia

Many of the cytologic changes produced by external radiation, and described in samples from the female genital tract, are also seen in urinary samples containing irradiated cells. These changes may include cellular enlargement with preservation of the nuclear/cytoplasmic ratio in benign cells, nuclear hyperchromasia, multinucleation, and cytoplasmic vacuolization. However, these changes can also be seen in urothelial cells that have not undergone irradiation; these changes probably reflect a generalized reactive phenomenon. In a well-controlled study, Loveless[45] found that the most reliable change reflecting radiation effect on bladder epithelial cells was marked cellular enlargement. The distinction between radiation change in benign and malignant cells is based on the well-accepted nuclear criteria of malignancy.

Unusual Lesions

The limits of this text preclude a complete description of the variety of obscure lesions that may occur in the urinary tract. The interested reader is referred to the classic text of Koss[12] and other books relating to urinary cytology.

Squamous carcinoma and *adenocarcinoma,* both of which are infrequent cell types in the bladder, have the same characteristics in the urinary tract as they do elsewhere in the body. The microscopist should resist the temptation to call a urothelial lesion "squamous" or "glandular" when areas of squamous or glandular metaplasia are encountered in an otherwise clear-cut transitional cell carcinoma, as the treatment is much more aggressive for nontransitional cell lesions.

Renal cell carcinoma rarely sheds into the urine, and then only at a late stage, so that urinary cytology is not an appropriate screening test for that lesion. In our experience, cells of renal cell carcinoma, classically described as having very prominent nucleoli,[11,12] may not always present in such a clear-cut manner. The deceptively small and inconspicuous nucleoli that are often present in cells of this lesion can be very misleading (Fig. 10-21). Clinical setting

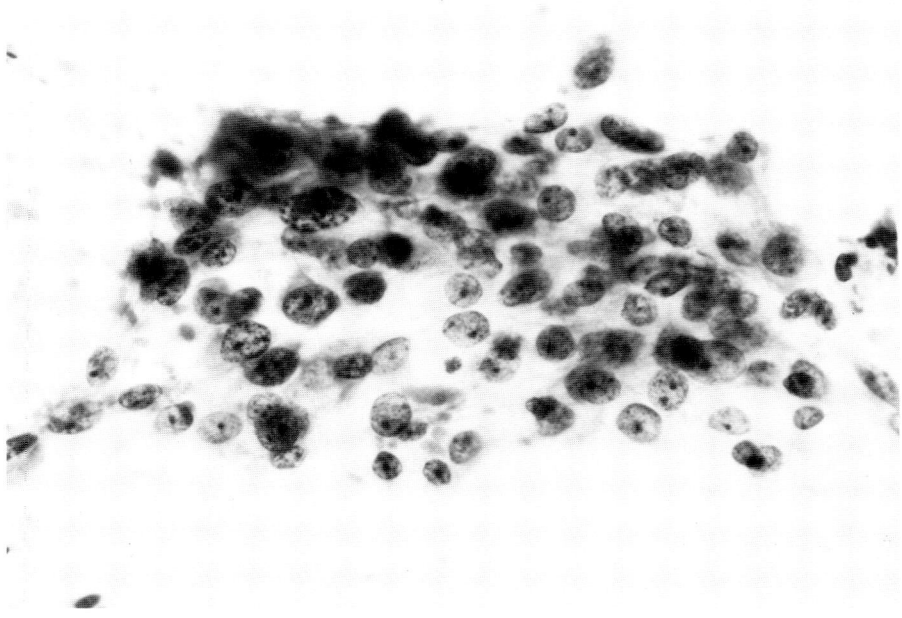

Fig. 10-21 Renal cell carcinoma metastatic to bone (FNA). Sheets of monomorphous cells with delicate cytoplasm could be from any epithelial malignant lesion. Contrary to popular teaching, renal cell carcinomas do not always have extremely prominent nucleoli. The clinical history must be determined before a definitive diagnosis is reached. (Papanicolaou stain, × 400.)

and index of suspicion are of great assistance in establishing an accurate diagnosis in such cases.

Metastatic lesions to the urinary bladder and ureters must immediately be considered when the history is consistent with such a diagnosis and when an unexpected cell population is found. The rectum, uterus, vagina, and prostate are contiguous, and may be a source of direct spread (Figs. 10-22 to 10-24). Drop metastases into the pouch of Douglas or on the dome of the bladder originate at distant sites; a complete and accurate history obviously is necessary to include such lesions in the differential diagnosis.

Correlation Between Cytology and Histology

In most organ systems from which specimens are obtained for both cytologic and histologic examination, there is a correlation between the cytologic and histologic diagnosis if the samples are obtained correctly. The urinary tract, on the contrary, is often a source of much frustration for both the clinician and the pathologist. In our experience and that of others,[6] a year may elapse between the initial "positive" cytologic diagnosis indicating a urothelial neoplasm and the confirming biopsy. In the interim, multiple negative biopsies may be obtained before the elusive source of the malignant cells is found. After a few such experiences shared by a confused urologist and an initially embarrassed pathologist, the urologist may well begin treatment of such patients based on the cytologic findings, even without a confirming tissue diagnosis. Such is the practice at UCLA.

Even more serious is the case in which there is cytologic evidence of an invasive lesion, evidenced by neoplastic cells, blood, and necrotic debris, but a tissue biopsy will not verify the diagnosis. Then, the

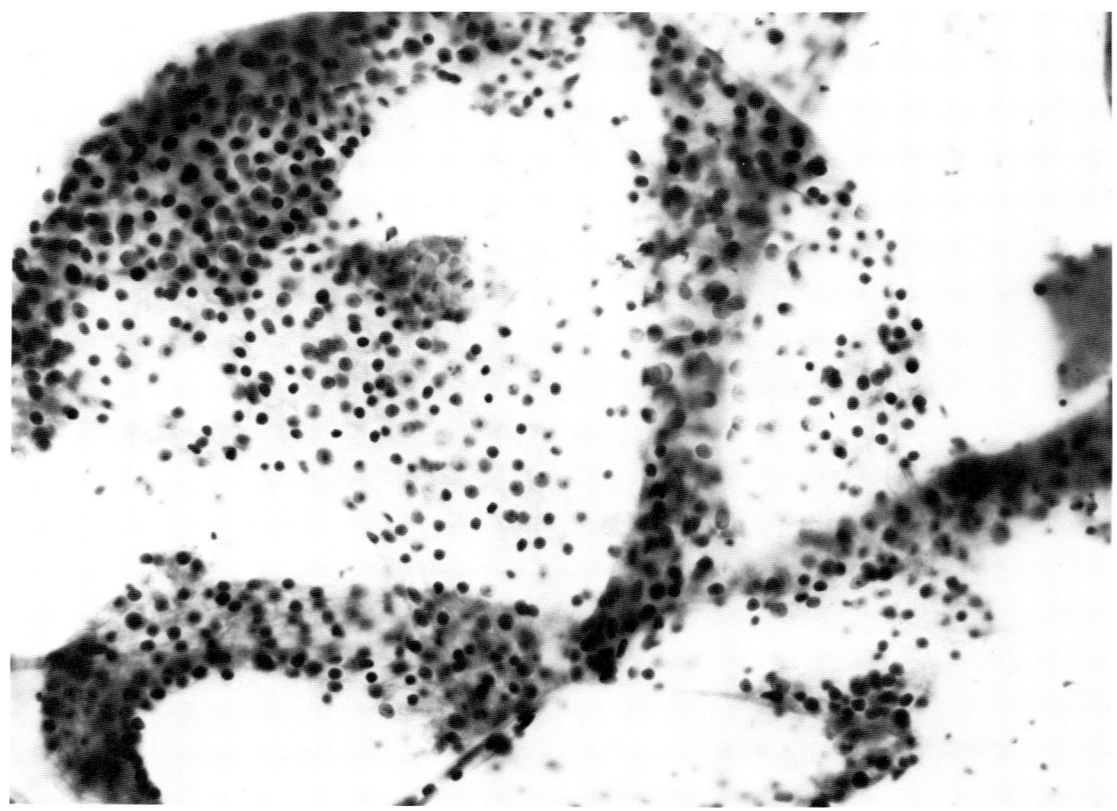

Fig. 10-22 Prostatic adenocarcinoma metastatic to the bladder (bladder washing). When carcinoma from elsewhere invades the bladder, the difference between those cells and the urothelial cells needs to be appreciated. The roundness of the nuclei is obvious on low power magnification, and is contrary to the oval nuclei expected in transitional carcinoma. (Papanicolaou stain, × 200.)

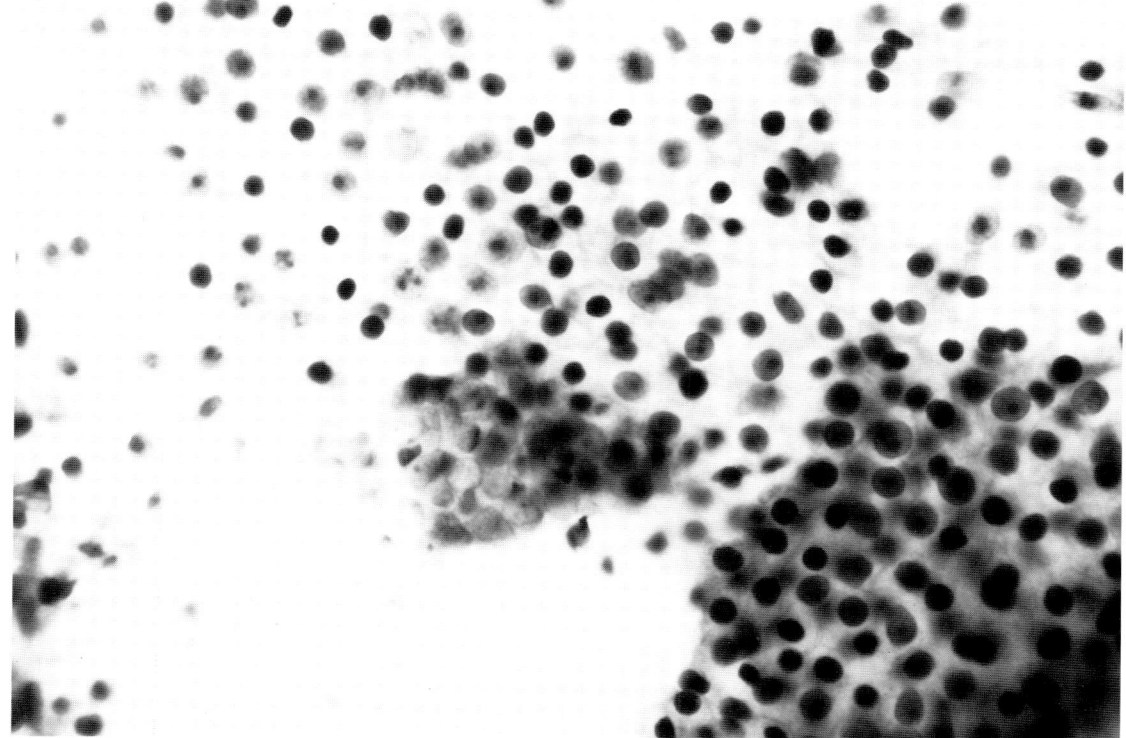

Fig. 10-23 Prostatic adenocarcinoma metastatic to the bladder (bladder washing). Although a honeycomb pattern is preserved, the enlarged, round nuclei with prominent nucleoli are quite unusual findings for transitional cell epithelium. (See Fig. 10-24.) (Papanicolaou stain, × 400.)

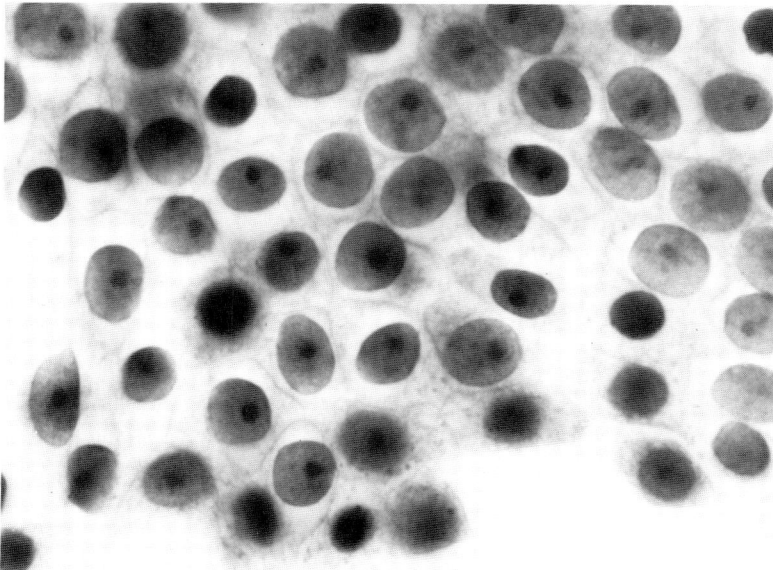

Fig. 10-24 Prostatic adenocarcinoma metastatic to the bladder (bladder washing). Inspection under oil discloses a uniformly fine chromatin, prominent nucleoli, a moderately high nuclear/cytoplasmic ratio, and a prominent honeycomb pattern. All of these are not expected from a neoplasm arising in the urothelium. These features are characteristic of prostatic adenocarcinoma. (Papanicolaou stain, × 1,000.)

ureters and upper tract should definitely be investigated, and if no radiologic evidence of a tumor is found, surgical exploration may be indicated. Thus, cytologic criteria must be very rigid and reliable.

Histologic and cytologic samples that are obtained at the same time or within temporal proximity should be examined together so that the source of any cytologic atypia can be determined. If the cytologic atypia is not accounted for, a comment to that effect should be included in the biopsy report so that the urologist knows that a further search must be conducted. As indicated earlier, a considerable amount of time may elapse between the discovery of significantly atypical cells in a urine sample and a final, verifying biopsy. Additionally, a biopsy from the bladder may reveal a low-grade lesion, whereas the cytology may suggest the presence of a high-grade lesion. Either a focus of CIS of the bladder must be sought, or a higher grade lesion within the upper tracts must be located. Therefore, an identical match between cytology and histology should be considered a "correlation." If even a moderate discrepancy is noted, the two diagnoses should be considered to be discordant.

Diagnostic Yield of Urinary Cytology

Perhaps the most well-summarized evaluation of the usefulness of urinary cytology in the detection of tumors of the urinary tract has been made by Farrow.[22] His data emphasize the low diagnostic yield obtained in low-grade papillary lesions, which contrasts with the excellent diagnostic yield for the high-grade lesions. Farrow further emphasizes the importance of correlating cystoscopic findings with cytologic changes to arrive at the optimal diagnosis for a given patient. Results from Farrow's study may be summarized as follows:

1. *Size of tumor*. The total surface area of a bladder tumor or tumors correlates with the cytologic result; that is, the greater the surface area, the more likely the diagnosis is to be "positive."
2. *Configuration of tumor*. Sessile (implying invasion) tumors and CIS lesions are more readily diagnosed than papillary tumors (a 73 percent "positive" rate for CIS or sessile versus a 37 percent "positive" rate for papillary lesions).
3. *Grade of tumor*. In 634 histologically confirmed tumors, the cytologic results were as follows:

   Grade I (98 patients)   22 percent "positive" results

   Grade II (291 patients)   62 percent "positive" results

   Grade III (215 patients)   84 percent "positive" results

   Grade IV (30 patients)   83 percent "positive" results

4. *Negative cystoscopy versus positive or suspicious cytology*. Most patients with initially negative results on cystoscopic examination and biopsy, but with significant cytologic atypia, were subsequently proven to have cancer somewhere in the urinary tract. The need for long-term follow-up of patients with abnormal urinary cytology should be emphasized.
5. *Overall reliability of urinary cytology for detection of bladder cancer*. The overall sensitivity rate was 66.6% (true positive results), and the overall specificity was 95.4% (true negative results).

Specimen Collection and Processing

Not to be minimized is the importance of the quality of the specimen submitted for microscopic examination. Each laboratory must decide the best way to collect and process specimens, depending upon the demands of the clinical setting.[46]

COLLECTION

The freshness of a specimen is the key to obtaining a urinary tract sample capable of providing a definitive diagnosis. If the clinical setting is not conducive to the immediate handling and processing of fresh specimens, then means should be provided for immediate fixation. Farrow[22] advocates the use of twice the volume of 70 percent ethyl alcohol to one volume of urine, with refrigeration if possible. No more than 8 hours should elapse before the specimen is processed. Patients should be instructed to empty their bladders before beginning the collection process. Hydration over a 2- to 3-hour period after the initial morning voiding (which is discarded) can produce a high-volume specimen of good quality provided processing is prompt. Some advocate that the patient jump up and down to agitate the cells, thereby facilitating an abundant collection of cells.

The collection of samples over a prolonged period, such as in 24-hour collections, results in a useless specimen, as cells deteriorate in the toxic urine within a very short period of time. Specific instructions for collection should be readily available in clinics and on wards so that optimal specimens are presented to the cytologist.

I acknowledge that catheterization carries some risk for infection. However, the value of obtaining a fresh catheterized specimen, especially in a female patient, far outweighs the risk of a urinary tract infection if the catheterization procedure is carefully performed.

Finally, if urinary cytology is to be diagnostic, the samples obtained by irrigation (washings) are definitely preferred in those patients in whom a neoplasm is suspected, either on the basis of clinical data or previous urine cytologic examinations. The difference between a carefully obtained, freshly prepared specimen from a bladder washing and a sample obtained from spontaneous voiding of urine is considerable.[47,48] In fact, I will not render a "positive" diagnosis on the basis of a voided urine unless the cytologic changes are so characteristic of a high-grade lesion and so unequivocal that a novice could make the diagnosis. On the other hand, reliable diagnoses, including those involving low-grade lesions, can be made using irrigation specimens from the upper tract.

PROCESSING

Rapid processing of unfixed specimens is mandatory. If specimens must be prefixed, fixation artifact and various changes produced by the technique should be considered when choosing an appropriate procedure.[49] Whether one chooses to smear the centrifuged sediment, utilize membrane filters, or Cytocentrifuge[50] (or any combination of those procedures), cell loss and staining techniques should be controlled carefully.

FINE NEEDLE ASPIRATION OF THE PROSTATE GLAND

Fine needle aspiration (FNA) of the prostate has been received with variable enthusiasm since Franzen invented a flexible transrectal needle and needle guide in 1960.[51] He and his colleagues at the Karolinska Institute have performed FNA with great success, but because of considerable controversy over the ultimate worth of the procedure to the patient, the prostate has not been subjected to FNA as often or as extensively as have other organs (e.g., the breast and thyroid).

Various methods exist for obtaining tissue from the prostate, including open perineal biopsy, transrectal and transperineal aspiration by thick needles, and transurethral resection. Prostatic massage to express exfoliated cells has not been considered to be a successful method of examining the prostatic epithelium. At UCLA, as well as in the hands of its proponents, FNA via the transrectal route (and as advocated by Franzen) has yielded excellent results, especially when one considers that the most significant lesions of the prostate occur in the posterior lobes and subcapsular areas, both of which are easily accessible to the transrectal FNA route.

Technical Aspects

For a complete description of the technique of transrectal FNA using the Franzen needle and guide, the reader is referred to the works of Linsk,[52] and Zajicek.[51] Suffice it to say that the technique requires practice, a thorough understanding of the anatomy involved, and experience with palpating prostatic masses. Most urologists, once convinced of the technique's worth, are easily trained to obtain good results. However, at UCLA, we still believe that the best results are obtained by those who perform a large number of FNAs; therefore, our pathologists obtain the samples at the request of the urologists.

Histologic Grading

Currently, the grading systems established for prostatic adenocarcinoma are quite complex, and are not necessary for an accurate cytologic diagnosis. We and others[19,53] have found that a simple grading sys-

324 PRACTICAL CYTOPATHOLOGY

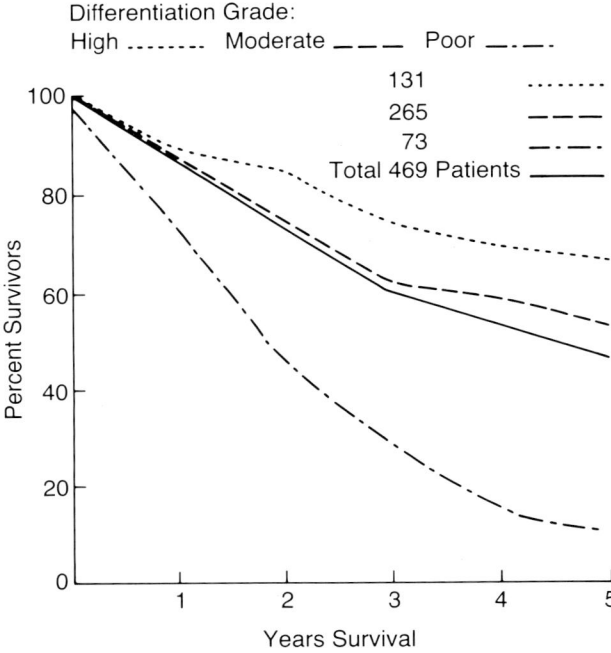

Fig. 10-25 Prostatic carcinoma (FNA) results. Graphic representation of the correlation between the ultimate outcome of patients and the grade of their prostatic carcinoma. The descriptive terms "high," "moderate," and "poor" mean "well-differentiated," "moderately differentiated," and "poorly differentiated," respectively. (From Willems and Löwhagen,[53] with permission.)

tem of I to III, representing well-differentiated, moderately differentiated, and poorly differentiated adenocarcinoma, categorizes the lesions commonly seen with prostatic FNA. In fact, Willems and Lowhagen,[53] who have correlated prognosis with a simple grading classification, have shown that the outcome of the patient is as predictable using this scheme as it is using the more complicated grading systems currently in vogue (Fig. 10-25).

The cytologic criteria for the three grades of prostatic adenocarcinoma are displayed in Table 10-3. Significant features to note, and those that correspond to increasing severity of grade on histologic examination, are the increased size and atypia of the nuclei, the increasing prominence of the nucleoli, and the loss of acinar pattern. These findings translate into the cytologic features described in the following section.

Cytologic Features

The most notable cytologic feature of prostatic carcinoma is the transformation within the smear pattern from uniform, small cells in microacini to disorganized epithelial groups of pleomorphic cells. Other features that are not appreciated on histologic examination relate to the pattern of distribution of the cells on the smear. In order to appreciate the transformation from benign to malignant, the benign lesions must be considered first (Table 10-4).

BENIGN PROSTATIC HYPERPLASIA

In cases of benign prostatic hyperplasia, the gross appearance of the aspirate on the slide is that of a watery fluid with some colloidal particles. Once stained, the prostatic epithelium assumes a monolayered pattern on the slide. These monolayers are delicate, diaphanous sheets of uniformly sized and dispersed epithelial cells (Fig. 10-26) with a very ob-

Table 10-3 Grading of Prostatic Adenocarcinoma

	Well-Differentiated	Moderately Differentiated	Poorly Differentiated
Microacinar pattern	+++	++	+/−
Dispersal of cells	+/−	+	++/+++
Nuclei			
Enlargement	+	++	+++
Polymorphy	+	++	+++
Nucleoli	+/−	++	+++

Table 10-4 General Microscopic Features of Prostatic Neoplasms

	Benign	Malignant
Pattern	Monolayers	Multilayers
Cytoplasm	Cohesive cells	Dispersed cells
	Well-defined borders	Ill-defined borders
	Red granules[a]	Vacuoles
Nuclei	Round or oval	Large and polymorphic
	Normochromatic	Hyperchromatic
	Intact	Fragile (smeared)
Nucleoli	Absent	Present

[a] Romanowsky-stained specimens.

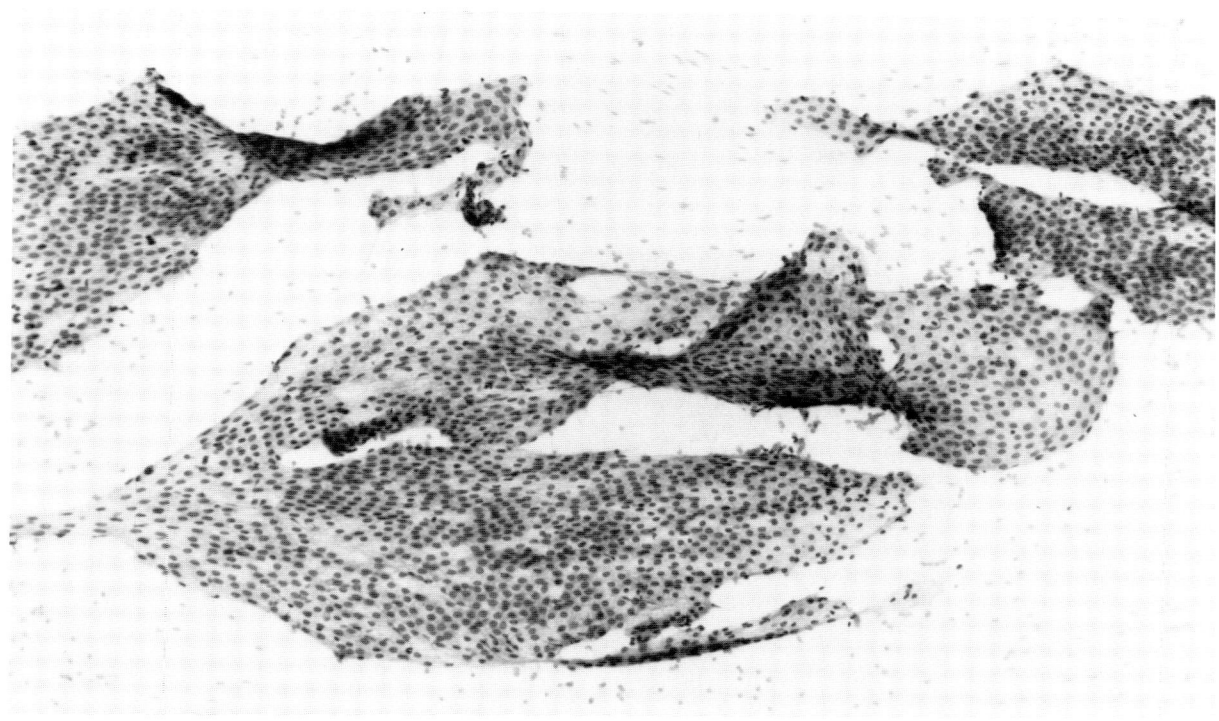

Fig. 10–26 Benign prostatic epithelium (FNA). Large, monolayered sheets of prostatic epithelial cells are characteristic of the epithelium of a benign mucosa. Only red blood cells are present in the background. (Papanicolaou stain, × 100.)

vious honeycomb pattern that corresponds to distinct cell borders, a finding that is characteristic of a benign lesion (Fig. 10-27). On Papanicolaou stain, the chromatin pattern is very fine, and nucleoli are absent or indistinct. On May-Grünwald-Giemsa (MGG) stain, cytoplasmic red granules may be seen, reinforcing a benign interpretation (Fig. 10-28).

ATYPICAL HYPERPLASIA

In all diagnostic schemes, cytologic atypia presents problems. The prostate is no exception, and the difficulty in distinguishing between atypical hyperplasia and well-differentiated adenocarcinoma is often impossible cytologically, as well as histologically. When such an equivocal cytologic diagnosis is rendered, a biopsy or repeat FNA within a short period of time is always a judicious recommendation. Cytologically, the difference between normal and atypical epithelium is most demonstrable in the crowding of the nuclei, which is produced by an increased nuclear/cytoplasmic ratio, and the three-dimensionality of cell groups in the latter. However, microacinar patterns should be absent, and nucleoli should not be discernible. If a microacinar pattern or micronucleoli are observed, a diagnosis of well-differentiated adenocarcinoma should be made.

PROSTATITIS

In cases of prostatitis, the gross appearance of the aspirate will vary depending upon how many inflammatory cells are present (Fig. 10-29), and it may resemble pus if the inflammation is severe. This type of situation is a contraindication for FNA. The microscopic appearance is that of an acute inflammatory reaction, similar to that which might be observed anywhere else in the body. The background is very dirty, being composed of neutrophils and, generally, some macrophages. The epithelium becomes atypical as it is involved in the inflammatory process (Fig. 10-30). Any diagnosis of cancer should be delayed until the inflammatory response resolves. If a diagnosis of adenocarcinoma is probable, either clinically or cytologically, urgent treatment is indicated, and a repeat biopsy following relief of the acute situation is a mandate.

Granulomatous Prostatitis

In granulomatous prostatitis, histiocytes, which are often multinucleated, are the prominent finding. (Fig. 10-31). Groups of fibroblasts and monocytes can also be aspirated in the sample. The epithelium may not be quite so atypical as in acute prostatitis, and the cell groups on the smears are usually fewer in number.

ADENOCARCINOMA

The gross appearance of the aspirate in cases of adenocarcinoma is textured, the result of small fragments of tissue suspended in a proteinaceous fluid. Table 10-3 presents the basic criteria for diagnosis of the various grades of adenocarcinoma. They can briefly be summarized as follows:

Grade I (well-differentiated) adenocarcinoma. Smears are cellular, with very few individual cells (Fig. 10-32). A microglandular pattern is variable but clearly evident (Figs. 10-33 and 10-34), and there are small, almost normal sized nuclei which are crowded. The honeycomb pattern is lost owing to indistinct cell borders. Nucleoli may be conspicuous, but are not necessarily large, and intracytoplasmic granules are usually absent.

Grade II (moderately differentiated) carcinoma. Cell cohesion is diminished, with an increased number of individual cells freely floating (Fig. 10-35). The reappearance of the monolayer (Fig. 10-36), as opposed to three-dimensional piling up of cell groups (as occurs in grade I), is apparent as cohesion is lessened, and the cells smear out more easily. Nuclei enlarge, the microacinar pattern is still present, and nucleoli become prominent.

Grade III (poorly differentiated) adenocarcinoma. Loss of cohesion is maximal, with many individual cells and very few cell groups present. Pleomorphism is prominent, nucleoli are large, and the honeycomb

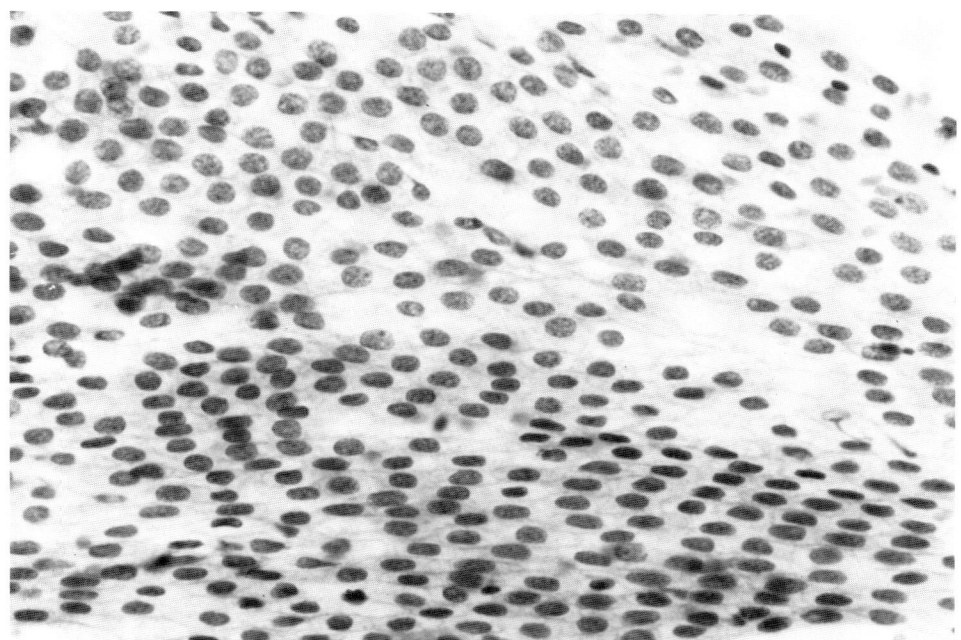

Fig. 10-27 Benign prostatic epithelium (FNA). A higher power view demonstrates the presence of a honeycomb pattern, as well as the uniformity of nuclear size and nuclear/cytoplasmic ratio. Nucleoli are inconspicuous, and a microacinar pattern is not evident. (Papanicolaou stain, × 400.)

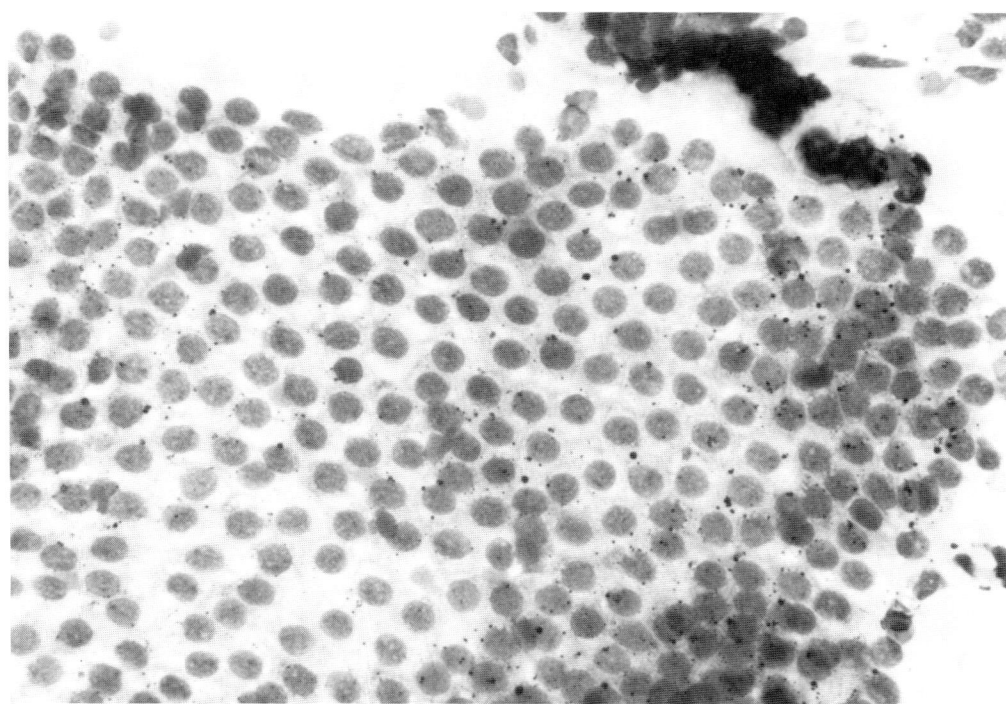

Fig. 10-28 Benign prostatic epithelium (FNA). The same benign epithelium as in Fig. 10-27, after air-drying and staining with MGG, demonstrates intracytoplasmic vacuoles, which stain red with MGG, a characteristic of benign prostatic epithelium. (MGG stain, × 400.)

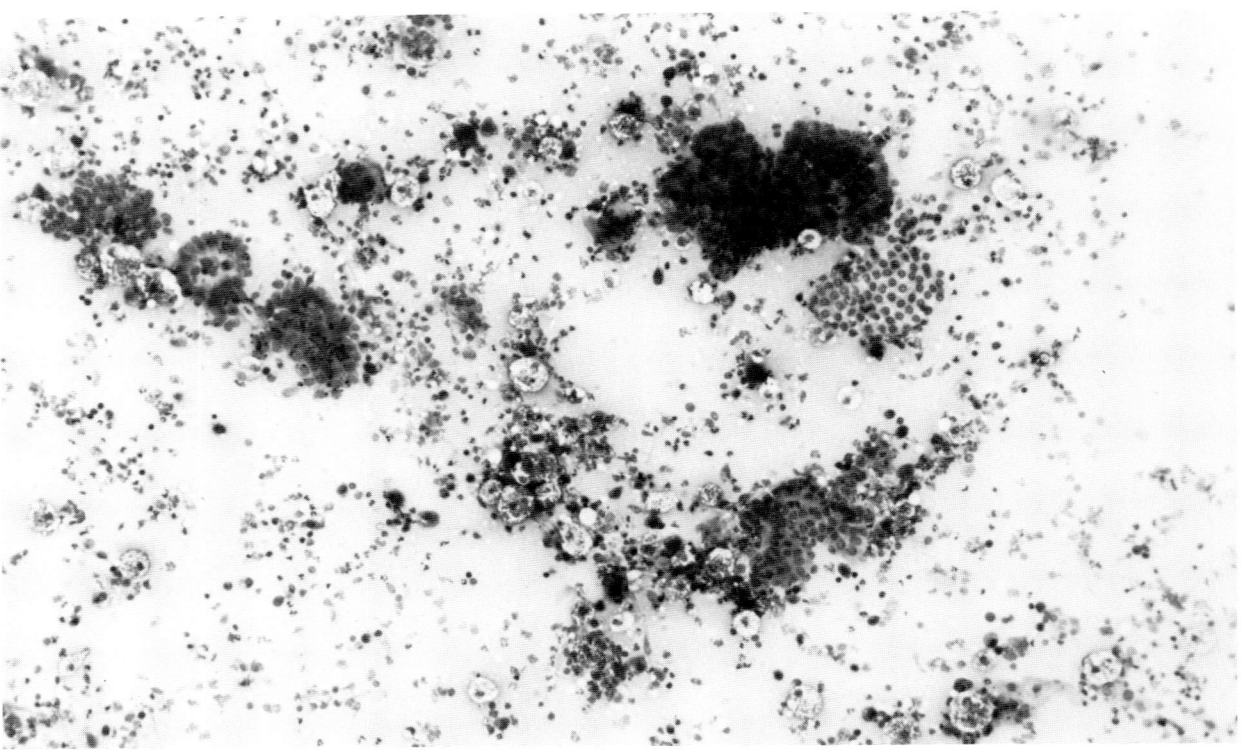

Fig. 10-29 Acute prostatitis (FNA). This highly cellular smear is characterized by large fragments of epithelium, numerous neutrophils, and foamy macrophages. (MGG stain, × 100.)

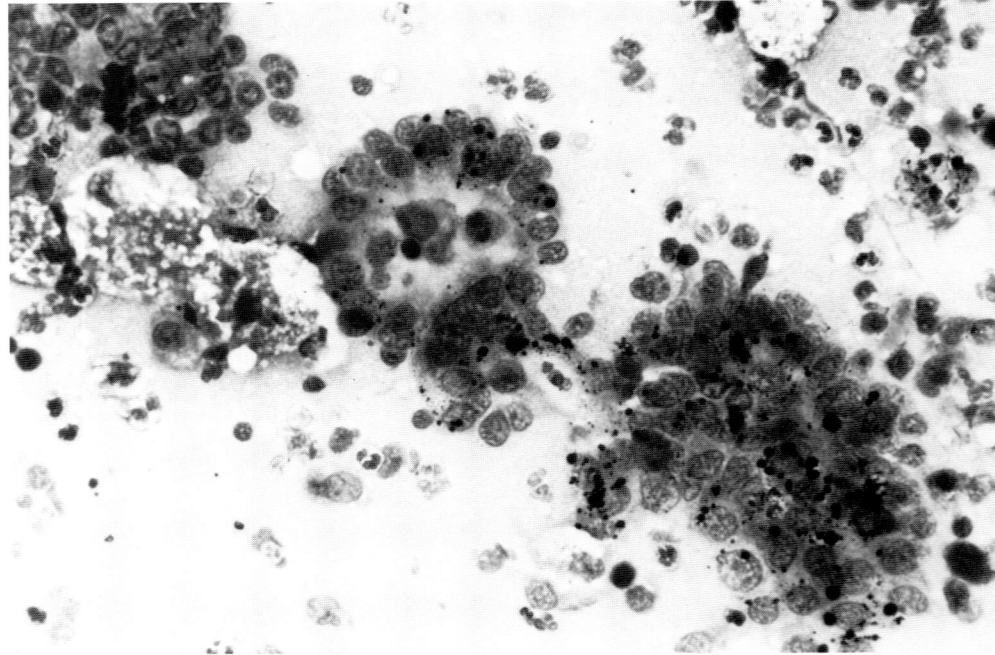

Fig. 10-30 Acute prostatitis (FNA). A higher power view demonstrates enlarged epithelial cells interspersed with intracytoplasmic granules, attesting to their benign nature. The foamy macrophages provide size contrast to the smaller neurophils. (MGG stain, × 400.)

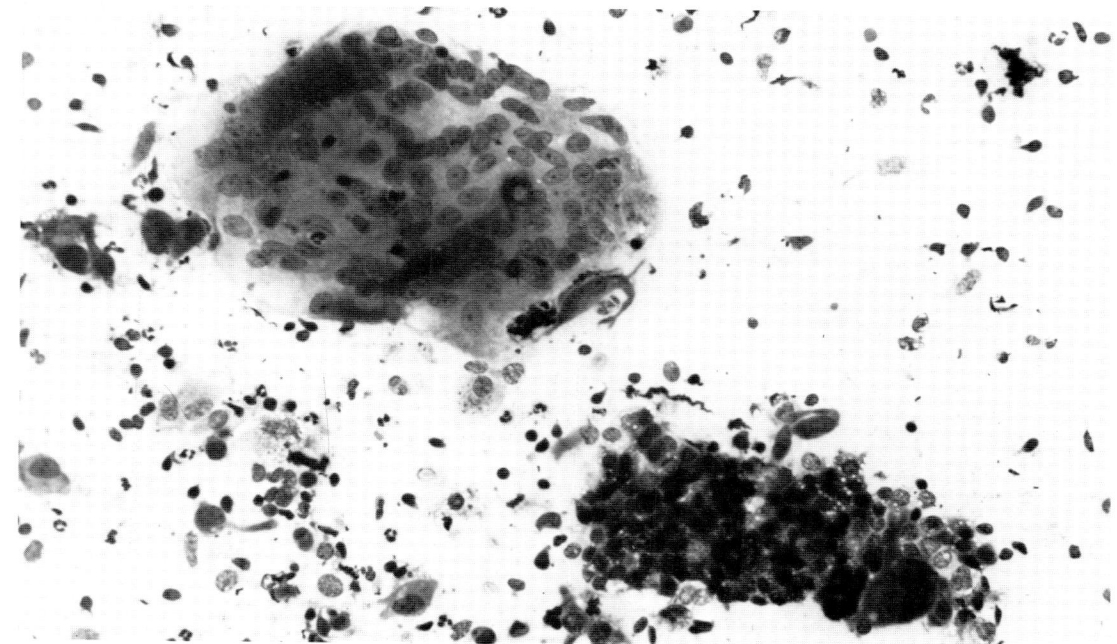

Fig. 10-31 Granulomatous prostatitis (FNA). This huge, multinucleated histiocyte indicates the correct diagnosis. Atypical epithelium, cell fragments, and a mixture of inflammatory cells complete the picture. Under no circumstances should a diagnosis of carcinoma be made when such profound inflammation is present (MGG stain, × 200.)

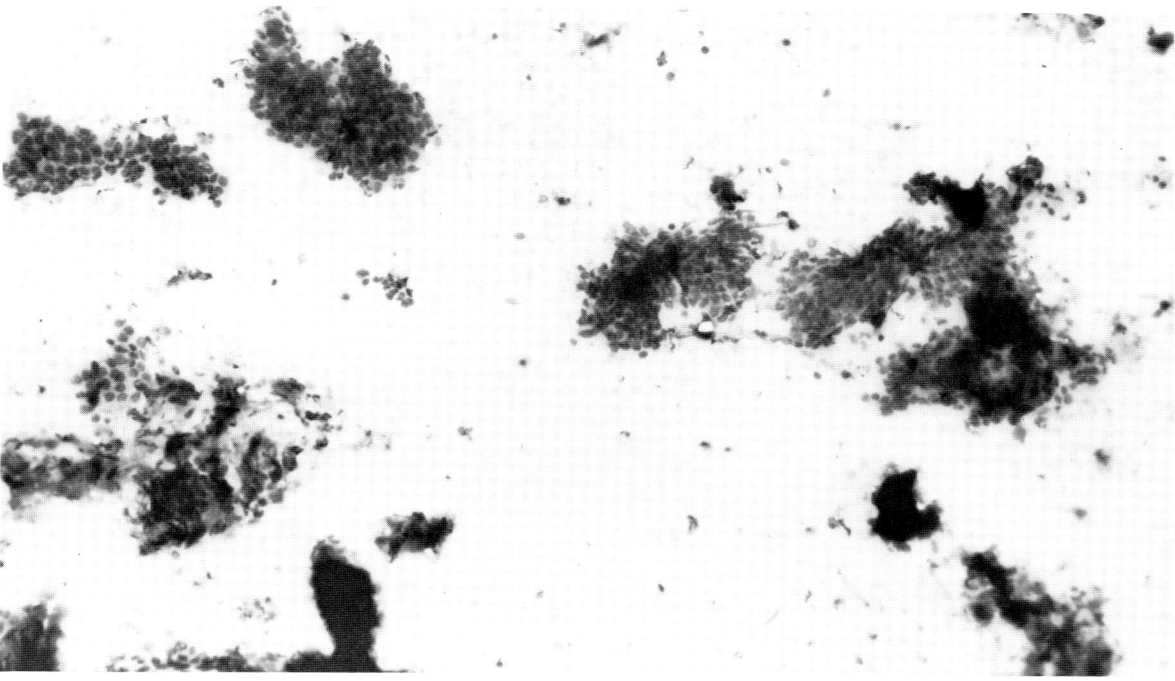

Fig. 10-32 Well-differentiated adenocarcinoma of the prostate (FNA). Against a bloody background are three-dimensional clusters of epithelial cells, with only a few scattered single cells or small groups of glandular cells. (MGG stain, × 100.)

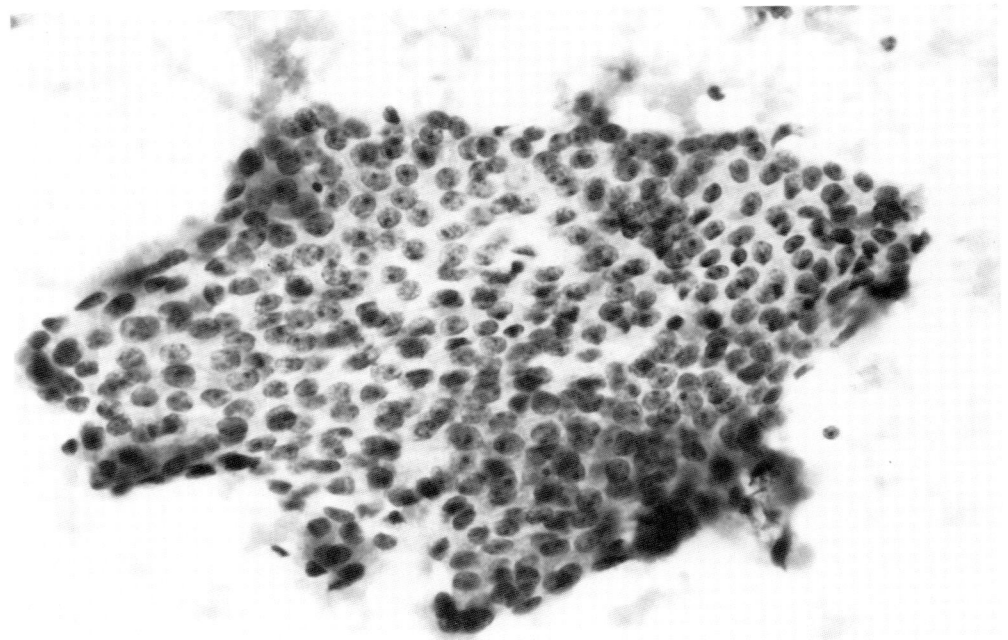

Fig. 10-33 Well-differentiated adenocarcinoma of the prostate (FNA). A higher power view of a tissue fragment from the sample shown in Fig. 10-23 demonstrates the enlarged nuclei, which are crowded and have prominent nucleoli. A microacinar pattern can be appreciated throughout the tissue fragment. (Papanicolaou stain, × 400.)

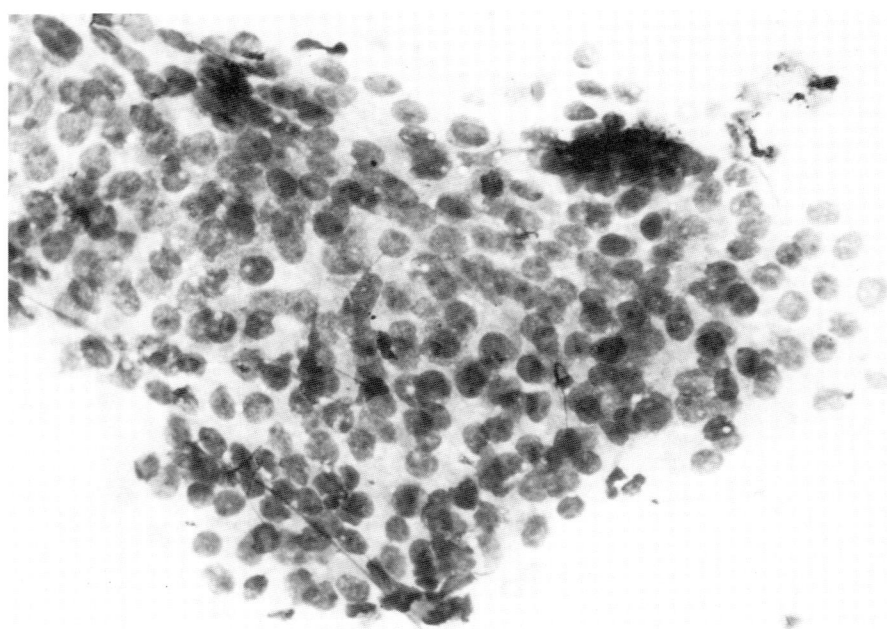

Fig. 10-34 Well-differentiated adenocarcinoma of the prostate (FNA). A fragment similar to that in Fig. 10-33, is air-dried and stained with a Romanowsky stain to exaggerate nuclear size and variability. The nuclei, because of air-drying, are larger than that seen in the Papanicolaou stain, but the other cellular features are still very prominent. Note the absence of intracytoplasmic granules. (MGG stain, × 400.)

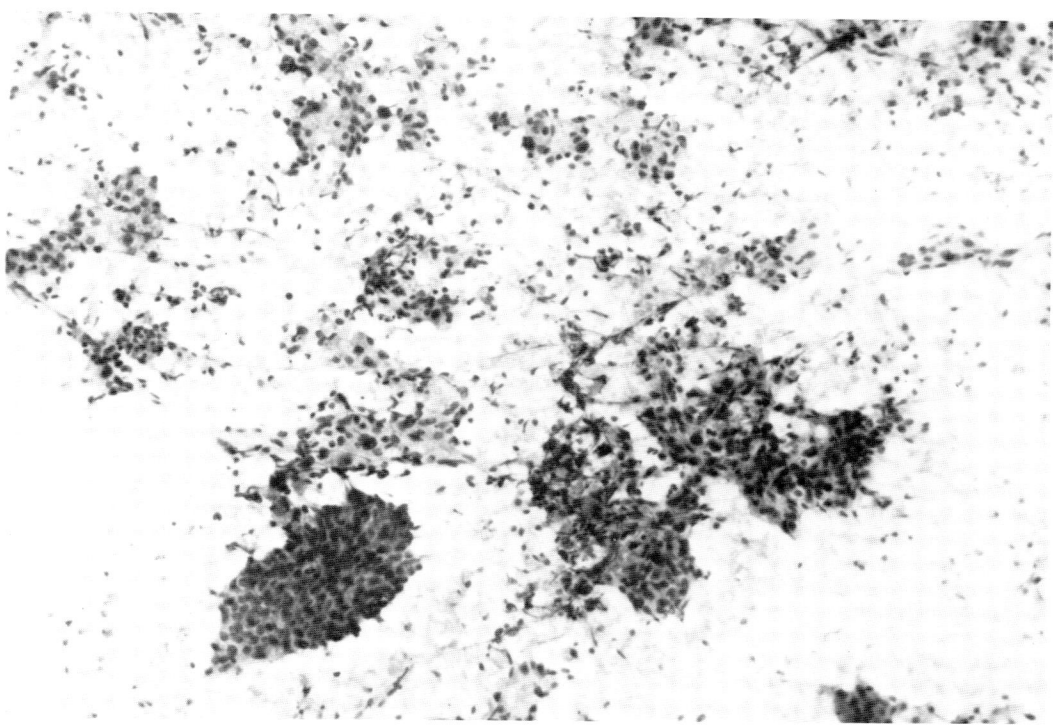

Fig. 10-35 Moderately to poorly differentiated adenocarcinoma (FNA). Note the cellularity of this smear, as well as the dispersal of the cell clusters. This smear pattern is as messy as that seen in inflammatory lesions, but on higher power, the nature of the dispersed cells (i.e., epithelial cells) can be appreciated in this cancerous lesion. (Papanicolaou stain, × 100.)

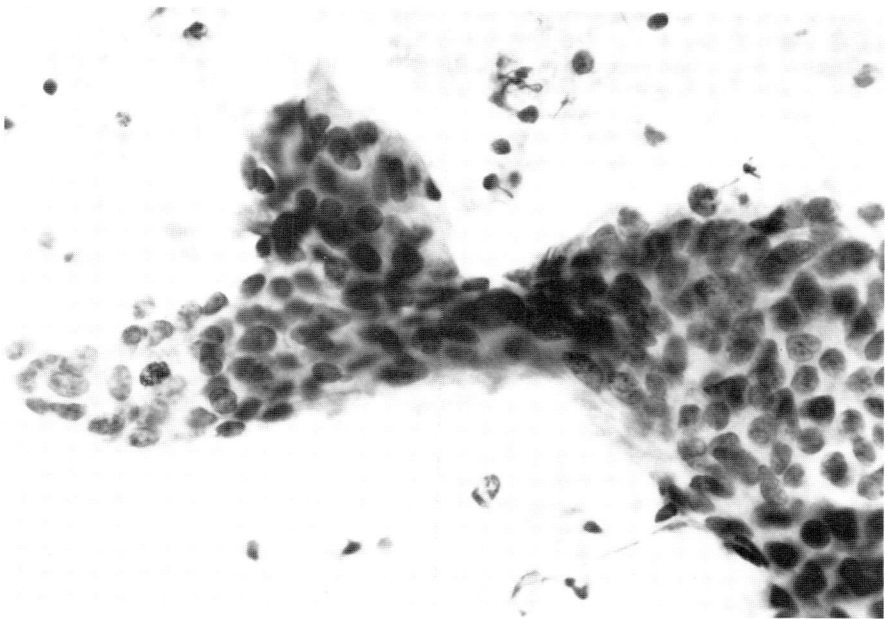

Fig. 10-36 Moderately to poorly differentiated adenocarcinoma (FNA). A higher power view of these neoplastic fragments discloses the three-dimensionality of the fragment, the irregular packing of the cells, and the presence of mitotic figures. In a higher-grade lesion, the microacinar pattern disappears, as does the order of the cell growth. (Papanicolaou stain, × 400.)

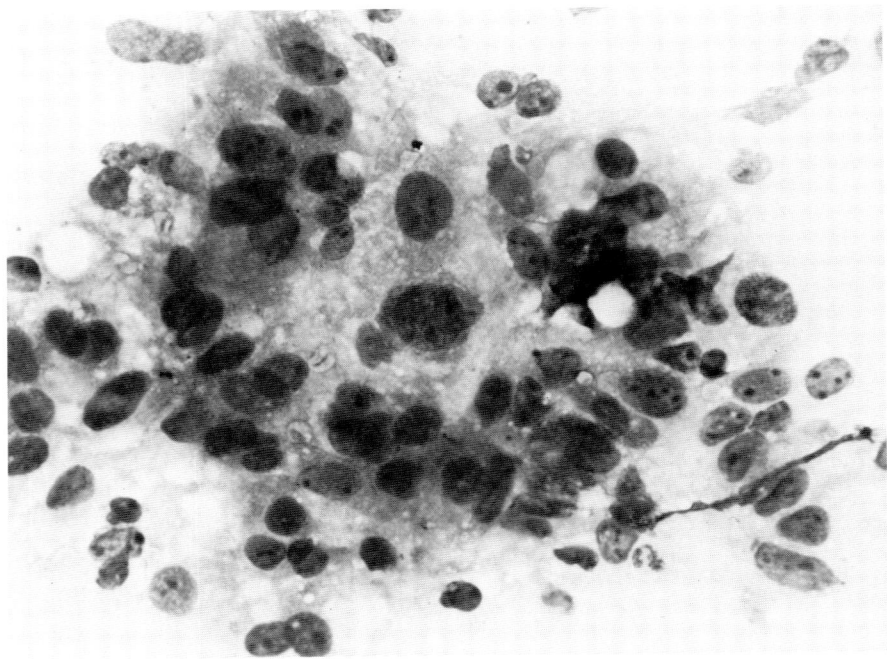

Fig. 10-37 Poorly differentiated adenocarcinoma (FNA). Considerable pleomorphism, complete disorganization, prominent nucleoli, and dispersal of the cells are all characteristic features of poorly differentiated carcinoma of the prostate. (MGG stain, × 400.)

pattern is replaced by a haphazard arrangement of enlarged, markedly atypical cells (Fig. 10-37).

Diagnostic Pitfalls

In addition to the atypia produced by prostatitis, cells from the seminal vesicles and rectal mucosa must also be considered (Table 10-5). Seminal vesicle cells tend to be highly atypical, as well as pleomorphic, but usually are accompanied by sperm and a fluid from the vesicles that produces a tigroid appearance in the smear background, especially on MGG stain. Lipofuscin granules are found in the cytoplasm of seminal vesicle cells, and stain a dark green-blue with MGG stain. Rectal mucosa is usually clearly evident, and is composed of tall cylindrical cells with more abundant cytoplasm than is characteristic of cells from the prostatic epithelium. Fecal material is sometimes present, providing an additional clue to the source of the cells.

Unusual Types of Carcinoma of the Prostate

Adenocarcinoma of the prostate constitutes approximately 97 percent of all prostatic cancers in most series. Cases of endometroid carcinoma and adenoid cystic carcinoma have also been reported.[19]

Table 10-5 Diagnostic Pitfalls Associated With Benign Prostatic Lesions

Rectum and anus	Columnar or squamous cells
	Mucin
	Bacteria
	Fecal debris
Seminal vesicle	Spermatozoa
	Large epithelial cells with hyperchromatic nuclei, dense cytoplasm, and lipofuscin granules
	Reticular ("tigroid") appearance of dried fluid

Table 10-6 Diagnostic Pitfalls Associated With Malignant Prostatic Lesions

Transitional carcinoma	Round to oval nuclei
	Nucleoli not prominent in low to moderate grade tumors
	No acinar patterns
	Clinical history
Metastatic tumor	Unusual cell features (e.g., very glandular patterns, as from rectal carcinoma; severe anaplasia)
	Clinical history

Table 10-7 Response to Treatment in Patients With Prostatic Adenocarcinoma

Response	Outcome/Cytologic Findings
Persistent tumor	Inaccurate grading
Good response	
Estrogen therapy	Atrophic (benign) clusters
	"Glycogenic" cells (metaplastic)
	Squamous cells
	Clear cytoplasm on MGG stain
	Clear or tan cytoplasm on Papanicolaou stain
Castration	Atrophic cells
	No "glycogenic" cells
Radiation therapy	Scanty smear
	Few clusters of atrophic cells
	No radiation atypia

Malignant lymphoma can involve the prostate, and leukemic cells can find sanctuary in the male genital glands, including the prostate. Sarcomas are usually rare, except in children, in whom rhabdomyosarcoma is not uncommon. In adults, possible prostatic sarcomas include leiomyosarcomas and fibrosarcomas; these have the same histology as when they occur elsewhere in the body.

Transitional cell carcinomas are relatively common (Table 10-6), and can coexist with prostatic adenocarcinoma. The cytomorphology of these carcinomas differs, and is illustrated in Figures 10-22 to 10-24—compare to Figures 10-10 to 10-12.

Stains

Most cytopathologists trained in the United States are familiar with the Papanicolaou stain and appreciate its advantages of transparency and nuclear detail. We have found the MGG stain to be a welcome addition in the diagnosis of prostatic lesions, complementing the features of the Papanicolaou stain. The MGG stain, using air-dried material, exaggerates nuclear detail, including nucleoli, and displays the cytoplasmic products, especially the presence of granules (a diagnostic feature of prostatic FNAs), more vividly than the Papanicolaou stain. With a little practice, even the most recalcitrant pathologist can learn to appreciate the advantages of using both stains.

Response to Treatment

HORMONAL THERAPY

Once the diagnosis of adenocarcinoma is made, treatment is prescribed (Table 10-7), which sometimes involves the use of hormones. If conservative treatment is chosen, either castration or estrogen therapy may be used. If castration is preferred, the only change noted in subsequent needle aspirates will be atrophy of the prostatic epithelium. However, if estrogen therapy is the preferred mode of treatment, not only will epithelial atrophy (including shrunken malignant cells) be obvious, but the formation of squamous metaplasia and glycogenated cells will be noted. These large, glycogen-filled, squamous epithelial cells are an indication that the hormonal therapy has been effective. If none is present, then other measures are indicated in order to confirm the efficacy of treatment. Even when tumor cells are present, if they are atrophic and if glycogenated cells are present, treatment is generally considered to be sufficient. Patients so treated are usually candidates for repeat FNA in order to evaluate their course. The challenge to the cytopathologist is great, and familiarity with these changes is mandatory.

RADIOTHERAPY

Radiation therapy produces the same changes in prostatic cells as are seen elsewhere in the body, including cellular enlargement, cytoplasmic and nuclear vacuolization, and maintenance of the nuclear/cytoplasmic ratio in benign cells. Irradiation is not commonly used unless the lesion is considered to be inoperable or too far advanced for other modes of treatment to be effective.

Table 10-8 Accuracy of Fine Needle Aspiration in Diagnosing Prostatic Lesions

False-negative Results (<5%–30%)	False-positive Results (% Unknown)

Possible causes
    Size of the carcinoma
    Inappropriate biopsy technique
    Inexperience
    Faulty handling of cell sample
    Inadequate diagnostic skill
	Possible causes
	    No accurate cytohistopathologic correlation study to date
	    Granulomatous prostatitis
	        Hypercellularity
	        Cell crowding
	        Anisonucleosis
	        Also, lymphocytes, plasma cells, histiocytes, multinucleated giant cells
	    Seminal vesicle samples
	        Clusters of 10–12 cells; abundant cytoplasm containing black pigmented granules
	        Large, hyperchromatic nuclei; anisonucleosis

Diagnostic Accuracy

Since the introduction of the thin needle technique by Franzen in 1960, results of this technique have been reported (Table 10-8).[51–54] Positive results are associated with a 66 to 97 percent sensitivity for the diagnosis of cancer. The false-negative rate has been reported to range from 1 to 30 percent, with the average being just less than 10 percent.[19] The lower the grade of prostatic cancer, the lower the diagnostic accuracy, as the well-differentiated adenocarcinomas are sometimes difficult to distinguish from atypical hyperplasia or benign epithelium. An important aspect of any technique is the number of unsatisfactory samples. This, of course, varies widely depending upon the experience of the operator; however, in the literature, the incidence of unsatisfactory specimens is usually less than 10 percent. Because the technique is well tolerated by patients, adequacy of the sample can be assessed while the patient is still present, and repeat aspirates can be performed, if necessary, to obtain sufficient material for an adequate diagnosis.

Complications

The complication rate of FNA of the prostate is very low—less than 1 percent—and includes epididymitis, transient fever (especially if the patient has had prostatitis), transient hematuria, and hemospermia. In general, prostatic FNA is contraindicated in patients with acute prostatitis because of the chance of fever and subsequent sepsis. Chronic prostatitis, which frequently presents as a mass lesion, is not a contraindication for this technique.

REFERENCES

1. Brannan W, Lucas TA, Mitchell WT: Accuracy of cytologic examination of urinary sediment in the detection of urothelial tumors. J Urol 109:483, 1973
2. Papanicolaou GN: Cytology of the urinary sediment in neoplasms of the urinary tract. J Urol 57:375, 1947
3. Papanicolaou GN: Atlas of Exfoliative Cytology. Harvard University Press, Cambridge, MA, 1963
4. Papanicolaou GN, Marshall JF: Urine sediment smears as a diagnostic procedure in cancers of the urinary tract. Science 101:519, 1945
5. Reichborn-Kjennerud S, Hoeg K: The value of urine cytology in the diagnosis of recurrent bladder tumors. Acta Cytol 16:269, 1972
6. Sarnacki CT, McCormack LJ, Kiser WS, et al: Urinary cytology and the clinical diagnosis of urinary tract malignancy: A clinicopathologic study of 1400 patients. J Urol 106:761, 1977
7. Schoonees R, Gamarra MG, Moore RH, et al: The diagnostic value of urinary cytology in patients with bladder carcinoma. J Urol 106:693, 1971
8. Wiggishoff CC, McDonald JH: Urinary exfoliative cytology in the diagnosis of bladder tumors. Acta Cytol 16:139, 1972
9. Say CC, Hori JM: Transitional cell carcinoma of the renal pelvis: Experience from 1940 to 1972 and literature review. J Urol 112:438, 1974
10. Bibbo M, Gill W, Harris M, et al: Retrograde brushings as a diagnostic procedure of ureteral, renal pelvic and renal calyceal lesions. A preliminary report. Acta Cytol 18:137, 1974
11. Koss LG: Diagnostic Cytology and Its Histopathologic Bases. 3rd Ed. JB Lippincott, Philadelphia, 1979
12. Koss LG: Urinary tract cytology. p. 405. In Wied GL, Koss LG, Reagan JW (eds): Compendium on Diagnos-

tic Cytology. 6th ed. International Academy of Pathologists, Chicago, 1988
13. Melamed MR: Introduction to cytology of the urinary tract. p. 401. In Wied GL, Koss LG, Reagan JW (eds): Compendium on Diagnostic Cytology. 6th ed. 1988
14. Eldidi MM, Patten SF, Jr: New cytologic classification of normal urothelial cells: An analytical and morphometric study. Acta Cytol 26:725, 1982
15. Coleman DV: The cytodiagnosis of human polyomavirus infection. Acta Cytol 19:93, 1975
16. Koss LG: Tumors of the urinary bladder. p. 24. In Firminger HI (ed): Atlas of Tumor Pathology. Armed Forces Institute of Pathology, Washington, DC, 1975
17. Peterson RO: Urologic Pathology. JB Lippincott, Philadelphia, 1986
18. Lerman RI, Hutter RV, Whitmore WF: Papilloma of the urinary bladder. Cancer 25:333, 1970
19. Orell SR: Transitional cell epithelioma of the bladder: Correlation of cytologic and histologic diagnosis. Scand J Urol Nephrol 3:93, 1969
20. Esposti PL, Moberger G, Zajicek J: The cytologic diagnosis of transitional cell tumors of the urinary bladder and its histologic bases. Acta Cytol 14:145, 1970
21. Esposti PL, Zajicek J: Grading of transitional cell neoplasms of the urinary bladder from smears of bladder washings. Acta Cytol 16:529, 1972
22. Farrow GM: Urine cytology of transitional cell carcinoma: Diagnostic efficacy. p. 410. In Wied GL, Koss LG, Reagan JW (eds): Compendium on Diagnostic Cytology. 6th ed. International Academy of Pathologists, Chicago, 1988
23. Foot NC, Papanicolaou GN, Holmquist ND, Seybolt JF: Exfoliative cytology of urinary sediments. Cancer 11:127–137, 1958
24. Holmqvist ND: Diagnostic Cytology of the Urinary Tract. Monographs in Clinical Cytology. Vol. 6. S Karger AG, Basel, 1977
25. Johnson WD: Cytopathological correlations in tumors of the urinary bladder. Cancer 17:867, 1964
26. Kalnins ZA, Rhyne AL, Morehead RP, et al: Comparison of cytologic findings in patients with transitional cell carcinoma and benign urologic diseases. Acta Cytol 14:254, 1970
27. Kern WH: The cytology of transitional cell carcinoma of the urinary bladder. Acta Cytol 19:420, 1975
28. Naib ZM: Exfoliative Cytopathology. 2nd ed. Little, Brown, Boston, 1976
29. Devonec M, Darzynkiewicz Z, Kostyrka-Claps ML, et al: Flow cytometry of low stage bladder tumors: Correlation with cytologic and cystoscopic diagnosis. Cancer 49:109, 1982
30. Allegra SR, Broderick PA, Corvese NL: Cytologic and histogenic observations in well differentiated transitional cell carcinoma of bladder. J Urol 107:777, 1972
31. Wolfson WL, Rosenthal DL: Cell clusters in urinary cytology. Acta Cytol 22:138, 1978
32. Murphy WM, Crabtree WN, Jukkola AF, Soloway MS: The diagnostic value of urine versus bladder washing in patients with bladder cancer. J Urol 126:320, 1981
33. Flanagan MJ, Miller A III: Evaluation of bladder washing cytology for bladder cancer surveillance. J Urol 119:42, 1978
34. Harris MJ, Schwinn CP, Morrow JW, et al: Exfoliative cytology of the urinary bladder irrigation specimen. Acta Cytol 15:385, 1971
35. Cooper PH, Waisman J, Johnston WH, Skinner DG: Severe atypia of transitional epithelium and carcinoma of the urinary bladder. Cancer 31:1055–1060, 1973
36. Eriksson O, Johansson S: Urothelial neoplasms of the upper urinary tract. Acta Cytol 20:20, 1976
37. Koss LG, Bartels PH, Sychra JJ, Wied GL: Diagnostic cytologic sample profiles in patients with bladder cancer using TICAS system. Acta Cytol 22:392, 1978
38. Zajicek J: Papillary carcinoma of the bladder. p. 421. In Wied GL, Koss LG, Reagan JW (eds): Compendium on Diagnostic Cytology. 6th ed. International Academy of Pathologists, Chicago, 1988
39. Murphy WM, Irving CC, Crabtree WN: Developing carcinoma (dysplasia) in the mammalian urinary bladder. Acta Cytol 24:63, 1980
40. Yamada T, Yokogawa M, Mitani G, et al: Two different types of cancer development in the urothelium of the human bladder with different prognosis. Jpn J Clin Oncol 5:77, 1975
41. Koss LG, Tiamson EM, Robbins MA: Mapping cancerous and precancerous bladder changes. A study of the urothelium in ten surgically removed bladders. JAMA 277:281, 1974
42. Yamada T: Cytopathology in precancerous and metaplastic lesions of the urinary tract. p. 417. In Wied GL, Koss LG, Reagan JW (eds): Compendium on Diagnostic Cytology. 6th ed. International Academy of Pathologists, Chicago, 1988
43. Malmgren RA, Soloway MS, Chu EW, et al: Cytology of ileal conduit urine. Acta Cytol 15:506, 1971
44. Forni AM, Koss LG, Geller W: Cytological study of the effect of cyclophosphamide on the epithelium of the urinary bladder in man. Cancer 17:1348, 1964
45. Loveless KJ: The effects of radiation upon the cytology of benign and malignant bladder epithelia. Acta Cytol 17:355, 1973

46. Pearson JC, Kromhout L, King EB: Evaluation of collection and preservation techniques for urinary cytology. Acta Cytol 25:327, 1981
47. Schwinn CP, Harris MJ: Exfoliative cytology of the urinary bladder irrigation specimen. p. 425. In Wied GL, Koss LG, Reagan JW (eds): Compenium on Diagnostic Cytology. 6th ed. International Academy of Pathologists, Chicago, 1988
48. Trott PA, Edwards L: Comparison of bladder washings and urine cytology in the diagnosis of bladder cancer. J Urol 110:664, 1973
49. Bales CE: A semi-automated method for preparation of urine sediment for cytologic evaluation. Acta Cytol 25:323, 1981
50. Bobbitt D, Silverman M, Ng A et al: Centrifugal cytology of urine. Acta Cytol 24:61, 1980
51. Zajicek J: Aspiration Biopsy, Cytology. Part II. Cytology of Infradiaphragmatic Organs. Monographs in Clinical Cytology. Vol. 7. S Karger, AG, Basel, 1979
52. Linsk JA, Franzen S: Clinical Aspiration Cytology. JB Lippincott, Philadelphia, 1983
53. Willems J-S, Lowhagen T: Transrectal aspiration biopsy of the prostate. p. 556. In Wied GL, Koss LG, Reagan JW (eds): Compendium on Diagnostic Cytology. 6th ed. International Academy of Pathologists, Chicago, 1988
54. Orell SR, Sterrett GF, Walters MN-I, Whitaker D: Manual and Atlas of Fine Needle Aspiration Cytology. Churchill Livingstone, Edinburgh, 1986

11
Cytology of Body Cavity Fluids

Bernard Gondos

ANATOMY AND HISTOLOGY OF BODY CAVITIES

The pleural, pericardial, and peritoneal cavities are referred to as the body cavities. These three cavities are structurally similar, consisting of a space lined by a thin double membrane. The inner layer covering the organs contained within the space is called the visceral layer, whereas the layer that lines the outer wall of the cavity is called the parietal layer. Under normal conditions, the visceral and parietal layers are separated only by a small amount of fluid; therefore, the body cavities are not true cavities, but are virtual cavities.

The body cavities are lined by a single layer of mesothelial cells that are derived from embryonic mesoderm (Fig. 11-1). The mesothelial lining cells of the different cavities have a similar appearance as a result of their common embryologic origin. The mesothelium is supported by connective tissue containing nerves and blood vessels.

CLASSIFICATION OF EFFUSIONS

The term effusion refers to the presence of fluid in a body cavity. Because a small amount of fluid is normally present, it is only when there is significant fluid accumulation that the term effusion indicates a pathologic condition. Under these circumstances, the body cavity becomes a true cavity.

Terminology

Several different terms are used to indicate the site and character of effusions. The terms pleural effusion and pericardial effusion are self-explanatory. Presence of fluid in the peritoneal cavity is referred to as *ascites*. The fluid may be thin and watery (serous), bloody (sanguinous) or partially bloody (serosanguinous). In the presence of blood, the prefix *hemo-* is used (e.g., hemopericardium). When the fluid has a milky or chylous character, the prefix *chylo-* is used. For pleural effusions, the suffix *-thorax* is often used to designate the chest cavity (e.g., hemothorax, chylothorax). Penetration of air into a body cavity is indicated by the prefix *pneumo-* (e.g., pneumothorax).

The procedures used for withdrawal of fluid from the pleural, pericardial, and peritoneal cavities are referred to, respectively, as thoracentesis, pericardiocentesis and abdominal paracentesis or, simply, paracentesis.

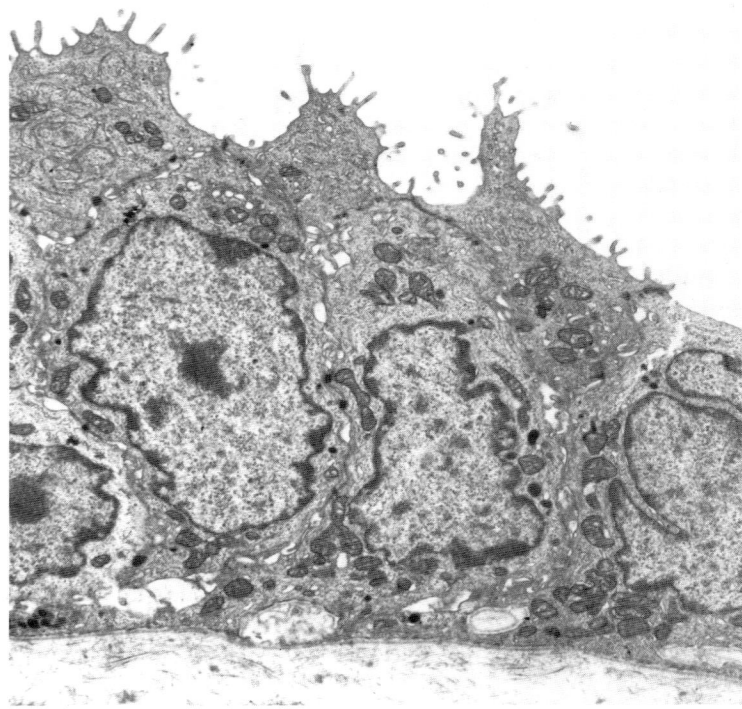

Fig. 11-1 Electron micrograph of peritoneal mesothelium showing columnar cells with prominent microvilli. ($\times$ 3,500.)

Types

Effusions may be classified as either transudates or exudates on the basis of protein content and specific gravity. *Transudates* are characterized by low protein content (<3 g%) and low specific gravity (generally less than 1.015). The accumulation of transudates is a result of passage of blood serum through vessel walls into the body cavity. The fluid includes mesothelial cells and macrophages (histiocytes). Small numbers

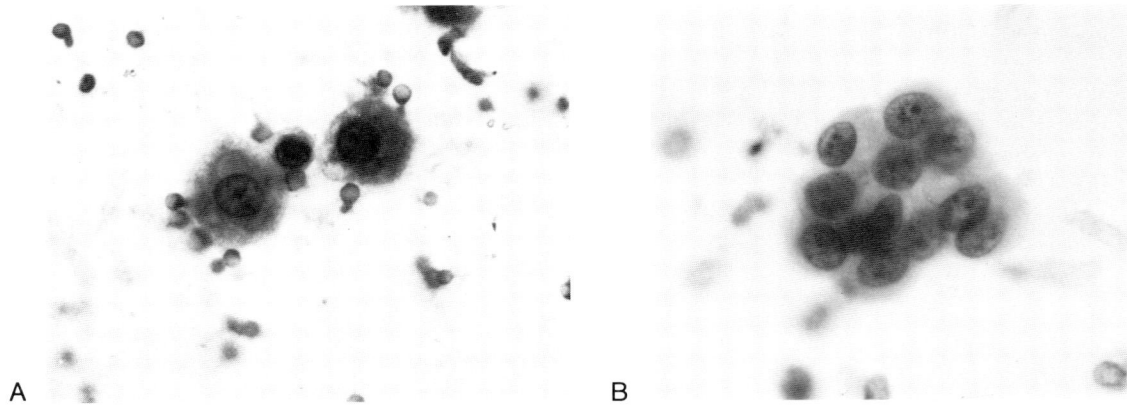

Fig. 11-2 (A) Individual mesothelial cells with central, round nuclei and dense cytoplasm. **(B)** Group of mesothelial cells, some of which are closely attached.

of red blood cells, neutrophils, and lymphocytes may also be present. The fluid typically has a serous character.

Exudates are characterized by a high protein content (usually >3 g%) and a correspondingly high specific gravity. The presence of an exudate generally indicates an inflammatory or neoplastic condition affecting the organs within the body cavity or the lining tissue, or both. The exudate is associated with damage to the walls of blood vessels. The cellular composition of the fluid depends on the underlying abnormality.

Causes

Effusions can result from both benign and malignant conditions. The principal role of diagnostic cytology in relation to effusions is the identification and classification of malignant tumors. Cellular findings can be used to indicate the presence of a malignant tumor and, in many cases, to establish a specific diagnosis as to tumor type. In benign conditions, the findings are most often nonspecific; in some instances, however, identification of particular abnormalities may help to support a specific clinical diagnosis. Benign disorders associated with effusions include inflammatory conditions, circulatory diseases, metabolic disorders, autoimmune diseases, treatment effects, and idiopathic effusions.[1]

CYTOLOGY OF BODY FLUIDS IN BENIGN CONDITIONS

The principal cellular component of body cavity fluids is the mesothelial cell. When an effusion occurs, the mesothelial lining becomes disrupted, with exfoliation of individual mesothelial cells into the body cavity. In some circumstances, there may be proliferation and distortion of the mesothelial lining, resulting in accumulation of groups of mesothelial cells in the fluid.

Macrophages, or histiocytes, represent the other major component commonly found in effusions. They appear as mononuclear cells that are similar in size to mesothelial cells. They usually occur singly, but may appear in loosely arranged clusters. Macrophages are ubiquitous cells found in effusions under a variety of conditions.

Mesothelial Cells

Individual mesothelial cells in body fluids are usually round or oval, measuring 10 to 20 μm in diameter (Fig. 11-2). Nuclei are large and centrally located, with finely granular, evenly distributed chromatin. Nucleoli may often be prominent, but are generally small and compact.

The cytoplasm of mesothelial cells often has a characteristic biphasic staining pattern. The portion nearest the nucleus is dense and heavily stained, whereas the peripheral portion has a thin, relatively clear appearance. The cell surface is generally smooth, although an appearance suggesting a brush border may be present. By electron microscopy, mesothelial cells show a prominent microvillous border[2] and complex intercellular junctions between adjacent cells.[3] These features are difficult to appreciate at the light microscopic level.

Mesothelial cells occurring in clusters are flat and closely attached to one another. The clusters are most often made up of small numbers of cells, although occasionally, large aggregates may be seen. The uniformity of nuclear size and cellular appearance in such aggregates is helpful in confirming their mesothelial origin when differentiation from malignant tumors is a consideration. Sometimes, adjacent mesothelial cells are separated by a small space or lumen. When this occurs, the cells do not overlap or exhibit the dense arrangement that is characteristic of malignant cell groups. Mesothelial cells may also form papillary clusters occasionally, and in these instances, the lack of variability in nuclear structure is useful in differentiating them from cells derived from papillary malignant tumors.

Macrophages

Macrophages in effusions are characterized by their oval shape, eccentric nucleus, and foamy cytoplasm (Fig. 11-3). The cytoplasm may contain numerous, small vacuoles or some distended, large vacuoles. These features are not always helpful in identifying macrophages, as similar changes can occur in mesothelial cells. Binucleation also is seen in both cell types. Macrophages usually have a cell border that is less sharply defined than that of mesothelial cells seen in the same field.

With electron microscopy, the distinction between

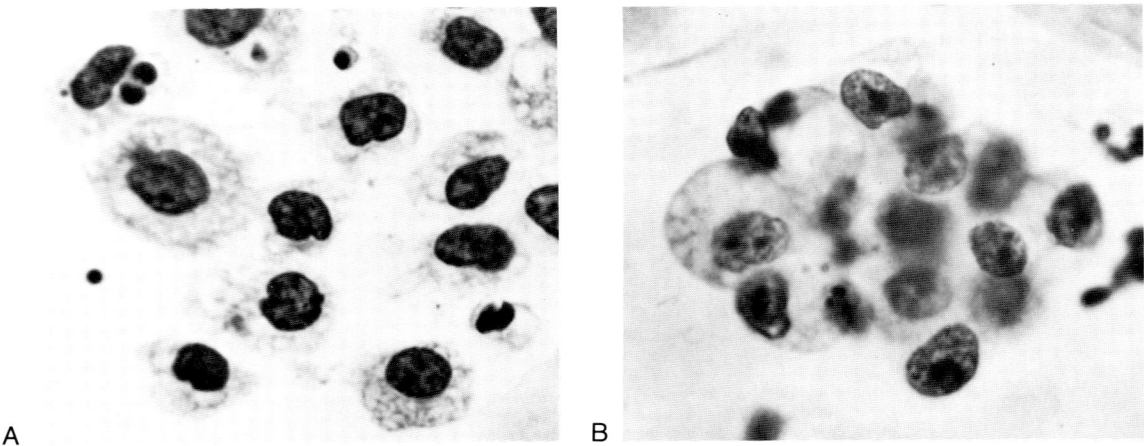

Fig. 11-3 (A) Macrophages have eccentric nuclei and prominent, vacuolated cytoplasm. **(B)** Group of macrophages with irregular nuclei.

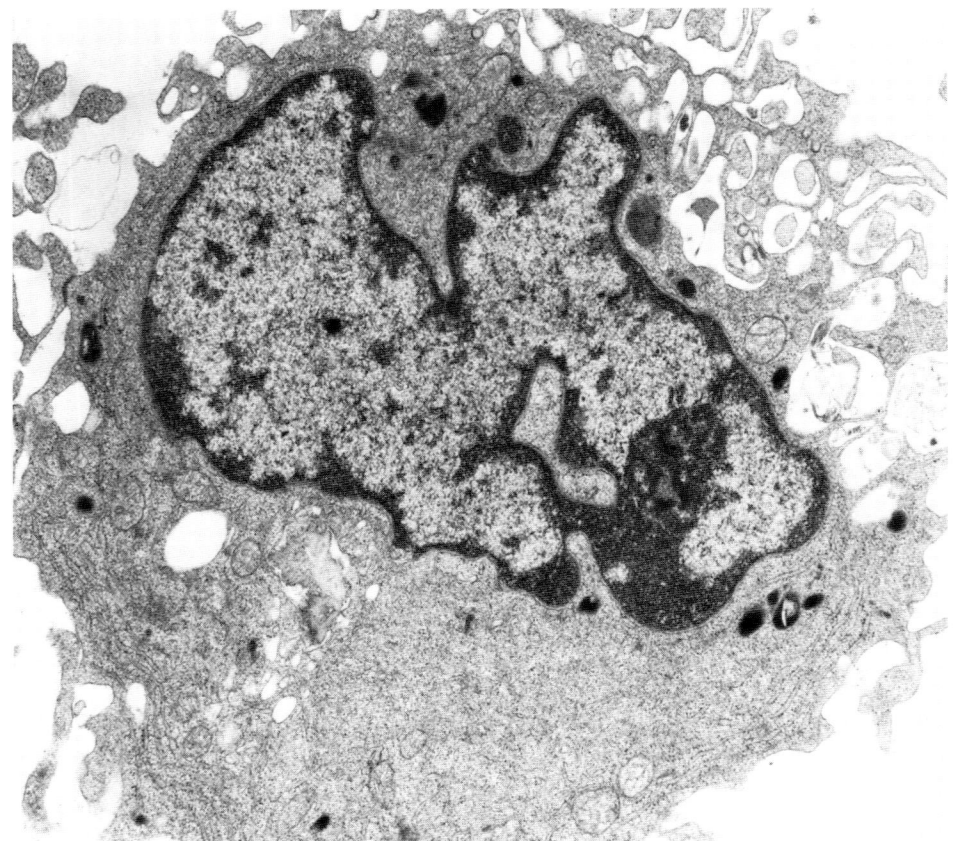

Fig. 11-4 A macrophage at the ultrastructural level demonstrates extensive surface irregularity resulting from multiple cytoplasmic projections. (× 12,000.)

the two cell types is easily made. Macrophages have prominent lysosomal structures in their cytoplasm and demonstrate marked cell surface irregularities, including numerous elongated cytoplasmic projections (Fig. 11-4). These features are not found in mesothelial cells (Fig. 11-5). Distinction at the light microscopic level may be difficult, but is generally of no practical importance, as both cell types are seen in a variety of benign and malignant conditions.

Other Benign Cells

Other cells that may be encountered in benign effusions include neutrophils, lymphocytes, eosinophils, Langhans giant cells, and other types of multinucleated giant cells. In lupus serositis, lupus erythematosus cells may be found,[4] and in rheumatoid disease, granular amorphous material can be seen in association with elongated spindle cells and multinucleated giant cells.[5] If an organ is penetrated during the aspiration procedure, parenchymal cells can be seen (e.g., liver cells in ascitic fluid). Rarely, parasitic organisms may be identified.

Many benign conditions can cause effusions. In acute and chronic inflammatory processes, such as pleuritis, pericarditis, and peritonitis, the characteristic leukocytic infiltrate indicates the type of inflammation. When there is extensive lymphocytic infiltration, differentiation between lymphoma and leukemia is necessary. Tuberculous effusions can be associated with an abundance of lymphocytes.

In the presence of cirrhosis of the liver, ascites is a frequent occurrence. The cell population includes mesothelial cells and macrophages. Papillary formations of mesothelial cells with nuclear atypia and enlarged, occasionally multinucleated macrophages

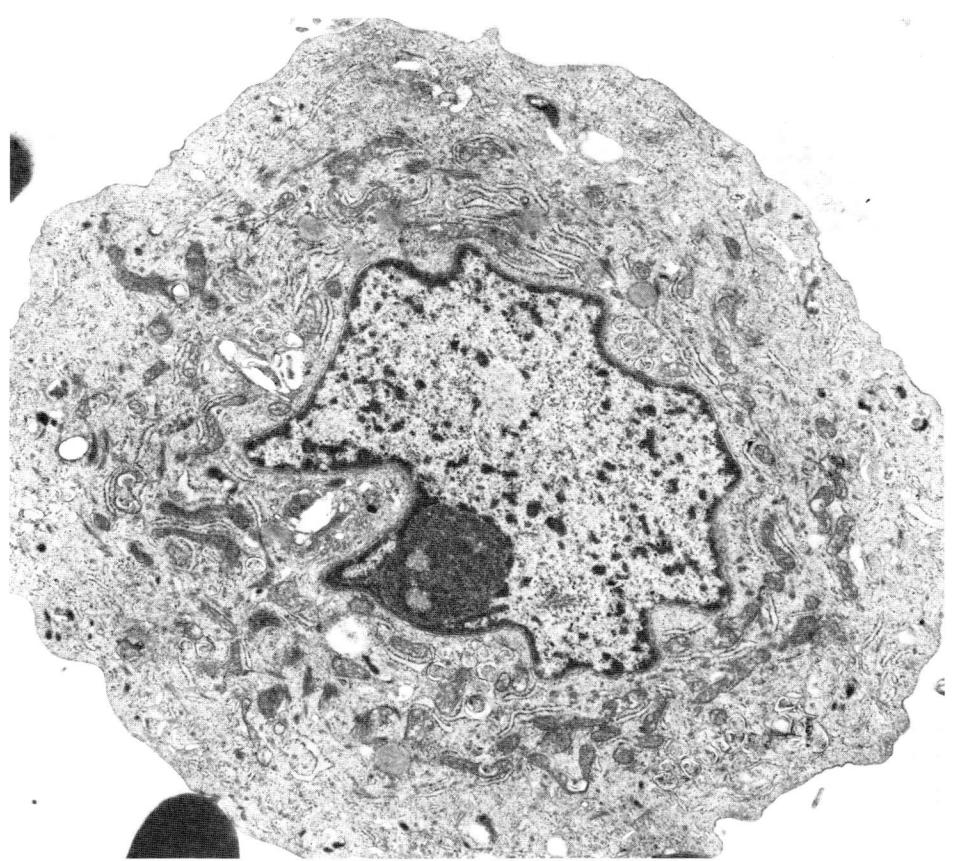

Fig. 11-5 Electron micrograph of a mesothelial cell showing perinuclear concentration of organelles. (× 9,500.)

may be encountered in association with active cirrhosis and should not be misinterpreted as indicating a malignant process.

Pulmonary infarction may lead to a pleural reaction, with resultant effusion. In such fluids, alterations in proliferating mesothelial cells can be significant, and may result in sheets and clusters of apparently atypical cells. This is, however, an unusual occurrence in infarcts, which generally are not associated with effusions.

Congestive heart failure is a common cause of pleural effusion. Pericardial effusion and ascites may also occur. The fluid is a transudate which does not pose any diagnostic problems in the interpretation of the cellular findings.

Effusions occur in a variety of other benign conditions. In most instances, there is no need to submit the specimen to the cytology laboratory. However, if there is reason to suspect malignant disease, careful cytologic evaluation and correlation with clinical findings should be undertaken.

CYTOLOGY OF MALIGNANT TUMORS IN BODY FLUIDS

Malignant cells in body fluids may come from primary tumors, such as mesotheliomas, or from metastatic tumors. Malignant effusions are most often a result of secondary involvement, as mesotheliomas are relatively rare tumors. Metastatic carcinoma is the most frequent tumor encountered. Lymphoma and leukemia may also involve the serosal surfaces and produce effusions. Metastatic sarcoma in association with malignant effusion is a rare occurrence.

Mesothelioma

Mesotheliomas are tumors derived from the body cavity linings. Special interest in these tumors has been generated by the observation of their increased frequency in relation to asbestos exposure,[6] which may be occupational, environmental, or both. In communities with high levels of asbestos, such as in shipbuilding areas, the incidence of mesothelioma is particularly high. Both pleural and peritoneal mesotheliomas are associated with asbestos exposure.

Cytologic diagnosis of mesothelioma is especially important in populations at risk. In addition, cytology laboratories in general are increasingly confronted with the consideration of mesothelioma in the evaluation of pleural and peritoneal fluids. Even with extensive experience, however, the diagnosis remains a difficult one, both in terms of recognizing the cells as malignant, and also in identifying them as mesothelial.[7]

Mesotheliomas may be epithelial or fibrous. Those that are detected by cytologic examination are predominantly epithelial, as this is the most frequent type and fibrous mesotheliomas exfoliate few, if any,

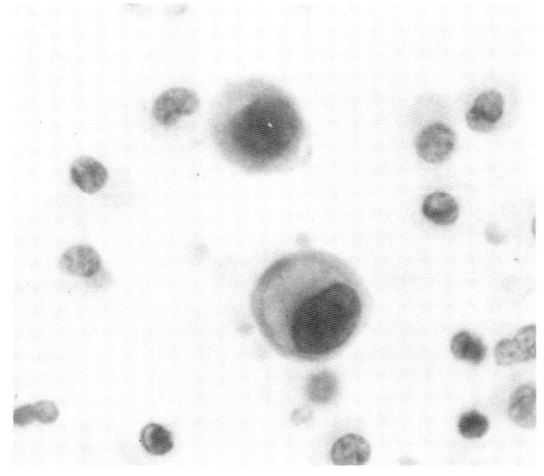
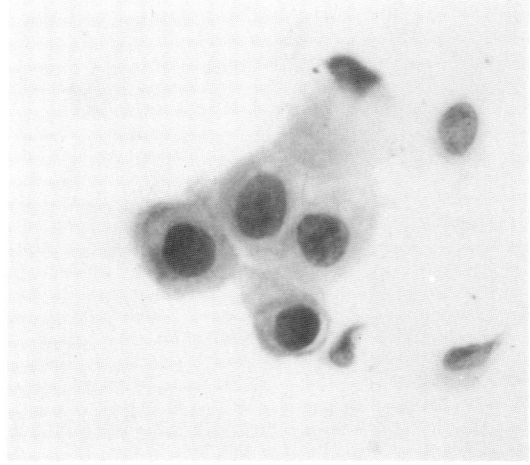

Fig. 11-6 Cells from pleural mesothelioma. **(A)** An individual cellular arrangement resembles mesothelial cells. **(B)** A group of cells with central nuclei and distinct cell borders is demonstrated.

tumor cells into effusions. Carcinomatous mesotheliomas often shed abundant malignant cells. The cells may be arranged singly (Fig. 11-6) or in clusters (Fig. 11-7, Plates 11-1 to 11-4); in most cases, both patterns are found.

The presence of numerous papillary clusters of cells in an effusion from a patient without a known primary tumor should suggest the possibility of a mesothelioma.[8] Malignant cells may show marked pleomorphism with bizarre forms. More often, however, they have the general features of mesothelial cells, including abundant, occasionally vacuolated cytoplasm, a sharp cell border, and a small, somewhat hyperchromatic nucleus. Distinguishing such

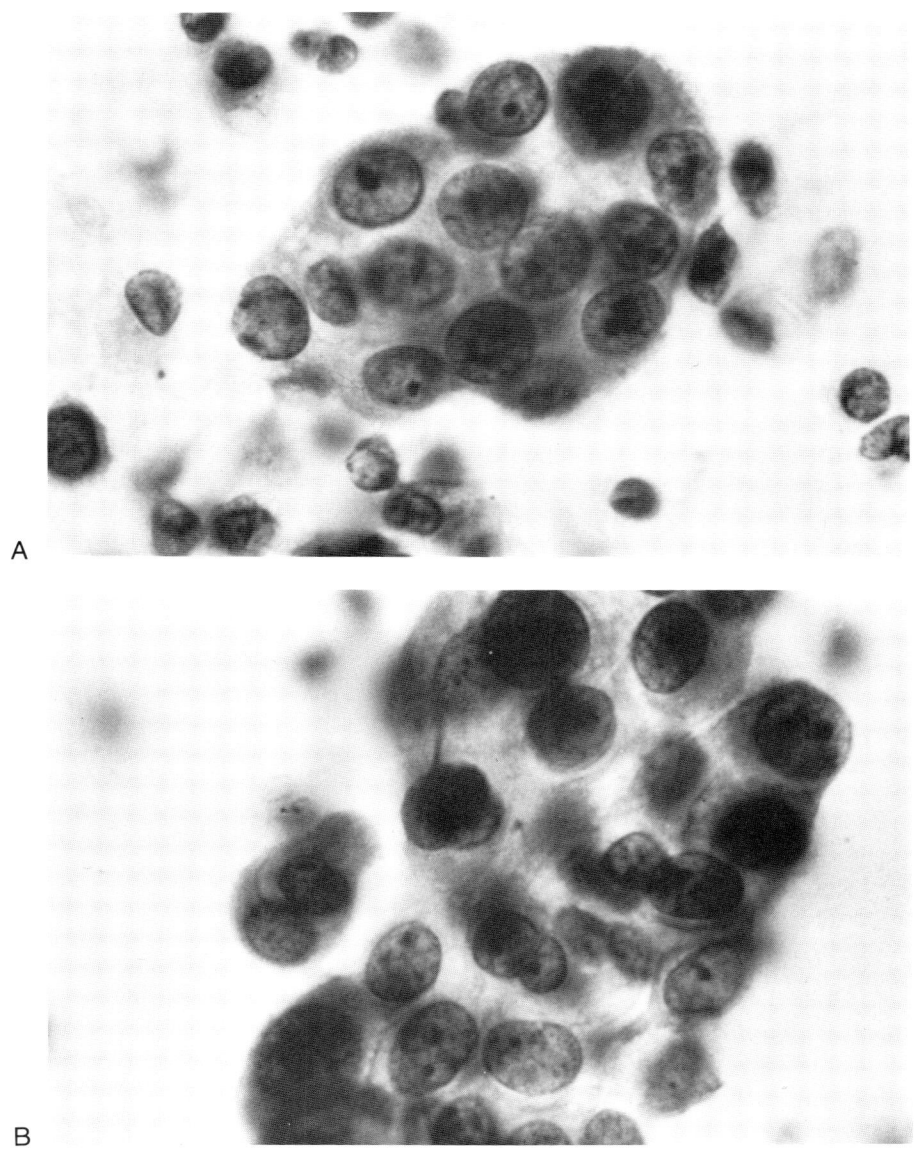

Fig. 11-7 (A) Peritoneal mesothelioma in a patient who formerly worked as an asbestos pipe coverer and insulator in a naval shipyard. Note the tight cluster of cells. (See Plate 11-1.) **(B)** Group of loosely attached cells in ascitic fluid from the same patient. (See Plate 11-2.) (*Figure continues.*)

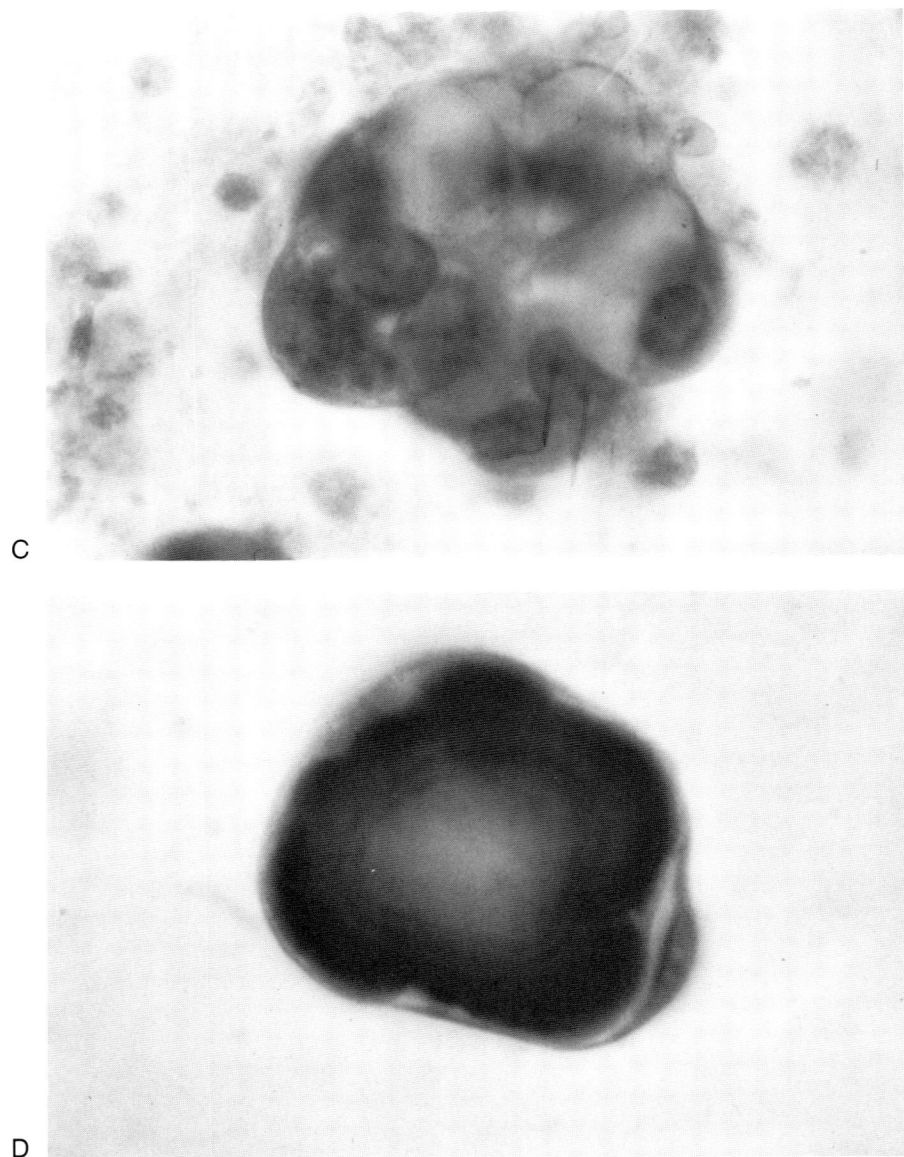

Fig. 11-7 (*Continued*). **(C)** Ascitic fluid from a patient with malignant ovarian tumor exhibits an abundant, clear cytoplasm indicating the presence of mucin. (See Plate 11-3.) **(D)** Psammoma body, papillary adenocarcinoma of the ovary. The presence of psammoma bodies does not always signify malignant disease as they may also occur in benign conditions, but there is a high incidence of associated papillary adenocarcinoma. (See Plate 11-4.)

cells from benign mesothelial cells can present a significant diagnostic problem.[9]

Differentiation between mesothelioma and metastatic adenocarcinoma is another source of difficulty in the diagnosis of effusions. Similarities in cytologic presentation include bizarre cell forms, glandlike structures, large nucleoli, and nuclear irregularities. The diagnosis of adenocarcinoma may be facilitated if mucin is demonstrated. Mesotheliomas are usually negative or weakly positive for mucin. Additional special stains, such as periodic acid-Schiff (PAS), Alcian blue, and colloidal iron stains, with and without hyaluronidase, can also be helpful as the presence of hyaluronic acid is associated with a mesothelial origin. In many cases, the distinction is difficult on the basis of cytologic evaluation alone, and information on clinical history, radiologic findings, and anatomic distribution is required in order to establish a definitive diagnosis.

Because of these problems, special techniques have been utilized to provide more specific information. One such technique is electron microscopy (see the section on special procedures), as certain ultrastructural features have been found to be particularly helpful in supporting a diagnosis of mesothelioma.[10]

One noteworthy finding in mesothelioma is the abundance of microvilli on all free surfaces (Fig. 11-8). This finding sets the lesion apart from most adenocarcinomas in which prominent microvilli are found principally on the apical surface. Another ultrastructural feature that is characteristic of benign and malignant mesothelial cells is the perinuclear concentration of cytoplasmic organelles. This is not a constant finding in the malignant cells, but when present, it is strongly suggestive of a mesothelial origin. The occurrence of bundles of intermediate filaments, abundant glycogen, and intracytoplasmic lumen formation in mesothelioma is quite distinctive. Although these features can all be found in adenocarcinoma, their combined presence in individual cells is particularly characteristic of mesothelioma.

In addition to electron microscopy, recent reports have cited the usefulness of immunohistochemical studies in the diagnosis of mesothelioma.[11]

Metastatic Carcinoma

The role of the cytology laboratory in the diagnosis of metastatic carcinoma in effusions is threefold: (1) documenting the presence of malignant cells; (2) classifying the type of carcinoma; and (3) determining, if possible, the primary site of origin.

Identification of malignant cells in effusions depends on the same principles that apply to cytologic

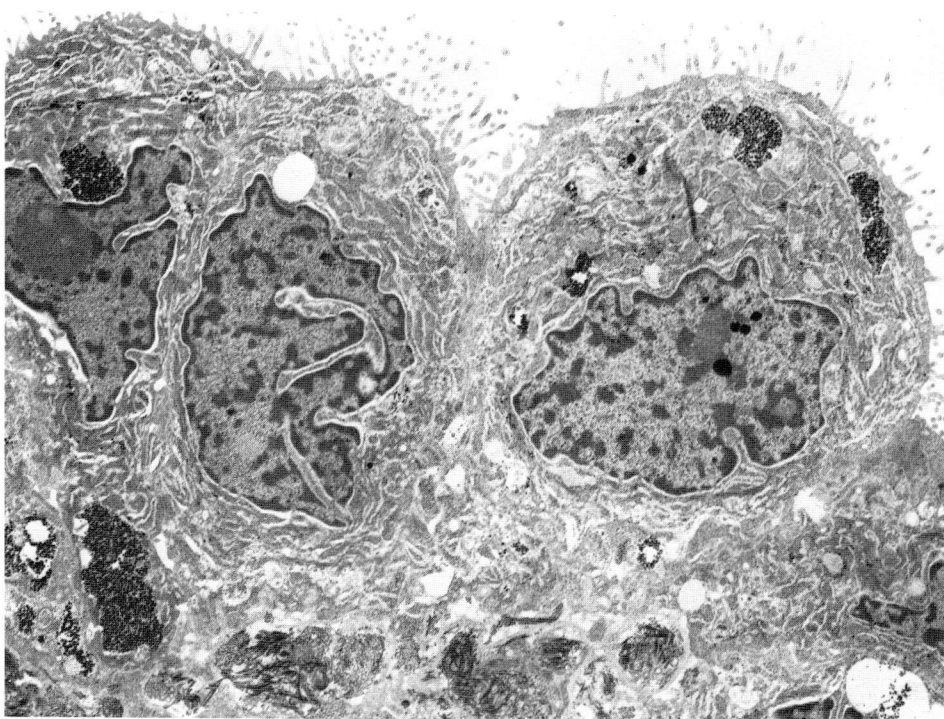

Fig. 11-8 Electron micrograph of a mesothelioma demonstrating abundance of microvilli and prominent accumulation of glycogen. The nuclei are markedly irregular, with dense collections of chromatin. ($\times$ 3,200.)

diagnosis in other areas of the body. The presence of abnormal cells with large, hyperchromatic nuclei, irregular nucleoli, and abnormal chromatin patterns is indicative of malignant disease. Arrangement of cells in papillary clusters, sheets, or glandlike formations indicates an epithelial origin. Caution must be exercised, however, as it is not unusual for mesothelial cells to exhibit some degree of nuclear alteration in long-standing effusions. Shedding of mesothelial cells in clusters, either in papillary groups or sheets, may also occur under such circumstances, simulating carcinoma. Therefore, strict adherence to criteria for malignant disease must be observed before rendering a diagnosis of metastatic carcinoma. In general, the extent of nuclear change in such mesothelial groups is minimal, and there is overall uniformity in appearance. By contrast, carcinomatous cells in effusions demonstrate varying degrees of abnormality and significant pleomorphism.

Classification of the type of metastatic carcinoma in effusions is usually readily accomplished. Arrangement in papillary groups, acinar formations, or glandular structures suggests a diagnosis of adenocarcinoma (Fig. 11-9). Additional findings, such as signet ring cells, mucin production, prominent vacuolization, and psammoma bodies, are helpful supportive features (see Fig. 11-7). On a statistical basis, adenocarcinoma is the most frequent diagnosis. This is because, of the tumors that are associated with malignant effusions, those of glandular origin are the most numerous.

Squamous cell cancers are uncommonly observed in effusions. When such tumors do appear in body fluids, their identification is relatively easy. Anucleated cells or elongated, spindle-shaped cells with pale, rectangular nuclei and pearl formation may be observed. Metastatic transitional cell carcinoma that originates in the urinary tract is a rare occurrence. In such situations, the cells are generally quite anaplastic and classification depends on awareness of the site of origin. Small cell carcinomas are usually readily identified in fluids as they retain various characteristic cytologic features, including small hyperchromatic cells with scant to absent cytoplasm and molding of adjacent cell borders. Occasionally, precise classification may require ultrastructural examination (see below).

The primary site of origin for metastatic carcinomas in effusions can be determined only in certain cases. Most adenocarcinomas that arise in different parts of the body show fundamental similarities in cellular appearance; therefore, specific patterns in metastatic locations will not be evident. Fortunately, this is usually not a problem as the primary site is generally well established on the basis of clinical data. However, when there is an unknown primary lesion or a questionable relationship to a pre-existing tumor, the cytologist may be asked to determine the most likely origin of malignant cells in an effusion.

Such a determination is often not possible, but some general observations can be made. For example, the presence of papillary formations is consistent with ovarian or thyroid origin (Fig. 11-10). In metastatic breast carcinoma, the cells are typically ar-

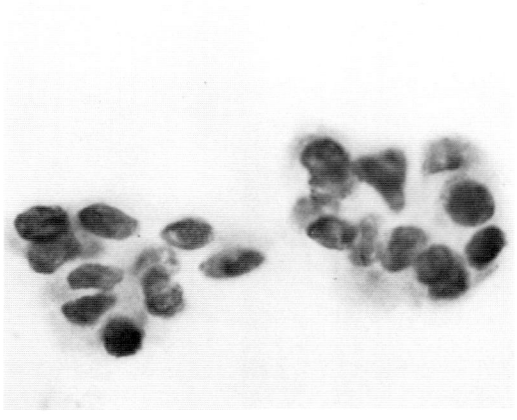
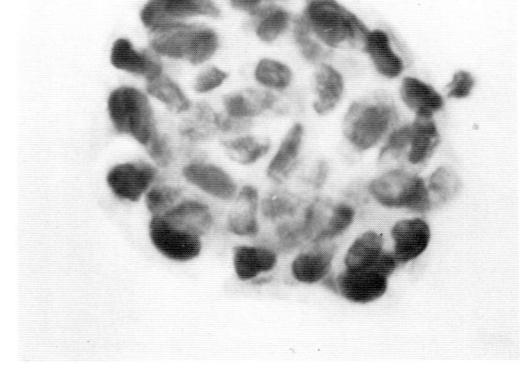

Fig. 11-9 **(A)** Papillary formation, adenocarcinoma. **(B)** Acinar grouping, adenocarcinoma of endometrium.

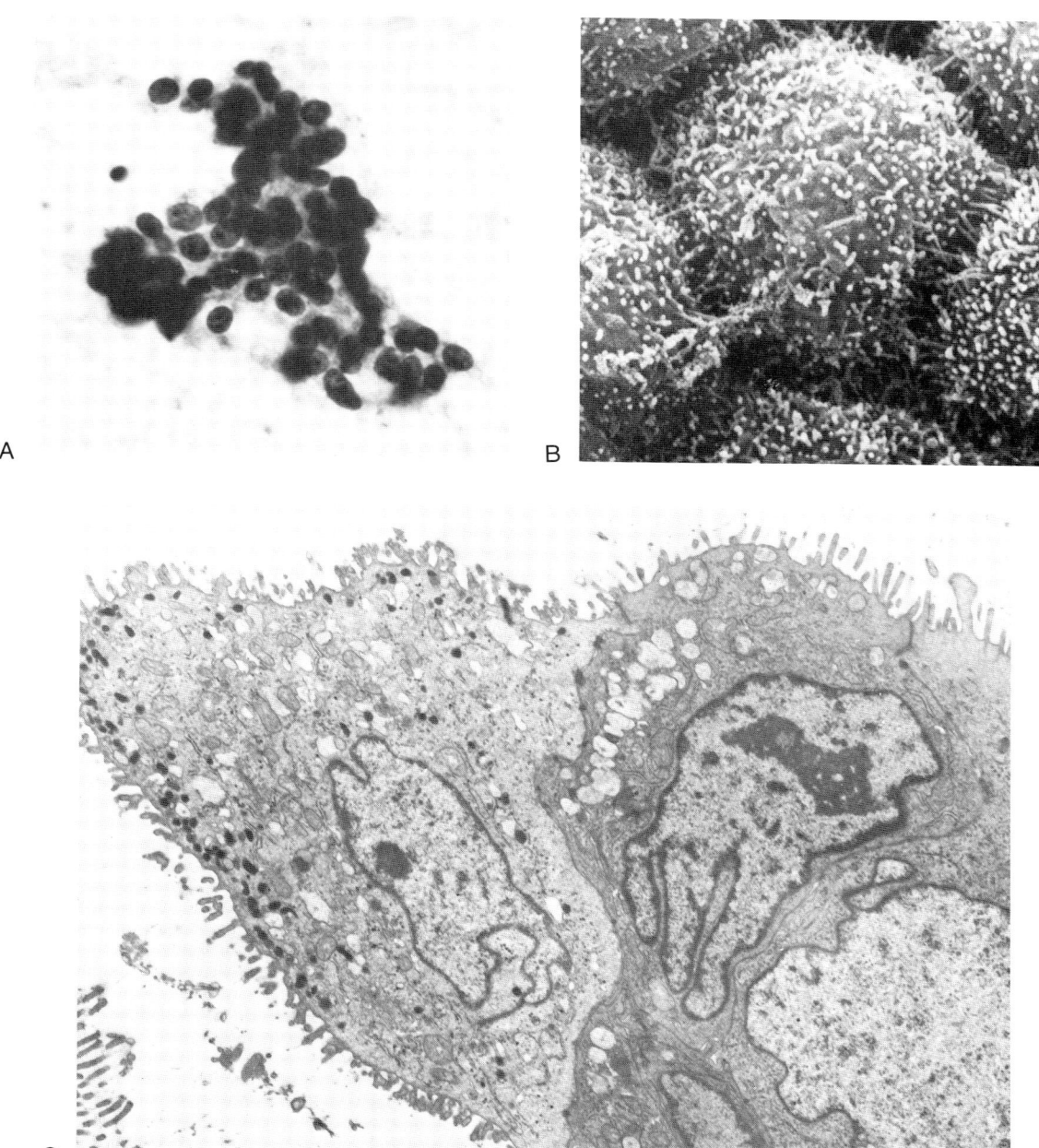

Fig. 11-10 (A) Sheet of cells in papillary formation obtained from a sample of ascitic fluid in a patient with adenocarcinoma of the ovary. **(B)** Deep, intercellular grooves and irregular, elongated microvilli are seen in this scanning electron micrograph of cells from ovarian adenocarcinoma. (× 6,500.) **(C)** Transmission electron micrograph, papillary cystadenocarcinoma of the ovary. (× 6,300.)

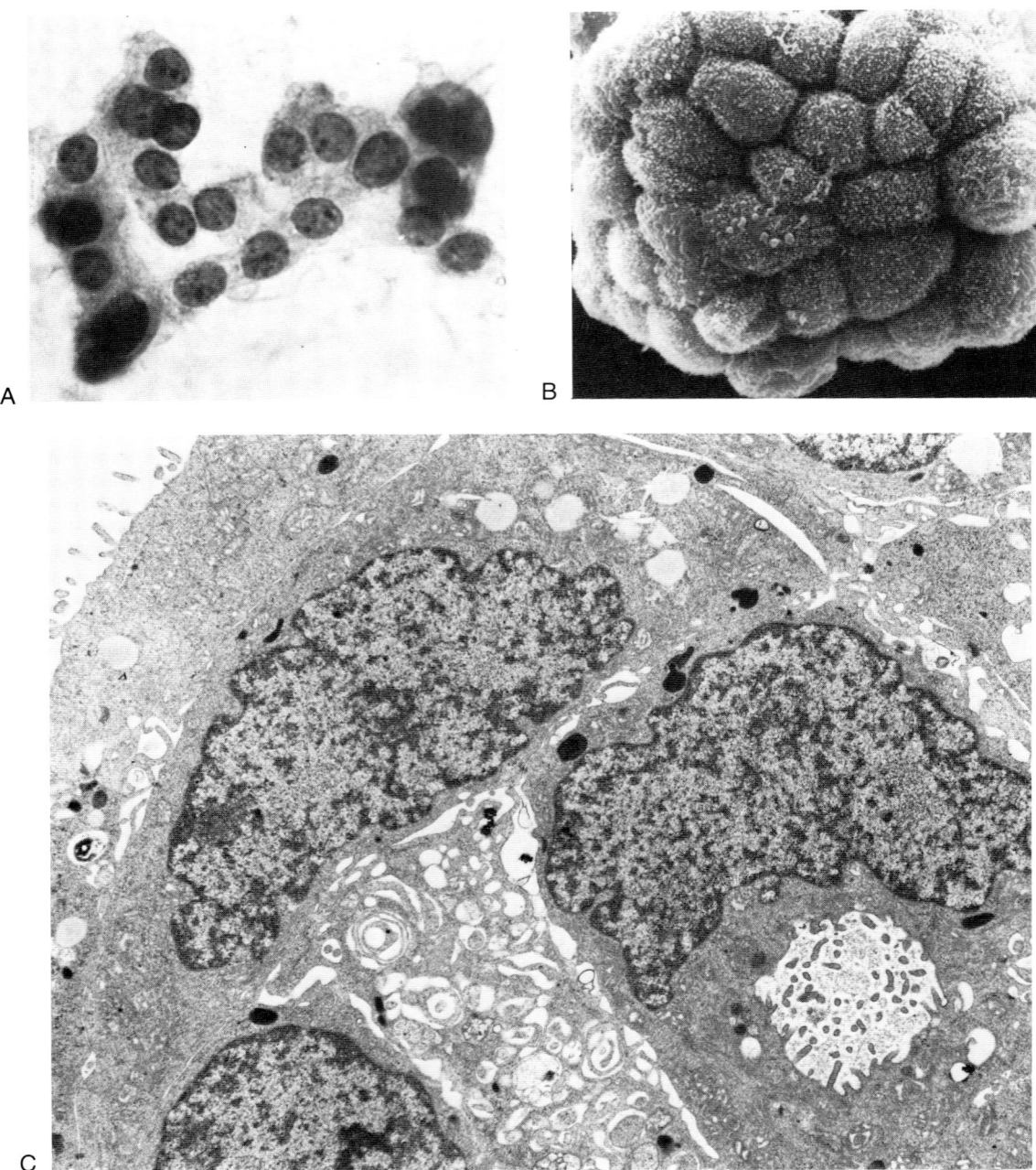

Fig. 11-11 **(A)** Metastatic breast carcinoma, pleural fluid. Note the arrangement of the cells in rows, which is characteristic of infiltrating ductal carcinoma. **(B)** A scanning electron micrograph reveals a ball-like arrangement of cells in a patient with adenocarcinoma of the breast. (× 1,600.) **(C)** Transmission electron micrograph, pleural fluid, from a patient with metastatic breast carcinoma. Note the irregular chromatin condensation. (× 7,500.)

ranged in a ball-like configuration or in rows, and they exhibit minimal pleomorphism and subtle, but definite, chromatin abnormalities (Fig. 11-11). Metastatic carcinoma of the prostate is characterized by tight clusters of glandular cells. It should be noted, however, that these findings are not specific, and represent only the most commonly occurring patterns. When the existence of a previous primary tumor is known, it is of particular importance that the findings be compared with the original slides. In metastatic adenocarcinoma of unknown origin, it is likely that the cytologic findings alone will not allow the site of origin to be determined.

Electron microscopy may be helpful in some cases, as some types of metastatic adenocarcinoma have ultrastructural features that are distinctive. For instance, the presence of microvilli with dense-core microfilaments that extend as long rootlets into the apical cytoplasm and glycocalyceal bodies is characteristic of colonic adenocarcinoma;[12] numerous intracytoplasmic channels lined by microvilli and abundant lipid are typical of carcinoma of the breast;[13] abundant lipid and glycogen are common findings in renal clear cell carcinoma;[14] extensive glycogen aggregates occur in clear cell carcinoma of the female genital tract;[15] lamellar inclusions are characteristic of pulmonary alveolar cell carcinomas;[16] mucin droplets are evident in certain tumors of the ovary, colon, and other sites; and secretory granules may be associated with certain tumors of the ovary, thyroid, pancreas, and other sites.

In most of these instances, the findings are of limited specificity and must be correlated with other data. The use of electron microscopy should therefore be restricted to carefully selected cases. In the future, immunohistochemical studies utilizing monoclonal antibodies may have increasing application in determining the site of origin of metastatic tumors in effusions. (See Ch. 14.)

Lymphoma

Leukocytes are often found in body fluids. In the presence of long-standing effusion, lymphocytes may predominate. If they are numerous, and particularly if neutrophils and other white blood cells are not present, the possibility of lymphomatous involvement should be considered.

Careful correlation of cytologic findings with clinical data is imperative in such cases. It is highly unusual for lymphoma to appear in an effusion without evidence of disease elsewhere, although it is possible.[17] Conversely, even with a previous diagnosis of lymphoma, the presence of lymphocytes in a body fluid specimen might still be attributable to an inflammatory process. Therefore, caution must be exercised in establishing a diagnosis.

In lymphomas, the malignant cells are individually distributed (Fig. 11-12), a pattern that allows differentiation from metastatic carcinoma. Even when there are large numbers of malignant cells in a lymphomatous effusion, cohesive aggregates are not seen.

The differential diagnosis of lymphoma and inflammatory conditions in effusions depends as much on clinical data as on cytologic findings. In some cases, the malignant nature of the cells is obvious, but in others, it may be difficult to distinguish malignant cells from benign lymphoid elements. A helpful feature in benign conditions is the mixed pattern of white blood cells, which is generally lacking in effusions of lymphomas. Comparison of findings with available tissue specimens is also important.

Leukemia

Leukemic cells may be identified in effusions. Because effusions in patients with leukemia must be differentiated from inflammatory reactions, the earlier comments pertaining to lymphoma also apply in this instance. It is extremely unusual for patients with leukemia to develop effusions in the absence of a previous clinical diagnosis. Thus, the main role of the cytology laboratory is to determine the extent of the disease for the purposes of deciding on appropriate treatment protocols.

Myeloma

Effusion in association with multiple myeloma is an unusual finding that generally occurs late in the course of the disease.[18] Occasionally, cytologic detection is a diagnostic problem. A distinction must be made from chronic inflammatory conditions and other types of malignant tumors. Generally, the diag-

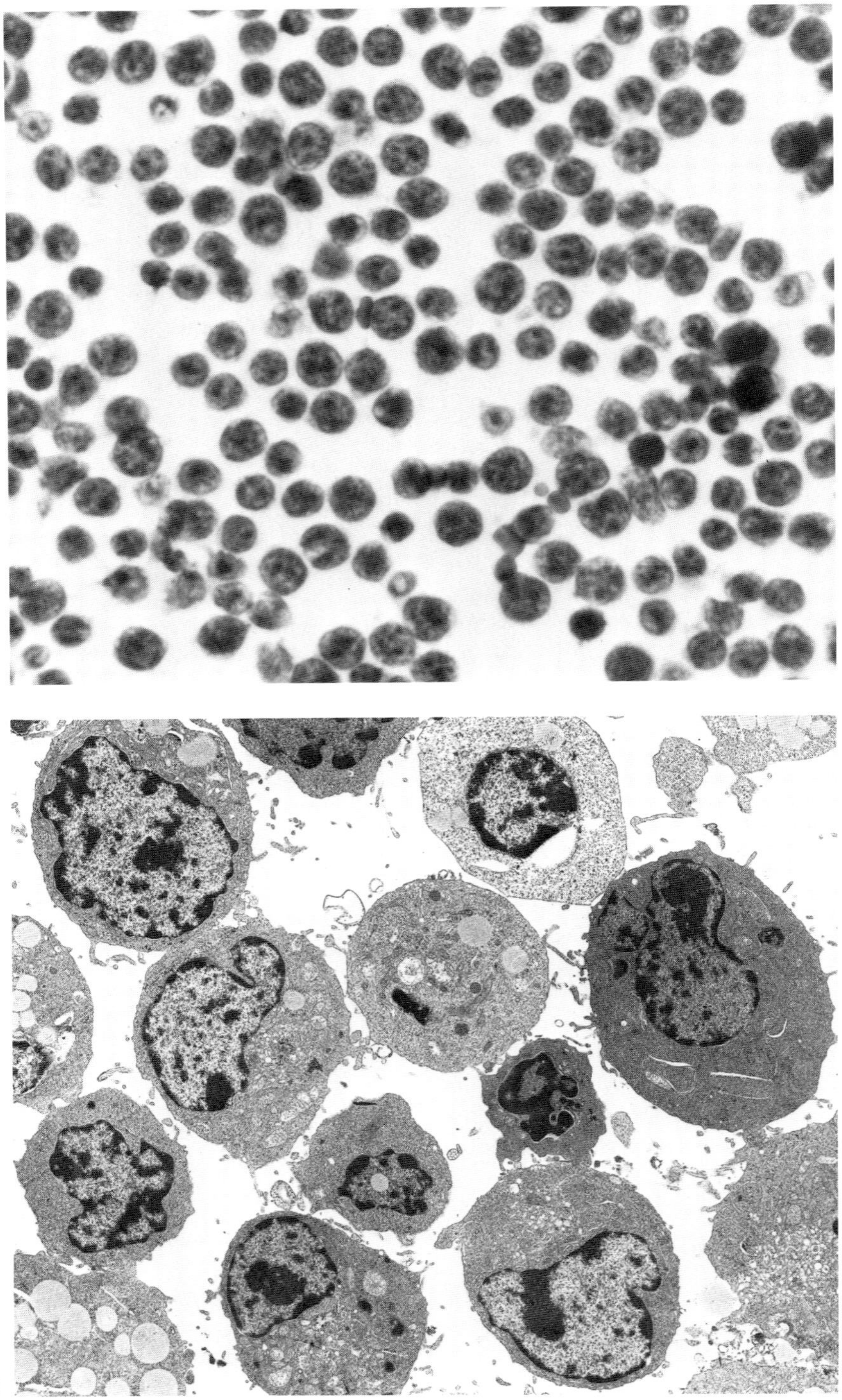

Fig. 11-12 **(A)** Lymphoma, pleural fluid. Note the individual arrangement of cells. Numerous malignant cells are present without attachment or overlapping. **(B)** Electron micrograph, lymphoma, pleural fluid. Cells are densely distributed, but junctional attachments are absent. (× 3,800.)

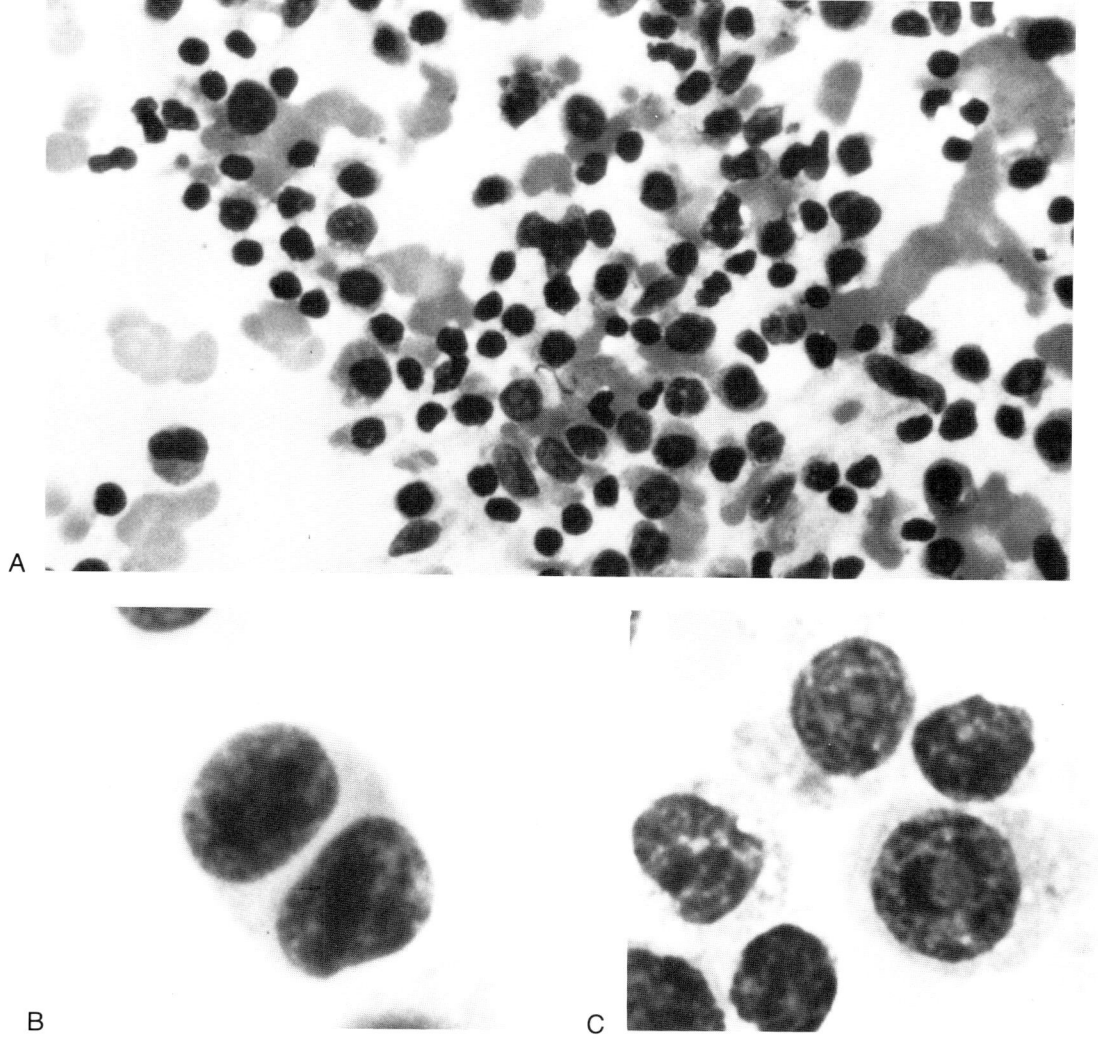

Fig. 11-13 **(A)** Multiple myeloma involving the pleura. Note the abundance of plasma cells in varying stages of differentiation. **(B)** Binucleated cell from the pleural fluid in a patient with metastatic myeloma. **(C)** Immature plasma cells, peritoneal fluid specimen.

nosis can readily be established on the basis of clinical features, fluid characteristics, and cytologic findings. In myeloma, the fluid has a high specific gravity and high protein content. Plasma cells predominate to the exclusion of other cell types, and varying stages of differentiation are present (Fig. 11-13). In difficult cases, additional procedures that may facilitate establishment of a definitive diagnosis include methyl green pyronine stain, fluid electrophoresis, and electron microscopy.

Other Tumors

Additional metastatic tumors that may be found in effusions include melanoma,[19] germ cell tumors,[20] neuroblastoma,[21] and various types of sarcomas.[22] These are all unusual occurrences, but such tumors should be considered in the differential diagnosis when abnormal cells of uncertain origin are detected in fluids (Fig. 11-14). Specific information on clinical presentation is essential in such cases.

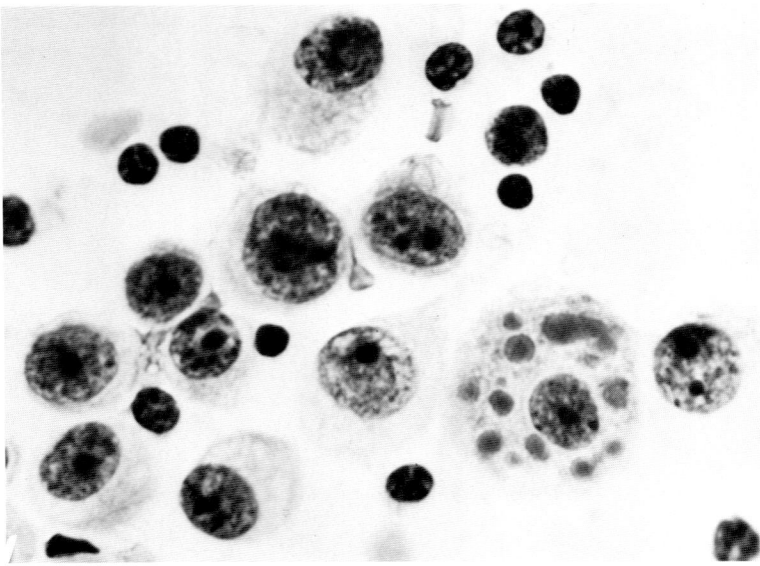

Fig. 11-14 Metastatic melanoma, characterized by cells with large, vesicular nuclei, prominent nucleoli, and evidence of pigment formation.

PRACTICAL CONSIDERATIONS

Differential Diagnosis

Arriving at a correct diagnosis in the analysis of an effusion does not usually present difficulties. In most cases, either the absence of cellular abnormalities will clearly point to a benign effusion or, alternatively, obviously malignant cells resembling those in a previously diagnosed tumor will indicate metastatic disease. However, in some instances, the findings require consideration of more than one possibility. In these cases, careful evaluation and a thorough understanding of diagnostic criteria are critical.

A frequent and particularly important problem arises with the distinction between atypical mesothelial cells and malignant cells. As indicated earlier, mesothelial cells in long-standing effusions occasionally exhibit considerable cytologic atypia. Misinterpretation of atypical mesothelial cells as malignant is a serious error which must be avoided. The following factors should be considered when attempting to distinguish between mesothelial and malignant cells: the clinical findings (previous tumor, presence of a benign condition associated with effusions); the character of the fluid (appearance, specific gravity); the cellular arrangement (individual, grouped, type of grouping); the chromatin pattern; the nuclear variability; and comparison with previous cytologic and histologic specimens. Because there is some degree of overlap in the cytologic appearance of severely atypical mesothelial cells and well-differentiated malignant cells, all available information should be utilized in problem cases.

A less serious but often more difficult problem involves the distinction between different types of malignant tumors. If the primary tumor is not known, or if different sources for the metastatic disease are being considered, specific interpretation of the findings in the fluid may be critical for diagnosis and treatment. The following considerations are important in such cases: the age and sex of the patient; the radiologic findings; the location of the effusion; the cellular arrangement (e.g., papillary, ball-like, individual, etc.); the cytoplasmic characteristics (e.g., the presence of mucin, melanin, cross-striations, etc.); and comparison with previous specimens. In addition, certain special procedures, such as electron microscopy and immunologic techniques, may be helpful (see below).

Cytohistologic Correlations

Examination of body fluid specimens should include both smear and cell block preparations whenever sufficient sediment is available to prepare a cell block. The smears provide details of individual cell characteristics. With the Papanicolaou stain, chromatin pattern, general nuclear structure, and cytoplasmic appearance can be studied. Other staining procedures, such as the Wright or Giemsa stain for the evaluation of hematologic cell types, should also be employed as indicated.

Cell block preparations enable evaluation of architectural arrangement and comparison with biopsy material. Using the standard hematoxylin and eosin (H&E) stain, the overall histologic pattern can be determined. Additional special stains can also be utilized as required. Of special importance in difficult diagnostic problems is the comparison of the histologic appearance in cell block preparations with available biopsy specimens. Cytologic characteristics of the smears should also be compared with biopsy material. Because the findings derived from smear and cell block preparations may not always be similar, each has to be evaluated thoroughly, and the diagnosis should be based on whatever significant changes are found.

Clinical Correlations

Every effort should be made to utilize clinical findings and other available information in the evaluation of effusions. There are several situations in which clinical correlation is critical in the establishment of a correct diagnosis. The following examples indicate the importance of such correlations.

LYMPHOCYTES IN EFFUSION

The presence of numerous lymphocytes in an effusion could be a result of lymphoma, leukemic involvement, or inflammation. Although the cytologic findings may indicate clear-cut malignant changes in some specimens, in most instances, this is not the

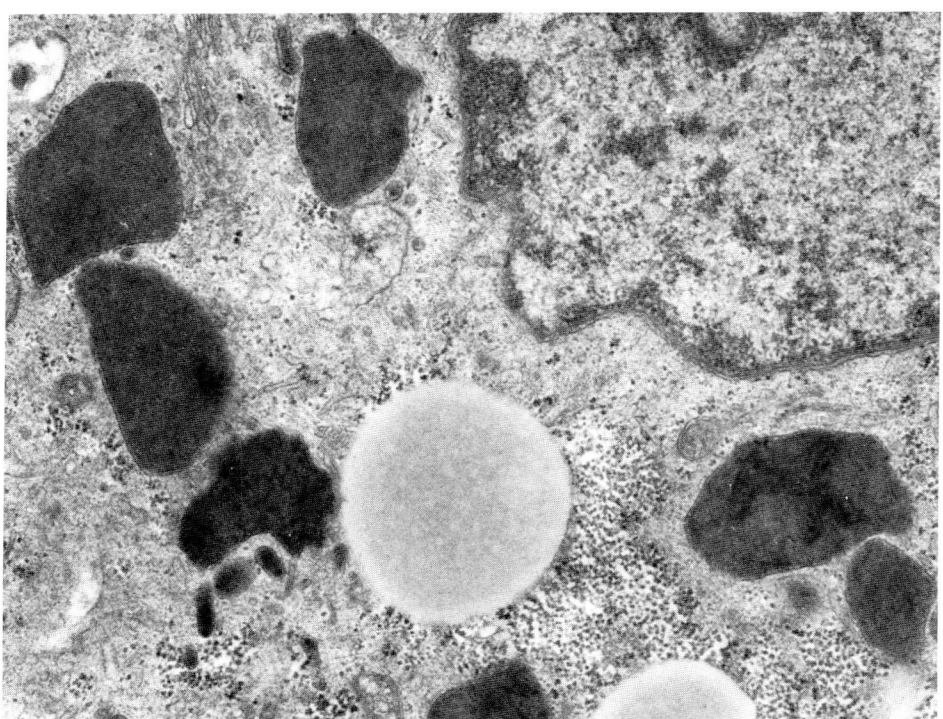

Fig. 11-15 Electron micrograph showing melanosomes in a case of metastatic melanoma, pleural fluid. (× 21,000.)

case. Consequently, interpretation will rest heavily on clinical findings.

MESOTHELIOMA VERSUS METASTATIC CARCINOMA

There is considerable overlap in the cytologic presentation of mesothelioma and metastatic carcinoma. Because the clinical findings in mesothelioma are usually quite distinctive, they carry special weight in determining a definitive diagnosis. In the absence of findings that are consistent with mesothelioma, establishment of a specific diagnosis will depend strongly on evidence of tumor elsewhere.

BENIGN EFFUSIONS

Among the most common causes of effusions are benign conditions, such as hepatic cirrhosis, which may be associated with significant cellular atypia and, therefore, with the potential for false-positive diagnoses. Awareness of the underlying clinical findings will help in avoiding this pitfall.

Special Procedures

Ancillary procedures designed to enhance the diagnostic capability of the cytology laboratory should be utilized whenever indicated. Because of the time, expense, and specialized personnel required, selective application of such procedures is important. In certain situations, they may be essential for establishing the diagnosis.

ELECTRON MICROSCOPY

The indications for performing electron microscopy on body cavity fluid specimens relate to the type of information sought.[23] Electron microscopic evaluation should be utilized to identify specific structures and to classify cell types (Fig. 11-15) rather than to distinguish between benign and malignant cells, which is generally not possible by this method. Electron microscopy has been found to be useful in diagnosing tumors with secretory granules, such as small cell carcinoma and neuroblastoma, as well as tumors with characteristic cytoplasmic inclusions, such as melanoma and bronchiolo-alveolar carcinoma; in differentiating between mesothelioma and adenocarcinoma; in identifying the primary site in metastatic adenocarcinoma; and in diagnosing special tumors, such as germ cell tumors, myeloma, and sarcomas.[24] In any individual case, the usefulness of electron microscopy has to be determined on the basis of routine light microscopic findings, as well as other clinical and laboratory data.

CYTOCHEMISTRY

Diagnosis of serosal involvement by leukemia can be facilitated by cytochemical studies of effusions. Identification of leukocytes in body cavity fluid specimens is achieved by use of air-dried smears and cytocentrifuged specimens stained with Wright-Giemsa and Sudan black B stains, as well as by evaluating nonspecific esterase, chloracetate esterase, and peroxidase reactions.[25]

IMMUNOCYTOCHEMISTRY

Microscopic examination of fluids can be further enhanced by the immunologic demonstration of cell-specific or tissue-specific markers. Carcinoembryonic antigen (CEA) is found in a wide variety of epithelial tumors and thus can be helpful in the diagnosis of metastatic carcinoma.[26] Differentiation between mesothelioma and metastatic carcinoma may be accomplished by certain immunocytochemical methods.[27] Alpha-fetoprotein (AFP) is a useful marker for certain germ cell and liver tumors.

Increasing attention has been directed toward intermediate filament typing using either conventional or monoclonal antibodies to distinguish cells of epithelial, mesenchymal, muscle, glial, and neuronal origin. Thus, carcinomas may be identified using keratin antibodies since their cells are keratin-positive. Melanomas, lymphomas, and nonmuscle sarcomas contain vimentin, whereas muscle tumors are characterized by the presence of desmin. Glial fibrillary acidic protein can be demonstrated in some tumors of glial origin, and most tumors of neural origin contain neurofilaments. Tumor cells evidently retain the intermediate filament characteristic of their cell of origin and, in general, do not acquire new filament types in metastases.[28]

OTHER METHODS

Additional methods, such as chromosome analysis[29] and fluorescent banding techniques,[30] have also been employed in the examination of effusions. However, clinical application has not yet been assigned to these methods.

SUMMARY

The evaluation of body cavity fluids requires a systematic process that includes consideration of clinical history, the appearance of the specimen, microscopic examination, differential diagnosis, and utilization of special procedures as indicated.

Pertinent clinical information should be provided with the specimen to enable proper evaluation. Clinical findings that may be important include age, sex, relevant history, physical findings, type and duration of effusion, amount of fluid present, radiologic findings, and other laboratory findings. When previous cytologic or histologic material is available, all such specimens should be reviewed. It is usually helpful and often advisable to discuss the clinical findings directly with the patient's primary physician.

The appearance of the specimen should be recorded, including its color, consistency, and specific gravity. Although such findings are not specifically diagnostic, they may be useful as points of correlation with other findings. A thorough examination of a body fluid specimen requires recording of this type of information.

Microscopic examination involves a thorough evaluation of smears and cell blocks that are prepared according to the procedures established by the individual laboratory. Diagnosis depends on standard cytologic criteria for determining the presence or absence of malignant changes. Particular consideration should be given to characteristic features of mesothelial cells and to the distinction between changes in mesothelial cells and malignant cells. Care must be taken to avoid false-positive diagnoses when atypical mesothelial cell groups are present and false-negative diagnoses when only sparse malignant cells are present.

Differential diagnosis requires an understanding of the cytologic presentation of different types of benign and malignant conditions in effusions. In evaluating cellular abnormalities in body cavity fluid specimens, the different conditions that might produce the changes identified must be fully considered. In addition, correlation with clinical findings and other laboratory findings is essential. When indicated in difficult diagnostic problems, special procedures may be utilized to arrive at a specific diagnosis.

REFERENCES

1. Koss LG: Diagnostic Cytology and Its Histopathologic Bases. 3rd Ed. JB Lippincott, Philadelphia, 1979
2. Andrews P, Porter KL: The ultrastructural morphology and possible functional significance of mesothelial microvilli. Anat Rec 177:408, 1973
3. Simionescu M, Simionescu N: Organization of cell junctions in the peritoneal mesothelium. J Cell Biol 74:98, 1977
4. Metzger AL, Coyne M, Lee S, Kramer LS: In vivo LE cell formation in peritonitis due to SLE. J Rheumatol 1:130, 1974
5. Boddington MM, Spriggs AI, Morton JA, Mowat AG: Cytodiagnosis of rheumatoid pleural effusions. J Clin Pathol 24:95, 1971
6. Selikoff IJ, Lilis R, Nicholson WJ: Asbestos disease in United States shipyards. Ann NY Acad Sci 330:295, 1979
7. Spriggs AI, Boddington MM: The Cytology of Effusions. 2nd Ed. Heinemann, London, 1968
8. Klempman S: The exfoliative cytology of diffuse pleural mesothelioma. Cancer 31:691, 1972
9. Kawai T, Suzuki M, Kageyama K: Reactive mesothelial cells and mesothelioma of the pleura. Virchows Arch[A]393:251, 1981
10. Kobzik L, Antman KH, Warhol MJ: The distinction of mesothelioma from adenocarcinoma in malignant effusions by electron microscopy. Acta Cytol 29:219, 1985
11. Szpak CA, Johnston WW, Roggli V, et al: The diagnostic distinction between malignant mesothelioma of the pleura and adenocarcinoma of the lung as defined by a monoclonal antibody (B72.3). Am J Pathol 122:252, 1986
12. Posalaky A, McGinley DM, Posalaky IP: Electron microscopic identification of the colorectal origin of tumor cells in pleural effusions. Acta Cytol 27:45, 1983
13. Spriggs AI, Jerrome DW: Intracellular mucous inclu-

sions. A feature of malignant cells in effusions in the serous cavities, particularly due to carcinoma of the breast. J Clin Pathol 28:929, 1975
14. Sun CN, Bissada NK, White HJ, Redman JF: Spectrum of ultrastructural patterns of renal cell adenocarcinoma. Urology 9:195, 1977
15. Ohkawa K, Amasaki H, Terashima Y, et al: Clear cell carcinoma of the ovary: Light and electron microscopic studies. Cancer 40:3019, 1977
16. Woyke S, Domagala W, Olszewski W: Alveolar cell carcinoma of the lung: An ultrastructural study of the cancer cell detected in the pleural fluid. Acta Cytol 16:63, 1972
17. Spriggs AI, Vanhegan RI: Cytological diagnosis of lymphoma in serous effusions. J Clin Pathol 34:1311, 1982
18. Gondos B, Miller TR, King EB: Cytologic diagnosis of multiple myeloma and macroglobulinemia in effusions. Ann Clin Lab Sci 8:11, 1978
19. Yamada T, Itou U, Watanabe Y, Ohashi S: Cytologic diagnosis of malignant melanoma. Acta Cytol 16:70, 1972
20. Kapila K, Hajdu SI, Whitmore WF, et al: Cytologic diagnosis of metastatic germ-cell tumors. Acta Cytol 27:245, 1983
21. Farr GH, Hajdu SI: Exfoliative cytology of metastatic neuroblastoma. Acta Cytol 16:203, 1972
22. Hajdu SI, Hajdu EO: Cytopathology of Sarcomas and Other Nonepithelial Malignant Tumors. WB Saunders, Philadelphia, 1976
23. Gondos B, McIntosh KM, Renston RH, King EB: Application of electron microscopy in the definitive diagnosis of effusions. Acta Cytol 22:297, 1983
24. Bewtra C, Greer KP: Ultrastructural studies of cells in body cavity effusions. Acta Cytol 29:226, 1985
25. Yam LY, Lin DG, Janckila AJ, Li CY: Immunocytochemical diagnosis of lymphoma in serous effusions. Acta Cytol 29:833, 1985
26. Walts AE, Said JW, Banks-Schlegel S: Keratin and carcinoembryonic antigen in exfoliated mesothelial and malignant cells: An immunoperoxidase study. Am J Clin Pathol 80:671, 1983
27. Battifora H, Kopinski MI: Distinction of mesothelioma from adenocarcinoma: An immunohistochemistry approach. Cancer 55:1679, 1985
28. Altmannsberger M, Osborn M, Droese M, et al: Diagnostic value of intermediate filament antibodies in clinical cytology. Klin Wochenschr 62:114, 1984
29. Dewald G, Dines DE, Weiland LH, Gordon H: Usefulness of chromosome examination in the diagnosis of malignant pleural effusions. N Engl J Med 295:1494, 1976
30. Benedict WF, Porter IH: The cytogenetic diagnosis of malignancy in effusions. Acta Cytol 16:304, 1972

12
Cytology of the Central Nervous System

Dorothy L. Rosenthal

Cell samples from the central nervous system (CNS) require expert interpretive skills of the cytopathologist, as such specimens may provide the only diagnosis upon which therapy and prognosis are based.[1-3] Origins of many of the cells found in cytologic specimens from the CNS are not always obvious,[4,5] considerable confusion exists in the literature as to the identification and naming of cells found therein, and confirmatory biopsies are rare. The cytopathologist, therefore, is well-advised to establish ground rules for the collection, preparation, and diagnostic assessment of CNS cell samples.

The guidelines presented in this chapter are derived from the examination of more than 700 CNS samples submitted annually to the Cytology Service at the University of California, Los Angeles (UCLA) Medical Center. Diagnostic categories utilize the cytologic pattern, the age and history of the patient, and other test results, to eliminate or indicate certain diagnostic choices.

CNS cytology is not a screening procedure but, rather, a tool for evaluating conditions for which a tissue correlation is not usually available. Patients in whom CNS cytology is performed either have symptoms related to a CNS disease or are candidates for CNS involvement by a metastatic neoplasm. The type of disease requiring cytopathologic examination will depend on the clinical emphasis and population of patients seen in a particular hospital or clinic.[6]

CLINICAL HISTORY

Accurate patient information is vital in reaching a valid diagnosis. These data are best gathered by close communication between the clinician and the laboratory. Of greatest import are (1) the clinical diagnosis; (2) the symptoms and physical findings; (3) all results from tests done within recent months that involve the CNS, including invasive procedures (pneumoencephalogram, myelogram, and arteriogram) and noninvasive procedures (computerized tomography [CT] scan and magnetic resonance imaging [MRI]); (4) previous therapy, including intrathecal medication, irradiation to the brain or spinal cord, or the presence or insertion of shunts; (5) surgical history, including fine needle aspiration (FNA), brain biopsy, or cyst drainage; (6) source of cerebrospinal fluid (CSF) (e.g., lumbar space, cisternum, ventricle, or parenchymal cyst); and (7) the temporal relationship of the specimen to therapy, surgical intervention, invasive diagnostic procedures, or a previous spinal tap, all of which will provoke reactive cellular responses additional to the cytopathology of the disease itself.

SPECIMEN COLLECTION

The collector of CSF should be expert enough to avoid a bloody tap or aspiration of solid material, such as the nucleus pulposus, which can lead to a false-positive diagnosis. Speed in delivery to the laboratory and immediate processing are imperative, as spinal fluid is not a good environment for these fragile cells. Indeed, diagnostic material may disintegrate in less than an hour, yielding a false-negative assessment. Fixation with alcohol or alcohol/carbowax (Saccomanno fixative) are less than ideal as these agents harden the cells and shrink them; if fixation is needed, the Saccomanno method is the preferred option.

FNA of solid tissue should be performed by an experienced neurosurgeon, utilizing controlled localizing techniques (e.g., CT scan or MRI).[7] Smears must be prepared more rapidly than with FNA in other sites because of the accelerated clotting time of brain tissue. As with frozen section analysis, immediate microscopic assessment for specimen adequacy and a preliminary diagnosis, using a rapid stain, should be provided to the clinician whenever possible.

Tissue ("crush") preparations or smears made from stereotactic brain biopsies are finding greater use at many medical centers in the diagnosis of neoplasms and other conditions of the CNS.[7a]

SPECIMEN PREPARATION

Total cell recovery with good detail are two prime requisites for any method of specimen preparation; relative expense and ease of handling also should be considered. The methods available include the various filtration methods (e.g., Nuclepore and Millipore); sedimentation or centifugation directly onto a glass slide; and centrifugation with smear transfer of the sediment onto a glass slide.[8] At UCLA, the cytocentrifuge is currently believed to be the optimal method. Two spins are prepared, one that is air-dried and stained with Wright stain, and one that is other alcohol-fixed and stained with Papanicolaou stain. Both stains complement each other, and the Wright-stained sample is available for discussion of contentious cases with the hematologists.[9]

SPECIAL STUDIES

With the current availability of immunochemical procedures,[10,11] extra slides should be prepared whenever possible to allow such tests to be performed. Glial fibrillary acidic protein, neuron-specific enolase, and common leukocyte antigen are frequently helpful in identifying the cell line, especially when faced with a small cell neoplasm. The epithelial membrane markers (carcinoembryonic antigen [CEA], epithelial membrane antigen, and milk fat globule) are useful in distinguishing carcinomas from high-grade astrocytomas. Occasionally, the tumor-specific antibodies, such as prostate-specific antigen and alpha-fetoprotein (AFP), will determine in which primary tumor the CNS metastasis originated, if the prostate and liver are possibilities. Simultaneous staining of available tissue from the suspected parent neoplasm is important to ensure that the original tumor is also antigen-positive.

PHYSIOLOGY OF CEREBROSPINAL FLUID

CSF is an ultrafiltrate of plasma that is produced by the choroid plexuses. It flows from the ventricles to the subarachnoid spaces; both areas comprise the so-called CSF compartment. Reabsorption occurs through arachnoidal villi into the venous sinuses. The blood–brain barrier, located at the capillary level, prohibits certain substances from entering the CSF compartment. This is an important factor in chemotherapy, and necessitates intrathecal medication for effective treatment. The total fluid contained in the CSF compartment is 150 ml; a quantity of 500 ml is produced in a 24-hour period, representing a turnover rate of approximately 14 percent.[9]

FACTORS INFLUENCING CELL EXFOLIATION

Contact of tumor with the CSF compartment will increase cell recovery. Therefore, the tumors that are anatomically most likely to shed cells are meningioma, metastatic carcinoma, medulloblastoma, ependymoma, and sarcoma.[6,12] Meningioma occurs in the subarachnoid space, but rarely exfoliates. The ability of a tumor to shed depends on the cohesiveness of the tumor. Metastatic squamous cell carcinoma and adenocarcinoma appear in the CNS in about equal numbers; however, squamous cell carcinoma in the CSF is rare.[19]

In deep-seated tumors, cells probably enter the CSF by direct extension or via a perivascular cuff of tumor cells in Virchow-Robin spaces, with migration along the meninges. Secondary tumors may be found in the subarachnoid space by erosion of a metastatic nodule or by way of meningeal metastases. Usually, very few diagnostic cells will be recovered in the CSF sample. If many neoplastic cells are found, then extensive leptomeningeal involvement (also termed meningeal carcinomatosis and carcinomatous meningitis) is probably present.[9,12,13]

CELLULAR PATTERNS

As in histopathology and other types of cytologic specimens, CNS cell samples present with a variety of cell patterns (Figs. 12-1 and 12-2). Although a designation of "positive" or "negative" is sometimes considered to be adequate, more significant information can be gleaned from most cellular samples.[9,14] Consider the importance of distinguishing between an inflammatory/infectious process (Figs. 12-3 and 12-4) and a reactive one[15] (Figs. 12-5 and 12-6, Table 12-1). The difference between obstetrical head

Table 12-1 Non-Neoplastic Cells in Cerebrospinal Fluids

"Normal" cell population
    Lymphocytes: only a few; really the only cell allowable in a "negative" fluid
    Leptomeningeal cells: very infrequent; possibly ependymal cells or "free" cells
    Monocytes: very infrequent; also known as pia-arachnoid mesothelial (PAM) cells, monocytoid cells
    Ependymal cells: particularly expected in a ventricular tap; otherwise, rare

Inflammatory conditions
    Neutrophils: acute conditions, acute bacterial meningitis, also early tuberculosis, and early viral meningitis
    Lymphocytes: viral meningitis, late bacterial meningitis, tuberculosis
    Plasma cells: syphilis, tuberculosis, other immune responses
    Eosinophils: sometimes appearing with parasites, in allergic situations, or in subacute meningitis
    Monocytes/macrophages, including multinucleated histiocytes: tuberculosis, fungi; also seen postoperatively after placement of shunts and Ommaya reservoirs

Reactive conditions (e.g., following CNS investigative procedures or, CNS therapy or as a result of underlying tumor)
    Increased numbers of 'normal' cells, especially leptomeningeal cells and monocytes
    Astrocytes
    Neurons: rare

Macrophages (may contain ingested material)
    Fat: post-oil myelogram, secondary to trauma, infarct, or parenchymatous destructive disease
    Blood pigment: following intracranial hemorrhage (not fresh blood, as in a bloody tap)
    Melanin: not pathognomonic for melanoma; as a rare benign condition, termed melanosis cerebri, can shed melanin pigment; other pigmented tumors
    "Pneumoencephalogram" (PEG) plaques: clusters of bare, oval, bland nuclei that appear following air ventriculography (PEG), probably from arachnoid or pial membranes, or from degenerated astrocytes

Contaminants (cartilage, bone marrow elements, debris, talc)

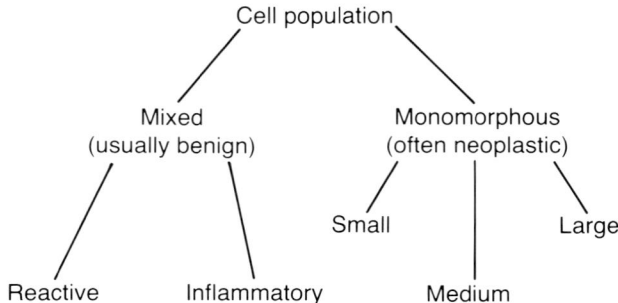

Fig. 12-1 Diagnostic choices when "normal" inflammatory reactive, tumor-related (primary/metastatic), and leukemic/lymphomatous cellular changes are found.

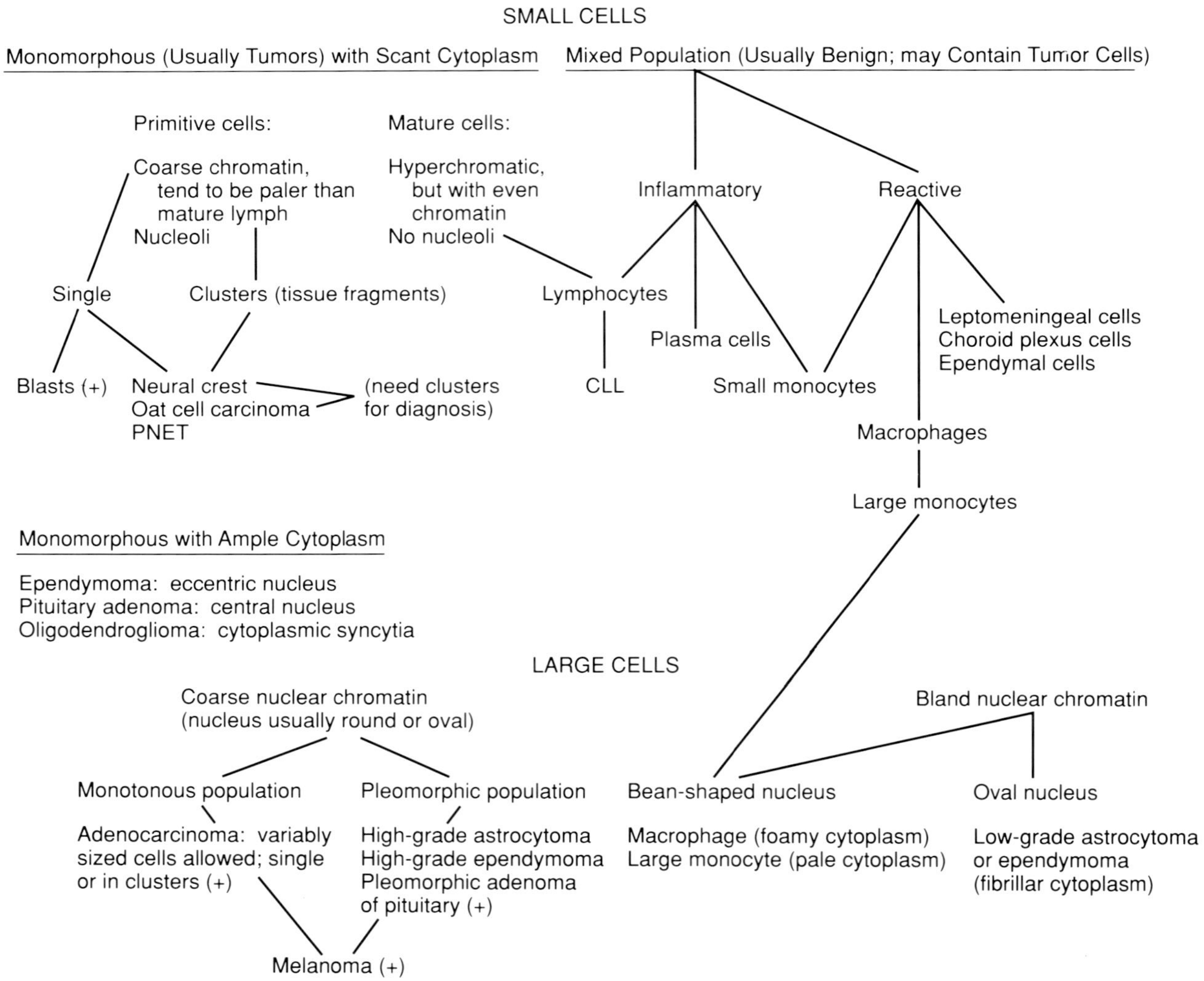

Fig. 12-2 Diagnostic decision tree based on cytomorphologic characteristics of cells found in the CNS. (PNET, primitive neuroectodermal tumor; +, prominent nucleolus; CLL, chronic lymphocytic leukemia).

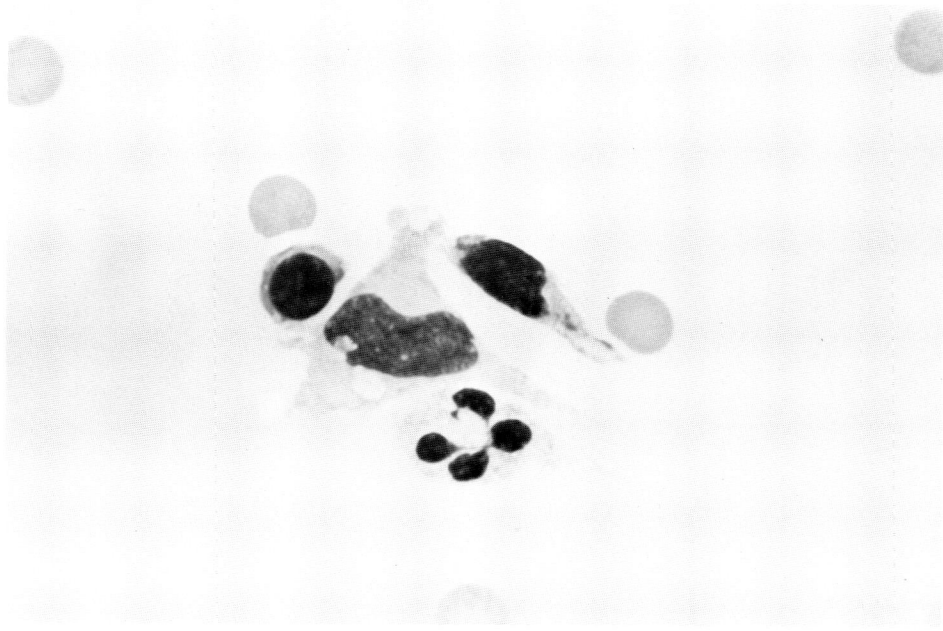

Fig. 12-3 A monocyte, accompanied by other inflammatory cells. (Cytospin, Wright stain, × 1,000.)

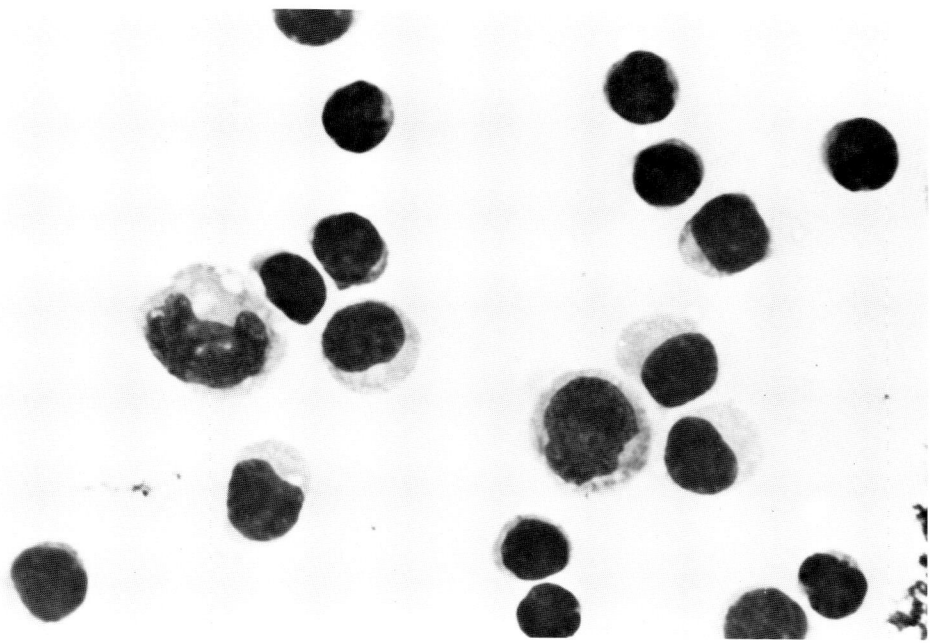

Fig. 12-4 Chronic meningitis, etiology undetermined. The absence of nucleoli, and predominantly dense nuclear chromatin imply a benign diagnosis. However, a hematologic work-up is indicated in this situation. (Cytospin, Wright stain, × 1,000.)

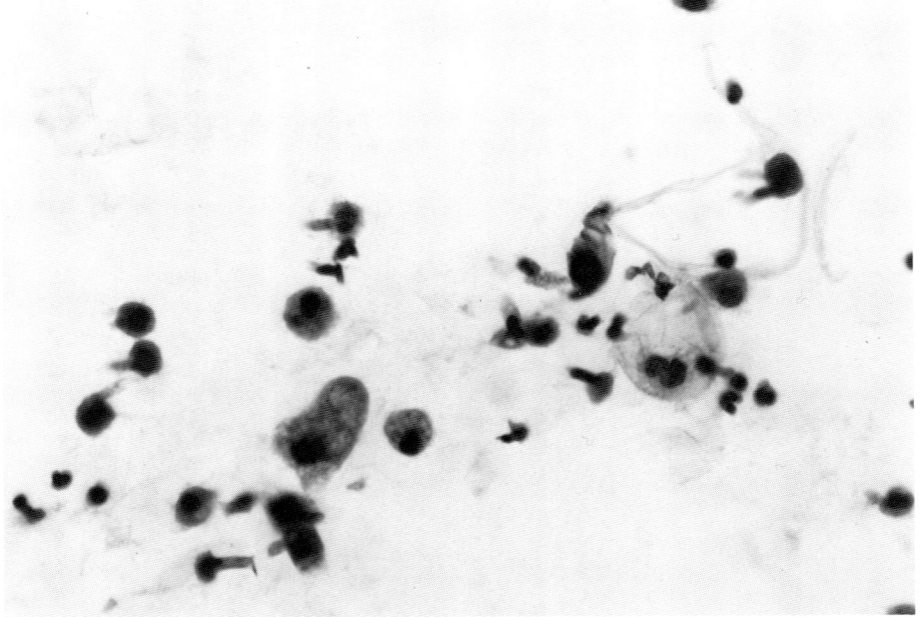

Fig. 12-5 Cerebral histiocytosis in a 13-year-old girl. The benign-appearing cells in the second spinal tap of this patient followed invasive diagnostic procedures. Reactive elements accompany these macrophages. (Nuclepore filter, Papanicolaou stain, × 400.)

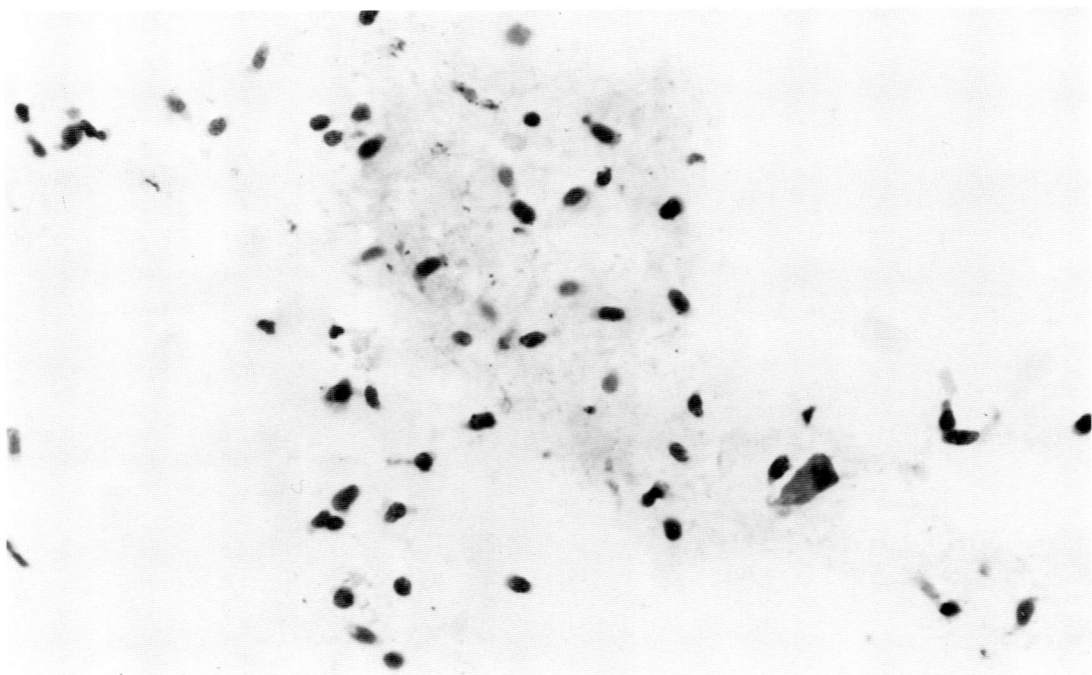

Fig. 12-6 Reactive pleocytosis secondary to tumor work-up. Leptomeningeal cells are the predominant cell in this reaction to a work-up for brain tumor. Elongated, small cells are comparable in size to lymphocytes, but the eccentric flair of the cytoplasm and the occasional blepharoplast differentiate them from the lymphoid group. (Nuclepore filter, Papanicolaou stain, × 400.)

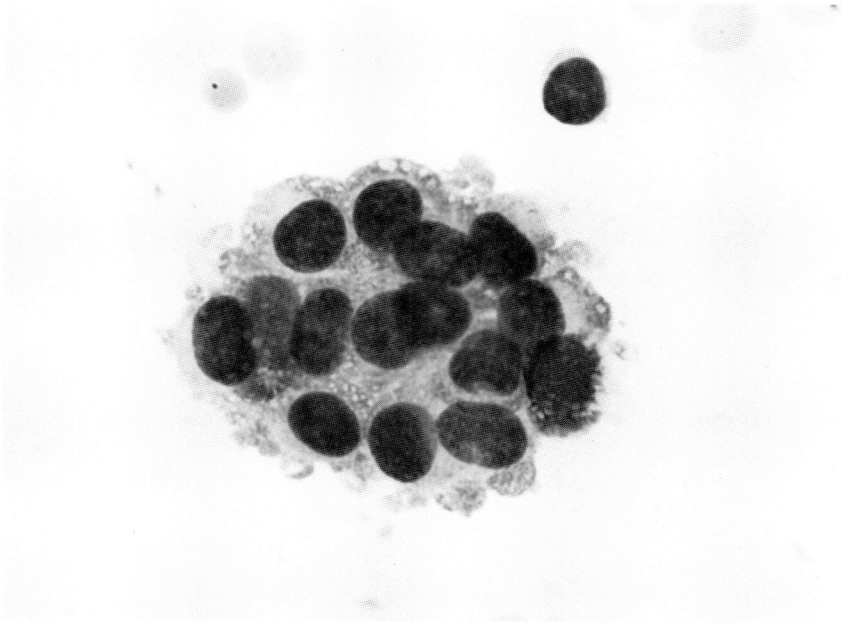

Fig. 12-7 Choroid plexus cells in neonatal head trauma. The abundant cytoplasm that is evident contrasts with that found in cells of a neural crest tumor, which in the latter is essentially invisible. The uniform chromatin and lack of nucleoli distinguish these cells from an adenocarcinoma cluster. (Cytospin, Wright stain, × 1,000.)

trauma (Fig. 12-7) and an infectious meningitis in the neonate is critical to the care of the patient, and is readily reflected in the cytologic interpretation of the CSF. The schema to follow take full advantage of cell identification and correlation with the clinical setting to arrive at a diagnosis that reflects the origin of the cells. Clearly, conscientious communication with the clinicians caring for the patient is paramount, both in terms of increasing one's experience with these specimens and arriving at a logical conclusion.

TUMORS OF THE CENTRAL NERVOUS SYSTEM

Because general experience with cytologic samples containing neoplastic cells is limited, certain rules of thumb are helpful. If the cell population is mixed, the lesion will usually be benign; if the cells are monomorphous, a neoplasm is probably present. However, lymphocytes frequently accompany tumor cells as a host response, so their presence should not infer that the mixture of cells is a benign process (Figs. 12-8 and 12-9). The diagnostic decision tree shown in Figure 12-2 is based on the size of tumor cells. Specific morphologic characteristics are described in Tables 12-2 to 12-5.

Primary Brain Tumors

Primary brain tumors account for 1 percent of all deaths and 9 percent of all neoplasms of the CNS. In the child, 70 percent of these lesions are infratentorial; in the adult, 70 percent are supratentorial. Primary tumors are less likely to exfoliate than are metastatic tumors. Gliomas are, by far, the most common primary brain tumors in both adults and children. Anatomic site is important to cell recovery in the CSF; the number of cells in a cytologic sample is usually small. Medulloblastomas, ependymomas, and leukemias shed the greatest amount of material.[16-18]

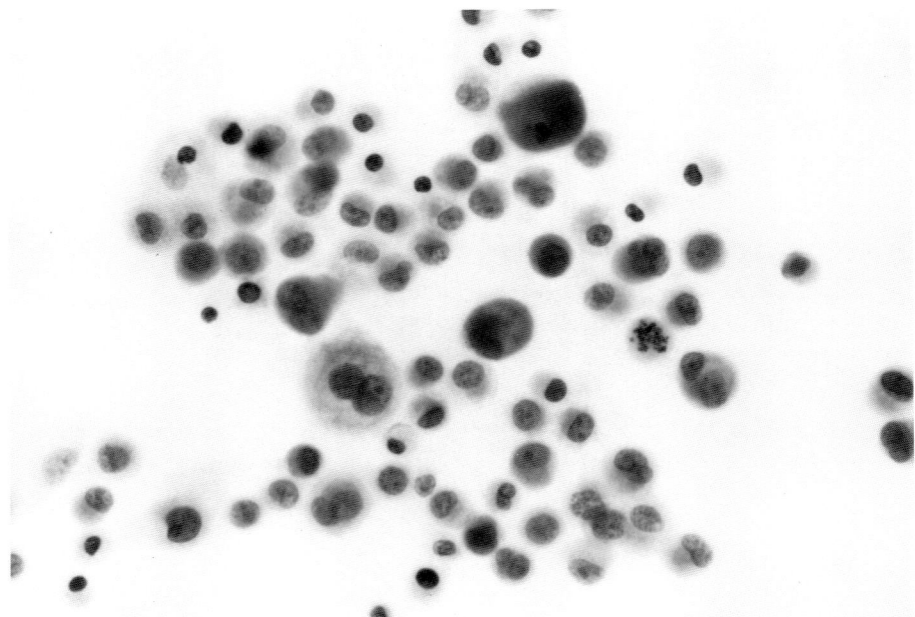

Fig. 12-8 Metastatic adenocarcinoma from the gallbladder. The enormous cellularity of this specimen with almost exclusively malignant cells immediately suggests a diagnosis of meningeal carcinomatosis. Compare the size of the tumor cells with the small inflammatory cells to appreciate their extraordinary size. Also note the mitotic figure. (Millipore filter, Papanicolaou stain, × 400.) (Courtesy of Dr. Torsten Löwhagen, Karolinska Institute.)

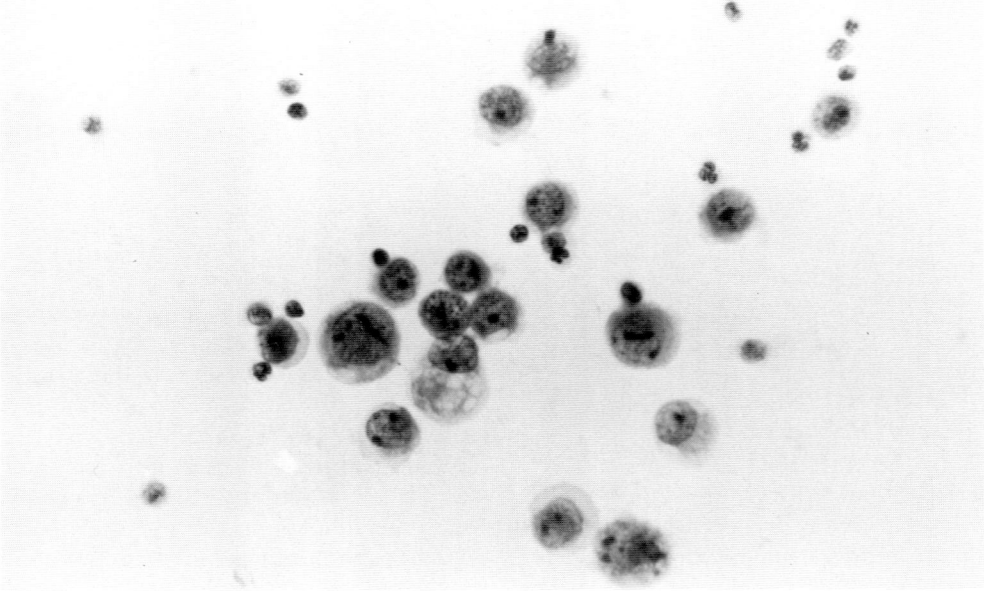

Fig. 12-9 Metastatic adenocarcinoma from the breast. In addition to the tumor cells, note the mononuclear cells that represent a response to the presence of tumor. The small cells are good indicators of the relatively large size of the tumor cells. (Nuclepore filter, Papanicolaou stain, × 400.)

Table 12-2 Cytomorphologic Characteristics of Neoplastic Large (>20 μm) Cells in CSF

Cellular Characteristics	Type of Tumor
Hazy cytoplasmic outline; single mass on CT scan; affecting child or adult; Crisp nuclear chromatin	Primary tumor, especially all glial tumors
Distinct cytoplasmic outline; multiple masses on CT scan; usually affecting adults; nuclear chromatin often blurred	Secondary tumor, especially adenocarcinoma or melanoma
Many cells; no parenchymal lesion detected on CT scan	Meningeal carcinomatosis

Table 12-4 Cytomorphologic Characteristics of Neoplastic Cells in CSF Small-to-Medium Cells (12–20 μm)

Cellular Characteristics	Type of Midline Tumor
Anterior	
Size: larger than in neuroectodermal tumors (NETs)	Pituitary adenoma
Chromatin: fine	
Nuclear outline: round or oval	
Nucleoli: small but visible	
Cytoplasm: abundant; often appearing syncytial	
Posterior	
Size: larger than in NETs	Germinoma
Chromatin: finely granular	
Nuclear outline: round	
Nucleoli: very prominent	
Cytoplasm: abundant	
Often accompanied by small lymphocytes	
Very similar to NETs	Pineoblastoma

GLIOMAS

Astrocytoma is the most common primary brain tumor occurring in both children and adults. It may be of low or high grade (glioblastoma multiforme) (Fig. 12-10). The anatomic location is important to survival. Cell presentation varies depending on the grade of the tumor. Cells often look epithelial and benign. The higher the grade of the tumor, the more pronounced is the associated hyperchromasia and multinucleation. Nuclei are round to oval. Nucleoli are indistinct with bland chromatin in low-grade lesions. High-grade neoplasms demonstrate severe nuclear hyperchromasia and variation in cytoplasmic shape (Fig. 12-11). The cytoplasm may be opaque or lacy; cell borders may be distinct or hazy (Table 12-2). Glial fibrils (cytoplasmic extensions) are apparent in Papanicolaou-stained smears of needle aspirates (Figs. 12-12 and 12-13) and touch preparations; immunochemistry for glial fibrillary acidic protein can be used to confirm the glial nature of the cells.[19] Cell aggregates are common, especially in cystic lesions, and may be confused with cell balls of a metastatic adenocarcinoma.

Ependymomas and choroid plexus papillomas originate in the ventricular system. These tumors are easily recovered in CSF because of cell accessibility to the CSF compartment. Ependymoma is the most common tumor of the spinal cord, with cells that bear a striking resemblance to the columnar epithelial cells of benign lesions (Fig. 12-14) or, when atypical, that resemble cells from an adenocarcinoma. Nucleoli are inconspicuous, and chromatin is usually fine. Rosettes can occasionally be recognized (Fig. 12-15), but should not be confused with those indicating a neural crest tumor (Fig. 12-16).

Oligodendrogliomas (Figs. 12-17 and 12-18) are rare tumors that affect adults. The cells are monoto-

Table 12-3 Cytomorphologic Characteristics of Neoplastic Cells in CSF Small Cells (<15 μm)

Nonhematopoietic Origin/Cellular Characteristics	Tumor Type

Size: larger than a lymphocyte
Chromatin: clumped, coarse, smudged
Nuclear outline: round to polygonal, no notches, clefts, or "noses," molding is a characteristic feature
Nucleoli: indistinct
Cytoplasm: minimal, best seen in clusters
	Neuroectodermal (neural crest) tumor (NET) in children or young adults
	    Medulloblastoma,
	    Retinoblastoma, primitive NET
	Small cell undifferentiated (oat cell) carcinoma in older adults

366 PRACTICAL CYTOPATHOLOGY

Table 12-5 Comparative Cytomorphology of Benign versus Malignant Lymphoid Cells in CSF Small Cells (<15 μm)

Hematopoietic Origin/Cellular Characteristics	Tumor Type

Benign lymphoid cells
  Cytoplasm: small amount
  Chromatin: maximum hyperchromasia; smooth even if clumped
  Nuclear borders: smooth
  Nucleoli: absent or rare
	Mature lymphocytes indicating *virus* or *chronic lymphocytic leukemia* (very rare)

Malignant lymphoid cells
  Size: larger than mature lymphocytes
  Chromatin: paler and coarser than lymphocytes
  Nuclear borders: irregular, with notches, clefts, and "noses"
  Nucleoli: often multiple
	Monotonous nuclear shape indicates *leukemic blasts;* variable shape and size indicate *lymphoma*

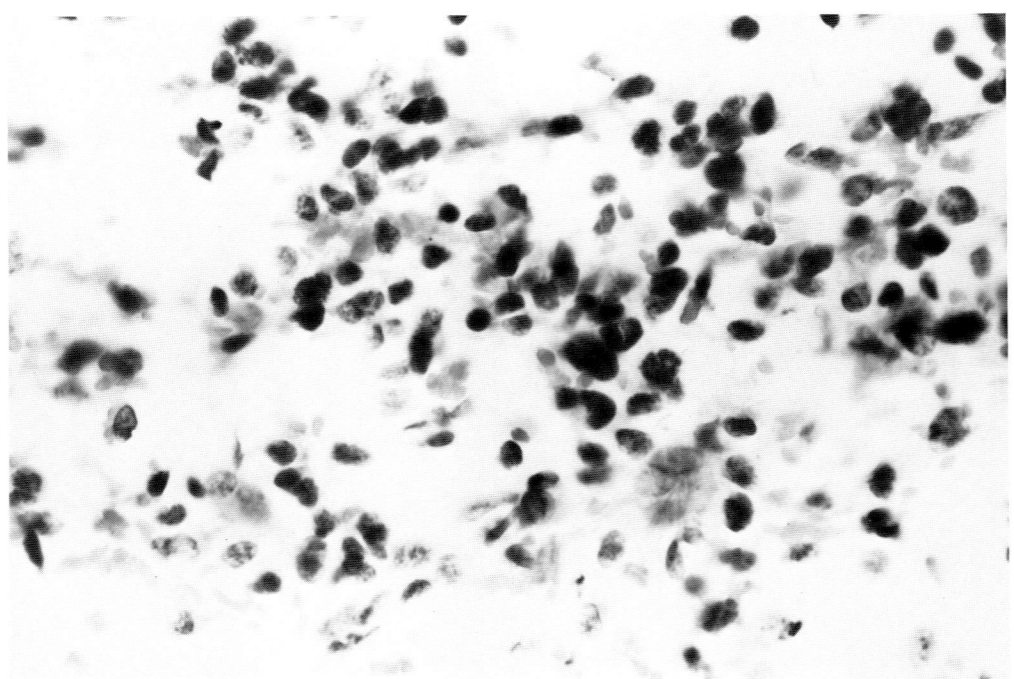

Fig. 12-10 Astrocytoma, grade IV. Nuclear hyperchromasia, anisonucleosis, and pleomorphism are characteristic of high-grade gliomas. Note the lack of intercellular connections and the singularity of the cells. Such a pattern could be mistaken for an anaplastic epithelial tumor. (Sediment smear, Papanicolaou stain, × 200.)

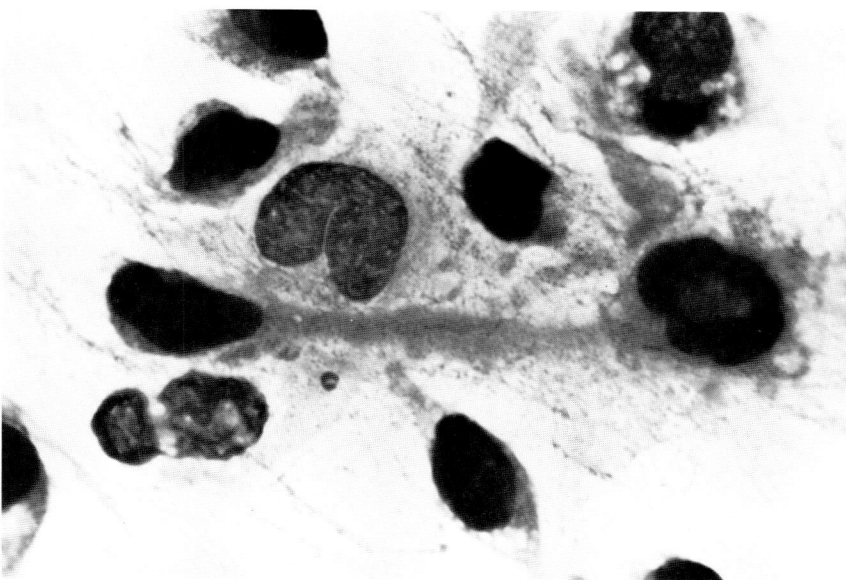

Fig. 12-11 Astrocytoma, grade IV. The great variation from one cell to another in the high-grade astrocytomas is evident. Not only do the size and shape vary, but the chromatin content and pattern are inconsistent from one cell to the other. (FNA, MGG stain, × 1,000.)

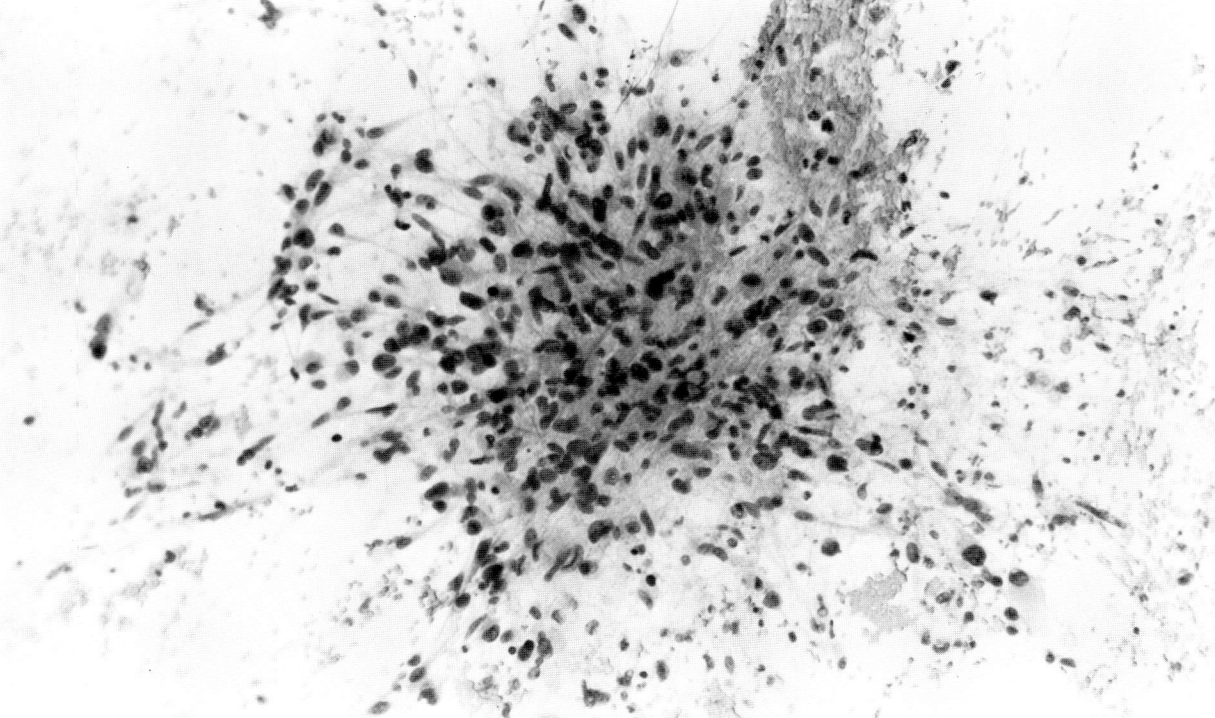

Fig. 12-12 Astrocytoma, grade IV. This low-power view of the yield of an FNA shows the generous quantity of material that can be obtained by this procedure. (FNA, H&E stain, × 100.)

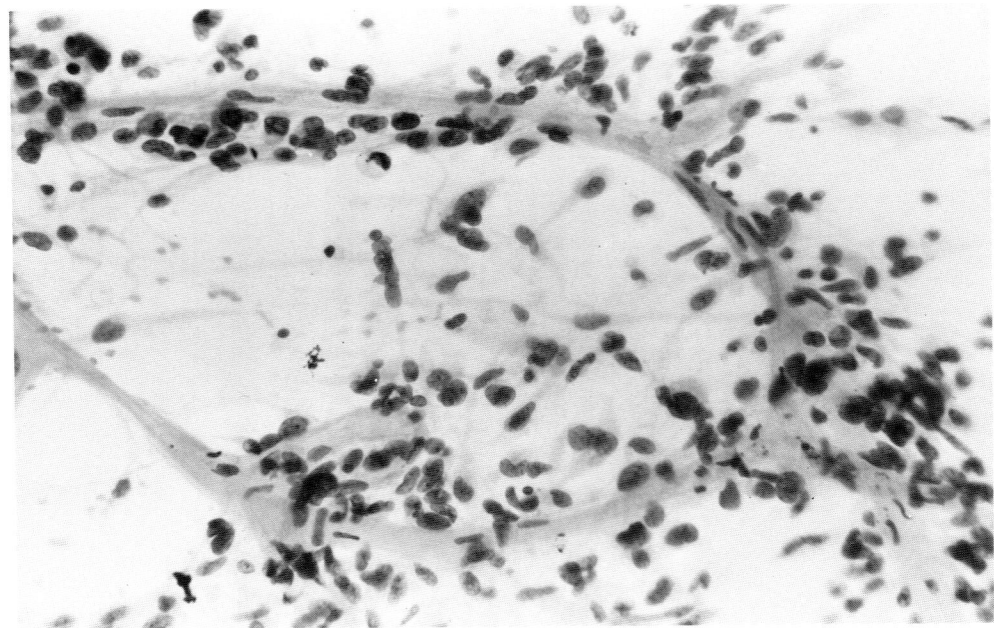

Fig. 12-13 Astrocytoma, wet-fixed smear. The nuclear detail is clearly visible, but cytoplasmic components and fibrillar extensions are better appreciated with air-dried, MGG-stained material. (FNA smear, H&E stain, × 200.)

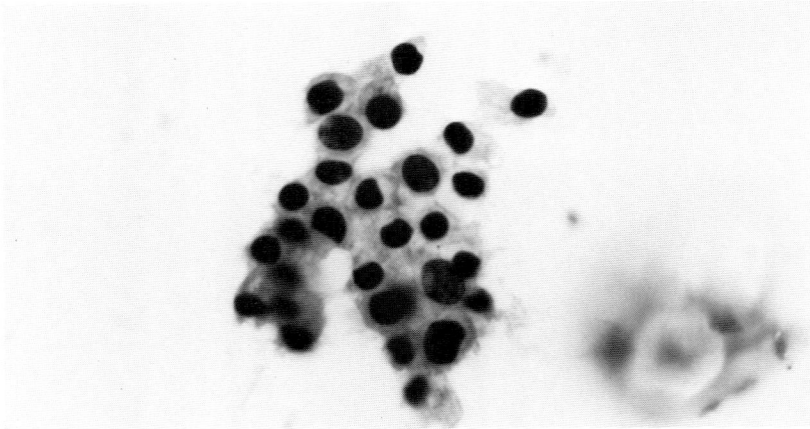

Fig. 12-14 Ependymoma. The almost uniformly round nuclei are unusually hyperchromatic, probably as a result of degeneration. The honeycomb and distinct cytoplasmic outlines are characteristic of this tumor. Note the talc crystal that is located to the right of the group. (Nuclepore filter, Papanicolaou stain, × 1,000.)

CYTOLOGY OF THE CENTRAL NERVOUS SYSTEM **369**

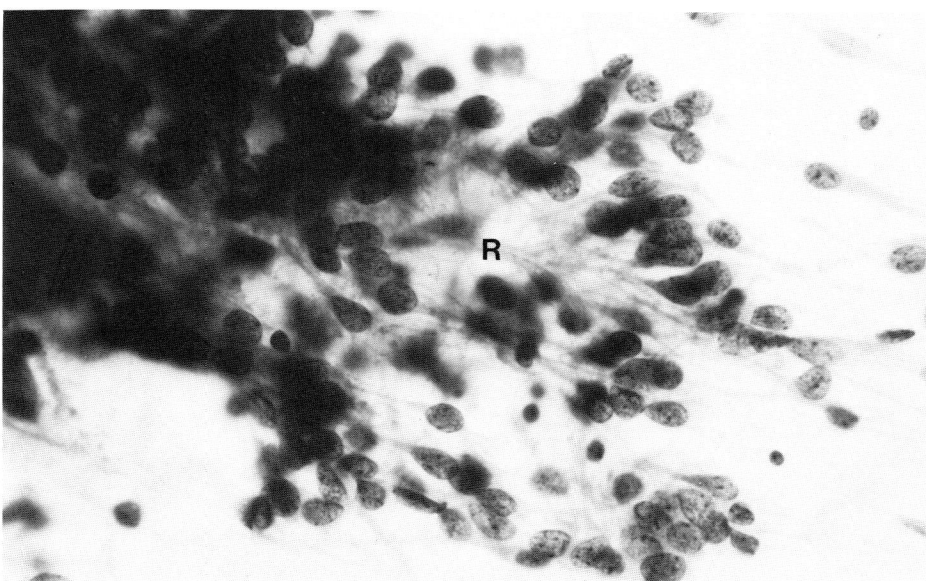

Fig. 12-15 Ependymoma. The fibrillar extensions of cytoplasm, which have produced a rosette (R), are dramatically displayed here. (FNA smear, H&E stain, × 400.)

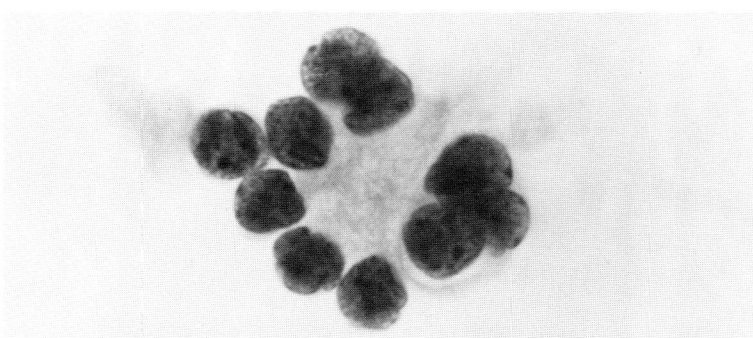

Fig. 12-16 Medulloblastoma. Both ependymomas and neural crest tumors form rosettes, but this neural crest rosette is distinguished by its lack of cytoplasm and hyperchromatic nuclei. Note also that the degree of molding is more prominent in neural crest tumors than in ependymomas. (Nuclepore filter, Papanicolaou stain, × 1,000.)

370 PRACTICAL CYTOPATHOLOGY

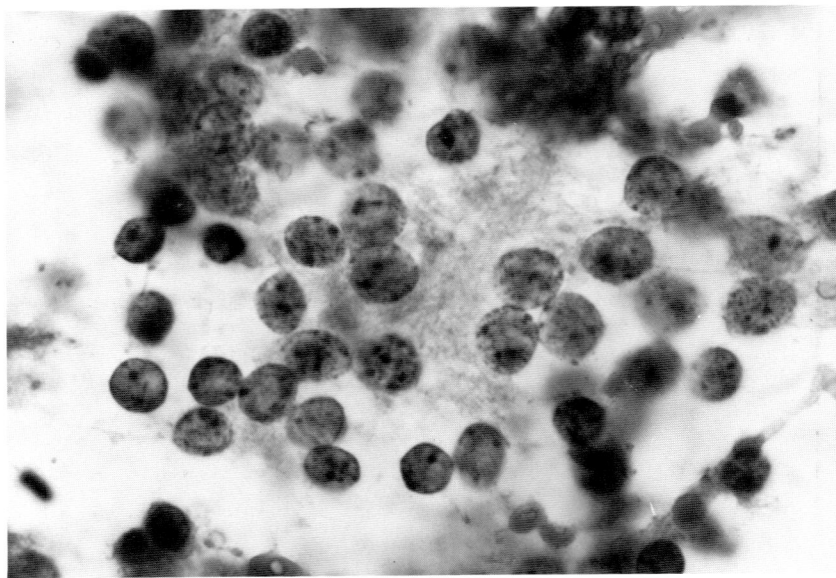

Fig. 12-17 Oligodendroglioma. The cytoplasm suspends the nuclei in a syncytial fashion. This appearance is distinct from that of other glial tumors in which fibrillary processes connect the cells. (Sediment smear, Papanicolaou stain, × 1,000.)

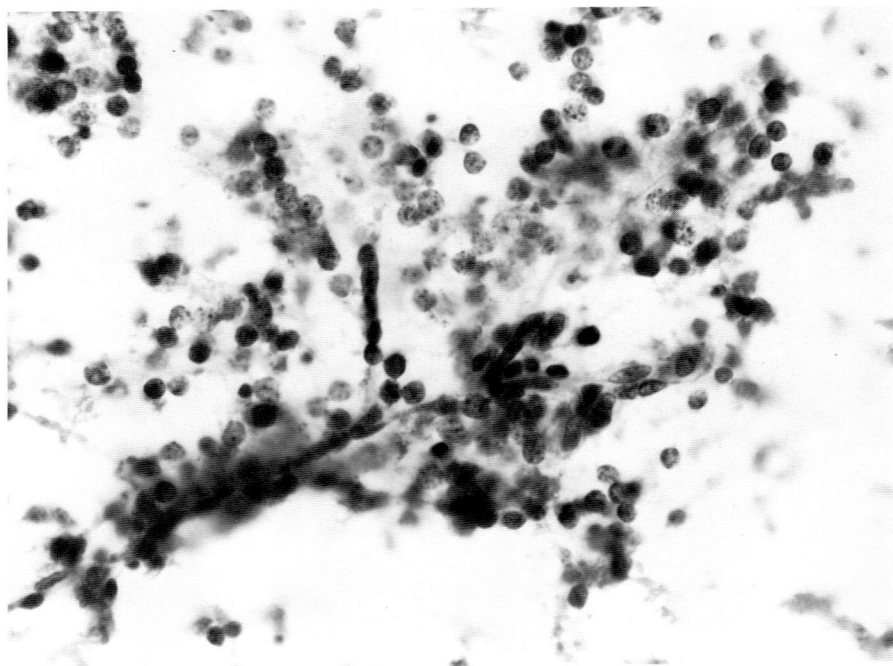

Fig. 12-18 Oligodendroglioma. In addition to the syncytial quality of the cytoplasm, note the right-angle branching of the capillary, a characteristic of this tumor. (Sediment smear, Papanicolaou stain, × 400.)

nous, with delicate cytoplasm that suspends the round nuclei in a transparent syncytial "wash" (Fig. 12-19). Chromatin is finely granular and nucleoli are indistinct.

NEURAL CREST TUMORS

Medulloblastomas, retinoblastomas, and neuroblastomas (Figs. 12-16, 12-20 and 12-21) occur in children and young adults. The cells of the lesions are small and hyperchromatic, and usually exfoliate in clusters (an essential criterion for diagnosis) (Table 12-3). Cytoplasm is very scant, and nuclei mold against each other. Chromatin is dark and smudged, and nucleoli are inconspicuous. Rosettes are rare. It is impossible to distinguish between these lesions by cytologic methods.[6,9,18] Careful attention to criteria, especially cell clusters, will help to differentiate these cells from those of leukemia (Fig. 12-22).

MIDLINE TUMORS

Pinealoma, a rare tumor of the pineal body that may affect both children and adults, is located at the end of the third ventricle under the corpus callosum. Tumors at this site are locally destructive. On cytologic examination, more than 50 percent of these tumors resemble the germinomas of the gonads, complete with accompanying lymphocytes (Fig. 12-23 and Table 12-4). The tumor cells are monomorphous and have round nuclei, moderate amounts of lacy cytoplasm, and prominent nucleoli. The cells of pinealoma are easily confused with those of oligodendroglioma or metastatic seminoma.

Pituitary adenomas constitute 10 percent of all intracranial growths in adults. They often produce abnormal endocrine activity. The cytomorphology of the lesion appears to be benign. A honeycomb or papillary pattern is frequently present. The nuclei are

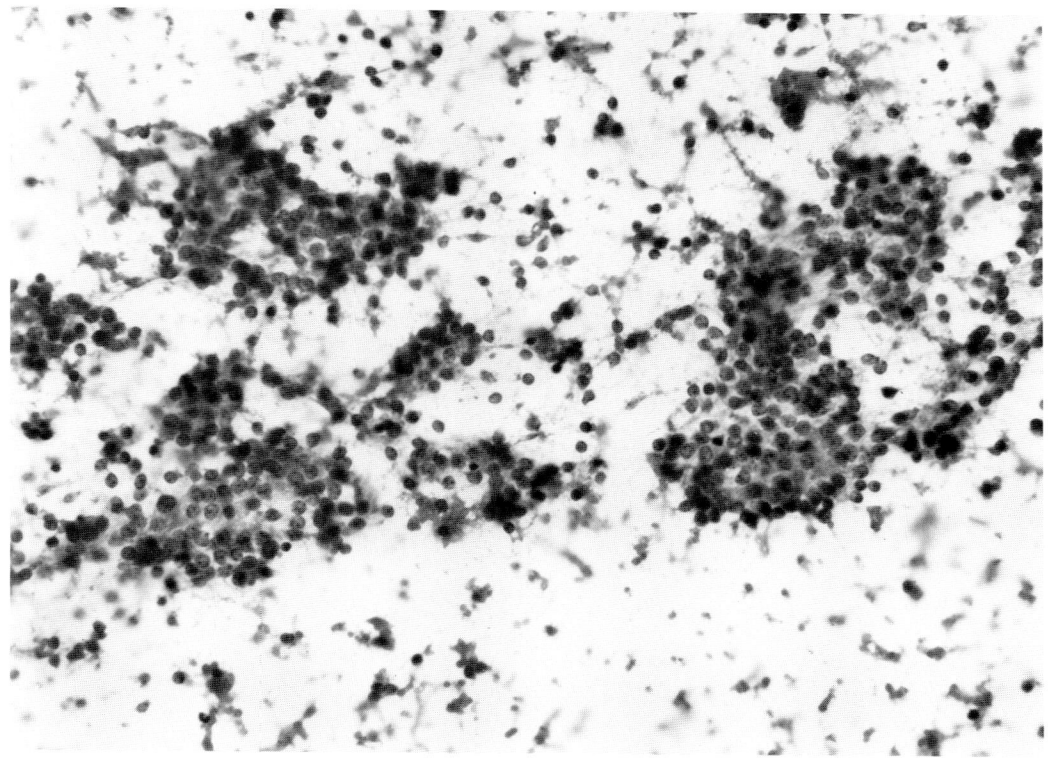

Fig. 12-19 Oligodendroglioma. In comparison to other glial tumors, note the absence of fibrillary processes. Instead, the cytoplasm forms a watery haze in which the very round nuclei are suspended. (FNA smear, Papanicolaou stain, × 200.)

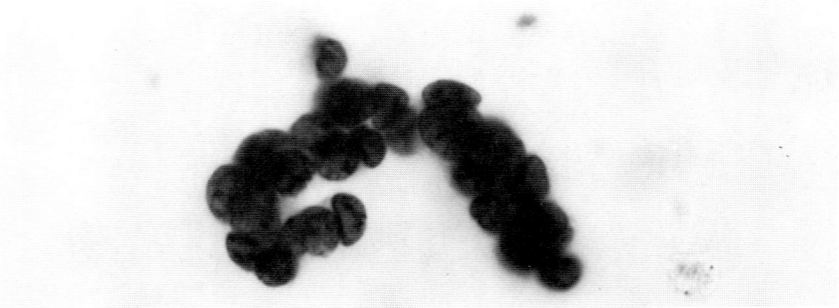

Fig. 12-20 Retinoblastoma. This cluster of cells in CSF cannot be distinguished cytologically from any of the other neural crest tumors. Note the nuclear molding and primitive appearance of these cells with their scanty cytoplasm. (Nuclepore filter, Papanicolaou stain, × 1,000.)

small and uniformly round, and chromatin is bland. Nucleoli are small, but may be prominent.

MENINGIOMAS

Meningiomas are tumors that affect young adults. They arise from the coverings of the brain, but rarely exfoliate. They are usually surgically resectable. The cells resemble small fibroblasts with oval nuclei and inconspicuous nucleoli, and grow in tight whorls (Fig. 12-24). Psammoma bodies may be seen. Most cytologic samples are needle aspirates; if cells exfoliate spontaneously, a meningiosarcoma should be considered.

Metastatic Tumors

Metastatic tumors account for 50 percent of all intracranial neoplasms. Lung (Figs. 12-25 and 12-26) and breast (Fig. 12-27) predominate among the common sites for adenocarcinomas that are metastatic to the brain.[13,16] Melanomas (Fig. 12-28) and choriocarcinomas, although uncommon, metastasize to the brain frequently. More than 80 percent of patients

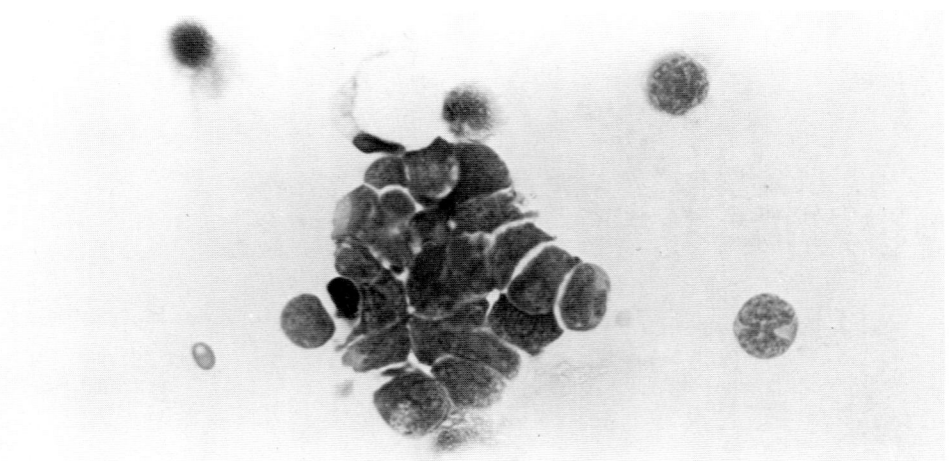

Fig. 12-21 Medulloblastoma. Note that this is a true tissue fragment, defined by tight cellular packing, sparse cytoplasm supporting the intercellular connections, and smooth outlines of the entire fragment. The cells appear to fit together much more closely than those of the lymphoma pictured in Figure 12-30. However, differential diagnosis is often difficult, and depends on a clinical history. (Cytospin, Wright stain, × 400.)

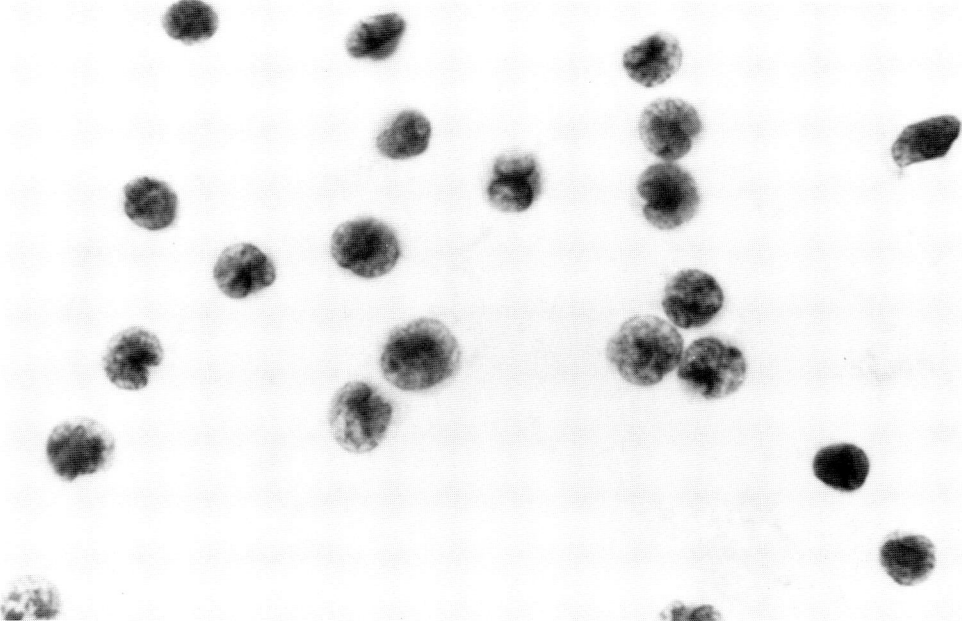

Fig. 12-22 Acute lymphocytic leukemia. These blasts may be difficult to differentiate from neural crest tumor cells, except that the blasts of acute lymphocytic leukemia usually have more convoluted nuclei and a rounder shape than do neural crest tumor cells, which tend to be more hyperchromatic and have angulated nuclear outlines. Clinical history is the most important deciding factor in diagnosis. (Nuclepore filter, Papanicolaou stain, × 1,000.)

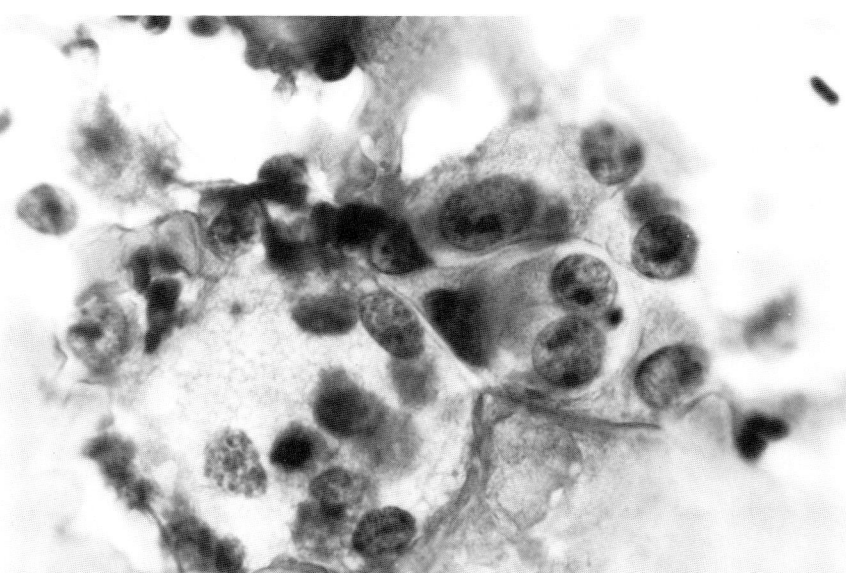

Fig. 12-23 Germinoma of the pineal area. This material was obtained from a hypothalamic tumor mass in a 12-year-old boy with a brief history of hydrocephalus. The material was obtained during a shunting procedure. Note the epithelial quality of some of the cells. The openness of the chromatin and the prominence of the nucleoli are characteristic of the germinoma group. (Sediment smear, Papanicolaou stain, × 1,000.) (Courtesy of Dr. Lilian Solt, Northwestern Memorial Hospital, Chicago, IL)

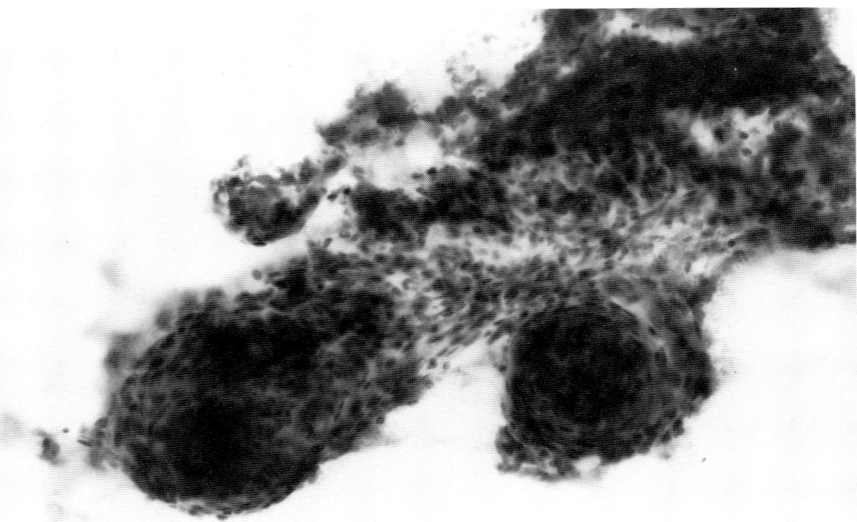

Fig. 12-24 Meningioma. These lesions rarely spontaneously exfoliate; this specimen was obtained prior to operative removal of the tumor. Note the tightly whorled, papillaroid groups. (Sediment smear, Papanicolaou stain, × 200.)

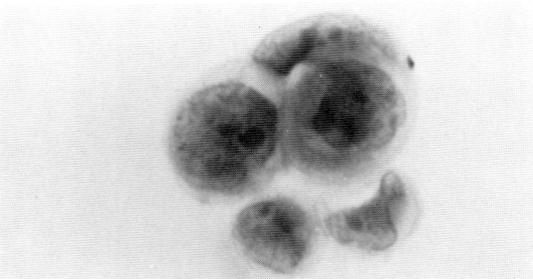

Fig. 12-25 Adenocarcinoma, CSF specimen. This patient had widely disseminated adenocarcinoma, the primary site of which was undetermined. (Nuclepore filter, Papanicolaou stain, × 1,000.)

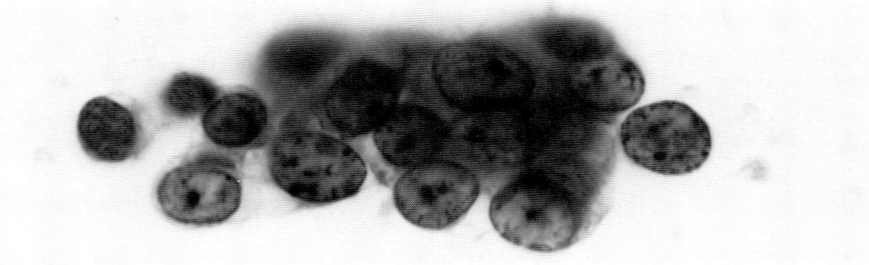

Fig. 12-26 Adenocarcinoma, sputum specimen. The diagnosis of alveolar cell carcinoma of the lung was suggested by both the cytomorphology of the sputum and the CSF, but was never confirmed as no autopsy was performed. (Sputum smear, Papanicolaou stain, × 1,000.)

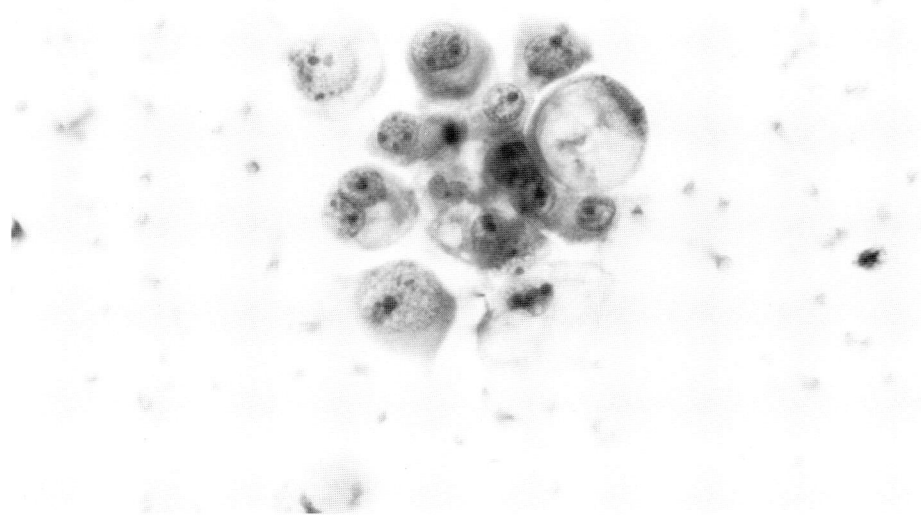

Fig. 12-27 Adenocarcinoma, breast. This lumar puncture was obtained prior to radiation therapy. Note the relative uniformity of the chromatin pattern and nuclear shape. (Nuclepore filter, Papanicolaou stain, × 1,000.)

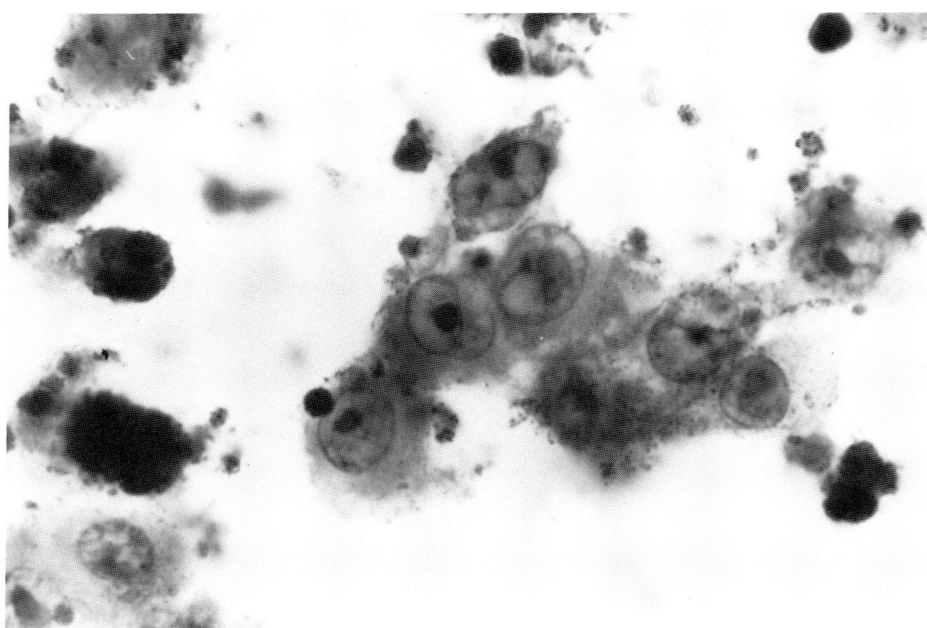

Fig. 12-28 Malignant melanoma. This specimen, obtained by FNA contains dark brown granular pigment, which is especially prominent within the macrophages. This, combined with a finding of definitely malignant cells, unquestionably establishes the diagnosis of melanoma. (FNA, Papanicolaou stain, × 1,000.)

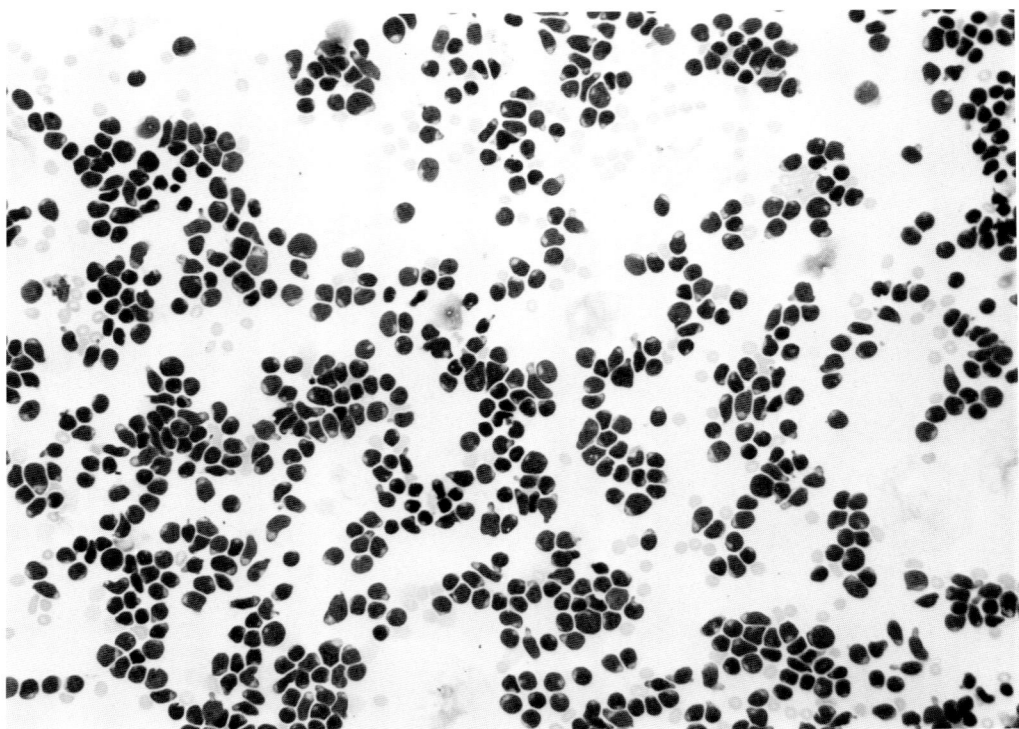

Fig. 12-29 Non-Hodgkin's lymphoma. This centrifuged sample could be derived from either a lymphoma or a leukemia, and is shown to illustrate the packing of cells in a cellular specimen. Although the denser areas display molding, neither the abundant solitary cells that are typical of malignant lymphoid forms, nor the outlines of the groups are as smooth as the tissue fragments from the medulloblastoma displayed in Figure 12-22. (Cytospin, Wright stain, × 200.)

with metastases to the brain have multiple lesions. Secondary tumors of the CNS usually shed more cells than do primary tumors (Figs. 12-8 and 12-9, Table 12-2). Knowledge of the patient's clinical history is crucial, for it is only rarely that the CSF is the first "positive" specimen; oat cell carcinoma of the lung and gastric adenocarcinoma are exceptions to this rule.[20] Comparison of the cytomorphology in the CSF with the histology of the primary tumor may be helpful; "second" primaries are becoming more the rule than the exception with increasingly successful treatment of "first" tumors. It must also be remembered that infections can present as tumor masses.

Leukemia/Lymphoma

Leukemic involvement of the CNS by hematopoietic tumors is common, especially if only systemic chemotherapy has been administered. As a rule, lymphomas shed greater numbers of cells (Fig. 12-29) than do leukemias. The cell type is usually difficult to identify; however, the diagnosis will already be established by the clinical history and bone marrow sample or lymph node biopsy. The role of the cytologist is to decide whether or not blasts are present in the CNS[13] (Table 12-5).

Since leukemias (Figs. 12-22) will have a clinically established diagnosis of cell type, the appropriate "positive" CSF diagnosis is "Blasts present, consistent with history." The number of blasts is sometimes minimal. Unless peripheral blood contamination is present, thereby invalidating any diagnosis, even a few blasts should be reported. Decisions regarding appropriate changes in therapy will be made by the clinician.

The CNS is a very vulnerable site for leukemic involvement without intrathecal therapy, and the chances of CNS involvement increase with survival.[21]

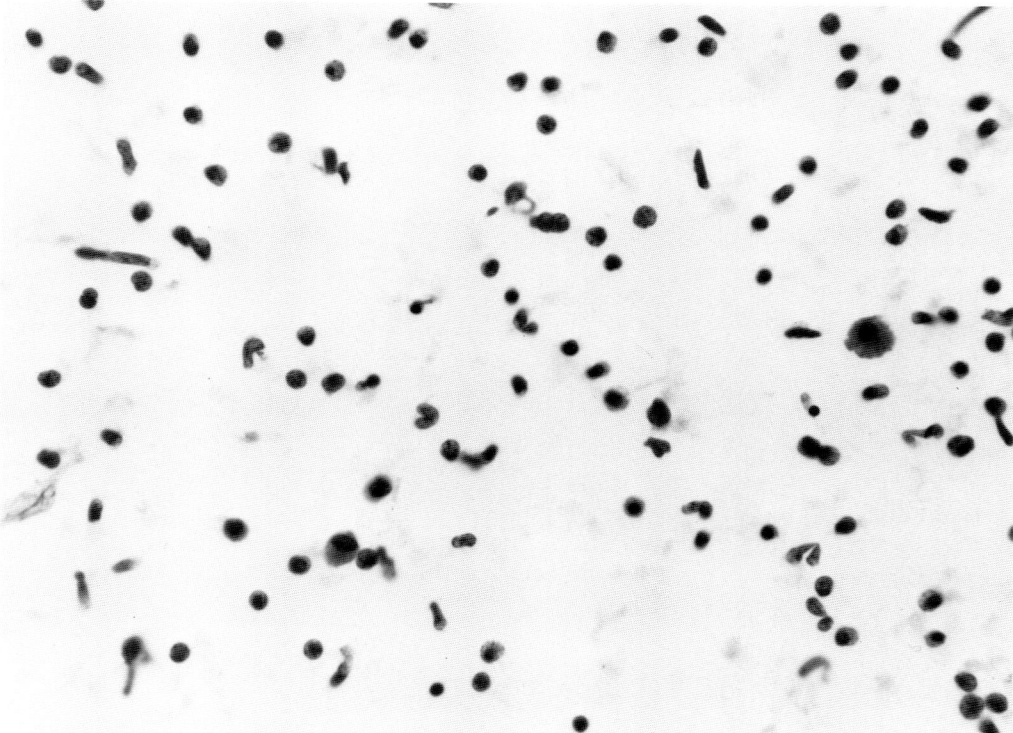

Fig. 12-30 Reactive pleocytosis in a patient with a history of acute lymphocytic leukemia. When a patient with leukemia has an increased CSF cell count, the question of a reactive versus an inflammatory versus a neoplastic process is often difficult to answer. Low-power magnification displays increased cellularity; note the variability in the size and shape of the cells. Higher power magnifications are necessary to determine the nature of the cells. (Nuclepore filter, Papanicolaou stain, × 200.)

Therefore, one usually develops a long-term familiarity with these patients as their treatment proceeds and the disease waxes and wanes. One must also be aware of reactive changes to intrathecal therapy (Fig. 12-30). To consider a specimen "positive," there should be well-preserved blasts in good numbers, distinct from reactive lymphocytes.[9] Close consultation with the clinicians and hematologists is vital.

REFERENCES

1. Kölmel HW: Atlas of Cerebrospinal Fluid Cells. 2nd ed. Springer-Verlag, New York, 1977
2. Naylor B: Cytologic study of intracranial fluids. Acta Cytol 5:198, 1961
3. Naylor B: The cytologic diagnosis of cerebrospinal fluids. Acta Cytol 8:141, 1964
4. Oehmichen M: Cerebrospinal Fluid Cytology. An Introduction and Atlas. WB Saunders, Philadelphia, 1976
5. Rich JR: A survey of cerebrospinal fluid cytology. Bull Los Angeles Neurol Soc 34:115, 1969
6. Hajdu SI, Hajdu EO: Cytopathology of sarcomas. p. 323. In Malignant Tumors of the Central Nervous System. WB Saunders, Philadelphia, 1976
7. Mouriquand C, Benabid AL, Breyton M: Stereotaxic cytology of brain tumors. Acta Cytol 31:756, 1987
7a. Chandrasoma PT, Apuzzo MLJ: Stereotactic brain biopsy. Igaku Shoin, New York, 1989
8. Gondos B, King EB: Cerebrospinal fluid cytology: Diagnostic accuracy and comparison of different techniques. Acta Cytol 20:542, 1976
9. Rosenthal DL: Cytology of the central nervous system. Monographs in Clinical Cytology. Vol. 8. Karger AG, Basel, 1984
10. Battifora H: Recent progress in the immunohisto-

chemistry of solid tumors. Semin Diagn Pathol 1:251, 1984
11. Vick WW, Wikstrand CJ, Bullard DE, et al: The use of a panel of monoclonal antibodies in the evaluation of cytologic specimens from the central nervous system. Acta Cytol 31:815, 1987
12. Bigner SH, Johnston WW: The cytopathology of cerebrospinal fluid. II. Metastatic cancer, meningeal carcinomatosis and primary central nervous system neoplasms. Acta Cytol 25:461, 1981
13. Bigner SH, Johnston WW: Cytopathology of the Central Nervous System. Masson Publishing USA, Paris, 1983
14. Glass JP, Melamed M, Chernick NL, Posner JB: Malignant cells in cerebrospinal fluid (CSF): The meaning of a positive CSF cytology. Neurology (NY) 29:1369, 1979
15. Mathios AJ, Nielson SL, Barrett D, King EB: Cerebrospinal fluid cytomorphology identification of benign cells originating in the central nervous system. Acta Cytol 21:403, 1977
16. An-Foraker SH: Cytodiagnosis of malignant lesions in cerebrospinal fluid. Acta Cytol 29:286, 1985
17. Balhuizen JC, Bots GTAM, Schaberg A, Bosman FT: Value of cerebrospinal fluid cytology for the diagnosis of malignancies in the central nervous system. J Neurosurg 48:747, 1978
18. Geisinger KR, Hajdu SI, Helson L: Exfoliative cytology of nonlymphoreticular neoplasms in children. Acta Cytol 28:16, 1984
19. Trojanowski JQ, Atkinson B, Lee VMY: An immunocytochemical study of normal and abnormal human cerebrospinal fluid with monoclonal antibodies to glial fibrillary acidic protein. Acta Cytol 30:235, 1986
20. Bigner SH, Johnston WW: The diagnostic challenge of tumors manifested initially by the shedding of cells into cerebrospinal fluid. Acta Cytol 28:29, 1984
21. Bigner SH, Johnston WW: The cytopathology of cerebrospinal fluid. I. Non-neoplastic conditions, lymphoma and leukemia. Acta Cytol 25:335, 1981

13
Cytopathology of Lymph Nodes

Robert W. Astarita

Lymph node aspiration cytology was employed during the early 1900s for the identification of trypanosomes in sleeping sickness.[1] Aspiration biopsy was practiced at Memorial Sloan Kettering during the 1930s,[2-4] with thin needle aspiration taking hold in Europe and Sweden in the 1950s and thereafter.[5-8] After several decades of apathy, fine needle aspiration (FNA) cytology diagnosis in the United States has recently attracted renewed interest. Its use has expanded dramatically to encompass a spectrum of reactive and malignant disorders, including those involving lymph nodes.[9-12] Familiarity with the cytologic features of benign and malignant conditions of lymph nodes has contributed substantially to the accuracy and precision of diagnosis both in FNA and in surgical biopsy specimens.

Indications for lymph node FNA (Table 13-1) include the diagnosis of malignant lymphoma, metastatic carcinoma, and infection in any patient presenting with persistent lymphadenopathy. FNA may be employed in staging of patients for non-Hodgkin's lymphoma (NHL), Hodgkin's disease (HD), and carcinoma. FNA also permits monitoring patient responses to therapy and assessment of disease progression. The simplicity and convenience of FNA expedite diagnosis and permit the clinician to proceed with therapy or surgical excision, if indicated.

Well prepared smears and cytospins from FNAs and imprints derived from surgical specimens yield technically optimal samples, ideally containing a monolayer of cells. Smears immediately fixed in 95-percent ethanol demonstrate crisp nuclear detail, while air-dried May-Grünwald-Giemsa (MGG)-stained preparations enhance cytoplasmic features. A variety of ancillary studies may be performed on cytologic specimens, including enzyme histochemistry, immunohistochemistry, electron microscopy, and flow cytometry in selected cases, although sample size and cost are obvious limiting factors. Some of these techniques are described in depth in Chapter 14. Additional material may be obtained in cases in which gene rearrangement studies appear indicated.[13,14]

A good way to become familiar with diagnostic cytologic criteria in lymph nodes is to prepare imprints from as many fresh specimens as possible, including those from normal tissue, inflammatory lesions, and benign and malignant tumors.[15,16] FNA technique and preparation of smears should be practiced on fresh or refrigerated surgical specimens before the first patient specimen is obtained.

Aspirate specimens may be processed in a variety of ways. Cytospin samples suspended in RPMI medium 1640 (Grand Island Biological, Grand Island,

Table 13-1 Indications for Lymph Node FNA

Patients presenting with persistent unexplained lymphadenopathy
Clinical suspicion of malignant lymphoma, metastatic carcinoma and infection
Staging of patients with Hodgkin's disease (HD), non-Hodgkin's lymphoma (NHL), and other known malignancies
Monitoring for response to therapy, disease progression, or recurrence
Providing samples for culture, immunocytochemistry, electron microscopy, and other ancillary studies
Determination of need for surgical biopsy/excision

NY) and fetal calf serum (FCS) and smears fixed in absolute alcohol, cold-buffered acetone, formal-acetone, or 95-percent ethanol may be used for most immunohistochemical studies. Some cytopathologists prefer to rinse the aspiration needle with Hank's balanced salt solution (HBSS) and 5 to 10 percent FCS for their cytospin preparations while others collect these specimens in phosphate buffered saline (PBS).

European-trained cytopathologists prefer MGG-stained smears, while those trained in the United States are more comfortable with Papanicolaou- and hematoxylin and eosin (H & E) stained smears. When possible, MGG stain should be combined with at least one other stain so that the advantages of each may be appreciated and correlated in the same sample. When an adequate sample is obtained, preparation of a cell block is sometimes useful in the assessment of tissue architecture and in the application of a variety of special stains.

In FNA, as is the case in surgical pathology, one can only diagnose what is on the slide. Adequate specimens must be obtained to achieve optimal diagnoses, and excellent technical preparations must be ensured. Ideally, the physician responsible for interpreting lymph node FNA should have a strong background in cytology, hematopathology, and surgical pathology. Also, the importance of clinical correlation cannot be overemphasized. For example, a history compatible with infectious mononucleosis, influenza, or drug hypersensitivity could explain an immunoblastic reaction that otherwise might be misdiagnosed as immunoblastic sarcoma (histiocytic lymphoma).

Identification of cohesive aggregates of cytologically malignant epithelial cells in an FNA specimen poses little diagnostic problem. A diagnosis of metastatic carcinoma is made with ease in most such cases.[17,18] Rarely in cases of micrometastases tumor may be missed in the FNA samples. Precise classification of metastatic neoplasms may prove more difficult in the less differentiated tumors, especially if there is no known primary site. The application of ancillary studies, including histochemistry, immunochemistry, and electron microscopy, often sharpens the diagnosis in these cases.

Cytologic diagnosis of lymphomas is most challenging. One pitfall is that FNA only samples a small percentage of the entire lymph node and therefore may not be representative of focal disease. However, multiple passes improve sampling and greatly reduce the number of false-negative results. Since most NHLs diffusely efface the lymph node, most samples adequately reflect the disease process.

Although tissue fragments are sometimes obtained in FNA specimens, tissue architecture is not discernible in most aspiration smears. Therefore, even if malignant lymphoma is diagnosed on FNA, assessment of a diffuse or nodular pattern still requires surgical biopsy. Despite this problem, lymphoma grading may be assigned in many cases without the need for surgical biopsy simply by correlating the grading in the National Cancer Institute (NCI) working formulation[19] with various modern classification systems (Tables 13-2 to 13-5). For example, according to the NCI working formulation, large cell malignant lymphomas, whether nodular or diffuse, are of intermediate grade, while large cell immunoblastic lymphomas, small noncleaved, and lymphoblastic lymphomas are classified as high grade.

Few pathologists feel comfortable making a primary diagnosis of malignant lymphoma on the basis of FNA without confirmatory surgical biopsy. Although lymph node FNA frequently yields an unequivocal diagnosis in conditions other than malignant lymphoma (e.g., metastatic carcinoma), in those aspirations in which malignant lymphoma is suspected, confirmatory surgical biopsy of the lymph node is the accepted practice at most centers. In experienced hands, however, an FNA primary diagnosis of malignant lymphoma may be made with confidence in selected cases. This is especially true in cases of large cell malignant lymphomas and in cases of HD in which the appropriate cell background and diagnostic Reed-Sternberg cells are identified. Furthermore, a combination of FNA and immunocyto-

Table 13-2 NCI Working Formulation of Non-Hodgkin's Lymphomas

Low grade
  Malignant lymphoma
    Small lymphocytic
      Consistent with CLL
      Plasmacytoid
  Malignant lymphoma, follicular
    Predominantly small cleaved cell
      Diffuse areas
      Sclerosis
  Malignant lymphoma, follicular
    Mixed, small cleaved and large cell
      Diffuse areas
      Sclerosis

Intermediate grade
  Malignant lymphoma, follicular
    Predominantly large cell
      Diffuse areas
      Sclerosis
  Malignant lymphoma, diffuse
    Small cleaved cell
      Sclerosis
  Malignant lymphoma, diffuse
    Mixed, small and large cell
      Sclerosis
      Epithelioid cell component
  Malignant lymphoma, diffuse
    Large cell
      Cleaved cell
      Noncleaved cell
      Sclerosis

High grade
  Malignant lymphoma
    Large cell immunoblastic
      Plasmacytoid
      Clear cell
      Polymorphous
      Epithelioid cell component
  Malignant lymphoma
    Lymphoblastic
      Convoluted cell
      Nonconvoluted cell
  Malignant lymphoma
    Small noncleaved cell
      Burkitt's
      Follicular areas

Miscellaneous
  Composite
  Mycosis fungoides
  Histiocytic
  Extremedullary plasmacytoma
  Unclassifiable
  Other

chemistry[20,21] may yield conclusive evidence of malignant lymphoma even in the more difficult mixed lymphocytic and histiocytic proliferations. Obviously, a lymph node FNA that is negative for malignancy does not exclude malignancy. In such cases repeat FNA or surgical biopsy is recommended should lymphadenopathy persist.

As more procedures are performed and greater experience is accrued in lymph node FNA, a positive diagnosis of malignant lymphoma will carry the same authority as it does in other organs. Furthermore, lymph node FNA currently provides useful information in the staging of patients previously diagnosed as having malignant lymphoma or HD and is helpful in monitoring patients for recurrent malignancy and for evolution of lymphomas from low-grade to higher-grade neoplasms.

Table 13-3 Rappaport Classification of Non-Hodgkin's Lymphomas

Nodular or Diffuse
  Lymphocytic well differentiated
  Lymphocytic poorly differentiated
  Mixed (lymphocytic-histiocytic)
  Histiocytic
  Undifferentiated

LYMPHOMA CLASSIFICATION

For clinicians and pathologists alike, lymphoma classification may closely approach the art of witchcraft. The problem has arisen as a result of imprecise subjective morphologic systems of the past and the

Table 13-4 Lukes-Collins Classification of Non-Hodgkin's Lymphomas

U-cell (undefined)

T-cell
    Small lymphocyte
    Convoluted lymphocyte
    Sézary cell-mycosis fungoides
    Immunoblastic sarcoma
    Lennert's lymphoma

B-cell
    Small lymphocyte
    Plasmacytoid lymphocyte
    Follicle center cell lymphoma (FCC)
        Follicular or diffuse with or without sclerosis
            Small cleaved
            Large cleaved
            Small noncleaved
            Large noncleaved
    Immunoblastic sarcoma
    Hairy cell leukemia

Histiocytic

logarithmic expansion of more modern classification systems during the 1970s and 1980s. Henry Rappaport's classification system (see Table 13-3) published in 1956[22] helped eradicate the confusion of past systems by recognizing two types of neoplastic cell: the lymphocyte and the histiocyte. Rappaport recognized lymphomas of well-differentiated and poorly differentiated lymphocytic type, a mixed lymphocytic and histiocytic type and an undifferentiated type of lymphoma. He also observed two patterns of lymph node involvement, diffuse and nodular, each of which correlates with biologic behavior and patient survival.

New functional classification systems were introduced during the 1970s by Lukes and Collins[23] (see Table 13-4) as well as by Lennert[24,25] (Table 13-5) and others, accompanying the rapid advances in immunology occurring at that time. The Lukes approach was based on two concepts: (1) morphologically similar small lymphocytes are composed of two cell types, B lymphocytes and T lymphocytes; and (2) small lymphocytes do not represent an end-stage cell but a cell that, under appropriate antigenic stimulation, undergoes transformation to a large functionally active cell, the immunoblast. The histiocytic lymphomas described by Rappaport were, in the main, recognized by Lukes and others as lymphomas of large transformed lymphocytes and lymphomas of immunoblasts, rather than as lymphomas of true histiocytes.

Neoplasms of the true histiocytic cells are in the minority, accounting for approximately 5 percent of the lymphomas now reported. A diagnosis of histiocytic lymphoma is a diagnosis of exclusion based on positive staining for α_1-antitrypsin, nonspecific esterase, antichymotrypsin, lysozyme, and monoclonal antibody (MoAb) phenotyping. The neoplastic histiocytes also are shown to lack the characteristic cytoplasmic or surface membrane markers of lymphocytes.

Functional classification systems are based on the assumption that lymphomas both morphologically

Table 13-5 Kiel Classification of Non-Hodgkin's Lymphoma

Low grade
    Malignant lymphoma lymphocytic
        B-CLL
        T-CLL
        Hairy cell leukemia
        Mycosis fungoides and Sézary's syndrome
        T-zone lymphoma
    Malignant lymphoma lymphoplasmacytic/lymphoplasmacytoid (LP immunocytoma)
    Malignant lymphoma plasmacytic
    Malignant lymphoma centrocytic
    Malignant lymphoma centroblastic/centrocytic
        Follicular
        Follicular and diffuse
        Diffuse
        With or without sclerosis

High grade
    Malignant lymphoma centroblastic
        Primary
        Secondary
    Malignant lymphoma lymphoblastic
        B-lymphoblastic (e.g., Burkitt's type)
        T-lymphoblastic (e.g., convoluted cell type)
        Unclassified
    Malignant lymphoma immunoblastic
        With plasmablastic/plasmacytic differentiation (B)
        Without plasmablastic/plasmacytic differentiation (B or T)

and biologically mimic their benign lymphoid counterparts, arising in, and homing to, the sites in which these benign lymphocytes normally reside. For example, malignant lymphomas of the B-lymphocytic type may be predicted to arise in or to home to lymph node follicles, bone marrow, hepatic portal tracts, and splenic malpighian bodies. By contrast, lymphomas of T lymphocytes are believed to arise in, or home to, lymph node paracortex, splenic periarteriolar sheath and to skin.

Once familiar with the cytomorphology of benign B and T lymphocytes, the clinician should have little difficulty in classifying most of the lymphomas composed of similar cells. For this reason, the B-cell areas of the lymph node, especially the secondary follicles, have been studied carefully and tracings (camera lucida) of the follicular center cells (FCC) and mantle zone cells prepared. The mantle zone is composed mostly of small lymphocytes and occasional dendritic reticulum cells. The cells in the follicular center are classified as small or large and as cleaved or noncleaved FCC. Classification of most B-cell lymphomas is based on the recognition of a preponderance of one of these morphologic lymphocytic cell types. Cytologic identification of T lymphocytes is more difficult, except in the most florid examples of mycosis fungoides and large cell T-immunoblastic sarcoma. Cerebriform nuclei, cytoplasmic pallor, interlocking cell membranes, and a background containing increased numbers of endothelial cells, eosinophils, and histiocytes are some of the features suggesting T-cell origin.[26,27] Confirmatory marker and/or gene rearrangement studies are critical to the diagnosis of most T-cell lymphomas.

DIFFERENTIAL DIAGNOSIS IN LYMPH NODE CYTOLOGY

In the evaluation of lymph node aspiration samples, the adequacy and satisfactory technical quality of the preparation must be ensured. Paucity of cells, bloody smears, nuclear crush artifact, overly thick smears, and air-drying artifact (e.g., ethanol-fixed smears) preclude the diagnosis in most cases. The slide is then viewed at low power to assess the overall arrangement of cells. Are the cells dispersed (Fig. 13-1, Plate 13-1), noncohesive and isolated, or are there cell aggregates (Fig. 13-2, Plate 13-2), sheets, and cell balls? Noncohesive cells almost always reflect a lymphoreticular or hematologic process. The presence of lymphoglandular bodies (background

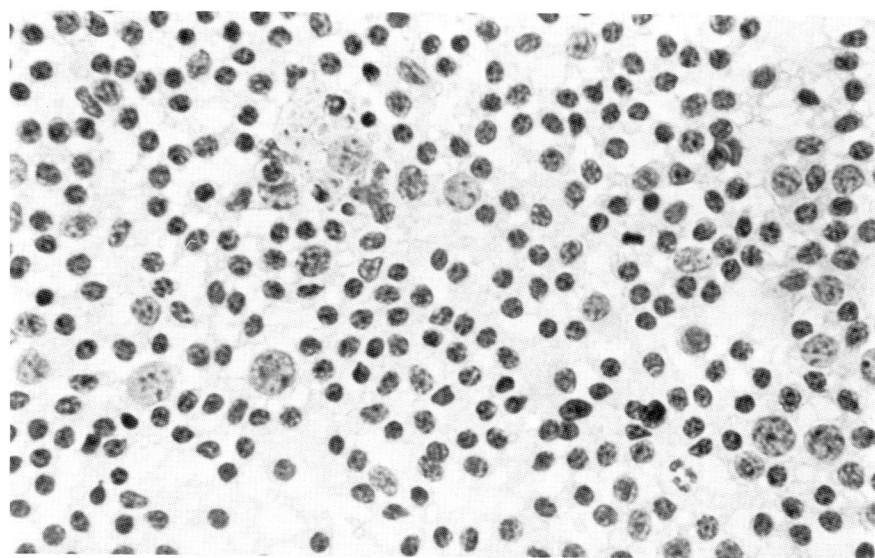

Fig. 13-1 Smear from lymph node FNA showing a spectrum of small lymphocytes, transformed follicular center cells, and tingible body macrophages indicative of a benign reactive process. The dispersed cellular smear is characteristic of lymphoid tissue. (Papanicolaou stain, × 125.) (See Plate 13-1.)

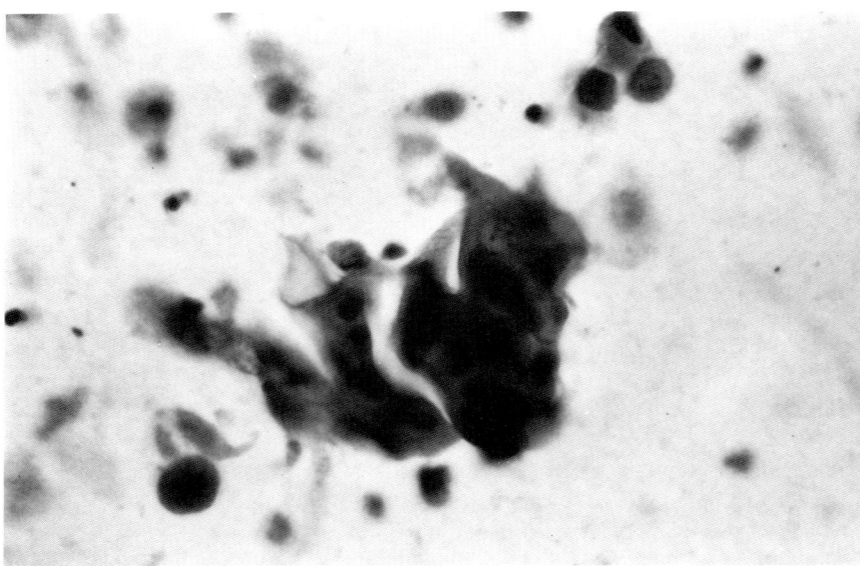

Fig. 13-2 Lymph node FNA specimen containing cell groups and aggregates in a case of metastatic squamous carcinoma. (Papanicolaou stain, × 200.) (See Plate 13-2.)

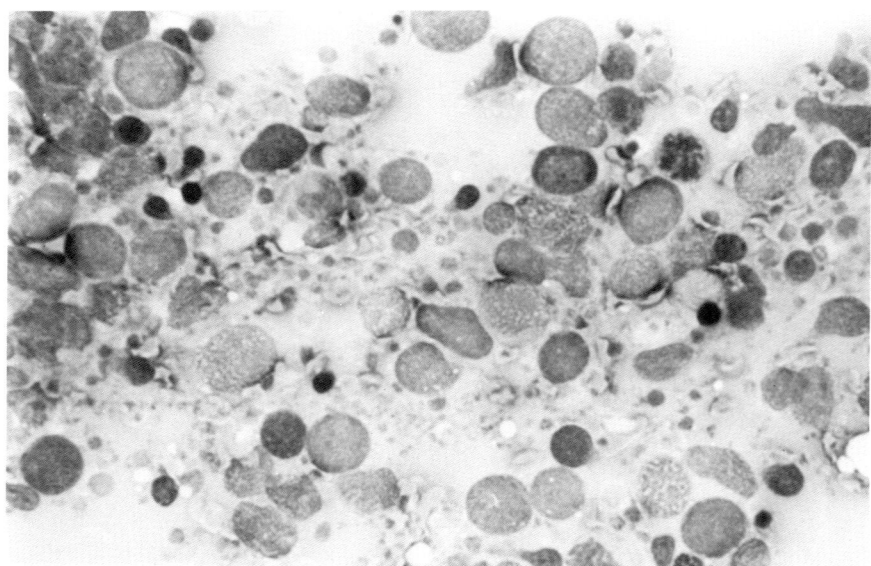

Fig. 13-3 Lymph node FNA smear from patient with malignant lymphoma of the large noncleaved FCC type (centroblastic) showing relatively monomorphous population of large transformed follicular center cells and prominent lymphoglandular bodies (fragments of lymphocytic cytoplasm) characteristic of lymphoid proliferations. (May Grünwald Giemsa stain, × 250.) (See Plate 13-3.)

blue gray cytoplasmic fragments) argues in favor of a benign or malignant lymphocytic proliferation (Fig. 13-3, Plate 13-3). Lymphoglandular bodies are seen best in air-dried MGG smears in lymphoid proliferation of large transformed lymphocytes and immunoblasts. Malignant cohesive cell aggregates usually represent metastatic carcinoma. The slide is then screened for loose aggregates and cords of atypical small cells that could correlate with small cell carcinomas or rarely with Merkel cell tumor.[28] Monotonous ribbons and uniform small cell cords and aggregates correlate with carcinoid, islet cell, and similar tumors of the APUD or neuroendocrine group. Clusters, sheets, and/or isolated large atypical cells suggest metastatic carcinoma or HD.

Recognition of a necrotic background is suggestive of metastatic carcinoma, high-turnover lymphoma, nodular sclerosing HD, nodes draining suppurative infections, infarct, and cases of necrotizing granulomatous lymphadenitis. Epithelioid histiocytes (EH) may be seen in granulomatous conditions such as sarcoid (in the absence of necrosis) (Fig. 13-4) and toxoplasmosis (in which there are associated monocytoid cells). EH are also found in tuberculosis (with caseating background), in cat-scratch disease, and in lymphogranuloma venereum (accompanied by ne-

Table 13-6 Diagnostic Criteria for Non-Hodgkin's Lymphoma

Dispersed cellular smear
Lymphoglandular bodies
Relatively monomorphous lymphoid population
Confirmatory immunocytochemistry or gene rearrangement studies

crosis and neutrophils). Eosinophils and epitheloid histiocytes are identified in some cases of HD and in certain T-cell lymphomas (e.g., Lennert's lymphoma).

When almost all the cells are lymphoid, a relatively monomorphous population argues in favor of a diagnosis of malignant lymphoma (Table 13-6). The clinician should then determine whether the majority of cells are small lymphocytes, large lymphocytes, or mixtures of these cells. An attempt should be made to estimate the proportion of lymphocytes of varying cell size. Generally greater than 75 percent small cleaved FCC are seen in small cleaved FCC lymphomas (poorly differentiated lymphocytic lymphomas), while 25 percent to 50 percent of large cells are correlated with large cleaved, and large noncleaved FCC malignant lymphomas (mixed lymphocytic and his-

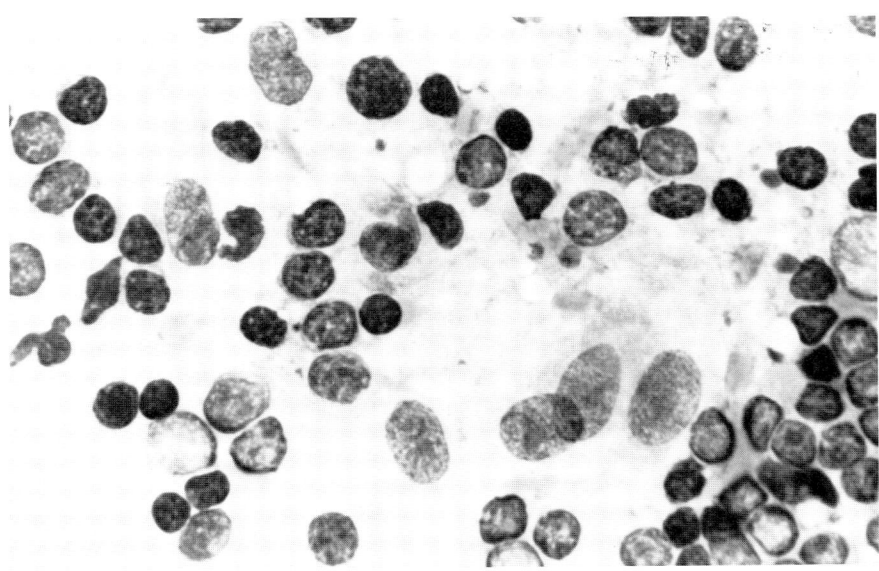

Fig. 13-4 Lymph node FNA in a patient with sarcoid. Note the aggregates of epithelioid histiocytes and the lymphocytic background. (Wright-Giemsa stain, × 200.)

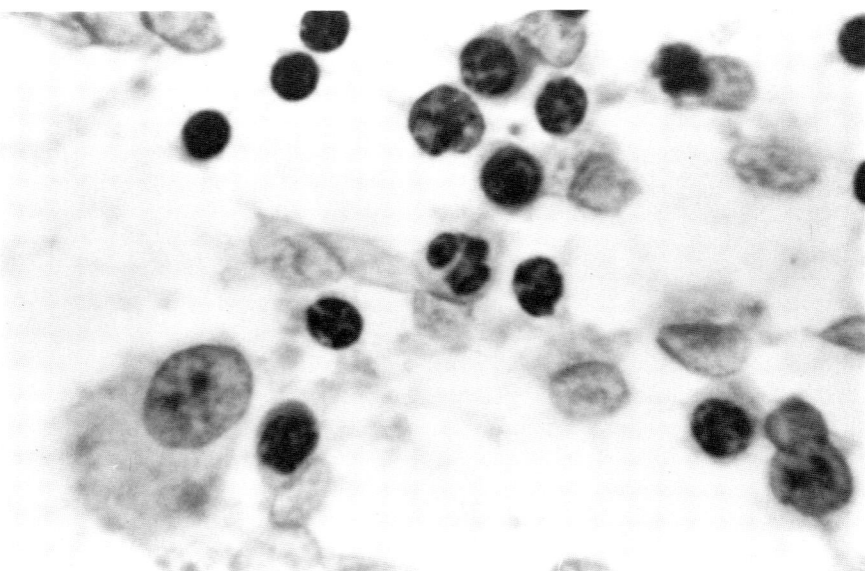

Fig. 13-5 Lymph node FNA consistent with reactive lymphoid hyperplasia. There are mixtures of cell types including small lymphocytes, transformed lymphocytes, plasma cells, histiocytes, and neutrophils. (H&E stain, × 250.) (See Plate 13-4.)

tiocytic lymphomas). Lymphomas composed of more than 50 percent large transformed lymphocytes are diagnosed as malignant lymphomas of large cell type. Immunoblastic sarcomas (immunoblastic lymphomas) are composed predominantly of immunoblasts. Although these criteria are not precise, they do serve as a broad guideline for classification.

Mixtures of cell types (Fig. 13-5, Plate 13-4), including lymphocytes of variable size, immunoblasts, plasma cells, eosinophils, neutrophils, and tingible body macrophages (histiocytes containing phagocytozed cellular debris), are usually associated with benign reactive conditions (Table 13-7). One notable exception to this rule is Hodgkin's disease, which usually presents with a mixture of cell types in the background, interspersed with occasional Reed-Sternberg cells (or Reed-Sternberg variants). Sometimes an aspirate smear that is perfectly compatible with reactive lymphoid hyperplastia is seen in cases of HD focally involving interfollicular regions missed in the FNA. Like HD, mycosis fungoides and other T-cell lymphomas may exhibit a variety of cell types, including eosinophils and histiocytes, in addition to a spectrum of neoplastic T lymphocytes. Finally, metastatic carcinoma can involve a lymph node focally and occasionally be missed in an FNA sample.

Once an abnormal population of cells is recognized, the clinician can focus on the cytomorphology of these cells at high magnification. If the cells are lymphocytes, how does their size compare with the size of a benign histiocyte nucleus or that of a small mature lymphocyte or red blood cell (RBC) that may be present in the background? Lymphomas in which cells contain nuclei larger than the nucleus of a benign histiocyte (or greater than three or four small lymphocyte diameters) are classified as large cell lymphomas.

It is important to determine whether the nuclear chromatin is coarse or fine and to identify the presence or absence of prominent nucleoli, nuclear irregularities, and folds (clefts and/or convolutions), as well as the frequency of mitoses. For example, small cells exhibiting homogeneous salt-and-pepper chromatin, absent nucleoli, nuclear molding, and tumor

Table 13-7 Features of Reactive Lymphadenitis

Spectrum of lymphocytes mostly small, some transformed follicular center cells and immunoblasts

Heterogeneous cell population: lymphocytes, plasma cells, tingible body macrophages, eosinophils, and occasional neutrophils; epithelioid histiocytes and multinucleated giant cells in granulomatous lymphadenitis

diathesis are most compatible with a diagnosis of undifferentiated small cell carcinoma (oat cell). By contrast, small lymphocytic lymphomas demonstrate cells containing coarse granular checkerboard chromatin and rare mitoses. These cells are noncohesive, lack nulcear molding, and show little, if any, necrosis. Other metastatic small cell malignancies that may involve the lymph node include neuroblastoma, Ewing's sarcoma, Merkel cell tumor, and carcinoid tumors.

Neoplasms composed of loosely cohesive to noncohesive cells exhibiting prominent nucleoli and markedly increased mitoses are seen in small noncleaved FCC lymphomas (Burkitt's lymphoma or undifferentiated lymphoma, Burkitt and non-Burkitt types), large noncleaved FCC malignant lymphomas, and immunoblastic sarcomas. Convoluted and nonconvoluted T-cell lymphomas (malignant lymphoma lymphoblastic) often present as small to intermediate lymphoid proliferations containing fine stippled chromatin, increased mitoses, and so-called "chicken foot" nuclear convolutions. Large cell infiltrates exhibiting primitive chromatin, prominent nucleoli, and increased mitoses may reflect leukemic conditions such as acute lymphocytic leukemia (ALL) or blast crisis in chronic myelogenous leukemia (CML) (granulocytic sarcoma).

A definitive diagnosis of malignant lymphoma may be made on cytologic grounds in selected cases. Success is determined by the technical quality of the specimen and the expertise of the examiner. Even in experienced hands, a primary diagnosis of well-differentiated lymphoma of small lymphocytic cell type lymphocytic lymphoma/chronic lymphocytic leukemia and lymphomas of mixed lymphocytic and histiocytic type (large cleaved follicular center cell lymphomas/large noncleaved FCC lymphomas) is extremely difficult to make without the advantage of lymphocyte phenotyping studies or confirmatory biopsy.

Fine needle aspirations yielding mixtures of small and large lymphocytic cells present a diagnostic dilemma. Benign conditions such as follicular hyperplasia and granulomatous lymphadenitis may demonstrate a spectrum of FCC (both small and large), tingible body macrophages, epithelioid histiocytes, and plasma cells. Malignant lymphomas containing a mixture of small and large lymphocytes include mixed lymphocytic and histiocytic lymphoma of Rappaport (large cleaved FCC and large noncleaved FCC lymphomas of Luke's), certain T-cell lymphomas including Lennert's lymphoma (mixed small and large cell lymphoma with epithelioid cell component), and a small number of pleomorphic B- and T-immunoblastic sarcomas (histiocytic lymphomas of Rappaport). As noted, HD may also show a mixed cellular background, in addition to large polypoid Reed-Sternberg cells or Reed-Sternberg variants. Chloroma or granulocytic sarcoma in the early stages of leukemic infiltration may present with a mixture of large primitive leukemic cells as well as residual benign lymphoid cells.

Florid proliferations of large transformed lymphocytes and immunoblasts are identified in large cell malignant lymphomas and abnormal immune reactions (including infectious mononucleosis, viral infections, and drug reactions). Although such large cell proliferations may mimic immunoblastic sarcoma in the extreme, usually a mixture of other cells as well as a spectrum of transformed lymphocytes is seen. Lymphoid marker studies may prove useful in distinguishing a benign immunoblastic reaction from large cell malignant lymphoma. With rare exceptions,[29] a monoclonal B-cell population is equated with malignant lymphoma, while a polyclonal population is diagnosed as a benign reactive process.

The predominantly large cell malignant proliferations include malignant lymphomas of large transformed lymphocytes (large cleaved and large noncleaved FCC lymphoma), immunoblastic sarcoma (IBS) of B- and T-cell type, and true histiocytic lymphoma. These lymphomas are classified as histiocytic lymphomas in the traditional Rappaport classification. Lymphocyte-depleted HD and granulocytic sarcoma must also be considered, as well as a variety of undifferentiated carcinomas, sarcomas, and germ cell tumors. Malignant melanoma has earned its reputation as the great mimic, and always needs to be excluded.

CYTOPATHOLOGY OF LYMPHOMAS

Malignant Lymphoma of Small Lymphocytic Cells

A cellular monotonous proliferation of small lymphoid cells is the rule in malignant lymphoma of small lymphocytic cell type (well-differentiated lymphocytic lymphoma or its systemic counterpart, chronic lymphocytic leukemia) (Fig. 13-6A&B, Plates 13-5, 13-6). The small lymphocytes contain round nuclei and coarsely granular blocked checkerboard chromatin (best seen on 95-percent ethanol-fixed smears). Nucleoli and mitoses are vanishingly rare. One exception to these guidelines is the spectrum of cell size seen in cases of chronic lymphocytic leukemia in which proliferation centers are present. The lymphocytes in these areas contain more cytoplasm, more finely granular chromatin, increased mitoses, and nucleoli. Rare sinus histiocytes may be

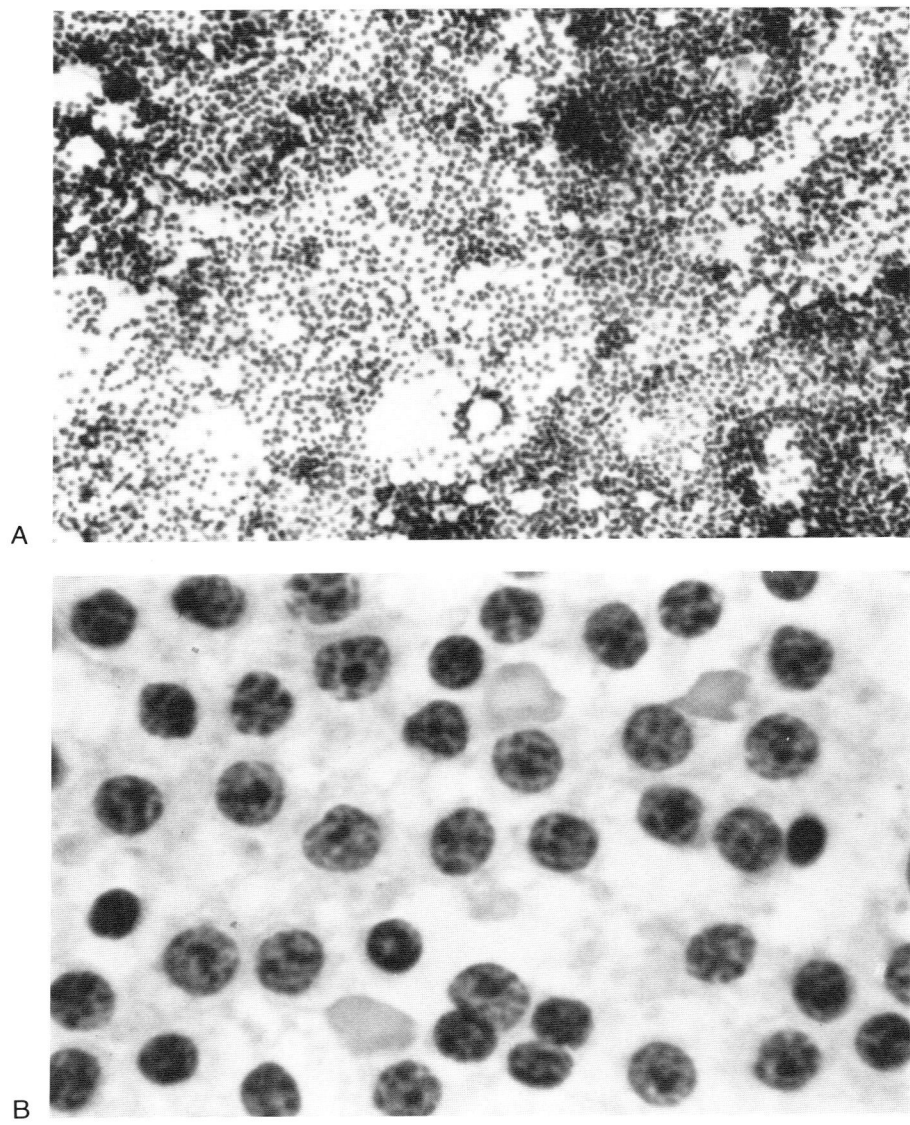

Fig. 13-6 (A) Lymph node imprint in patient with chronic lymphocytic leukemia. Note the monotonous population of small lymphocytes characteristic of both well-differentiated lymphocytic lymphoma and chronic lymphocytic leukemia. (Wright-Giemsa stain, × 50.) (See Plate 13-5.) **(B)** Lymph node imprint in case of chronic lymphocytic leukemia. Note the relatively uniform population of small lymphocytes, coarse checkerboard chromatin, and lack of mitoses. (H&E stain, × 250.) (See Plate 13-6.)

present, although tingible body macrophages are not seen.

When small lymphocytic proliferations are accompanied by plasmacytoid lymphocytes showing apparent intranuclear immunoglobin inclusions (PAS-positive) or Dutcher bodies, a diagnosis of plasmacytoid lymphocytic lymphoma, or Waldenström's macroglobulinemia, should be considered.

Small Cleaved Follicular Center Cell Lymphoma

Malignant lymphomas of small cleaved FCC (poorly differentiated lymphocytic lymphoma, malignant-lymphoma centrocytic) are markedly cellular and are composed of small lymphocytes and small cleaved FCCs in which nuclei are smaller than the histiocyte nucleus. These cells have scant cytoplasm and, granular chromatin and occasionally aggregate in Papanicolaou-stained material. Nuclear clefts and folds may be identified best in air-dried preparations (Fig. 13-7). Nucleoli usually are absent. A small percentage of larger transformed lymphocytes may be present, along with rare tingible body macrophages.

Small Noncleaved Follicular Center Cell Lymphoma

Small noncleaved FCC lymphoma (undifferentiated lymphoma, Burkitt's and Non-Burkitt's type, malignant lymphoma B lymphoblastic, Burkitt's type) has an exceptionally high mitotic rate and is an aggressive malignant tumor. In classic Burkitt's lymphoma, cells are uniform and monotonous. They are a little smaller than or equal to the size of a histiocyte nucleus, contain a scant cytoplasmic rim and multiple nucleoli (Fig. 13-8A&B, Plates 13-7, 13-8). Imprint preparations characteristically show small cytoplasmic vacuoles that stain positive for lipid when stained with Oil-Red-O. The cytoplasm of these cells contains a large amount of RNA that stains strongly pyroninophilic with methyl green pyronin (MGP). Necrotic debris usually is present in the back-ground as well as in the cytoplasm of histiocytes or tingible body macrophages. These are cells that contribute to the so-called "starry sky" effect seen in histologic sections (the lighter-staining macrophages are the "stars" set on a background of blue lymphoma cells). Non-Burkitt's lymphomas, or American Burkitt's lymphomas, have a somewhat different clinical and serologic profile than that in classic Burkitt's. On cy-

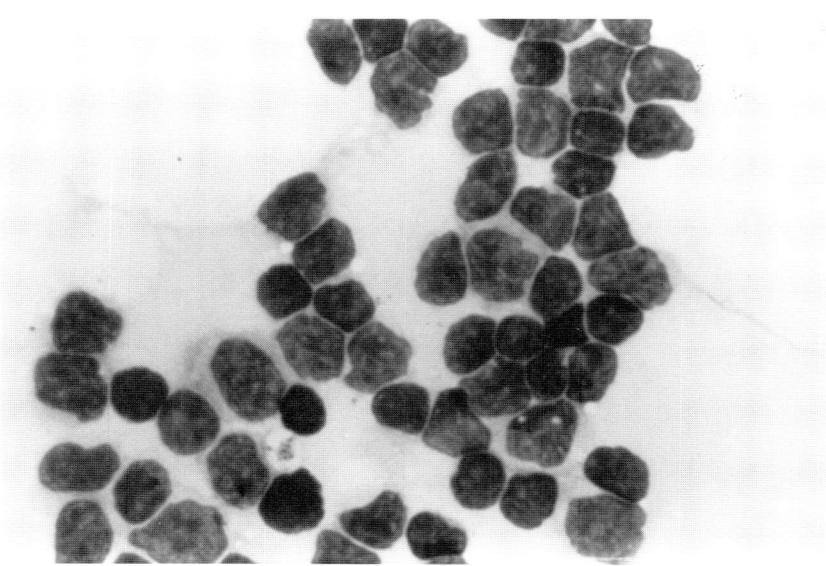

Fig. 13-7 Small cleaved follicular center cell lymphoma composed mostly of small to intermediate-sized lymphocytes, some of which show nuclear folds and clefts. (Wright-Giemsa stain, × 250.)

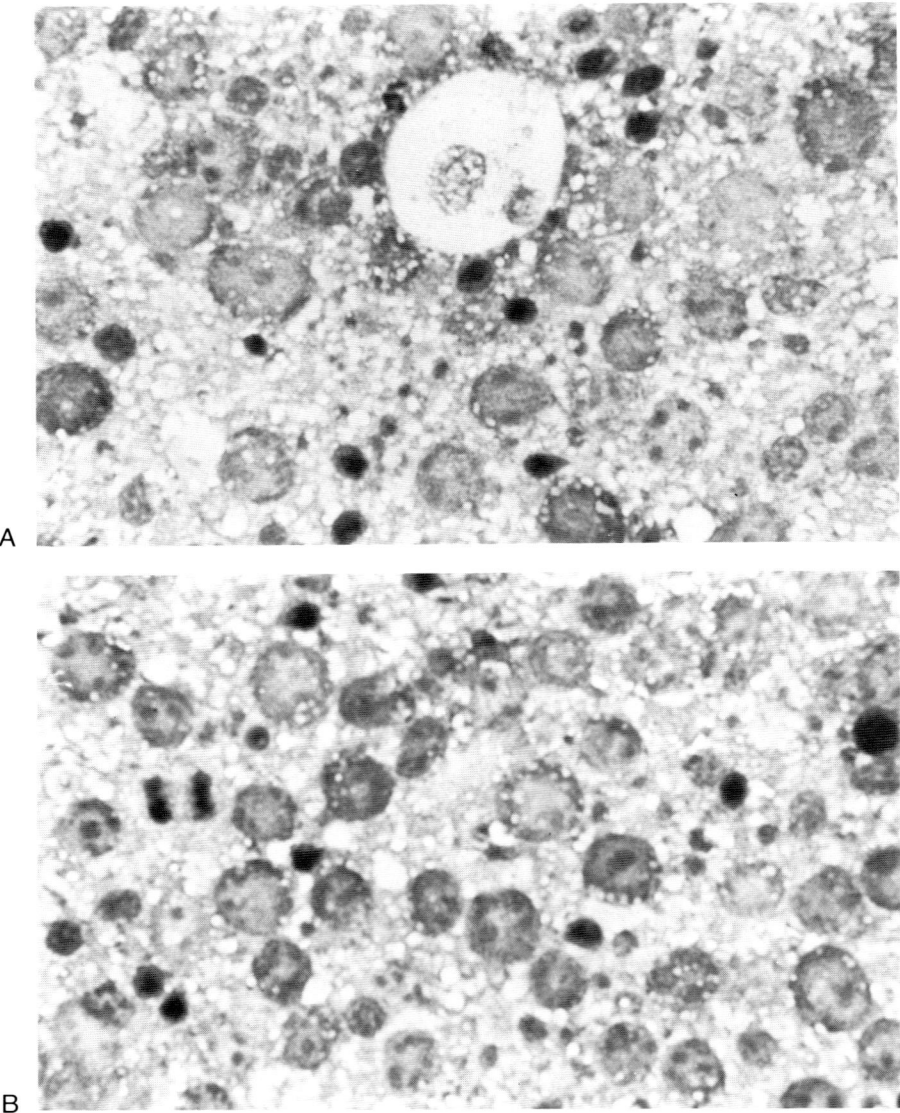

Fig. 13-8 (A) Lymph node FNA smear in patient with small noncleaved FCC lymphoma (malignant lymphoma, lymphoblastic, Burkitt type) showing cytoplasmic vacuolization, multiple nucleoli, deep blue cytoplasmic rims and "starry sky" histiocyte. FNA smears and lymph node imprints show more variable nuclear size and nuclear irregularity than in surgical biopsy sections. (May Grünwald Giemsa stain, × 350.) (Case courtesy of Edneia Tani, M.D., Karolinska Hospital, Stockholm, Sweden). (See Plate 13-7.) **(B)** Lymph node FNA from same patient showing vacuolated cytoplasm in relatively monomorphous population of intermediate-sized transformed lymphocytes (probably centroblasts), increased mitoses, and pyknotic cells. (May Grünwald Giemsa stain, × 250.) (See Plate 13-8.)

tologic grounds, non-Burkitt's lymphomas show more variability in cell shape and size, their cells containing more abundant cytoplasm than those in classic Burkitt's lymphoma. Clinically, it may present both in nodal and extranodal sites, developing into a leukemic phase more often than its African counterpart.

Large Cleaved Follicular Center Cell Lymphoma

Large cleaved follicular center cell (LCFCC) lymphoma (mixed lymphocytic and histiocytic lymphoma/histiocytic lymphoma, malignant lymphoma-centroblastic/centrocytic) produces a cellular specimen containing a mixture of small FCC and large transformed FCC (both large cleaved and large noncleaved FCC). Large cleaved FCC are the predominant cell, with large noncleaved follicular center cells constituting less than 25 percent of the cell population (Fig. 13-9; Plate 13-9). The large cleaved FCC contain large vesicular folded and irregular nuclei, do not display prominent nucleoli, and exhibit moderately increased mitoses. Plasma cells and tingible body macrophages are rare in these lymphomas.

Lymphomas composed of mixtures of large and small FCC are quite difficult, if not impossible, to diagnose on cytologic grounds alone because of the wide range of lymphocytic types that may be seen both in mixed lymphocytic and histiocytic lymphomas and in benign follicular and paracortical hyperplasia. In such cases, confirmation of the diagnosis of malignant lymphoma by surgical biopsy is recommended. The architectural features in the biopsy usually clarify the picture. Lymphocytic marker studies performed on snap-frozen biopsy specimens and/or cytologic smears also may be employed.

Malignant lymphoma of small and large lymphocytic cells, while usually of B-cell origin, sometimes represents a malignant lymphoma of T cells. Lymphocyte marker studies help resolve the question of cell type. Morphologically, T-cell lymphomas often contain a spectrum of lymphoid cells exhibiting irregular nuclear folds and convolutions. Eosinophils and epithelioid histiocytes may be prominent in T-cell lymphomas as well.

Large Cell Malignant Lymphoma

Large cell malignant lymphomas (large noncleaved FCC lymphoma, immunoblastic sarcoma of T cells, immunoblastic sarcoma of B cells, histiocytic lymphoma, malignant lymphoma-immunoblastic, and

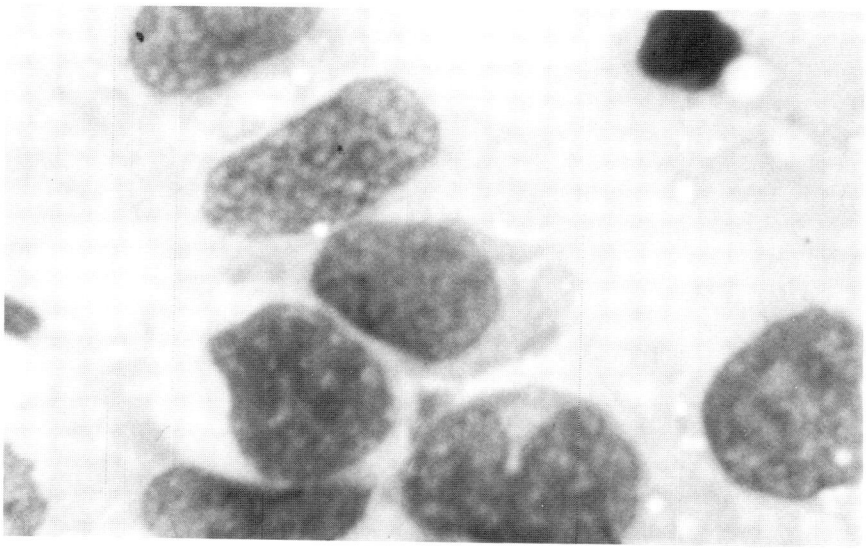

Fig. 13-9 Lymph node FNA in case of large cleaved follicular center cell lymphoma. Note the mixture of intermediate and large transformed follicular center cells in which large cleaved FCC lymphocytes predominate. (Wright-Giemsa stain, × 630.) (See Plate 13-9.)

true histiocytic lymphoma) are composed of cellular loose aggregates of large lymphocytes containing abundant cytoplasm, increased mitoses, prominent nucleoli, and lymphoglandular bodies. Tingible body macrophages may be abundant in any high-turnover malignant lymphoma/leukemia (small non-cleaved FCC/Burkitt and non-Burkitt, acute lymphocytic leukemias, convoluted T-cell lymphomas, malignant lymphoma lymphoblastic). Lymphocyte-depleted Hodgkin's disease, granulocytic sarcoma, germ cell tumors, nasopharyngeal carcinoma, and amelanotic melanoma all may mimic large cell lymphomas. Florid immunoblastic reactions (Fig. 13-10A&B, Plates 13-10, 13-11) such as those seen in

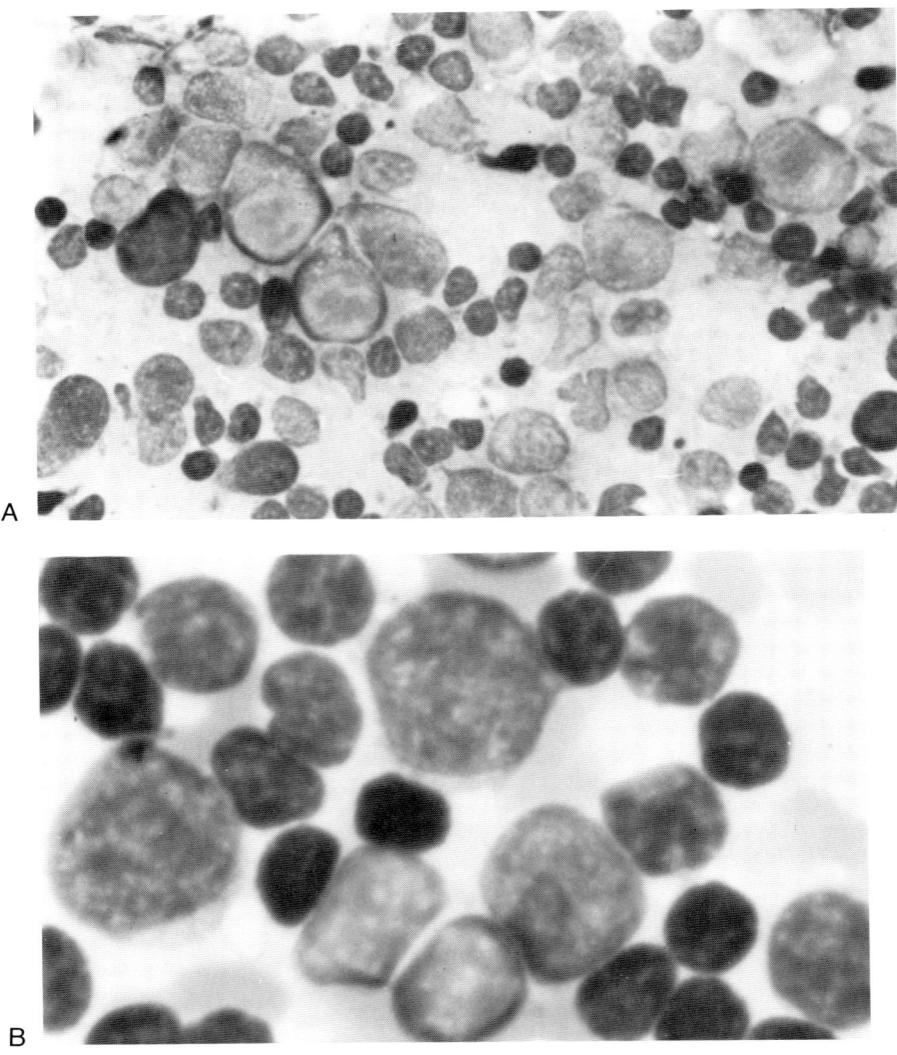

Fig. 13-10 (A) Reactive lymph node in a patient with proven infectious mononucleosis. Smear demonstrates a spectrum of cells including small and large transformed lymphocytes and occasional large immuonoblasts. The immunoblastic component may be marked in some cases so as to mimic malignant lymphoma. (May Grünwald Giemsa stain, × 220.) (Case courtesy of Edneia Tani, M.D., Karolinska Hospital, Stockholm, Sweden. (See Plate 13-10.) **(B)** Lymph node imprint in a patient with infectious mononucleosis showing a spectrum of lymphocytes including transformed follicular center cells and one or two immunoblasts exhibiting primitive nucleus and deep blue to purple cytoplasmic rim. (Wright-Giemsa stain, × 500.) (See Plate 13-11.)

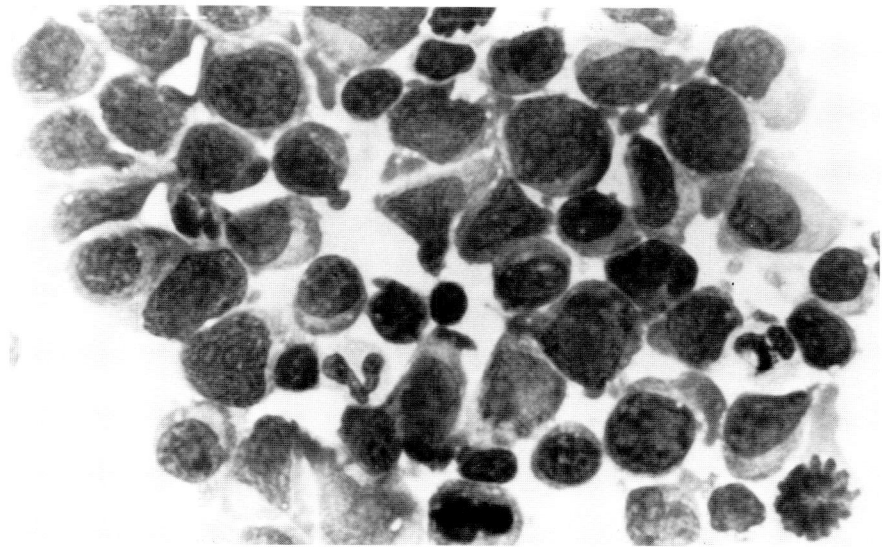

Fig. 13-11 Large noncleaved follicular center cell lymphoma. Note dispersed cellular smear containing a majority of large transformed lymphocytes exhibiting multiple prominent "dice-like" nucleoli and increased mitoses. (Wright-Giemsa stain, × 250.)

infectious mononucleosis, a variety of viral diseases, and drug reactions, may also be confused with large cell lymphoma, but these lack the homogeneous monomorphic lymphoid population seen in most of these lymphomas.

Distinctions among large noncleaved FCC lymphoma, B-IBS, and T-IBS may prove difficult. The presence of both large noncleaved FCC and lesser numbers of large cleaved follicular center cells is more consistent with a diagnosis of large noncleaved FCC lymphoma than of immunoblastic sarcoma, in which almost all the cells are immunoblasts. Large noncleaved follicular center cells (LNCFCC) usually contain multiple dice-like nucleoli situated subjacent to a relatively uniform nuclear membrane (Fig. 13-11). B-IBS contains rare FCC and may demonstrate spectacular plasmacytoid immunoblastic cells. The immunoblasts contain one or two centrally located prominent nucleoli and exhibit an irregularly thickened nuclear membrane (Fig. 13-12A&B, Plate 13-12). The cytoplasm of B-IBS cells stains more deeply in Giemsa-stained preparations than that of large noncleaved cells and T-IBS cells. The cytoplasm of B-IBS cells also stains more intensely with MGP than that of large noncleaved FCC and T-IBS cells. T-IBS cells (Fig. 13-13A,B,&C, Plate 13-13, Plate 13-14.) usually contain prominent nucleoli, a relatively uniform nuclear membrane, pale cytoplasm, and, frequently, irregular nuclear folds and convolutions best seen under oil immersion in Papanicolaou-stained smears. Immunohistochemical staining for T-cell membrane antigens may unmask the T-cell origin of the neoplastic cells (Fig. 13-13C).

The diagnosis of true histiocytic lymphoma is made on the basis of exclusion of other lymphomas after marker studies and enzyme histochemical studies are performed. True histocytic lymphoma cells stain positively for nonspecific esterase and are resistant to fluoride inhibition, stain positively for muramidase or lysozyme, and stain positively for α_1-antitrypsin and anti-chymotrypsin. Panels of monoclonal antibodies (MoAbs) that bind to histiocytic antigenic determinants are available commercially.

Hodgkin's Disease

Familiarity with the classic Reed-Sternberg cell and Reed-Sternberg cell variants as well as with the cellular background associated with these cells is critical to the diagnosis of HD.[30] Since HD may focally involve

394 PRACTICAL CYTOPATHOLOGY

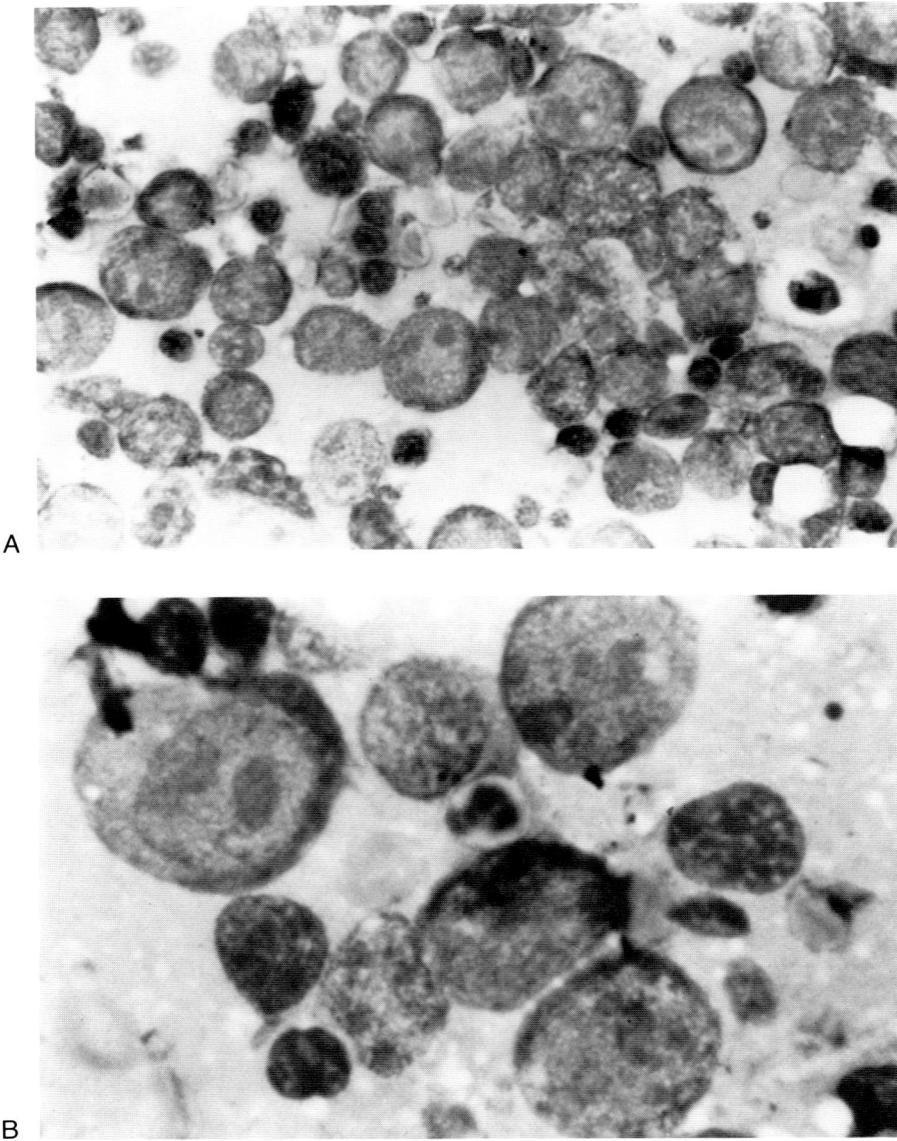

Fig. 13-12 **(A)** B-cell immunoblastic sarcoma characterized by large cells containing large nuclei, one or two prominent nucleoli, and irregularly thickened nuclear membrane. B-IBS may contain plasmacytoid immunoblasts with eccentric nuclei. (Wright-Giemsa stain, × 250.) **(B)** Lymph node imprint from B-cell immunoblastic sarcoma composed of large neoplastic immunoblasts exhibiting prominent nucleoli and plasmacytoid features. (Wright-Giemsa stain, × 500.) (See Plate 13-12.)

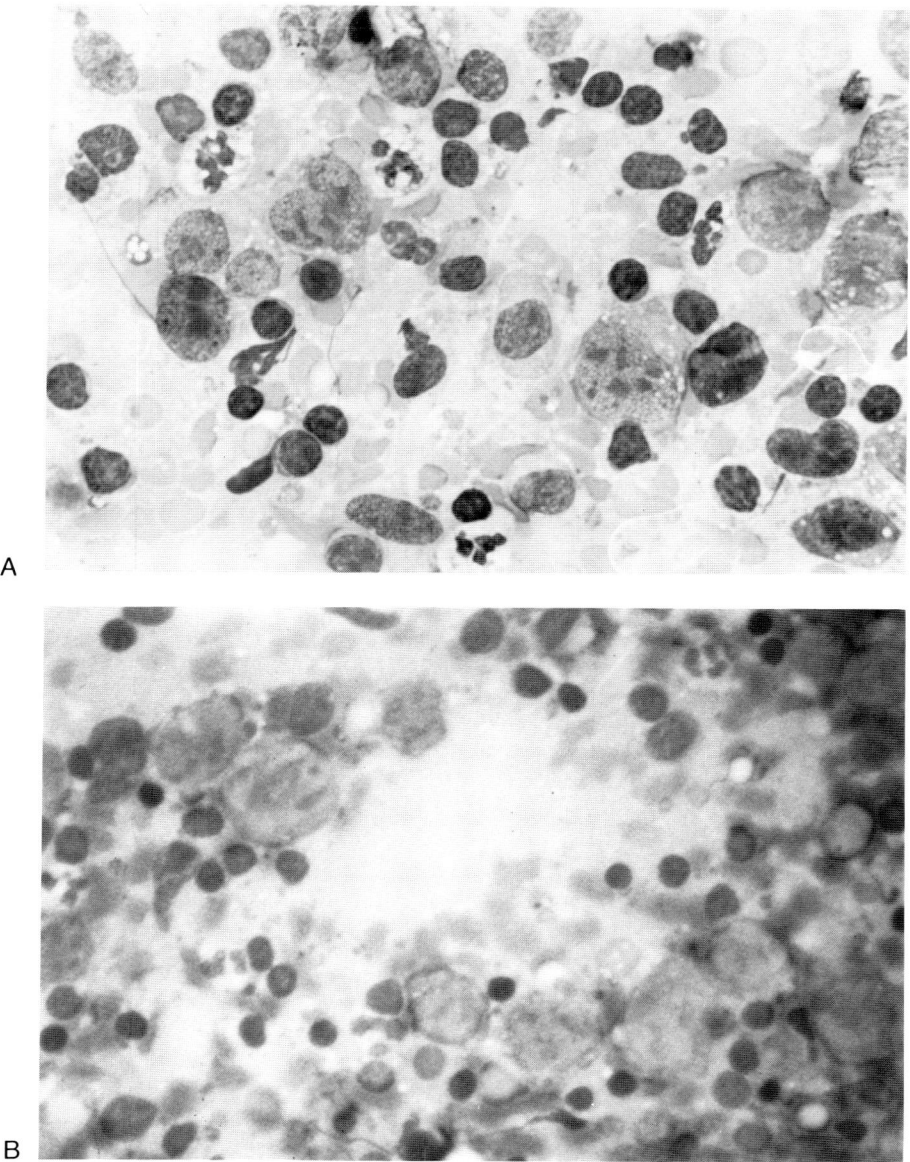

Fig. 13-13 (A) T-cell immunoblastic sarcoma containing immunoblasts of variable size, many of which demonstrate irregular nuclear folds and convolutions. Nucleoli are prominent and some cells show cytoplasmic pallor. (Wright-Giemsa stain, × 200.) **(B)** T-cell immunoblastic sarcoma showing large immunoblasts with irregular complex nuclear folding and cytoplasmic pallor. (Wright-Giemsa stain, × 160.) (See Plate 13-13.) (*Figure continues.*)

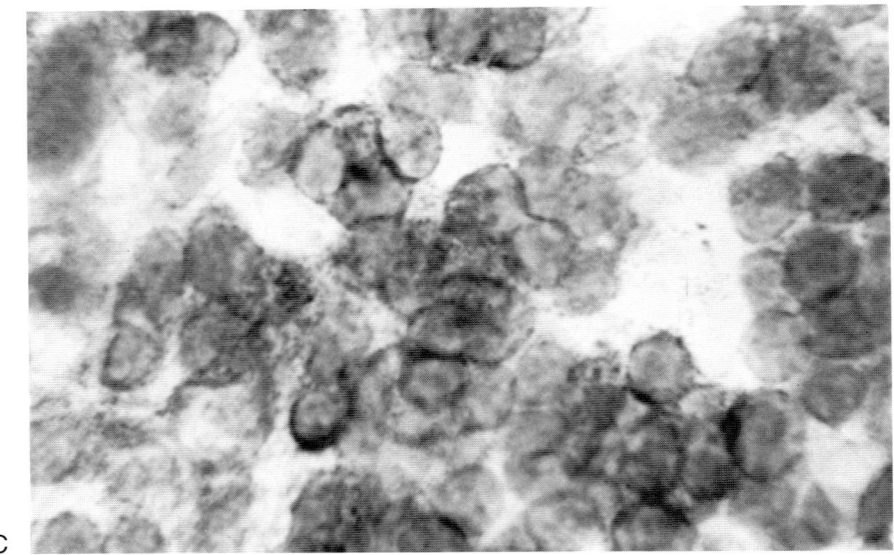

Fig. 13-13 (*Continued*). **(C)** An example of T-immunoblastic sarcoma in which T-cell origin is confirmed by strong staining of neoplastic cell membranes by a pan-T-cell antibody. Avidin-biotin-peroxidase complex. (× 160.) (See Plate 13-14.)

a lymph node (in mixed cellularity type, and in nodular sclerosing HD), FNA may miss the involved part of the lymph node. Samples obtained from lymph nodes showing interfollicular focal HD may also include cells derived from hyperplastic follicles. Too hasty and examination of the material from such a node may lead to the erroneous diagnosis of benign reactive lymphoid hyperplasia when, in fact, careful screening would have unmasked classic Reed-Sternberg cells or lacunar cells, as seen in nodular sclerosing HD.

In lymphocyte-predominent HD (L&H HD), the cellular background consists of small lymphocytes (L) small FCC, epithelioid histiocytes (H), and L&H variants of Reed-Sternberg cells (L&H cells). These cells contain large "popcorn kernel" lobated nuclei, scant pale cytoplasm, and small nucleoli. In contrast with lacunar cells, these cells have a high nuclear/cytoplasmic ratios. Occasional plasma cells and eosinophls are seen.

In mixed cellularity HD, there is a background population of small lymphocytes, eosinophils, plasma cells, occasional neutrophils (PMN), and epithelioid histiocytes. Classic Reed-Sternberg cells contains bilobated or multilobated nuclei exhibiting large, round, smooth nucleoli, usually measuring greater than 40 percent of the nuclear diameter (Fig. 13-14, Plate 13-15).

Often there is a clear zone about the nucleolus, and the nuclear membrane is thickened irregularly. Mononuclear cells containing large nucleoli (Hodgkin's cells) are seen quite often. These cells by themselves are suggestive, but not diagnostic, of HD. Identification of such cells dictates a diligent search for diagnostic Reed-Sternberg cells.

Nodular sclerosing HD[31] may show similar background cells as described above but in addition may exhibit areas of suppuration and necrosis. The classic lacunar cell, considered a Reed-Sternberg variant, is a large cell containing a highly lobated nucleus with ample pale cytoplasm and discrete, usually small, nucleoli (Fig. 13-15). These cells may be present in syncytia. In biopsy sections, they are seen about the periphery of acutely inflamed necrotic foci.

Lymphocyte-depleted HD of the diffuse fibrosis type yields a poorly cellular specimen containing small numbers of lymphocytes and eosinophils and rare Reed-Sternberg cells. The reticular type of lymphocyte-depleted HD may contain large numbers of classic Reed-Sternberg cells or pleomorphic bizarre cells resembling pleomorphic histiocytic lymphoma or anaplastic carcinoma.

CYTOPATHOLOGY OF LYMPH NODES 397

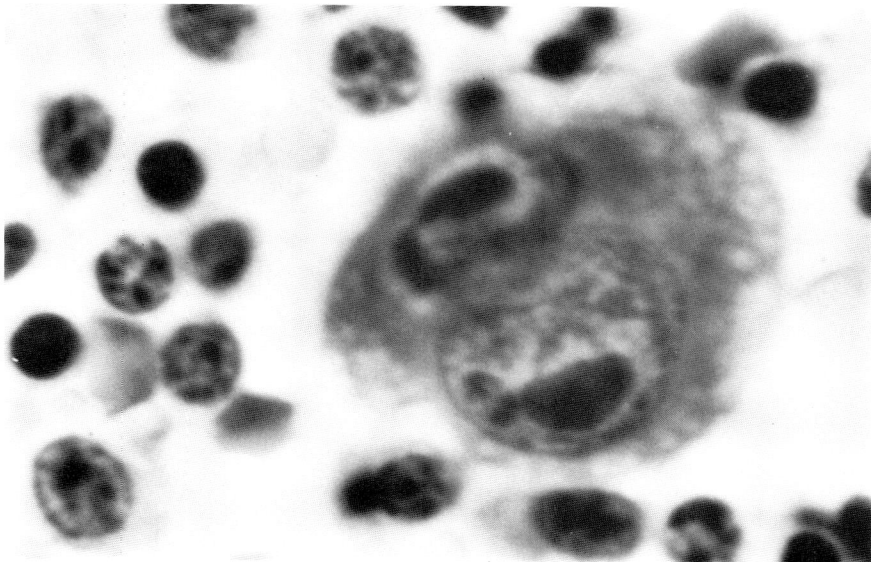

Fig. 13-14 Reed-Sternberg cell demonstrating large bilobed nucleus containing huge "owl's eye" nucleoli. Such cells are diagnostic of Hodgkin's disease in the appropriate cellular background. (Papanicolaou stain, × 400). (See Plate 13-15.)

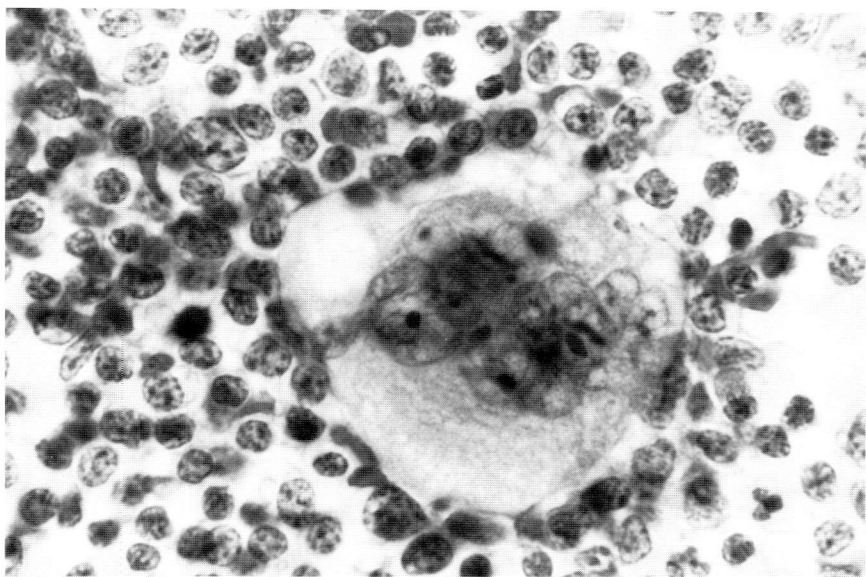

Fig. 13-15 Nodular sclerosing Hodgkin's disease smear showing "lacunar cell" containing multilobated nucleus, ample pale cytoplasm, and discrete small nucleoli. (× 400.)

FNA frequently is helpful in staging cases of HD that were previously diagnosed by surgical biopsy. Subclassification of HD on the basis of a FNA is difficult and not necessarily required. Pathologic staging and clinical assessment of symptoms determine therapy for these patients. A variety of monoclonal antibodies, including Leu-M-1 and KI-1, may help identify Reed-Sternberg cells in cytologic preparations as well as in paraffin-embedded surgical sections.[32-34] Unfortunately, while these antibodies are useful, they are not specific for the Reed-Sternberg cell.

Malignant Lymphoma-Lymphoblastic

Malignant lymphoma-lymphoblastic (including convoluted and nonconvoluted T-cell lymphoma, T-lymphoblastic-convoluted cell type)[35] exhibits a monomorphic population of intermediate to large lymphoid cells, some of which contain irregular nuclear convolutions (Fig. 13-16A&B, Plates 13-16, 13-17). Nuclei contain fine stippled salt-and-pepper chromatin and inconspicuous nucleoli. Mitoses are markedly increased, and tingible body macrophages may be seen in abundance. The lymphocytic cells are approximately the same size as histiocyte nuclei. Often so-called "chicken footprint" nuclear folds may be identified, although in some cases nuclei are round and lack obvious convolutions. The combination of increased mitoses, convoluted nuclear configurations, and lymphocytic marker studies in the appropriate clinical setting confirms the diagnosis. This lymphoma usually presents as a mediastinal mass in an adolescent male, but it also occurs in adults.

Granulocytic Sarcoma (Chloroma)

Granulocytic sarcoma (Chloroma) is a malignant neoplasm that may involve extramedullary sites such as lymph node, skin, perineural, epidural, paravertebral, and periorbital tissue. It usually reflects a rapidly deteriorating stage of acute myelogenous leukemia or blast crisis in chronic myelogenous leukemia. Occasionally, granulocytic sarcoma may present as an unknown neoplasm in a patient lacking hematologic evidence of myeloid leukemia. There have been some examples of cases in which such masses have antedated the clinical manifestations of leukemia by as many as 2 years.[36,37] The diagnosis of granulocytic sarcoma of the lymph node is usually missed by those unfamiliar with the clinical history and is often missed when such masses present as the initial manifestation of myelogenous leukemia. The most common incorrect diagnosis rendered in such cases is large cell lymphoma (histiocytic lymphoma).

Cytologically, large blast-like cells (Fig. 3-17A, Plate 13-18), are identified containing a rim of pale cytoplasm, a large nucleus, fine primitive chromatin, and prominent nucleoli. Myelocytes and metamyelocytes are sometimes seen. In blast-type proliferations, it is important to look for eosinophilic myelocytes as a clue to the cell of origin. Mitoses are increased, and tingible body macrophages may be seen in the background. When such a diagnosis is contemplated, myeloperoxidase stain, chloracetate esterase (CAE) stain, Sudan-Black, and other markers for myeloid cells should be considered. If a formalin-fixed cell button is available, CAE unmasks early myeloid precursors dramatically (Fig. 13-17B, Plate 13-19).

LYMPH NODE FNA IN PATIENTS AT RISK FOR AIDS

The dramatic increase in the number of patients at risk of acquired immune deficiency syndrome (AIDS) has brought with it a commensurate increase in the number of lymph node FNAs performed in patients presenting with persistent lymphadenopathy (lasting more than 3 months) without an obvious clinical explanation. Many of these patients show evidence of lymphoid hyperplasia, while others are diagnosed with mycobacterial infection, Kaposi's sarcoma, and non-Hodgkin's lymphoma.[38,39]

CONCLUSION

Lymph node FNA offers a convenient, rapid, economical, and accurate technique for diagnosing a variety of benign and malignant conditions. In cases in which interpretation proves elusive, conventional surgical biopsy and ancillary studies should enhance the accuracy of diagnosis.

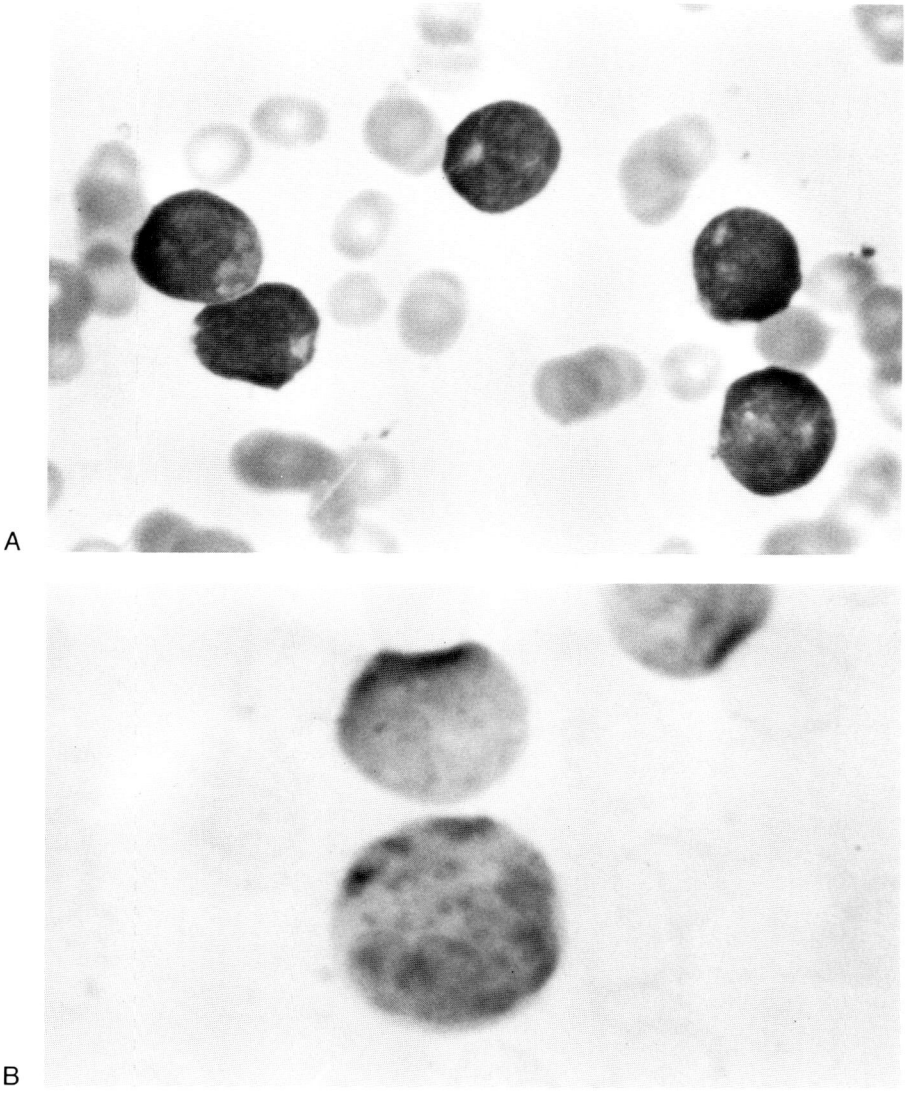

Fig. 13-16 (A) Convoluted T-cell lymphoma showing intermediate-sized primitive lymphoid cells (lymphoblasts) containing intricate nuclear folds and convolutions. (Wright-Giemsa stain, × 350.) (See Plate 13-16.)
(B) Convoluted T-cell lymphoma exhibiting positive intracytoplasmic acid phosphatase staining, suggesting T-cell origin. (Acid phosphatase stain, × 500.) (See Plate 13-17.)

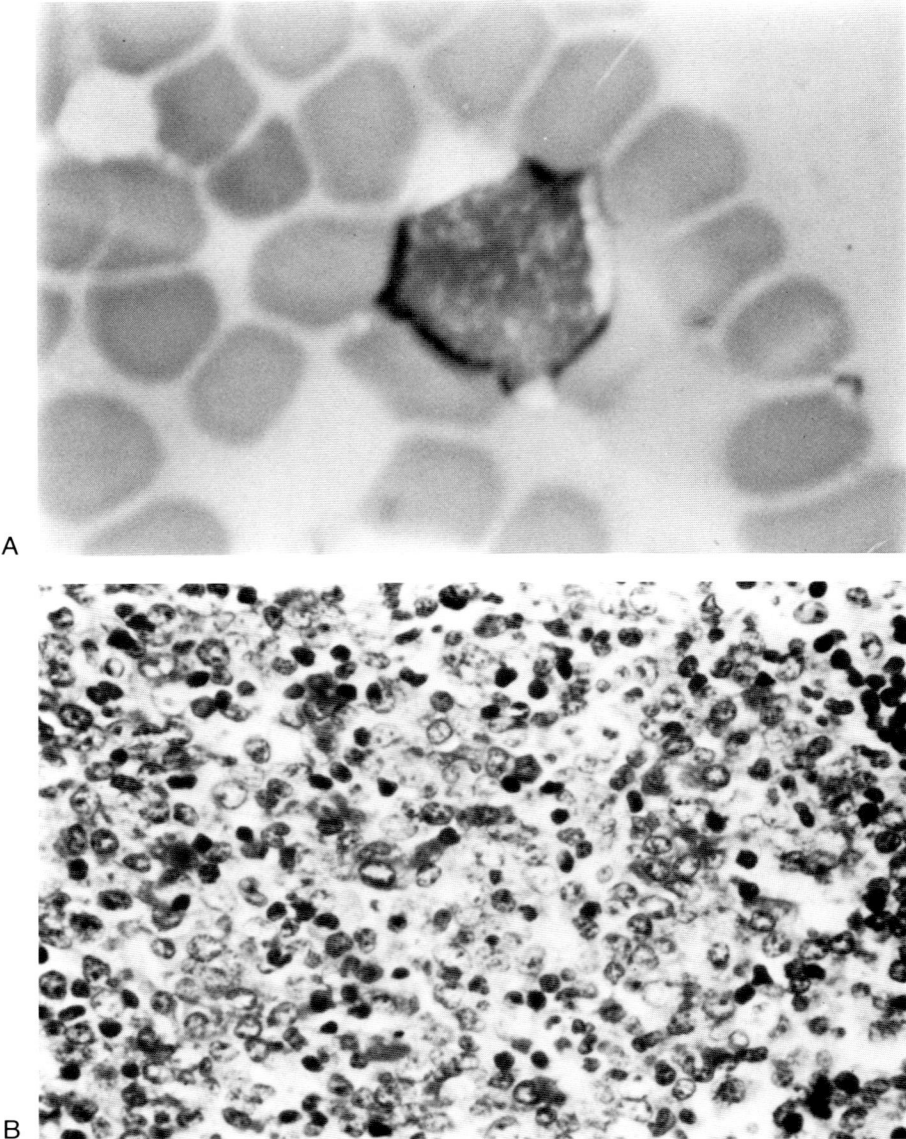

Fig. 13-17 (A) Primitive blast-like cell in a patient with granulocytic sarcoma or "chloroma." (Wright-Giemsa stain, × 500.) (See Plate 13-18.) **(B)** Paraffin-embedded, formalin-fixed section from enlarged lymph node in a patient with granulocytic sarcoma. Positive cytoplasmic staining (red) for chloroacetate-esterase (CAE) reveals the primitive myeloid origin of these cells. (Chloroacetate-esterase stain, × 100.) (See Plate 13-19.)

REFERENCES

1. Greig EDW, Gray ACH: Note on the lymphatic glands in sleeping sickness. Lancet 1:1570, 1904
2. Martin HE, Ellis EB: Biopsy by needle puncture and aspiration. Ann Surg 92:169, 1930
3. Coley BL, Sharp GS, Ellis EB: Diagnosis of bone tumors by aspiration. Am J Surg 13:215, 1931
4. Stewart FW: The diagnosis of tumors by aspiration. Am J Pathol 9:801, 1933
5. Lopez-Cardozo P: Clinical Cytology Using the May-Grunwald-Giemsa Stained Smear. 2 vols. L Staflen, Leyden, 1954
6. Franzen S, Giertz G, Zajicek J: Cytologic diagnosis of prostatic tumors by transrectal aspiration biopsy. A preliminary report. Br J Urol 32:193, 1960
7. Soderstrom N: Biopsy Used As a Direct Adjunct in Clinical Diagnostic Work. Grune & Stratton, Orlando, FL, 1966
8. Espositi PL: Aspiration Biopsy Cytology in the Diagnosis and Management of Prostatic Carcinoma. Stahl and Accidenstryck, Stockholm, 1974
9. O'Dowd JG, Frable WJ, Behm FG: Fine needle aspiration cytology of benign lymph node hyperplasias. Acta Cytol (Praha) 29:554, 1985
10. Qizilbash AH, Elavathil LJ, Chen V, et al: Aspiration biopsy cytology of lymph nodes in malignant lymphoma. Diagn Cytopathology 1:18, 1985
11. Ramzy I, Rone R, Schultenover S, et al: Lymph node aspiration biopsy. Diagnostic reliability and limitations—An analysis of 350 cases. Diagn Cytopathol 1:39, 1985
12. Stani J: Cytologic diagnosis of reactive lymphadenopathy in fine needle aspiration biopsy specimens. 31:8, 1987
13. Sklar J: DNA hybridization in diagnostic pathology. Hum Pathol. 16:654, 1985
14. Knowles D: The human T-cell leukemias: Clinical, cytomorphologic, immunophenotypic, and genotypic characteristics. Hum Pathol 17:14, 1986
15. Lee, TK: The value of imprint cytology in tumor diagnosis. Acta Cytol (Praha) 169, 1981
16. Shafir R, Hiss J: Imprint cytology in intraoperative diagnosis of malignant melanoma. Acta Cytol (Praha) 27:255, 1983
17. Engzell U, Jakobsson PA, Sigurdson A, et al: Aspiration biopsy of metastatic carcinoma in lymph nodes of the neck: A review of 1101 consecutive cases. Acta Otolaryngol 72:138, 1971
18. Bonfiglio TA, MacIntosh PK, Pattern SF Jr, et al: Fine needle aspiration cytopathology of retroperitoneal lymph nodes in evaluation of metastatic disease. Acta Cytol (Praha) 23:126, 1979
19. The Non-Hodgkin's Lymphoma Pathologic Classification Project: National Cancer Institute sponsored study of classification of non-Hodgkin's lymphomas. Summary and description of a working formulation for clinical usage. Cancer 49:2112, 1982
20. Martin SE, Zhang HZ, Magyarosy E, et al: Immunologic methods in cytology: Definitive diagnosis of non-Hodgkin's lymphomas using immunologic markers for T and B cells. Am J Clin Pathol 82:666, 1984
21. Chess Q, Hajdu SI: The role of Immunoperoxidase staining in diagnostic cytology. Acta Cytol (Praha) 30:1, 1986
22. Rappaport H: Tumors of the hematopoietic system. p. 270. In Atlas of Tumor Pathology, Section 3. Fasc. 8. Armed Forces Institute of Pathology, Washington DC, 1956
23. Lukes RJ, Collins RD: Immunologic characterization of human malignant lymphomas. Cancer 34:1488, 1974
24. Lennert K: Histopathology of Non-Hodgkin's Lymphomas (Based on Kiel Classification). Springer-Verlag, Berlin, 1981
25. Lennert K, Collins RD, Lukes RJ: Concordance of the Kiel and Lukes-Collins classification of non-Hodgkin's lymphomas. Histopathology 7:549, 1983
26. Levine, AM: Immunoblastic sarcoma of T-cell versus B-cell origin. Blood 58:52, 1981
27. Schneider DR, Taylor CR, Parker, et al: B and T cell immunoblastic sarcoma: Morphologic description and comparison. Hum Pathol 16:885, 1985
28. Mellblom, L: Aspiration cytology of neuroendocrine (Merkel-cell) carcinoma of the skin. (Report of a case.) Acta Cytol (Praha) 28:297, 1984
29. Levy N, Nelson J, Meyer P, et al: Reactive lymphoid hyperplasia with single class (monoclonal) surface immunoglobulin. Am J Clin Pathol 80:300, 1983
30. Lukes RJ, Butler JJ: The pathology and nomenclature of Hodgkin's disease. Cancer Res 26:1063, 1966
31. Banks PM: Sarcomatous lacunar cell Hodgkin's disease: A morphologic variant of the nodular sclerosing type. Lab Invest 44:3A, 1981 (abst)
32. Hsu M, Jaffe ES: Leu M-1 and peanut agglutinin stain the neoplastic cells of Hodgkin's disease. Am J Clin Pathol 82:29, 1984
33. Hou SM, Yang K, Jaffe ES: Phenotypic expression of Hodgkin's and Reed-Sternberg cells in Hodgkin's disease. Am J Pathol 118:209, 1985
34. Stein H, Gerdes J, Schwab U, et al: Identification of Hodgkin and Sternberg-Reed cells as a unique cell type derived from a newly-detected small-cell population. Int J Cancer 30:445, 1982

35. Das DK: Malignant lymphoma of convoluted lymphocytes: Diagnosis by fine-needle aspiration cytology and cytochemistry. Diagn Cytopathol 2:307, 1986
36. Mason TE, Demaree RS, Margolis CI: Granulocytic sarcoma (chloroma), two years preceding myelogeneous leukemia. Cancer 31:423, 1973
37. Pettinato G: Fine needle aspiration biopsy of a granulocytic sarcoma (chloroma) of the breast. Acta Cytol (Praha) 32:67, 1988
38. Ziegler JL, Beckstead JH, Volberding PA, et al: Non-Hodgkin's lymphoma in 90 homosexual men. N Engl J Med 311:565, 1984
39. Bottles K, Cohen MB, Brodie H, et al: Fine-needle aspiration cytology of lymphadenopathy in homosexual males. Diagn Cytopathol 2:31, 1986

14

Immunocytochemistry

Carlos W. M. Bedrossian

Cytopathology ranks high among the most eminently morphologic branches of pathology, but to think of cytopathology as purely morphologic constitutes a very shortsighted view of the subspecialty. Because of their shared basis on the visual recognition of structural alterations, surgical pathology is the natural accompaniment of cytopathology and the yardstick against which the accuracy of cytologic diagnoses is measured. As surgical pathology relies increasingly on structural-functional correlations, cytopathology progresses in the same direction. The mere recognition of cell types and cellular groupings carries functional connotations. When a cell is identified as squamous, it is implied that the cell function is to line a flat surface. Likewise, the recognition of vacuoles in a cell implies secretion; if not, it reflects either phagocytosis, which is another cellular function, or degeneration, itself an altered functional state of the cell. Thus, it is virtually impossible to separate a functional meaning from morphologic observations arrived at by cytologic examination.

Only when a meaningful assessment of the underlying altered function can be surmised is a cytologic diagnosis of any value to the physician treating the patient. Obviously, cytopathology would benefit from more detailed morphologic observation and a clearer understanding of the functional state of the cells. A natural evolution is to combine cytopathology with the same approaches that increased the clinical value of surgical pathology, namely, electron microscopy[1,2] and immunocytochemistry (ICC).[3,4] While the former vastly expands our ability to appreciate structural alterations, the latter brings totally new ways to look at the functions of the cell. Together, they add unlimited new dimensions to the practice of cytopathology. This chapter reviews mainly the application of ICC to cytologic specimens. Where pertinent, correlation is made between ICC and electron microscopy as applied to cytologic specimens.

TECHNICAL ASPECTS

The most significant factor affecting the success of ICC applied to cytologic specimens refers to having enough cells in the sample for meaningful results. In hypocellular specimens or in cellular specimens in which only a small proportion of cells are malignant, ICC has little to offer. Another factor of practical significance is preservation of antigenicity by choosing the proper fixative and a methodology most applicable to cytologic specimens.[5] In practice, the method yields best results in fine needle aspirates (FNA), body fluids, and touch imprints. However, it can be applied to smears from any source, including those of cervicovaginal, urogenital, broncho-pulmonary, gastrointestinal (GI), cerebrospinal, and other miscellaneous origins.[6] Fixation must be prompt but not excessive in time, not only for the preservation of antigenic sites but for the yield of impeccable morphologic detail. Both approaches are crucial to interpretation and often complement one another. Ten percent formalin (4 percent formaldehyde solution) is suitable for fixation of cell blocks and tissue sections. It preserves most antigens, but some loss of antigenicity is noted in the intermediate filaments. Alcohol-based fixatives such as Bouin's and Carnoy's are better at preserving the intermediate filaments, while a metallic fixative has the advantage of yielding better cytomorphologic detail. Ethanol-fixed smears are perfectly adequate for ICC.[7] However, prior staining by the Papanicolaou method may alter the results for certain markers.[8] For multiple antibody panels, cell suspensions from body fluids, FNA, or scrapes of surgical samples should first be centrifuged and made into cell pellets. These are aggregated by the addition of plasma and thrombin, which forms a clot that further concentrates the cells in a small volume. The cells may also be concentrated by capturing them in collodion bags, which yield a cell block easily sectioned for histologic evaluation. We recommend staining three levels with H&E and preparing four unstained sections of the cell blocks from body fluids and FNA specimens. If tumor cells are noted, the four unstained sections are used for an initial panel of four antibodies without further delay. This initial panel is usually sufficient to solve most diagnostic dilemmas; if additional antibodies are needed, one must be assured that deeper sections of the cell block contain tumor cells. This is not a problem, provided the initial cellularity of the specimen was high. In cases of low cellularity, or when a large number of immunostains are needed, multiple sections on the same smear can be walled off from each other by partitions etched with wax pencil. It is also possible to fraction a smear and transfer the cells to other slides for ICC staining with multiple antibodies.[9] Multiple antigens may also be searched for in the same smear, provided that the antibodies are raised in different species and different immunoenzymatic systems are used.

Various immunoenzymatic methods are applicable to cytologic specimens, but in practice the indirect unlabeled antibody techniques work best. The direct labeled antibody methods have their greatest application in hematopoietic samples and FNA smears for the quick separation between lymphoma and carcinoma. The three most common indirect methods, using unlabeled antibodies are (1) peroxidase-antiperoxidase (PAP), (2) avidin-biotin complex (ABC), and (3) alkaline phosphatase-antialkaline phosphatase (ALP) techniques (Table 14-1). The avidin-biotin technique is believed to offer improved sensitivity to certain antigens.[10] However, this possibility has not been investigated in cytologic specimens. If the chromogens used are of different colors, two or all three of these methods can be applied to the same specimen. We prefer DAB as the chromogen because it does not fade, but AEC provides a more vivid red color. The PAP and the ALP methods have equal sensitivity, slightly lower than that achieved with the

Table 14-1 Comparison of Unlabeled Antibody Methods Applicable to Cytologic Specimens

	PAP	ABC	AL-P
Chromogen	DAB (brown), AEC (red)	DAB (brown), AEC (red)	Fast blue, AS-MX Napthol
Enzyme	Horseradish peroxidase	Avidin biotinylated peroxidase complex	Alkaline phospatase
Middle bridge	Goat, sheep, or mouse peroxidase plus antigoat, antisheep, or antimouse IgG	Biotinylated goat antirabbit IgG	Rabbit antialkaline phosphosaphatase plus antirabbit IgG
Primary antibody	Monoclonal (mouse) or polyclonal (rabbit)	Monoclonal (mouse) or polyclonal (rabbit)	Monoclonal (mouse) or polyclonal (rabbit)

PAP, peroxidase-antiperoxidase; ABC, avidin-biotin complex; ALP, alkaline phosphatase-antialkaline phosphatase.

ABC technique. It is not clear whether they have different applications, depending on the tissues and the cells under study. Virtually all tissues have endogenous peroxidase, alkaline phosphatase and biotin activities resulting in high background.[11] This problem is minimized in cytologic preparations because the cells are disassociated from their intercellular connective tissue. Collagen itself creates a high background because of its positive electric charge, which tends to favor nonspecific immunostain. This too is obviated in cytologic preparations. The major problems in cytologic specimens pertain to (1) endogenous peroxidase activity of polys and macrophages, (2) nonspecific staining of degenerated or necrotic cells, (3) cross-reactivity among antibodies, and (4) variation of the patterns of staining between cytologic and histologic samples. It is therefore important to be certain that the cells displaying the positivity constitute the malignant elements one is after. This requires good morphologic definition of the nuclei, which, in turn, depends on excellent fixation of the cellular sample and the use of appropriate counterstains. We prefer postfixing our cell blocks in a mixture of B5, a mercury-based fixative and 10 percent formalin, and counterstaining with Lillie-Mayer hematoxylin, to accomplish these goals.[12] The counterstain need not be simply hematoxylin but can be any special stain that might complement ICC in better defining the cell type being investigated. Toluidine blue is excellent for demonstrating chromosomes, while an antibody to microfilaments highlights the spindle during mitosis (Fig. 14-1, Plate 14-1). In adenocarcinoma of the stomach, for instance, a combination of Alcian blue-carcinoembryonic antigen (CEA) will reflect mucin secretion in the form of punctate Alcian blue positivity, while the periphery of the cells will be positive for CEA. In carcinoid tumors, chromogranin is diffusely positive throughout the tumor, while mucicarmine is positive in scattered extracellular hollows indicating that the tumor is an adenocarcinoid. Other combinations are possible that define or clarify the various pathways of differentiation in tumors with mixed histology. ICC can also be combined with electron microscopy in the form of immunoelectron microscopy. The immunogold technique is an example of such an approach enjoying increasing popularity today.[13]

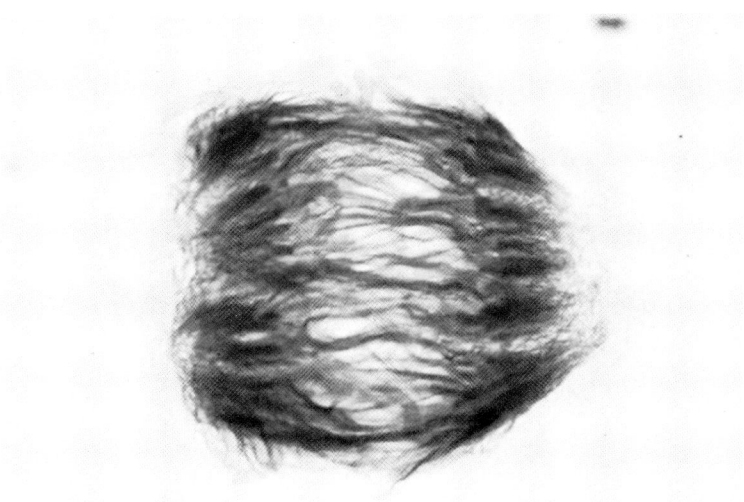

Fig. 14-1 Cell in mitosis. Microtubule spindle is stained red with rabbit antitubulin. Chromosomes are counterstained by toluidine blue. (Courtesy of Dr. S. Van Noorden.) (See Plate 14-1.)

INFECTIONS

One of the greatest applications of ICC is the specific diagnosis of infection in cytologic specimens. Various antibodies of restricted specificity are available that recognize viruses, bacteria, fungi, and protozoa in cellular samples (Table 14-2). The advantage of applying ICC to cytologic samples over using the same antibody by immunofluorescence is obvious; the latter does not appreciate cytomorphology, and it requires fluorescence microscopy.[9] However, as some antibodies are available only as fluorescent-labeled reagents, the direct method may be of help in some select cases.

The herpesvirus family includes several pathogens, among which are herpes simplex types 1 and 2 (HSV-1, HSV-2), cytomegalovirus (CMV), and Epstein-Barr virus (EBV). Among these, the detection of HSV[14,15] and CMV[16,17] has been extensively investigated in cytologic samples. Both the immunoperoxidase technique and in situ hybridization have been used for this purpose.[14] HSV, in fact, has been detected immunocytochemically in cervicovaginal[14,15] and pulmonary specimens.[18] In these cases the Lillie-Mayer counterstaining provides appreciation of the nuclear changes induced by herpes, which

Table 14-2 Antibodies Directed at Selective Infective Agents

Microorganism	Type of Antibody	Supplier
Viruses		
HSV (I, II)	Polyclonal	Biogenex
HSV I	Polyclonal	Biogenex
HSV II	Polyclonal	Biogenex
HPV	Polyclonal	Biogenex
CMV	Polyclonal	Biogenex
Rotavirus	Antiserum	Dakopatts
HBcAg	Monoclonal	Dakopatts
HBsAg	Monoclonal	Dakopatts
Bacteria		
Chlamydia	Monoclonal	Biogenex
Legionella	Antiserum	Dakopatts
E. coli	Antiserum	Dakopatts
M. tuberculosis	Antiserum	Dakopatts
M. paratuberculosis	Antiserum	Dakopatts
BCG	Antiserum	Dakopatts
Fungi		
Candida	Antiserum	Dakopatts
Aspergillus	Antiserum	Dakopatts
Protozoa		
Pneumocystis	Monoclonal	Dakopatts
Toxoplasma	Monoclonal	Chemicon
E. histolytica	Polyclonal	Clark
Trichomonas	Antiserum	CDC

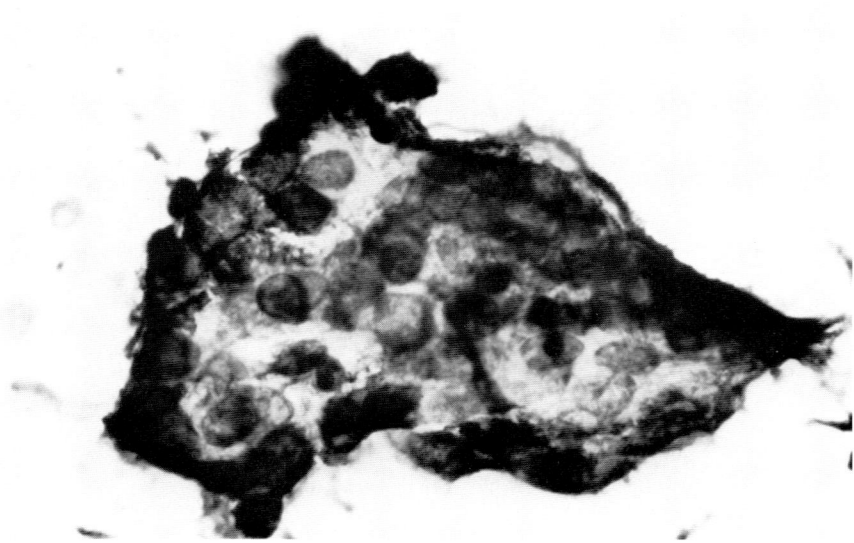

Fig. 14-2 Giant cell stained with HSV antibody. Notice positivity in the periphery of the cytoplasm and multinucleation typical of herpes. (See Plate 14-2.)

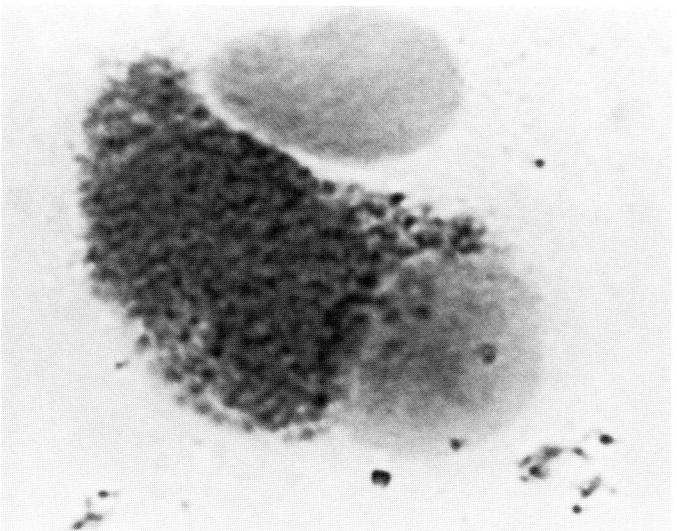

Fig. 14-3 Papanicolaou smear stained with anti-*Chlamydia* antibody. Note strong positivity of the cytoplasm pushing aside the nucleus. (Courtesy of Dr. T. Kobayashi.) (See Plate 14-3.)

serves as an internal control for the immunostaining of the cytoplasm (Fig. 14-2, Plate 14-2). In addition, *Trichomonas*[19] and *Chlamydia*[20,21] have been detected by ICC in cytologic smears. In the latter, ICC permits recognition of *Chlamydia* infection, even in the absence of morphologic alterations in affected cells[22] (Fig. 14-3, Plate 14-3). It is papillomavirus (HPV), however, that has received the greatest attention not only in tissue biopsies[23] but in cytologic specimens as well.[24] Most studies have used an antibody against structural proteins common to bovine and human papillomaviruses. However, it is possible to detect HPV also with synthetic antibodies directed at restricted HPV sequences. This method yields positiv-

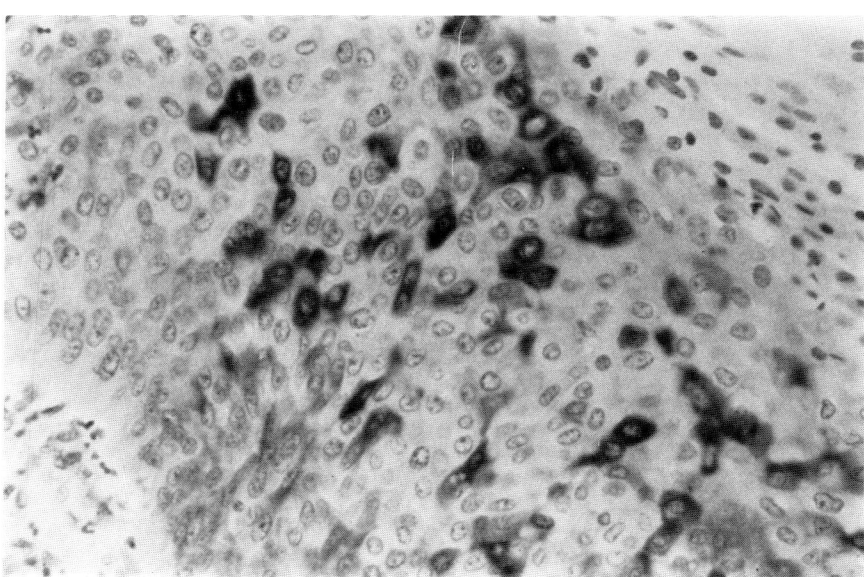

Fig. 14-4 Koilocytes stained by synthetic antibody that recognizes HPV-related DNA sequences. The positivity is noted mainly in the cytoplasm. (See Plate 14-4.)

ity not only in the koilocytes, but in neighboring cells as well[25] (Fig. 14-4, Plate 14-4). This approach is highly desirable because of the propensity of different HPV types to be associated with urogenital disease of variable malignant potential.

be further subdivided according to the tissues from which they were isolated: neurofilaments from neurons; glial filaments from astrocytes; vimentin from mesenchymal cells; keratin from epithelial cells; and desmin from muscle cells (Table 14-3).

CYTOSKELETAL DETERMINANTS OF CELL SHAPE

Cell shape is dictated by the composition and distribution of filament-shaped structural proteins within the cytoplasm. In this regard, they correspond to the meshwork that results from digesting the sap off certain fruits. The cytologist recognizes these as the lace-like configuration of the cytoplasm in non-keratinized cells, but in squamous cells, the richness in filaments is reflected mainly as an increased density of the cytoplasm. The advent of ICC has permitted characterization of the cytoskeletal components common to all mammalian cells, with resulting diagnostic applications in cytologic specimens.[26] With appropriate antibodies, it can be demonstrated that the cytoskeleton is composed of proteins and polypeptides arranged in a rich filamentous network, ranging in thickness from 6 nm (microfilaments) to 25 nm (microtubules). Those having a thickness intermediate between that of microfilaments and microtubules have been termed intermediate filaments (IF) and can

INTERMEDIATE FILAMENTS

At one time it was believed that a given cell expresses only one type of IF. However, it has become increasingly recognized that the coexpression of IF in tumors is very common and preferential in certain types of neoplasms[26-43] (Table 14-4). Rather than detract from the value of ICC in tumor diagnosis, this phenomenon adds greater value to it, since the patterns of IF coexpression may assume diagnostic significance with accumulated experience.

It is important for the cytopathologist to understand the value and limitations of IF typing, based on the use of antibodies raised against extracts of cell fractions. Tumor cells may be variably rich in the various types of IF, which look very similar under the electron microscope. The vast majority of the antibodies currently available are monoclonal and are produced by the hybridoma technique. In the characterization of these antibodies, they are applied mainly to frozen tissue specimens using the immunofluorescence technique, which has limited application in cytology. However, many monoclonal antibodies

Table 14-3 Intermediate Filaments of Diagnostic Interest in Cytopathology

IF Class	Protein Component and Molecular Weight	Occurrence in Cells	Expression in Tumors
1. Epithelial	Keratins (40 kDa (NF), 68 kDa)	Keratinizing and nonkeratinizing epithelium	Carcinomas some sarcomas
2. Neuronal	Neurofilament (68 kDa, 160 kDa, 200 kDa)	Neurons (CNS), peripheral nerve	Neuroblastoma, neuroendocrine carcinomas
3. Glial	GFAP (55 kDa)	Astroglial elements extra-CNS cells (i.e., salivary gld)	Astrocytotomas, pleomorphic adenomas
4. Muscular	Desmin (53 kDa)	Sarcomeric muscle (smooth, striated, cardiac)	Leiomyosarcoma, rhabdomyosarcoma
5. Mesenchymal	Vimentin (57 kDa)	Fibroblasts, chondrocytes, macrophages, endothelial cells	Sarcomas, some carcinomas

GFAP, glial fibrillary acidic protein.

Table 14-4 Tumors That Frequently Coexpress Two or More Intermediate Filaments

Filaments Coexpressed	Origin of Tumor	Histologic Type	Reference
Keratin and vimentin	Salivary gland	Pleomorphic adenoma	32
		Adenoid cystic carcinoma	30
	Kidney	Renal cell carcinoma	35
		Nephroblastoma	34
	Lung and pleura	Adenocarcinoma	33
		Mesothelioma	29
	Thyroid gland	Papillary carcinoma	36
		Hürthle cell tumor	37
	Ovary	Papillary serous carcinoma	26
Vimentin and desmin	Soft tissues	Rhabdomyosarcoma	38
		Leiomyosarcoma	31
Vimentin and GFAP	Brain	Astrocytoma	27
Keratin and NF	Skin	Merkel cell tumor	39
	Lung and GI tract	Carcinoid tumor, neuroendocrine carcinoma	24
			25
Keratin and desmin	Soft tissues	Leiomyosarcoma	28
Vimentin, keratin, and NF	Brain	Choroid plexus tumors	40

GFAP, glial fibrillary acidic protein; NF, neurofilament.

against IF exist that work well in alcohol-fixed smears and paraffin-embedded formalin-fixed cell blocks and tissue sections.

Keratin

Intermediate filaments are biochemically and immunocytochemically distinct; among these, the keratins constitute a complex family of fibrous proteins of different molecular weights.[44] As keratin can accumulate extracellularly, the term cytokeratin applies to the keratin that occurs in the cytoplasm of epithelial cells. Careful microdissection and immunoelectrophoretic studies have unraveled various types of keratin and classified them into two main groups, one acidic and one basic. Moll et al.[45] have further catalogued them into 19 families showing some tissue specificity that may be exploited for diagnostic purposes (Table 14-5). Antibodies can be raised to a mixture of naturally occurring keratins (polyclonal antisera) as well as to a more limited range of high- and/or low-molecular-weight keratins (monoclonal antibodies).[46] These chain-specific antibodies are highly specific for the cytokeratin they are intended to recognize, but they may lack sensitivity when applied to a carcinoma of unknown origin.[47] By carefully selecting appropriate panels that include various chain-specific keratin antibodies, it is possible to classify neoplasms in FNA of difficult interpretation, particularly carcinomas of various types.[48] The method is also applicable to soft tissue tumors[49] and to undifferentiated neoplasms arising in the retroperitoneum.[50] When used in combination with electron microscopy, the reliability of the various diagnoses appears to be considerably improved[51]; the method also seems to enhance the diagnostic accuracy of other types of cytologic samples,[51] including effusions.[52] There is generally good correlation between the results of keratin typing in cytologic and histologic preparations of neoplasms. In fact, since cytologic smears are fixed in alcohol, the preservation of IF antigenicity is particularly favorable in this type of specimen. Keratin is ubiquitous in all epithelial tumors, including small cell, large cell, pleomorphic cell, and spindle cell neoplasms (Fig. 14-5, Plate 14-5).

Table 14-5 Catalogue of Moll's Keratin Subfamilies in Human Epithelia

	Basic (B)		Acidic (A)	
	Moll #	kDa	kDa	Moll #
Skin	1,2	65—67	56—.5	10
Cornea	3	64	55	12
Esophagus	4	59	51	13
Other stratified epithelia	5	[a] 58	50	14, 15
	6	56	48	16
				17
Hepatocytes, pancreatic acini	7	54	46	
Other simple epithelia	8	52	45	18
			40	19

[a] Families expressed by many stratified epithelia.
kDa, kilodaltons.

Numerous attempts have been made at using very specific cytokeratin antibodies that might occur in one type of neoplasm but not in another.[53–55] Thus, it is possible to use antibodies such as the mixture AE1/AE3, which recognize, respectively, the acidic/basic subfamilies, in the diagnosis of carcinomas.[56] Other monoclonal antibodies exist, directed against a more restricted range of keratins of certain molecular weights, many of which are useful in diagnostic work. It is also possible to produce antibodies to just a pair or even a single member of a pair of cytokeratins.[57] Even though this approach has met with some degree of success, these chain-specific antibodies are not readily available for widespread diagnostic application. Consequently, verification of results under a wide variety of clinical situations and technical conditions has not been possible. Examples of chain-specific markers include antibodies RGE-53[57] and CK1-CK4[58] directed against Moll-18 cytokeratin, believed to recognize adenocarcinomas. In our practice, we use a broad spectrum of keratin antibodies, including (1) a polyclonal antibody raised against epidermis; (2) a monoclonal antibody of broad keratin specificity (IRL, Cambridge); (3) a monoclonal antibody (35B-H11) directed against low-molecular-weight cytokeratins (LMWK) 18 and 8; and (4) another monoclonal antibody (34B-E12) directed against high-molecular-weight cytokeratins (HMWK) 2 and 10. Table 14-6 compares a few other commercially available antikeratin antibodies.

Both squamous cell carcinoma and adenocarcinomas of various origins will express keratin and, by judicious use of LMWK and HMWK antibodies, one can classify or even derive the cell of origin these neoplasms. Thus, LMWK positivity is encountered in most adenocarcinomas, including those of the lung, kidney, liver, the GI tract, and the pancreas.[59] These neoplasms are negative for HMWK. Positivity for HMWK is indicative of squamous differentiation in neoplasms of the skin, esophagus, lung, anus, and vagina.[60] The pattern of staining is extremely variable

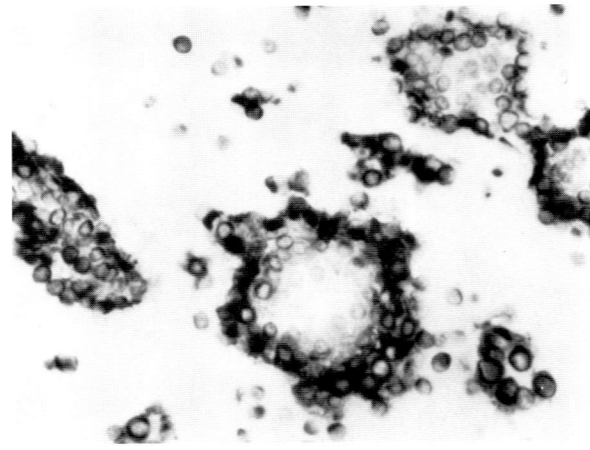

Fig. 14-5 Islet cell tumor of the pancreas stained for keratin with broad spectrum antibody. Note positivity in groups and in individual cells. (See Plate 14-5.)

Table 14-6 Comparison of Commercially Available Antikeratin Antibodies

Antibody	Molecular Weight Recognized		Antigenic Source
	Low	High	
AE1	40 - 48 - 50	51 - 56.5	Keratin from callus
AE3		58 - 65 - 67	Keratin from callus
CAM 5.2	39 - 43 - 50	52	Colorectal carcinoma
PKK 1	41	54 - 56	Kidney cell line
35 BH11	45	52	Hepatocellular cancer
34 BE12		57 - 66	Epidermis

and does not allow for a distinction between the various primary sites. As a rule, most neoplasms that express HMWK are not positive for LMWK, but many exceptions have been found. Mesothelioma is an example of such a neoplasm. The tumor is positive for a mixture of keratins, but the intensity of staining is greater for HMWK than for LMWK. Mesothelial cells are also unique in that they express vimentin, albeit focally, within the tumor and as a diffuse weak staining of the cytoplasm in cytologic preparations. By contrast, keratin creates a very dense perinuclear rim paralleling the neat endoplasmic-ectoplasmic demarcation demonstrated by mesothelial cells. The perinuclear rim of keratin positivity correlates well with the distribution of IF as noted by electron microscopy.[61] This is in contrast to the predominantly arborizing pattern of keratin positivity described for adenocarcinoma in effusion.[52] In our experience, the keratin pattern in adenocarcinoma is extremely variable. Most often, adenocarcinomas are negative for keratin in effusions. However, it may be positive, either peripherally or evenly distributed, but it is generally weaker than mesothelial cells. The cells of mesothelioma give a rim pattern, but the location of the rim ranges anywhere from perinuclear to peripheral, near, or at the edge of the cell. The combined use of HMWK and LMWK is also helpful in distinguishing keratinizing (stronger for HMWK) from nonkeratinizing (negative for HMWK) squamous cell carcinoma. Occasionally, in small cell carcinoma of the lung, IF will form dense tufts next to the nuclei, the significance of which is not clear. The same appearance is frequently noted in Merkel cell tumors. Some of these tufts have given a positive reaction to keratin, while in other instances neurofilament (NF) positivity was found.[62]

Vimentin

The distribution of vimentin by ICC correlates very closely with the appearance of various cell types when visualized cytologically and by electron microscopy. Thus, spindle-shaped mesenchymal cells show parallel intermediate filaments that curve to surround the nucleus and fuse at both ends of the cell. Most sarcomas, melanoma, and lymphoma express vimentin, while squamous cell carcinoma and adenocarcinoma generally do not, except for the coexpressant tumors already alluded to. The cells of sarcoma are usually more strongly positive than those of melanoma and lymphoma. The mesenchymal cells will invariably stain for vimentin and, depending on the direction of their differentiation, for other IF as well. Coexpressant carcinoma cells stain less predictably for vimentin, but they are usually focally or weakly positive. In contrast to thyroglobulin, vimentin is positive only in the cytoplasm of neoplastic cells of follicular carcinoma, without staining the colloid. (Fig. 14-6, Plates 14-6 and 14-7.) Some epithelial cells are negative for vimentin in a primary site but are positive in metastases, effusions, and tissue culture.[63] It is therefore possible that vimentin shares some epitome configurations with other intermediate filaments and that they are variably exposed, depending on the milieu in which the cell finds itself. Azar[64] believes that vimentin is an ancestral IF, sort of a nonsecretory CEA that will be expressed by epithelial and other nonmesenchymal cells when they un-

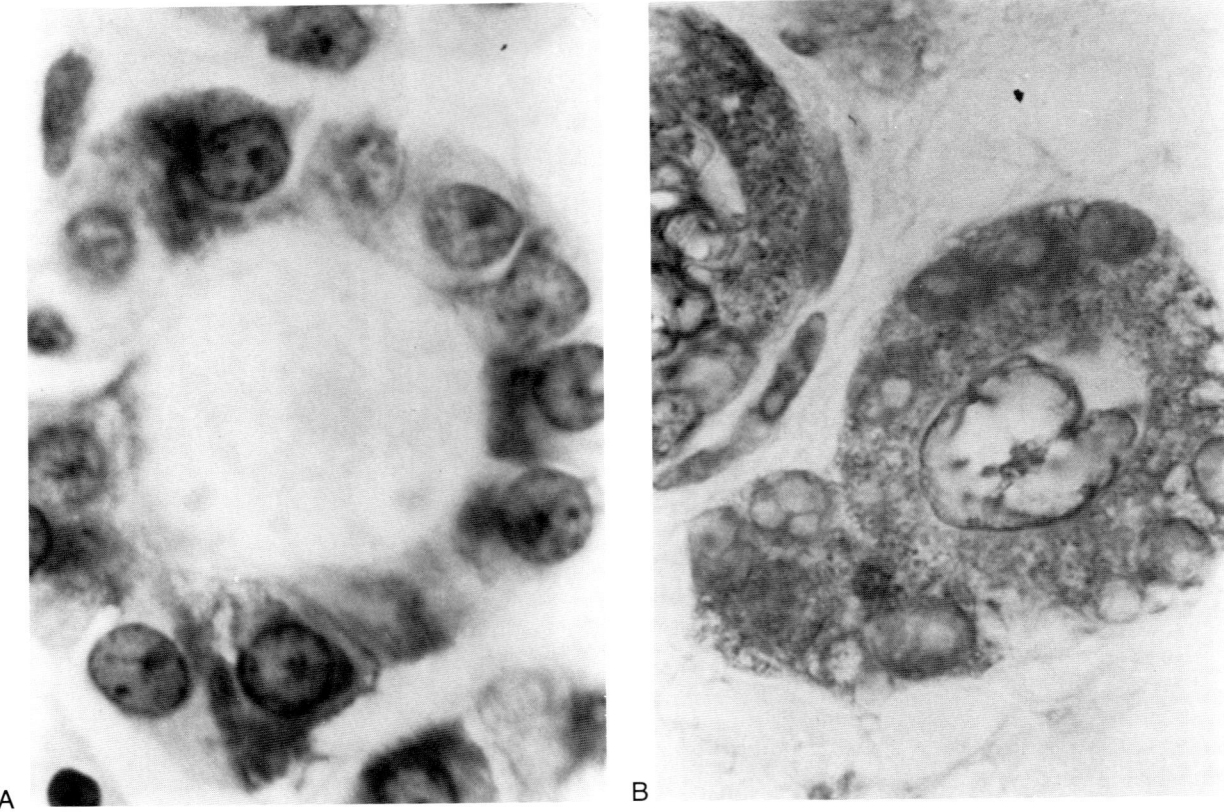

Fig. 14-6 Immunocytochemistry of follicular carcinoma of the thyroid. **(A)** Note variable intensity vimentin in tumor cells and negativity of the colloid. (See Plate 14-6.) **(B)** Thyroglobulin is strongly positive, both in follicle cells and in the colloid. (See 14-7.)

dergo malignant transformation.[64] Vimentin-positive cells should be tested for keratin, desmin, S100, and leukocyte common antigen (LCA) in order to establish the true lineage of the cell under scrutiny. Thick and thin filaments also accompany vimentin in a number of cell types. Actin is the main protein of the thin microfilaments, while myosin is the prototype of thick filamentous proteins. Neither protein, however, is helpful in diagnostic work, because both are ubiquitous in a variety of cell types.

Neurofilament

Neurofilament spans a wide range of molecular weights and is expressed by neuronal tumors of the central and peripheral nervous systems. There are antibodies that recognize three related NF proteins of molecular weights 68 kDa (NF-L), 160 kDa (NF-M), and 200 kDa (NF-H), respectively, which occur as NF triplets.[65] Even though it has been possible to produce antibodies specifically against each member of the triplet, ICC studies have shown that the three often coexist in the same cell. Consequently, most commercial antibodies recognize the three molecular weights of NF indistinctively of their relative proportion. This renders the NF antibody extremely sensitive in the recognition of even partially expressed neural differentiation.[66] Antibodies against NF can be applied to cerebrospinal (CSF) specimens and aid in the recognition of oligodendroglioma, as they are not expressed by lymphocytes, ependymal cells, or metastatic carcinomas.[67] However, cells from the choroid plexus express NF and at times mimic malignancy in a cytologic specimen.[68] NF-positive cells should be tested for neuron-specific enolase (NSE) and other markers of neuroendocrine differentiation. NF positivity is found in neuroblastomas of the pediatric and adult age group,[69] a large proportion of neuroendocrine carcinomas,[70] Merkel cell tumors,[71] and other peripheral neuroectodermal tumors.[72,72] Antibodies against NF are extremely useful in the differential diagnosis of small blue round cell tumors because they are negative in Ewing's sarcoma, embryonal rhabdomyosarcoma, lymphoma, and Wilms' tumor (Table 14-7).

The presence of NF in small cell carcinoma and other neuroendocrine tumors of the lung is hotly disputed.[74–76] While some investigators claim that keratin[74] is the IF of oat cell carcinoma, others believe it is NF.[75] Still others have found both.[76] This is due in part to the differences in the antibodies employed in the various studies but may also be related to the method of fixation and cytopreparation of the cells. For instance, fresh, frozen, and alcohol-fixed cells demonstrate NF more readily than cells fixed in formalin and the B5-formalin mixture. In our hands, not a single oat cell carcinoma has shown NF positivity in cell blocks fixed in B5-formalin. If this trend is proved correct, it would lend further support to the theory of non-neural crest derivation for lung neoplasms. In fact, compelling current evidence suggests that all lung tumors, carcinoids included, derive from the same precursor: immature, small granular mucous cells, the true reserve cells of the bronchial mucosa.[77] These cells are totipotential, capable of evolving into ciliated, goblet, Kulchitsky-like, and metaplastic cells, explaining the marked heterogeneity found in lung carcinoma. Other tumors that frequently express multidirectional differentiation are those derived from salivary glands, uterus, ovaries, and pancreas. The exact clinical significance of this heterogeneity is the object of increasing attention.[78]

Glial Fibrillary Acidic Protein

Glial fibrillary acidic protein (GFAP) is the typical IF of glial tissue and glial neoplasms and as such enjoys a lot of applications in diagnostic workups.[79] This protein is poorly characterized, and yet antibodies against GFAP are extremely useful in the recognition of astrocytic neoplasms.[80] The GFAP antibody works equally well by immunofluorescence as a rapid diagnostic procedure to document embryologic defects in the amniotic fluid[81] and by the immunoperoxidase technique for tumor diagnosis in the CSF.[82,83] Not only gliomas and ependymomas, but extracranial neoplasms such as teratoma, renal cell carcinoma,[84] and salivary gland tumors,[85] may be positive for GFAP. The greatest application of GFAP is in the differentiation between a meningeal sarcoma and glioblastoma multiform, which can be very difficult by cytologic means alone.[86] GFAP positivity

Table 14-7 Differential Diagnosis of Small Blue Round Cell Tumors

Tumor Category		NE	Ker	NF	Hormone	LCA	LN1/LN2	ACT	VIM
Neuroendocrine									
Epithelial	Carcinoid	+	+	+	+	–	–	–	–
	Intermediate	+	+	+	+	–	–	–	–
	NE carcinoma	+	+	+	–	–	–	–	–
Neural	Neuroblastoma	+	+	+	–	–	–	–	–
	Pheochromocytoma	+	+	+	–	–	–	–	–
	Paraganglioma	+	+	+	–	–	–	–	–
Non-neuroendocrine									
Lymphohistiocytic	Lymphoma	–	–	–	–	+	+	+/–	+/–
	Plasmacytoma	–	–	–	–	–	+	–	+/–
	Histiocytic	–	–	–	–	+	+/–	+	+
Mesenchymal	Wilms' tumor	–	–	–	–	+	+/–	+	+
	Ewing's sarcoma	+/–	+/–	–	–	–	–	–	+
	Rhabdomyosarcoma	–	–	–	–	–	–	–	+

NE, neuroendocrine marker; Ker, keratin; NF, neurofilament; LCA, leukocyte common antigen; ACT, antichymotrypsin; VIM, vimentin.

extends to ependymal cells but not to neurons or Schwann cells.[87] The antibody can be used not only in FNA and in the CSF, but also in imprints of brain neoplasms removed at surgery[88] and in malignant effusions.[89] GFAP-positive cells should be tested for keratin and vimentin in order to clarify their lineage further. In tissue specimens, GFAP positivity should be interpreted with caution because it occurs in reactive gliosis and in reactive ependymal cells that may be intimately associated with brain neoplasms. This antibody is also expressed by a small proportion of cells of medulloblastomas, suggesting a tendency toward glial differentiation in these primitive neural tumors.

Other Cytoskeletal Components

Microtubules and microfilaments complement IF in providing the cytoplasm with a cytoskeleton. These structures are easily visualized by electron microscopy, but their recognition by ICC in cytologic preparations has not been adequately explored. Antibodies against tubulin have been used in the recognition of cytoplasmic fibrils believed to represent arrays of microtubules.[90] These antibodies have been used in the study of cells in tissue culture but not in clinical cytologic material. Most studies with antibodies against microfilaments recognize actin-like proteins in the cytoplasm of various cell types.[91] Smooth muscle actin (SMA) is particularly helpful in the recognition of myoepithelial cells in various types of breast carcinoma.[92] HHF-35, a marker believed to recognize actin, is positive in adenoid cystic carcinoma of the salivary gland[93] but is not demonstrated in prostatic carcinoma, suggesting that the basal cells in the prostate are not myoepithelial in origin.[94]

INDICATORS OF HISTOGENESIS AND DIFFERENTIATION

Cytoplasmic organelles dispersed within the meshwork of IF provide clues as to the origin of the cell, its degree of differentiation, as well as its functional state. Since the cytoskeleton is very similar, if not identical, among a wide range of cells, these distinctive organelles actually define the cell type. An example of this are the parallel stacks of rough endoplasmic reticulum (RER), indicative of immunoglobulin synthesis, which characterize and define plasma cells. The greater the degree of plasmacytic differentiation the greater is the amount of RER in the cytoplasm. However, in order to be sure one is dealing with plasma cells, they should be positive for immunoglobulins. Fibroblasts are another cell type that display prominently dilated cisternae of RER when actively synthesizing collagen, but not while in a quiescent state. This property is shared by any mesenchymal cell engaged in the production of their respective extracellular material, that is, collagen, osteoid, or chondroid. So, by itself, abundant RER is not sufficient to distinguish fibroblasts from other mesenchymal cells. Often such distinction can only be accomplished by determining the biochemical composition of the extracellular matrix surrounding the individual cell. It is no surprise, therefore, that the spindle cells of fibrosarcoma, osteosarcoma, and chondrosarcoma are very difficult to distinguish from one another in cytologic specimens. Even at the ultrastructural level, these primitive mesenchymal cells are shared by virtually all neoplasms of the soft tissues. Consequently, one must look for other organelles not shared by all mesenchymal elements, in order to classify the various types of sarcomas. Examples of organelles that occur only in cells already committed to a restricted pathway of differentiation include (1) the contractile proteins in myogenous cells; (2) pinocytotic vesicles, typical of endothelial cells; (3) a high lipid content found in lipoblasts; (4) enzymes and proteins of the protease-antiprotease system, such as lysozyme, α_1-antitrypsin (A_1AT) and α_1-antichymotrypsin (A_1ACT) present in histiocytes; and (5) keratin and a few secretory products in epithelioid mesenchymal cells. A much greater array of differentiation pathways exist in epithelial cells and form the basis of their cytologic, ultrastructural, and immunocytochemical recognition.

Until very recently, it was customary to classify tumors according to putative cell or tissue of origin, (e.g., osteogenic sarcoma). Presently, the preferred terminology is osteosarcoma (indicative of osteoid differentiation, independent of the site of origin) because the concept of differentiation is gaining greater credence at the expense of histogenesis.[95] This has the advantage of explaining the presence of heterologous elements in neoplasms of mixed histologic appearance and the occurrence of neoplasms of a given cell type where a normal counterpart does not exist. When a tumor cell expresses a marker that is no longer present in the differentiated mature state, it is said to have dedifferentiated.[96] However, evidence for such a change in vitro has not been produced. There are, nevertheless, numerous substances, proper of the oncofetal stage that are expressed in neoplasms but not in the mature tissues, suggesting that gene derepression may accompany the neoplastic process. Even though the finding of such substances was once heralded as a marker of neoplastic transformation, it is now used more within the context of differentiation/dedifferentiation.

Oncofetal Markers

During the neoplastic process, cells regress to a very primitive stage, rendering their histogenesis impossible to discern by morphologic means. Hand in hand with neoplastic transformation, synthesis of abnormal proteins takes place, recapitulating embryonic protein synthesis. CEA is the classic example of one such protein believed to be a tumor marker. Because CEA was first detected in colonic neoplasms, it was initially believed to be specific for this type of tumor. We know now that CEA occurs in other tumors, particularly adenocarcinomas, regardless of the site of origin.[97] Other oncofetal markers, including alpha-fetoprotein (AFP), β-human chorionic gonadotropin (BhCG), and human placental lactogen (HPL) are also expressed by a wide variety of neoplasms. In our experience, CEA is a good marker to distinguish epithelial cells from cells of lymphocytic or histiocytic derivation in lymph node FNA and epithelial cells from cells of mesothelial origin in malignant effusions.[97] CEA has been applied to sputum specimens,[98] CSF,[99] needle aspirates,[100] washes of various organs,[100,101] bone marrow,[102] and effusions.[60,97,100,103] Both the immunofluorescence and the immunoperoxidase techniques serve well in demonstrating CEA, but the latter is preferred because of good appreciation of cytologic detail. The antigen is widely expressed by a variety of neoplasms, including carcinomas of the colon,[99] lung,[103] stomach,[104] breast,[105] and ovary.[106] By contrast, mesotheliomas are invariably negative for CEA.[107] By the immunogold technique, the marker is easily demonstrable attached to the glycocalyceal system of the tumor cells.[108,109] Even though monoclonal CEA antibodies are more specific than polyclonal CEA antibodies, their sensitivity in detecting the same type of neoplasms is slightly lower.

Oncofetal markers are expressed in various proportions in different types of germ cell tumors (Table 14-8). They reliably permit the identification of these neoplasms in gonadal and extragonadal sites and, to a certain extent, their subclassification into dysgerminoma/seminoma, embryonal carcinoma, and choriocarcinoma.[110] Thus, dysgerminoma is not associated with either AFP or BhCG. The mononuclear cells in embryonal carcinoma contain AFP, but not BhCG, and the syncytiocytotrophoblastic giant cells of choriocarcinoma are positive for BhCG, but not AFP.[111] In the endodermal sinus tumor, mononuclear cells show no immunostaining for BhCG, and the positivity for AFP is focal rather than diffuse, as noted in embryonal carcinoma.[111] The use of markers has shown greater cellular heterogeneity in germ cell tumors than was previously realized. Some neoplasms express one marker predominantly but may show positivity for numerous other markers focally.[112] AFP and BhCG, for example, are both very commonly positive in the same tumor but in different cell types.[112] The exact significance of this phenomenon

Table 14-8 Oncofetal Markers and Their Distribution in Human Neoplasms

	CEA	AFP	BhCG	SP1	PLP	A_1AT	PLAP
Metastatic carcinoma	+	+/−	+/−	−	−	−	−
Dysgerminoma seminoma	−	−	+/−	−	−	−	+
Embryonal carcinoma	−	+	−	−	−	−	+
Choriocarcinoma	+	−	+	−	−	−	+
Endodermal sinus tumor	−	+	−	−	−	+	+

CEA, carcinoembryonic antigen; AFP, alpha-fetoprotein; BhCG, β-chorionic gonadotropin; SP1, pregnancy-specific glycoprotein; PLP, human placental lactogen; A_1AT, α_1-antitrypsin; PLAP, placental variant of alkaline phosphatase.

is not clear but, with rare exceptions, the positivity for AFP has directed us to recognize the tumor as of endodermal sinus differentiation[113] (Fig. 14-7, Plate 14-8). BhCG on the other hand, in general indicates a choriocarcinomatous differentiation[114] (Fig. 14-8, Plate 14-9). The same is true of pregnancy-specific glycoprotein (SP1), but BhCG, SP1, placental variant of alkaline phosphatase (PLAP), and AFP may all occur in nontrophoblastic malignancies such as extragonadal carcinomas.[104,115] This seems to indicate that oncofetal markers are expressed by carcinomas as part of the neoplastic process which derepresses metabolic pathways unavailable in the adult tissues. Consequently, careful interpretation of these markers is required. This is particularly true at sites in which both germ cell neoplasms and carcinomas are likely to occur. Accordingly, the presence of oncofetal markers in a mediastinal tumor is not proof of extragonadal germ cell derivation.[116] A lung neoplasm should be ruled out, since lung carcinomas can occasionally be positive for BhCG and AFP[117] and are frequently positive for A_1AT, another marker present in germ cell tumors.[118] In the retroperitoneum and in the liver, AFP positivity is not equivalent to germ cell origin either, because hepatocellular carcinomas are frequently positive for this marker.[119] A_1AT, too is frequently expressed by carcinomas arising in the liver and in the lung.[120] We find that interpretation of this stain is always problematic, if not outright misleading, particularly in poorly differentiated large cell tumors of the mediastinum or retroperitoneum. A_1AT may also be positive in effusions that contain neoplastic cells.[121] In such cases, A_1AT positivity will not help distinguish among liver, lung, germ cell, or histiocytic origin of the large cell neoplasms. The precise classification of these tumors usually involves a comprehensive antibody panel[121] and the use of electron microscopy.

Epithelial Membrane Antigens

The epithelial nature of neoplastic cells may be demonstrated by their richness in cytoplasmic membrane systems. This feature is a more sensitive indicator of epithelial origin than evidence of mucin secretion, as the latter occurs only in well-differentiated adenocarcinomas. Demonstration of epithelial membrane antigens (EMA) is also more sensitive than

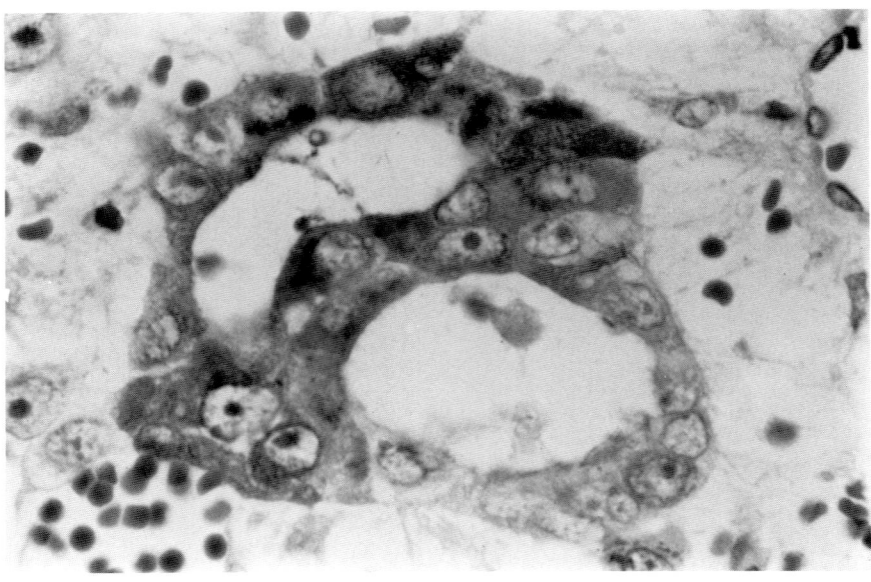

Fig. 14-7 Embryonal carcinoma stained for alphafetoprotein. Diffuse positivity is noted in the cytoplasm of the tumor cells. (See Plate 14-8.)

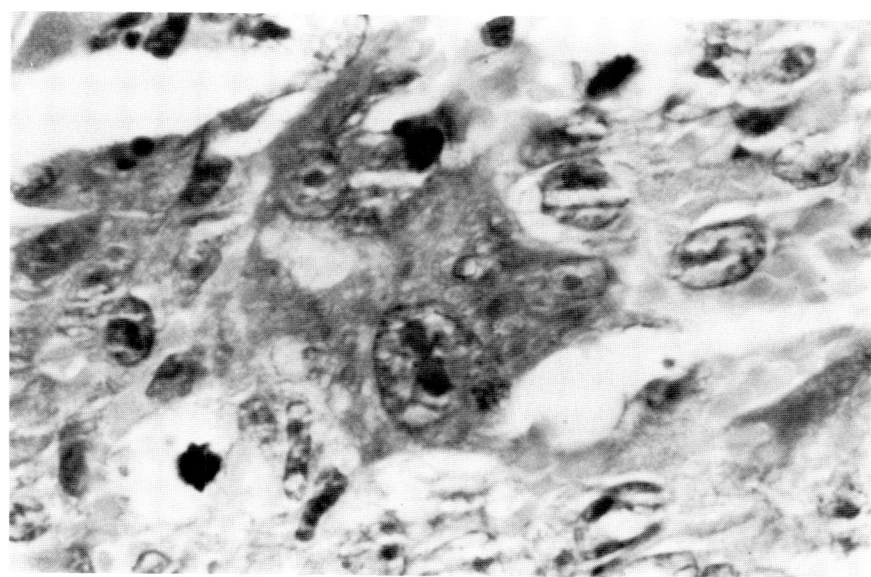

Fig. 14-8 Choriocarcinoma stained for BHCG. Diffuse positivity is noted in the cytoplasm of a syncytiocytotrophoblastic giant cell. (See Plate 14-9.)

demonstration of CEA because not all neoplasms show regression to an oncofetal stage. Consequently, EMA has emerged as a very reliable marker of epithelial origin and is frequently positive in a wide variety of carcinomas.[122] Most EMA preparations derive from membranous cell fractions, and many commercial sources are available. Several of these have been well characterized, particularly antibodies raised against membranes from human milk fat globule, known as HMFG-1 and HMFG-2.[123] A combination of CEA, EMA, and keratin antibodies is helpful in distinguishing mesotheliomas from carcinomas in surgical specimens.[124] EMA in particular is very effective in detecting malignant epithelial cells in effusions (Fig. 14-9, Plate 14-10). EMA stains preferentially malignant epithelial cells with no staining of macrophages and only a weak, if at all, positive staining of the cytoplasm of mesothelial cells.[125,126] The generic antibody against EMA clearly delineates the apical cell membrane as well as the intracytoplasmic lumina of many carcinomas, including those arising in the breast.[97,127] This feature, however, cannot be used to exclude mesothelioma, since this tumor may exhibit a strong linear pattern of immunostaining with EMA. By immunoelectron microscopy, EMA is not restricted to the glycocalyceal apparatus but deposits diffusely beneath the plasma membrane of neoplastic epithelial cells.[128] When using EMA preparations, one should be familiar with the range of specificity of the antibody, its properties under various conditions of fixation, and its distribution within positive cells.[129] With this in mind, both HMFG and generic EMA can be very useful in the study of breast and other carcinomas in histologic and cytologic material.[130,131]

Another antibody with wide application in cytology was raised against a membrane fraction, from a breast cancer cell line, known as TAG 72.3.[132] The antibody thus obtained, B72.3, seems to be a very sensitive marker for breast carcinoma. However, many other carcinomas are positive for B72.3 making it a pancarcinoma marker of broad specificity.[133] The marker seems to work equally well in tissues,[134,135] effusions,[136,137] and needle aspirates.[138,139] The staining pattern of B72.3 in tissue sections of breast carcinoma combines apical staining with a distribution more akin to that of CEA, resulting in diffuse positivity of the cytoplasm.[140] Other less frequently used examples of EMA antibodies have been very successful in immunophenotyping of human neoplasms. However, their usefulness is limited because they are not commercially available.

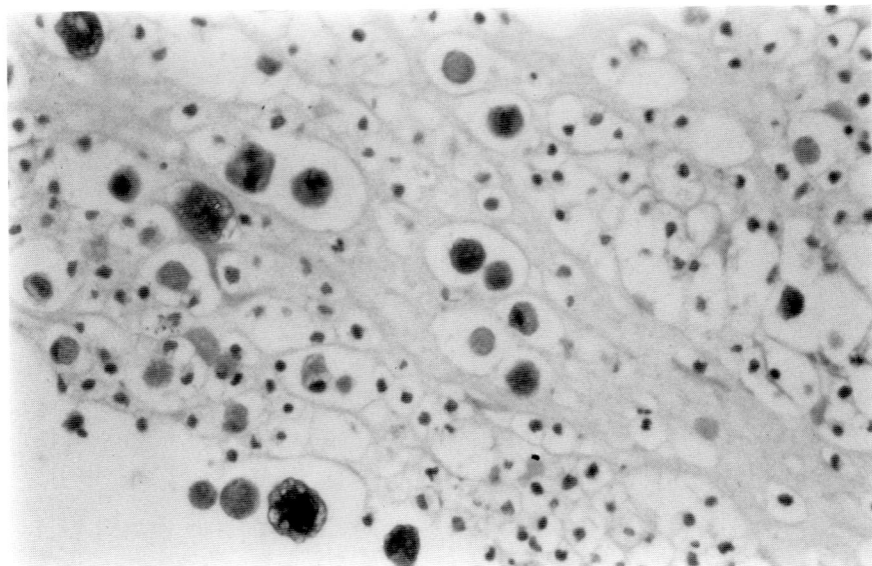

Fig. 14-9 Pleural effusion stained for EMA. Malignant cells stand out prominently from the negative mesothelial cells in the background. (See Plate 14-10.)

Hormones

Endocrine tumors produce hormones typical of their parent gland (Table 14-9). In general, the first step when dealing with a tumor arising in the endocrine organs is to decide whether it is a primary neoplasm or a metastasis. This is particularly crucial in the adrenal gland, where a primary tumor will express keratin, CEA, and EMA and also coexpress vimentin.[141] These tumors produce various hormones, such as aldosterone, glucocorticoids, and the sex steroids, which may be detected in the serum. However, their small molecules make detection in cytologic and histologic material very unpredictable. Neoplasms of the adrenal medulla are indistinguishable from their counterparts arising in the dispersed neuroendocrine system.[142,143] Pheochromocytomas, exceptionally, may present with very large pleomorphic cells that can be recognizable by cytologic criteria.[144] These cells display an abundance of granules by electron microscopy and stain for NSE, NF and norepinephrine by ICC.[145]

Papillary and follicular carcinomas of the thyroid gland are easily recognized by their typical cytologic appearance. These tumors are positive for thyroglobulin and negative for calcitonin and CEA. However, the staining of colloid is extremely variable from neoplasm to neoplasm, so that positivity of the tumor cells is a more reliable marker of thyroid derivation (Fig. 14-10, Plate 14-11). Medullary carcinomas, on the other hand, are positive for calcitonin and CEA and negative for thyroglobulin[146] (Fig. 14-11, Plate 14-12). These tumors show evidence of neuroendocrine differentiation and are capable of ectopically secreting other hormones besides calcitonin.[147,148]

Neoplasms arising in the adenohypophysis are usually benign. The various pituitary adenomas are classified by ICC according to their predominant cell types into somatotroph, lactotroph, corticotroph, gonadotroph, and null cell adenomas.[149] Cytologically, however, these cell types are difficult to distinguish from one another and, not infrequently, pituitary adenomas are capable of multiple hormonal secretion.[150] Gliomas can be distinguished from pituitary adenomas in needle aspirates by the use of GFAP. Pituitary tumors arising in the neurohy-

Table 14-9 Immunocytochemical Detection of Hormones and Other Markers in Endocrine Neoplasms

Site of Origin	Tumor Type	Useful Markers
Adrenal cortex	Cortical adenoma, carcinoma	Steroids (aldosterone, glucocorticoids, sex hormones)
Adrenal medulla	Pheochromocytoma, neuroblastoma	NSE, syntaptophysin, S100, chromogranin, Leu-enkephalin
Thyroid follicles	Papillary and follicular carcinoma	Thyroglobulin, keratin, vimentin
Thyroid C cells	Medullary carcinoma	Calcitonin, CEA, somatostatin
Neurohypophysis	Pituitary adenomas, gliomas	GFAP, vasopressin, oxytocin, S100 protein, neuroendocrine markers
Adenohypophysis	Pituitary adenomas	Growth hormone, prolactin, ACTH, FSH, LH, TSH, neuroendocrine markers
Ovary	Granulosa-theca	Estradiol, progesterone, testosterone
Testis	Sertoli-Leydig cell tumors	Testosterone, progesterone
Parathyroid	Parathyroid adenomas, carcinoma	PTH, parathyroid secretory protein
Pancreatic islets	Islet cell tumor, carcinoid tumor	Insulin, glucagon, gastrin, somatophysin, VIP, motilin, neurotensin, PP, cholecystokinin

ACTH, adenocorticotropin; CEA, carcinoembryonic antigen; FSH, follicle-stimulating hormone; GFAP, glial fibrillary acidic protein; LH, luteinizing hormone; NSE, Neuron-specific enolase; PTH, parathyroid hormone; TSH, thyroid-stimulating horone; PP, pancreatic polypeptide; VIP, vasointestinal peptide.

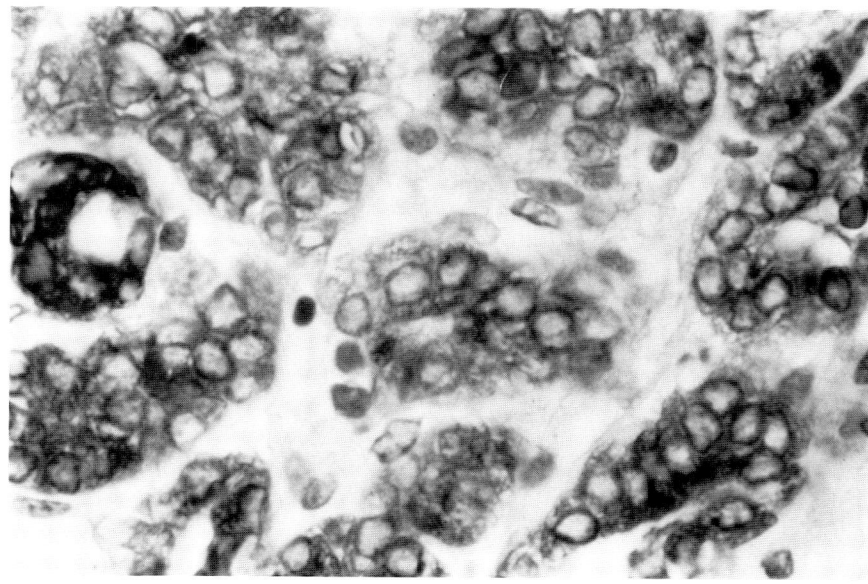

Fig. 14-10 Follicular variant of papillary carcinoma stained for thyroglobulin. Tumor cells are clearly positive against the negative staining of the background. Note margination of the chromatin in the malignant ("optically clear") nuclei. (See Plate 14-11.)

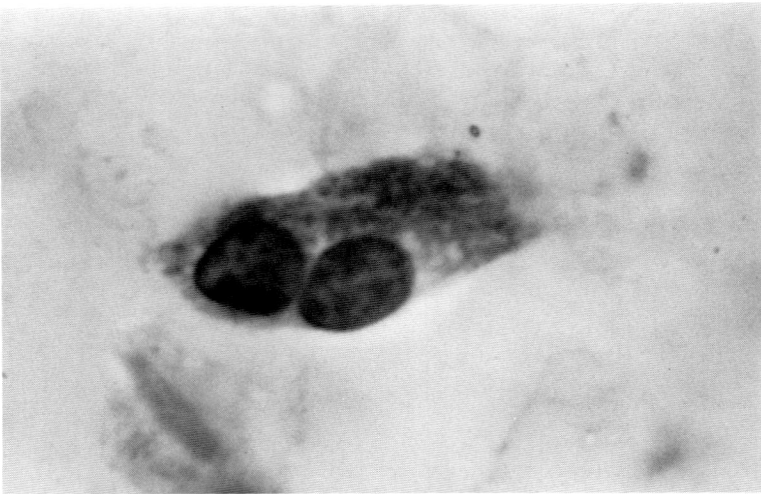

Fig. 14-11 Neoplastic C-cells stained for calcitonin. Note diffuse, strong positivity of the abundant, square-shaped granular cytoplasm. (See Plate 14-12.)

pophysis will secrete vasopressin and oxytocin,[151] but they may actually be ganglioneuromas. These tumors are usually positive for S100 and the neuroendocrine markers.

The cytologic diagnosis of hormone-producing gonadal neoplasms is only seldom accomplished.[152] In surgically resected specimens, ovarian tumors are very similar to their male counterparts. Both Sertoli-Leydig cell and granulosa-theca cell tumors share common pathways of hormonal synthesis and consequently secrete the same types of hormones.[153,154] Because the expression in individual tumors may be extremely variable, ICC alone is not capable of accurately classifying these neoplasms. Parathyroid tumors exhibit a wide range of neoplastic potential from hyperplasia to adenomas to carcinomas.[155] These tumors express parathyroid hormone, a helpful feature in distinguishing them from thyroid tumors in FNA and surgical biopsies.[156] Needle aspirates are frequently used in the evaluation of pancreatic tumors, yielding small blue round cell tumors of difficult interpretation. Very often these are simply classified as nonexocrine or neuroendocrine with islet cell/carcinoid differentiation.[157] These tumors express the various nonhormonal neuroendocrine markers plus serotonin, in the case of carcinoid, and any of the islet cell hormones, in the case of islet cell tumors.[158] Not infrequently, these tumors are plurihormonal in their pattern of immunostain.

Tumors outside the endocrine glands are capable of ectopic hormonal secretion, a very common phenomenon in tumors showing neuroendocrine differentiation. A small proportion of exocrine neoplasms may also exhibit this same property, even though neuroendocrine differentiation is not readily apparent. A classic example is squamous cell carcinoma of the lung, which may ectopically secrete parathormone (PTH). The measurement of a hormone in the serum requires a biologically active molecule, and antigenic sites in the cells or tissue must be intact for ICC detection. With these many variables, there is usually poor correlation between the serum level of the hormone and its demonstration by ICC. The greatest application of antibodies against hormones is in the recognition and classification of small cell neoplasms in FNA from lymph nodes and the liver. In the liver, it is not uncommon for the differential diagnosis to be between carcinoid and islet cell tumor of the pancreas. As previously noted, both tumors will be positive for a nonspecific marker of neuroendocrine differentiation, such as NSE or chromogranin. Islet cell tumor, however, will also display positivity for hormones such as gastrin, insulin, glucagon, and, rarely, other polypeptides.

Secretory Markers

Based on the presence of secretory vacuoles, one recognizes glandular differentiation. Further subtyping of the adenocarcinoma can be accomplished by identifying the nature of the secretory product. A classic example of this approach is the subclassification of bronchioloalveolar carcinoma into three main types according to the nature of their secretory granules.[159] Mucinous neoplasms show granules with a fluffy matrix by EM, whereas Clara cell-derived neoplasms display large electron-dense granules limited by a single membrane. Type II cell neoplasms—the rarest of the three variants of bronchioloalveolar carcinoma—contain lamellated inclusion bodies typical of the surfactant substance they produce.[160] Since surfactant is not produced by the other subtypes, an antibody against surfactant apoprotein is specific for type II cell-derived neoplasms.[161]

Evidence of secretory differentiation may be demonstrated by well-performed routine cytologic stains (Fig. 14-12, Plate 14-13). These secretory products can also be demonstrated by histochemical and immunocytochemical methods applied to cellular samples. CEA is a good indicator of glandular differentiation and is present in virtually all adenocarcinomas, particularly colon and lung (Fig. 14-13, Plates 14-14 and 14-15). Mucicarmine and alcian blue positivity are typical of well-differentiated adenocarcinomas, as is periodic acid-Schiff (PAS) positivity following diastase digestion. Mucicarmine can easily be applied to cytologic smears, which may obviate the use of ICC for the diagnosis of adenocarcinoma (Fig. 14-14, Plate 14-16). In my own material, CEA was positive in 90 percent of adenocarcinomas and alcian blue in 71 percent of cases[97] when both stains were used in combination (Fig. 14-15, Plate 14-17). As previously noted, markers that delineate the secretory apparatus, even in the absence of secretion, are useful markers for poorly differentiated adenocarcinomas. Some of these, such as EMA, HMFG-2, and B.72.3, have been used extensively in cytology. Others have not been as thoroughly investigated, but preliminary explorations are promising. Secretory piece, first described in breast carcinoma, is one marker used in tissue specimens for the identification of adenocarcinomas.[162] The marker is not as consistently positive as CEA, even though it is positive in 90 percent of colon carcinomas, 50 percent of breast carcinomas, and 40 percent of lung carcinomas.[163] Ovarian, prostatic, pancreatic, and gastric carcinomas are consis-

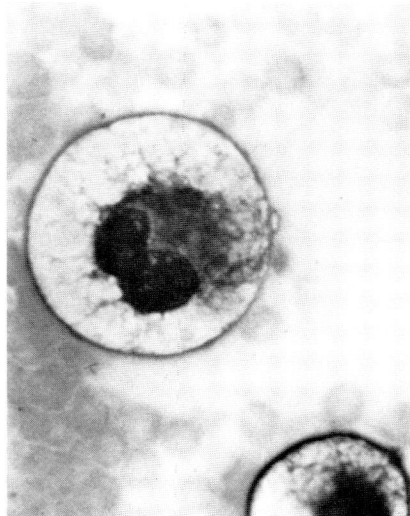 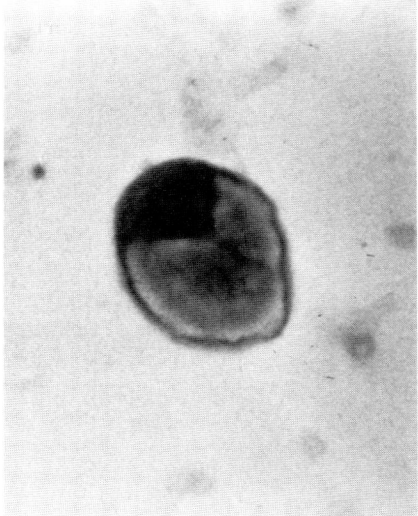

Fig. 14-12 Adenocarcinoma, by routine cytologic stains. (Left) With MGG, mucin appears clear and floculent. (Right) With Papanicolaou the secretory product is retracted from the cell membrane and surrounded by a halo. (See Plate 14-13.)

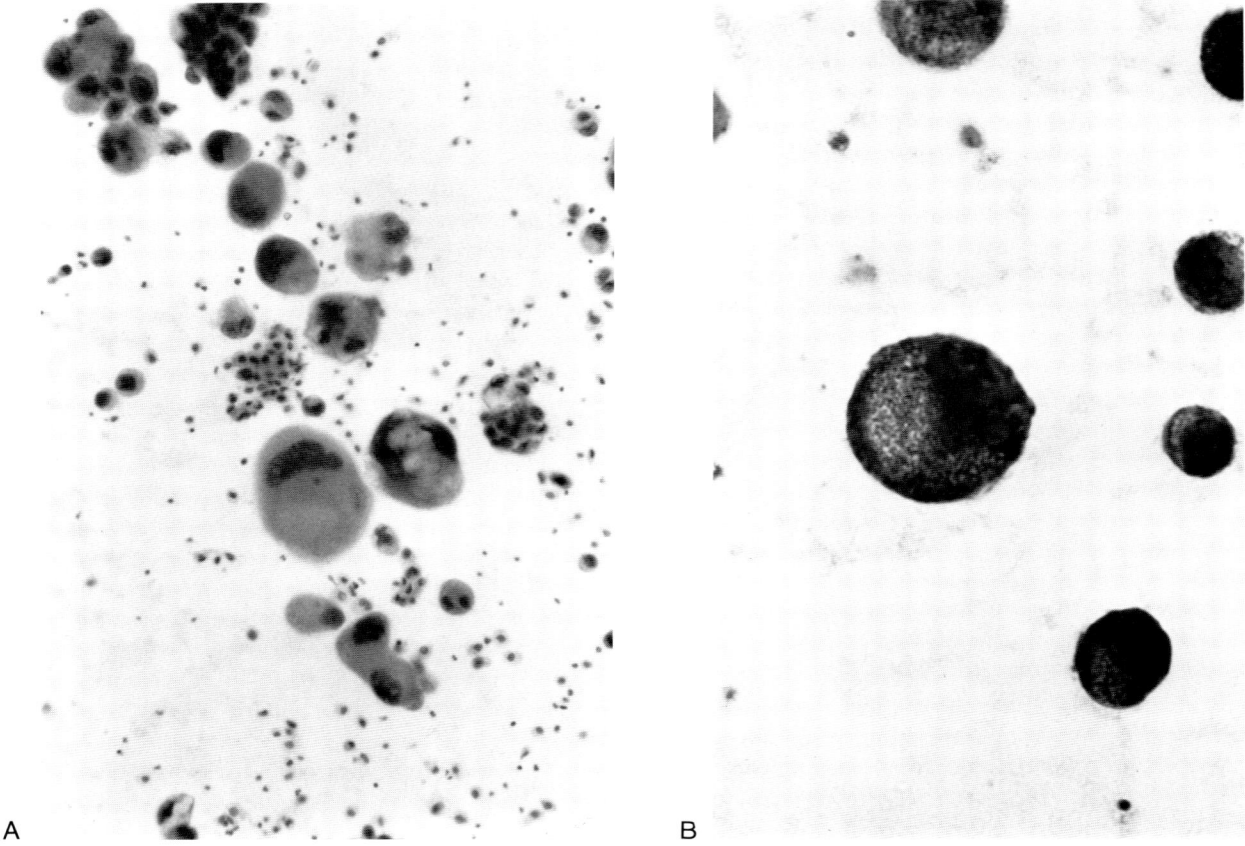

Fig. 14-13 Metastatic adenocarcinoma. **(A)** The large tumor cells show partial vacuolization of the cytoplasm with the Papanicolaou stain. (See Plate 14-14.) **(B)** Positivity of the CEA immunostain is evenly distributed throughout the cytoplasm. (See Plate 14-15.)

tently negative for secretory piece, and renal cell carcinomas give a peculiar interstitial pattern of positivity. By electron microscopy, renal cell carcinomas demonstrate abundant glycogen and lipid droplets.

Leu M_1 was initially developed as a lymphohistiocytic marker useful in the recognition of lymphomas including Hodgkin's disease[164] and mycosis fungoides.[165] By experimentation, it was soon realized that the marker stains nonhematopoietic malignancies, particularly adenocarcinoma.[166,167] Leu M_1, actually discriminates between the cells of adenocarcinoma (frequently positive) and mesothelial cells (usually negative) and is therefore useful in the diagnosis of mesothelioma.[168] The distribution of positive cells in the peripheral sinusoids of lymph node helps in the distinction between metastatic carcinoma and lymphoma. The marker is positive in anaplastic carcinomas, including those arising in the breast, lung, colon, thyroid, pancreas, and stomach.

Other markers of adenocarcinomatous differentiation include specific secretory products, such as thyroglobulin (TGb), prostatic-specific antigen (PSA), ovarian carcinoma product (OCP-125), and pancreatic specific antigen (CA-1) (Table 14-10). TGb and the prostatic antigens are highly reliable in cytologic and histologic material, while the other secretory markers await confirmation of their specificity in clinicopathologic studies. However, it should be remembered that the chemotherapy for various types of adenocarcinoma remains similarly dismal. Consequently, the cost of establishing a primary site has to be weighed carefully against the other clinical data in

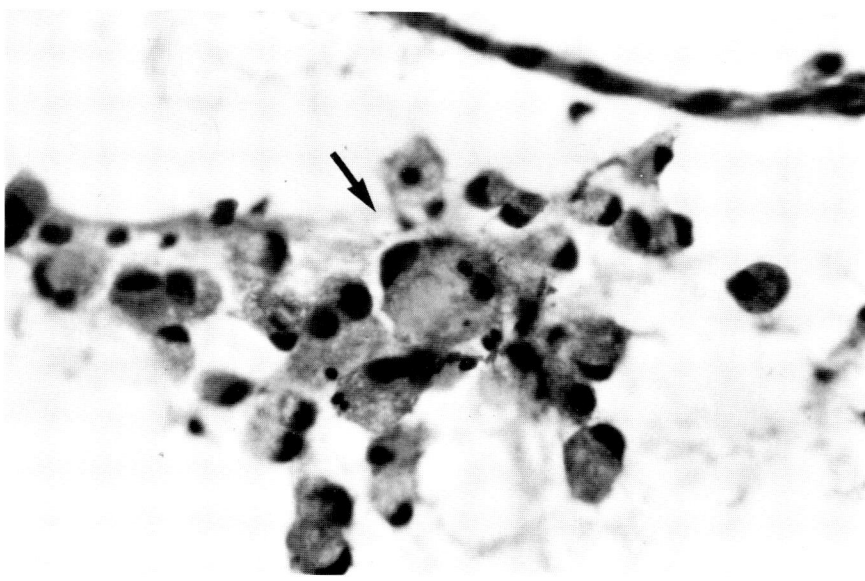

Fig. 14-14 Mucicarmine stain of adenocarcinoma cells. Strong positivity is noted, and faint positivity within tumor cells (arrow). (See Plate 14-16.)

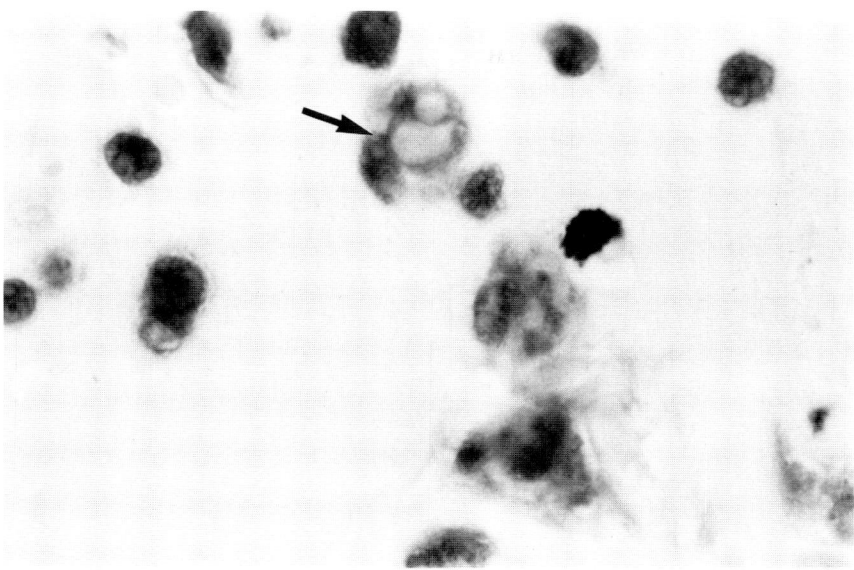

Fig. 14-15 Two markers of glandular differentiation combined in the same stain. The CEA appears brown while alcian blue delineates mucin droplets in the cytoplasm (arrow). (See Plate 14-17.)

Table 14-10 Markers of Adenocarcinomatous Differentiation

Morphologic
    Gland or acinar formation
    Signet ring configuration
    Cytoplasmic vacuolization
    Tridimensional cell groups
Histochemical
    PAS with diastase digestion
    Mucicarmine (neutral mucin)
    Alcian blue pH 1.5 (acid mucin)
Immunocytochemical
    CEA
    EMA
    Secretory piece
    Leu M1
    B72.3
    HMFG-1
    "Organ-Specific" markers (TGb, PSA, CA-1, Ca-125, etc.)
Ultrastructural
    Surface microvilli
    Intracytoplasmic lumina
    Terminal bars
    Secretory granules

PAS, periodic acid-Schiff. CEA, carcinoembryonic antigen; EMA, epithelial membrane antigen; HMFG-1, human milk fat globule; TGb (thyroglobulin).

each individual case. Because adenocarcinoma is mainly treatable by chemotherapy, while squamous cell tumors may respond to radiotherapy, it is important to decide between these two lineages in metastatic sites.

ORGAN-SPECIFIC MARKERS

The initial impetus to ICC was its potential to identify specifically the precise origin of neoplasms. As should be clear by now, very few markers exist that are specific for one cell type and none has the title role as the mythical magical marker. Most antibodies have an imperfectly defined specificity and are not capable of solving diagnostic dilemmas single handedly. However, when used in conjunction with cytomorphologic and clinical data a few organ-specific panels have been useful to the cytopathologist.

Prostate

Prostatic markers were the earliest and now rank among the most specific in the current armamentarium of the immunocytopathologist.[169] Both prostatic acid phosphatase (PSAP)[170] and prostatic specific antigen (PSA)[171] are very useful in the evaluation of FNA of neoplasms of putative prostatic origin. These two markers are usually positive, regardless of the degree of differentiation of the prostatic neoplasm (Fig. 14-16, Plate 14-18). However, slightly greater sensitivity is obtained with PSAP (93 percent) than with PSA (81 percent).[171] In conjunction with CEA and EMA, these markers aid in the distinction between prostatic and metastatic neoplasms in the pelvic lymph nodes.[94] They also help in the differential diagnosis among prostatic, colonic, and urothelial neoplasms in the urinary bladder.[172] The presence of a two-layered epithelium in benign prostatic hyperplasia has found diagnostic application in cytologic specimens because of the difference in staining properties between basal cells and acinar cells.[173]

The basal cells are positive for some of the keratin antibodies, while acinar cells are negative for most. An intertwined pattern of keratin positivity suggests that the aspirated fragment has an involucrum of basal cells and consequently is benign.[174] In those instances in which well-differentiated carcinomas are positive for keratin, acinar cells show a diffuse and weak pattern of positivity, and no basal cells are identified. These features are better demonstrated when the FNA material is collected and processed as a cell suspension rather than pressed and smeared between two glass slides.[94]

Thyroid

Thyroglobulin is a very specific marker for the recognition of thyroid follicular cells.[175] This marker is expressed in hyperplastic, benign, and malignant follicular cells, but it does not allow for the distinction between them. In cytologic and histologic preparations, TGb fails to discriminate between follicular and papillary tumors, but positivity for thyroglobulin excludes medullary carcinoma from diagnostic consideration.[176] The marker works equally well in tissue sections[176,177] and in cytologic preparations[177,178] but is of no help in distinguishing follicular

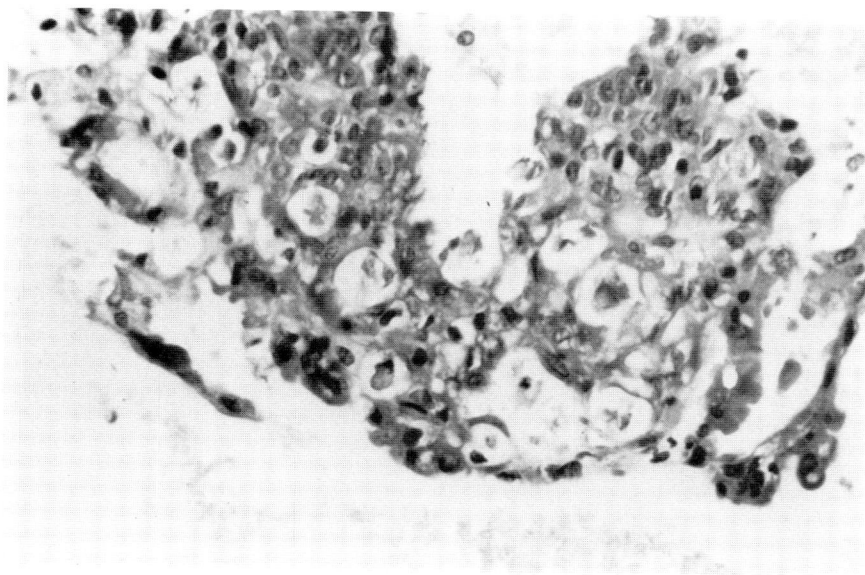

Fig. 14-16 Bone FNA stained with PSA. Strong immunopositivity and small gland pattern indicates a prostatic origin for this metastatic neoplasm. (See Plate 14-18.)

adenomas from follicular carcinomas (Fig. 14-6). Small transfer proteins, such as lactoferrin, lactalbumin, and ferritin, were once believed to accomplish such distinction,[179] but recent evidence failed to demonstrate any difference in the invariably negative expression of lactoferrin in adenomas and carcinomas.[180]

Ovary

OC-125 is an excellent serologic marker for the diagnosis, monitoring, and prognostication of ovarian carcinoma in clinical practice. In frozen sections, the marker will immunostain ovarian carcinomas much more consistently than will other types of carcinoma.[181] However, stainability is less predictable in pronase-digested, formalin-fixed, paraffin-embedded material.[182] The marker is more useful in the serous variety than in the mucinous variety of ovarian carcinoma, but this phenomenon may be influenced by the type of fixative used and the use of protease digestion.[183] In cytologic material, CA-125 may show preferential staining of cilia in serous tumors of the ovary (Fig. 14-17, Plates 14-19 and 14-20). Other markers reputed to show preferential staining of ovarian carcinomas in relationship to other types of carcinoma include CA-19.9,[184] Mov 2,[185] and 1D3/1D5.[186] The latter antibodies recognizes the mucinous variety of ovarian cystadenocarcinoma, which is particularly difficult to distinguish from mucinous tumors of endocervical, GI, or pulmonary origin. Ovarian tumors are variably positive for CEA, EMA, and keratin, particularly the LMWK variety.

Breast

Carcinoma of the breast is the most frequent neoplasm found in malignant effusions of female patients. This may occur at the time of presentation or may appear many years after surgery and hormonal manipulation have eradicated the tumor in its primary site. In these instances, it is important to rule out a second primary, even though, cytologically, carcinoma of the breast may be difficult to distinguish from carcinomas arising in the lung, ovary or stomach. Certain proteins are secreted mainly by the mammary epithelium, including α-lactalbumin,[187]

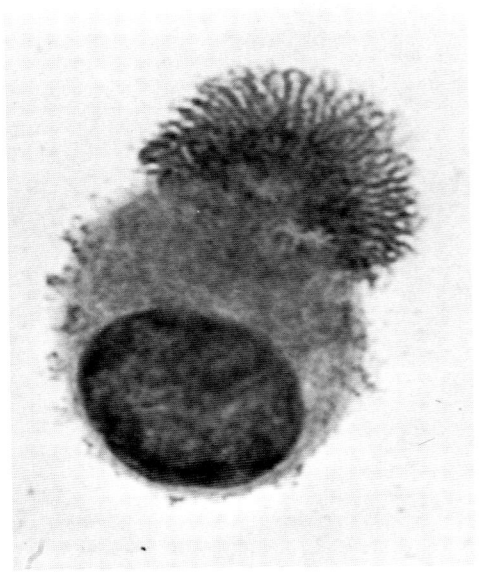 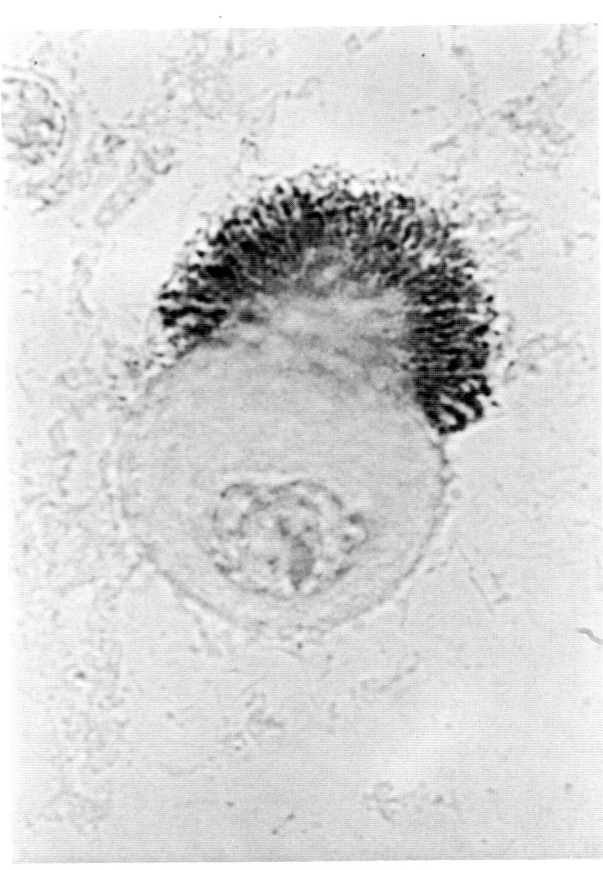

Fig. 14-17 Serous cystadenocarcinoma of the ovary. **(A)** With the Giemsa stain, a tuft of cilia is noted in the apex of the cell. (See Plate 14-19.) **(B)** Immunostain with anti-CA-125 antibody clearly delineates a ciliary tuft. (Courtesy of Dr. T. Kobayashi, M.D.) (See Plate 14-20.)

lactoferrin,[188] and casein.[189] All have been tried as markers of breast carcinoma with variable degrees of success.

Positivity for lactalbumin ranges anywhere from 60 to 70 percent of cases[190] (Fig. 14-14, Plate 14-16). If the marker is strongly positive, a breast primary is very likely, but negativity does not rule out origin in the breast. Positivity for estrogen receptor is also highly suggestive of a malignant breast origin and has the advantage of identifying the most likely responders to tamoxifen.[191] The proteinaceous content of breast cysts has been used as an immunogen in the recognition of breast carcinoma with apocrine features.[192] A combination of linear and arborizing pattern of EMA positivity together with a predominance of single cells in a malignant effusion should prompt the search of the breast as a likely primary site. A number of monoclonal antibodies are reactive with breast carcinoma, but their specificity is still under investigation.[193,194]

Lung

Lung carcinomas are rather common tumors presenting in metastatic sites and malignant effusions. The most frequent type found is an adenocarcinoma difficult to distinguish from similar neoplasms arising in the breast, ovary, and GI tract. These lung adenocarcinomas are negative for lactalbumin and CA-125, but they lack a specific marker indicative of their pulmonary origin. They are commonly positive for mucicarmine, alcian blue CEA, and EMA, but so

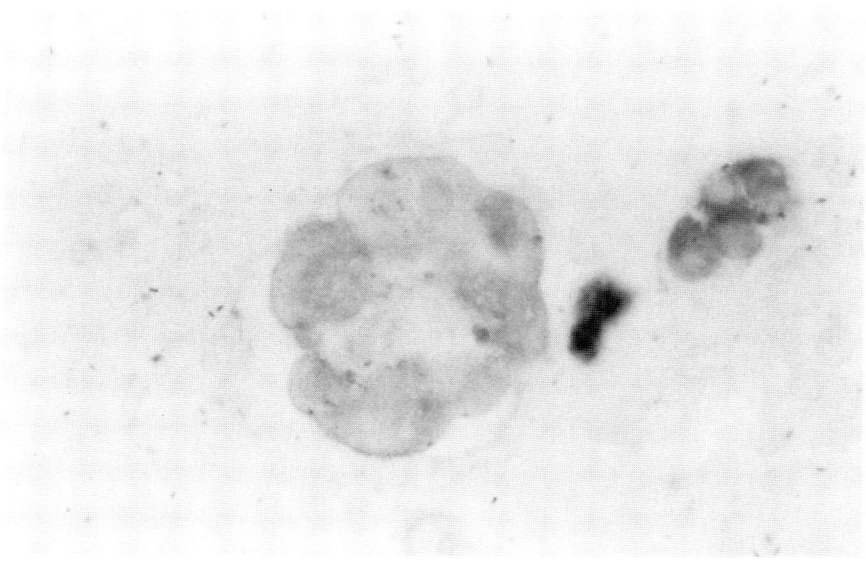

Fig. 14-18 Lung adenocarcinoma stained by alcian blue/CEA. Alcian blue positivity delineates a papillary cluster, while CEA is stronger in smaller groups of cells. (See Plate 14-21.)

are the vast majority of adenocarcinomas (Fig. 14-18, Plate 18-21). Only a small fraction of adenocarcinomas of the lung are positive for surfactant apoprotein, which is specific for origin from the type II alveolar epithelial cells.[195] Mesotheliomas are sometimes sampled by FNA and may be difficult to distinguish from adenocarcinoma.[196] An immunocytochemical panel, in conjunction with a few histochemical stains, may be helpful in this regard, since mesotheliomas are frequently negative for mucin, CEA, HMFG, and Leu M_1 and are variably positive for keratin and EMA.[107,124] At least one monoclonal antibody (44.3A6) has shown good results in recognizing lung adenocarcinoma in cytologic specimens.[197]

Liver

Hepatocellular carcinomas are rather distinctive cytologically, but their clinical presentation may mimic liver metastasis.[198] When large bizarre tumor cells display large eosinophilic nucleoli and intracytoplasmic lumen formation, the diagnosis of liver cell carcinoma should be suspected.[199] Frequent nuclear holes suggestive of cytoplasmic invaginations and PAS-positive inclusions in the cytoplasm are also supportive of the diagnosis of hepatocellular carcinoma (Fig. 14-19, Plates 14-22 and 14-23). For a more definitive recognition of hepatocellular origin, positivity for AFP, HBsAg, and A_1AT may be sought by ICC.[200] Both A_1AT and A_1ACT are positive in hepatocellular carcinoma.[201] However, it should be noted that the degree and extent of AFP positivity varies considerably from tumor to tumor and is subject to the methods of fixation and immunostaining used (Fig. 14-20, Plate 14-24). Consequently, the immunocytochemical results have to be correlated to cytomorphology and interpreted in light of clinical data. A useful confirmatory test is the level of AFP in the serum. CEA positivity in a cell block of a liver aspirate is not tantamount to metastatic carcinoma because hepatocellular carcinomas may occasionally be positive for CEA.[200] An intercellular distribution of the immunostain, the so-called canalicular pattern of CEA positivity, is characteristic of hepatocellular carcinoma.[202] Cholangiocarcinomas are negative for AFP and CEA but positive for keratin and EMA.[203]

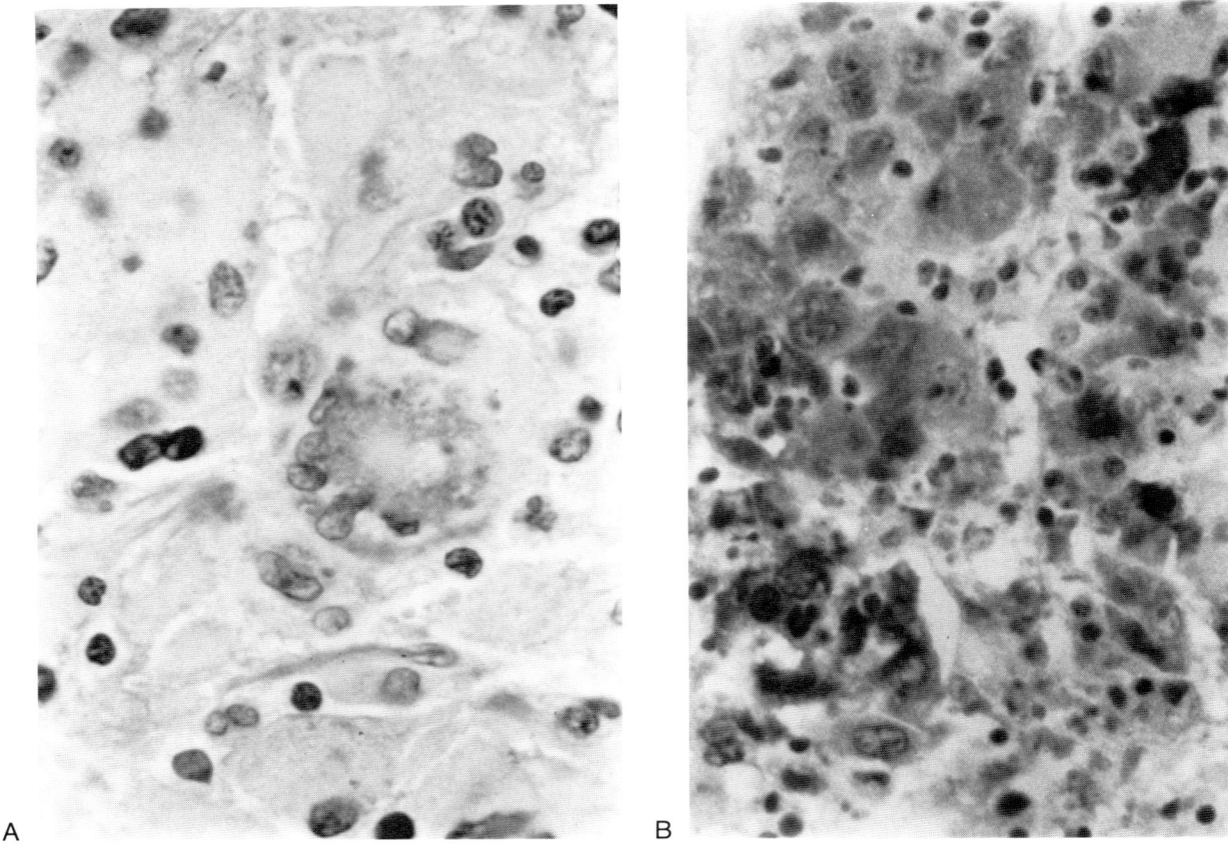

Fig. 14-19 Cell block from hepatocellular carcinoma. **(A)** Strongly PAS-positive inclusions are noted in the cytoplasm of tumor cells. (See Plate 14-22.) **(B)** Many of the bizarre tumor cells are positive for AFP. (See Plate 14-23.)

Pancreas

Several attempts have been made to identify a specific marker for a exocrine carcinomas of the pancreas.[204] To date the most promising seems to be DU-PAN-2, which showed reactivity to serum, tissue samples, and malignant cells in the ascitic fluid of patients with pancreatic carcinoma.[205] Certain monoclonal antibodies against glycoproteins with CEA-like properties have also been partially successful in identifying pleomorphic atypical pancreatic carcinomas.[206] Laminin has been used in an attempt to separate pancreatic carcinoma from ductal hyperplasia.[207] However, as no specific pancreatic markers are readily available, clinical trials involving cytologic material have not been performed to date. The same can be said of a number of antibodies against cells derived from colonic,[208] renal,[209] uterine,[210] and gastric carcinomas.[211]

Melanoma

The cells of malignant melanoma present as sheets or as single cells arranged in loose clusters. They may be large and pleomorphic with a peculiarly dusty or overtly pigmented cytoplasm.[212] Occasionally, however, they present as single cells of moderate size, minimal pleomorphism, and only slightly enlarged nucleoli. In these instances, they may be difficult to diagnose as malignant or may be mistaken for carcinoma.[213] The index of suspicion is raised when they are negative for keratin, CEA, and EMA, yet give a weak but positive reaction for vimentin. This should be followed immediately by a panel, including Fon-

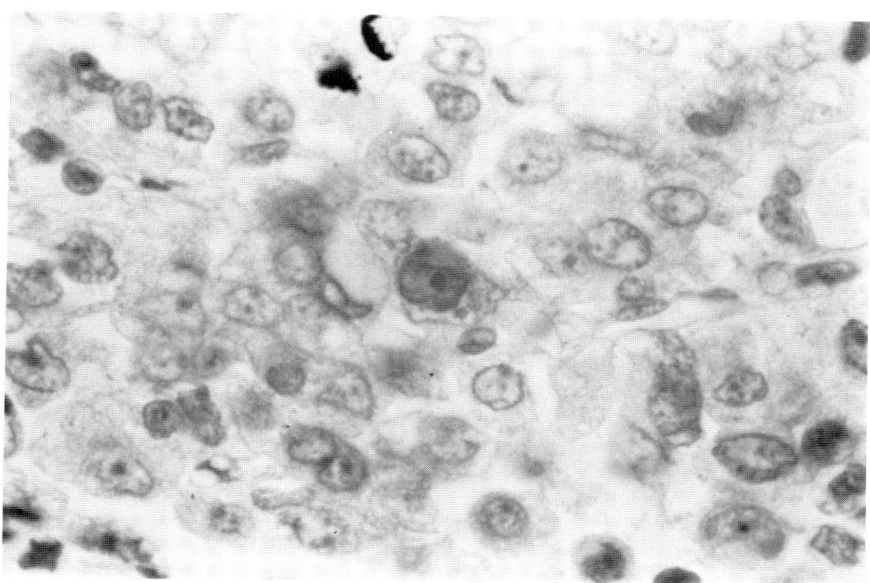

Fig. 14-20 HCC stained for A_1AT. Note variable positivity of individual tumor cells typical of this marker. (See Plate 14-24.)

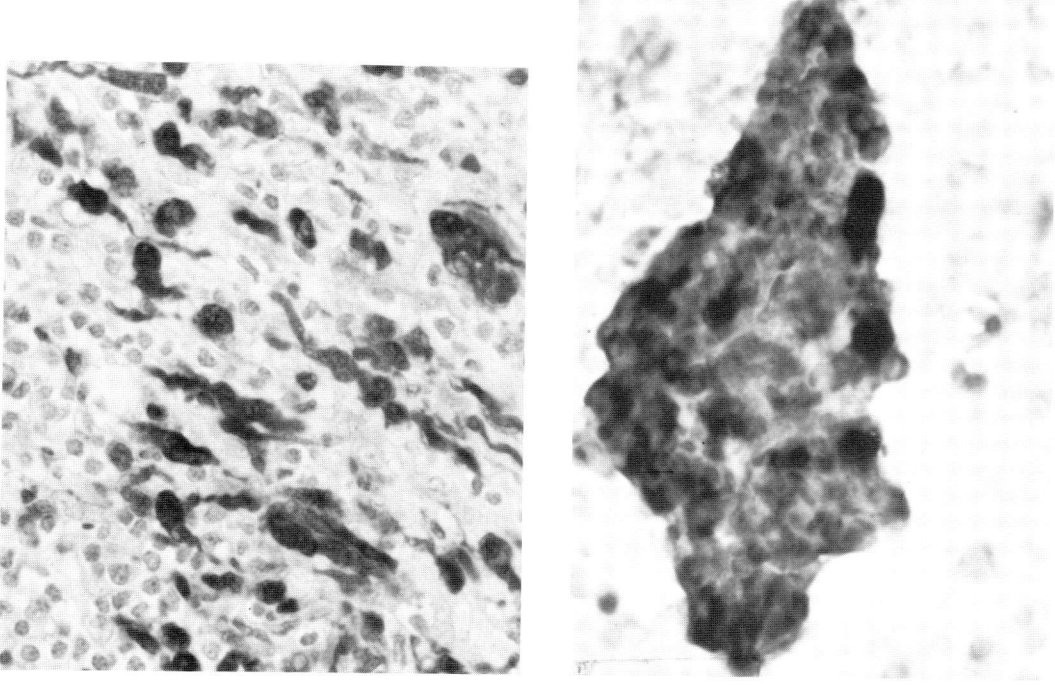

Fig. 14-21 S100 positivity in melanoma. (Left) Positive tumor cells are noted within a necrotic portion of the tumor. (Right) A cluster of tumor cells from the FNA shows strong cytoplasmic immunostaining. (See Plate 14-25.)

tana-Masson, S100, and HMB-45.[214] S100 is commonly positive in melanoma but, depending on the clinical setting, it is not at all specific (Fig. 14-21, Plate 14-25). By contrast, HMB-45 is considerably more specific, but its reliability in cytologic specimen is only now coming under investigation. Gentle digestion of the cell block with 0.1 percent pronase solution for 30 minutes increases the sensitivity of HMB-45 in melanoma as does suspension of the antibody in 0.02 M EDTA. Other monoclonal antibodies for melanoma exist, but they are not as readily available as HMB-45.[215,216]

NEUROENDOCRINE MARKERS

A large proportion of the small blue round cell tumors display neuroendocrine differentiation. The term "neuroendocrine" applies to these neoplasms of either neural (neuroblastoma, paraganglioma, pheochromocytoma) or epithelial (carcinoid, atypical carcinoid, neuroendocrine carcinoma) origin, which produce biogenic amines, polypeptides, and proteins capable of acting as hormones or neurotransmitters.[217] Evidence of such activity can be produced by the demonstration of dense-core neuroendocrine granules by electron microscopy or a variety of neuroendocrine markers by ICC (Table 14-11). NSE is the most sensitive marker of neuroendocrine differentiation, but the enzyme may be positive in a number of non-neuroendocrine neoplasms, so its specificity is of questionable value.[218] At the other end of the spectrum, the various hormones and polypeptides elaborated by endocrine cells are very specific for neuroendocrine differentiation. However, these markers are expressed only in a small proportion of neuroendocrine tumors and are difficult to correlate with the clinical setting (Fig. 14-22, Plate 14-26). Intermediate between NSE and the hormones are bombesin and chromogranin. Bombesin is a polypeptide expressed by a number of carcinoids and small cell carcinomas; it is also prevalent in various normal tissues from a number of animal species.[219] Even more pervasive are the chromogranins, a group of supportive proteins encountered in the matrix of neuroendocrine granules.[220] The value of this marker is based on

Table 14-11 Markers of Neuroendocrine Differentiation Useful in Tumor Classification

Marker (Antibody)	Component Recognized	Occurrence in Cells	Expression in Tumors
NSE	γ,γ-Enolase	Neurons, dispersed neuroendocrine cells	Neural tumors, neuroendocrine tumors
Chromogranin	NE granule matrix proteins	Adrenal medulla	Carcinoid tumor
Bombesin	Ancestral neuropeptide	Kulchitsky-like cells, neuroepithelial cells	Carcinoid tumor NE carcinoma
Synaptophysin (SY-38)	Presynaptic vesicle	Brain, spinal cord, adrenal medulla, islet cells	Neuroendocrine carcinoma
PGP 9.5	Protein gene product		
NF	Neurofilament triplets (NF-H, NF-L), NF-M)	Neurons, neuroendocrine cells	Neural tumors, neuroblastoma, certain NE carcinomas
NRY	Neuropeptide Y	Adrenal medulla, ganglion cells	Pheochromocytoma, ganglioneuroblastoma
S100 protein	Neural supportive elements	Astrocytes, meningeal cells	Neural, tumors, melanoma, some carcinomas
GFAP	Glial-type intermediate filaments	Astrocytes, ependymal cells	Astrocytomas, ependymomas
HNK-1 (Leu-7)	Myelin-associated glycoprotein	Natural killer cells, neuroendocrine cells	Melanoma, oat cell carcinoma

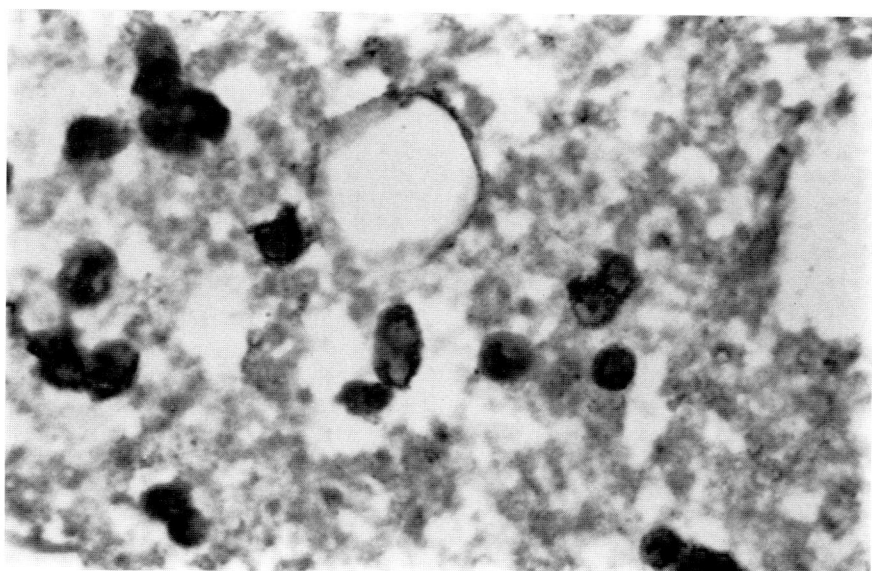

Fig. 14-22 Islet cell tumor stained for gastrin. The positivity for a hormone is often unpredictable and difficult to correlate with serum levels. (See Plate 14-26.)

the fact that its positivity is proportional to the density of granules in a given neoplasm. As such, chromogranins are quite prevalent in hormone-producing tumors.[221] Consequently, strong chromogranin positivity is an indicator of well-differentiated neuroendocrine activity, as noted in carcinoids, islet cell tumors, and medullary carcinoma of the thyroid. The marker can be used in conjunction with mucicarmine stain to identify the neuroendocrine and glandular differentiation of adenocarcinoids (Fig. 14-23, Plate 14-27).

Other recently described markers of neuroendocrine activity include PGP-9.5[222] and synaptophysin.[223] Both are detected by monoclonal antibodies of high specificity for neuroendocrine activity but that require optimal conditions of fixation and handling. NF is positive in the neuroendocrine tumors with more fully manifest neural differentiation. Another neural marker, S100 protein, is frequently present in neuroectodermal tumors and in a small proportion of neuroendocrine carcinomas. An unusual arrival in the arsenal of neuroendocrine markers is Leu 7, first used to recognize natural killer (NK) T cells in frozen tissues.[224] In paraffin sections, the antibody was found to be positive in melanoma and in neuroendocrine neoplasms,[225] a property extended to cell blocks.

The problem of classifying a neuroendocrine tumor persists even after the tumor has shown positivity for the neuroendocrine markers. Cytopathology can be very useful in this classification by demonstrating nuclear and cytoplasmic characteristics of the tumor cells.[226] In the lung, cytomorphology permits separation of tumors into carcinoids[227] and neuroendocrine carcinomas.[228] However, a more precise classification often depends on careful appreciation of histopathologic and ultrastructural features. The neuroendocrine nature of the neoplasm is manifested at the ultrastructural level by the presence of electron-dense secretory granules, typically limited by a double membrane. In carcinoid tumors, the neuroendocrine granules are very numerous and are found throughout the cytoplasm.[229] In oat cell carcinomas, they are less numerous and are preferentially distributed in the cytoplasmic projections just beneath the plasma membrane. Oat cell carcinomas show a greater tendency to crushing artifact in tissue samples and cytoplasmic fragility in cytologic specimens. As a result, NSE may play a crucial role not only in FNAs but in transbronchial and mediastinoscopic

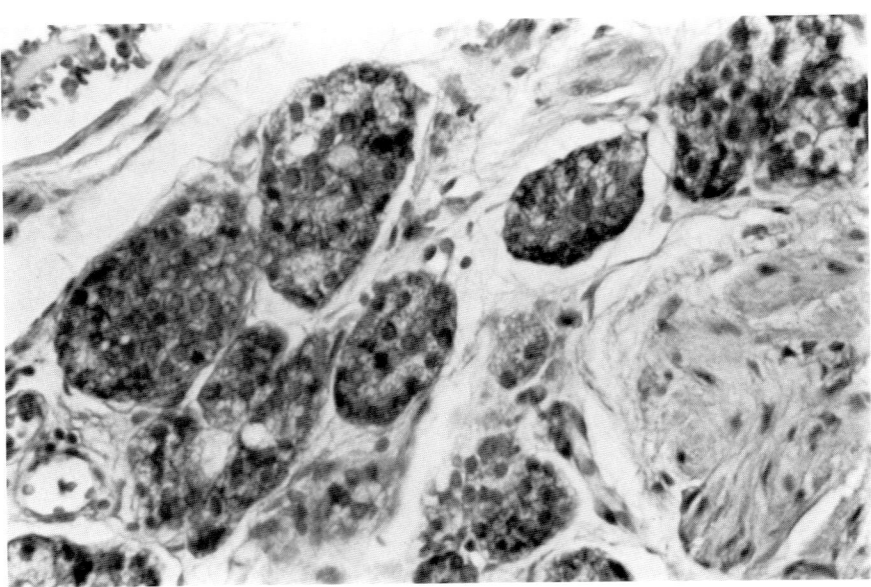

Fig. 14-23 Adenocarcinoid demonstrated by a combined stain. The rose mucicarmine stain demonstrated by PAS-D corresponds to glandular differentiation. Immunopositivity for chromogranin appears brownish and reticular. (See Plate 14-27.)

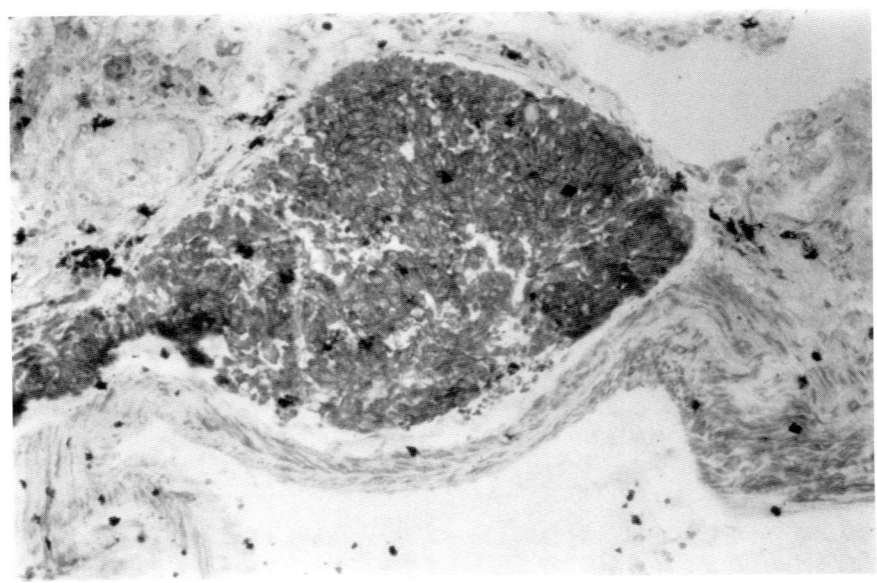

Fig. 14-24 Lymph node biopsy specimen stained for NSE. The positivity of the oat cell carcinoma in the center contrasts with the anthracotic pigment on the left and the negative lymph node on the right. (See Plate 14-28.)

biopsies as well (Fig. 14-24, Plate 14-28). These tumors shed smaller cells than do carcinoid tumors, but their cytologic characteristics are very similar. Neuroblastomas demonstrate neuroendocrine granules within the exuberant array of cytoplasmic extensions that contain microtubules.[230] A small proportion of neuroblastomas may express microtubule associated proteins in their cytoplasmic extensions.[231] These tumors may develop outside the adrenal and the paraganglia; they may even occur in adults.[232] Their neuroendocrine granules are indistinguishable from those of the other neuroendocrine neoplasms. Occasionally, the granules can be found in an extracellular location. This is important to explain the typical immunostaining of neuroendocrine neoplasms: a reddish-brown blush observed between neoplastic cells. The consistent intercellular pattern of stain observed with NSE and bombesin has also been described with chromogranin and should not be mistaken for high background. Classic studies with silver impregnation techniques divided carcinoid tumors as derived from the foregut, midgut, and hindgut, thus excluding nonendodermal organs. However, following the recognition that small cell carcinomas are histogenetically related to carcinoids a number of neuroendocrine neoplasms have been recognized in unusual sites. These include origin in the pancreas,[233,234] breast,[235] esophagus,[236] salivary gland,[237] kidney,[238] prostate,[239] bone,[240] soft tissues,[241] and many other sites[242-249] (Table 14-12).

LYMPHOHISTIOCYTIC MARKERS

The hematopathologist can recognize and classify lymphomas with a large number of antibodies against cell-surface antigens.[250] This approach is best applied to frozen sections or suspensions of unfixed cells, neither of which yields good cytologic detail.[251,252] The sample can either be concentrated onto slides by cytocentrifugation or dispersed further into a continuous flow of single cells paraded in front of the window of the flow cytometer. Cytocentrifuged preparations may be stained by direct immunofluorescence and examined under the ultraviolet (UV) microscope. Thus, rapid determination of immunoglobulins and clonality of the lymphoid cells is possible.[253] For concomitant phenotyping and better morphologic evaluation of effusions some of the cytospin preparations can be stained with Papanicolaou stain or Wright-Giemsa stain, while others are assayed by either immunoperoxidase,[254] avidin-biotin complex[255] or the alkaline phosphatase[256] techniques. Immunocytochemical markers allow the distinction between T-cell and B-cell lymphoma[257] and the further characterization of B-cell neoplasms,[258] plasmacytoid lesions,[258,259] and small cell lymphomas.[260] Even in surgically obtained biopsies, the preparations embedded in paraffin offer better cytologic detail than frozen sections. B5 fixation is crucial to preserve these cytologic features and permits the use of monoclonal antibodies that recognize T and B lymphocytes and monocytes.[261] This added feature permits appreciation of subtypes in B-cell[262] as well as T-cell[263] lymphomas by the judicious use of immunologic markers.

In flow cytometry, the individual cells, in single file, are first tagged with fluorescent probes. When excited by an argon or by a laser light source, the fluorescent content from each cell is measured and

Table 14-12 Sites of Origin for Neuroendocrine Neoplasms

Primary Site	References
Common	
Lung	217, 219
GI tract	227
Adrenal	142, 143, 145
Skin	204
Pancreas	233, 234
Pituitary	150, 151
Paraganglia	144
Prostate	259
Uncommon	
Thyroid	146, 148
Breast	139, 235
Esophagus	236
Salivary gland	237
Kidney	238
Bone	240
Soft tissue	241
Ovary	242
Thymus	243
Endometrium	244
Cervix	245, 246
Bladder	247, 248
Larynx	249

interpreted by a computer. Most often, cell surface markers for B-cell and T-cell subtyping are assayed by flow cytometry, but extension of the technology to solid tumors is imminent. If more than one light source is used, various fluorescent probes can be used for multiparameter evaluation.[264] The flow cytometer can also measure properties other than fluorescence with great sensitivity, objectivity, and high speed (10^5 cells/minute). However, since the tissue is architecturally disrupted, in order to obtain single cell suspensions, critics of flow cytometry contend that results are difficult to correlate with the underlying morphology of the lesion. Because needle aspirates yield suspensions of cells that are already disassociated, they are ideally suited for flow cytometry. Since a portion of the sample can be stained by Papanicolaou or one of the Romanowsky methods, they provide definition of cell morphology as an added advantage.

In cellular samples of lymphoid proliferations, it is frequently possible (1) to predict monoclonality by the uniform monotony of the cell population; (2) to distinguish small cell from large cell lymphomas by the size of the cells and their relative proportion[264]; (3) to identify predominantly cleaved as opposed to noncleaved proliferation by appreciating nuclear contours[265]; (4) to recognize certain plasmacytoid variants of lymphoma by the abundance of the cytoplasm and the characteristic chromatin distribution of the nuclei[266]; (5) to identify some special types of lymphoma with characteristic cytomorphologic features, such as convoluted T-cell,[267] lymphoblastic,[267] immunoblastic,[269] and the cerebriform (Sézary) variant of T-cell lymphoma[270]; (6) to recognize and occasionally classify Hodgkin's disease by the identification of Reed-Sternberg cells and different proportions of activated lymphocytes, plasma cells, and eosinophils[271]; and (7) to recognize reactive proliferation by the observation of a polymorphous cell population, including lymphohistiocytic aggregates and frequent tangible body macrophages.[272,273] In some cases, it is even possible to identify the etiology of benign hyperplasias.[274] However, cytomorphology alone falls short in attempts to separate nodular from diffuse lymphomas in FNA and to identify with certainty mixed cell lymphomas due to possible sampling artifacts. Consequently, every attempt should be made at maximizing the yield of diagnostic methods applicable to cytologic samples suspicious for lymphoma and leukemia.[275] Experienced hematopathologists are able to appreciate subtle morphologic variations that permit the recognition of Burkitt's, non-Burkitt's, Lennert's, and other rare types of lymphoma. There is no reason, therefore, that, with experience, cytopathologists cannot learn to identify these variants in Papanicolaou-stained preparations. One avenue to acquire this experience is the utilization of touch imprints of excisional biopsies[276,277] and to apply immunoperoxidase techniques to cytology specimens.[278]

Despite some limitations, monoclonal antibodies have been so entrenched in the study of lymphoma that the cytopathologist cannot ignore their value. In fact, by applying a combination of flow cytometry and monoclonal antibodies to cytologic specimens, it will be possible to establish a greater and more precise role for cytopathology in lymphomas. Some of the currently available antibodies recognize only the lymphoid origin of the cells, while others are lineage specific (Table 14-13). Since ICC results are best when correlated to cytomorphologic features in tissue or smears, cytomorphology plays a crucial role in the evaluation of lymphomas. Thus, positivity for a given monoclonal antibody by itself is not indicative of either malignancy or of a subtype of lymphoma. Malignancy is best determined by correlating the cytologic features of the cellular sample to the clues of clinical behavior and the architectural abnormalities in impeccably prepared histologic sections. The diagnosis of lymphoma is established when non-neoplastic and metastatic involvement of the lymph node is excluded by strict morphologic criteria, and the lymphoid proliferation emerges as the cardinal morphologic abnormality. In cytologic specimens, this can be accomplished by immediate examination of the sample at the time of the FNA or when the effusion first arrives in the laboratory. Thus, the specimen is triaged and handled especially for the diagnosis and classification of lymphoma.

Monoclonality, evidenced by expression of only one type of immunoglobulin and light chain is a highly regarded predictor of malignant transformation. However, it too, must be present in the proper clinical, cytomorphologic, and histopathologic setting, in order to be of value. The pattern of positivity of a panel of monoclonal antibodies in frozen sections and cell suspensions permits the subtyping of lymphomas. The use of monoclonal antibodies in paraf-

Table 14-13 Selective Lymphohistiocytic Markers Applicable to Cytologic Material

Antigen/Antibody	Cells Recognized	Diagnostic Applications
LCA (T29/33, PD7/26)	Lymphocytes, granulocytes, macrophages, monocytes	Lymphoid versus nonlymphoid neoplasms
LN-1	FCC lymphocytes, erythroid cells	FCC, lymphomas
LN-2[a]	Pan-B (except plasma cells), monocyte series	B-cell lymphomas, monocytic leukemias
L-26	Pan-B (includes mantle zone)	B-cell lymphomas
UCHL-1	Pan-T, macrophages, neutrophils, thymocytes	Peripheral T-cell lymphoma versus carcinoma
Anti-Ig (G,M,D,E)	Lymphoid and plasmacytoid cells (intracytoplasmic immunoglobulin)	Multiple myeloma, plasmacytoid lymphoma
κ, λ, and heavy chains	Lymphoid and plasmacytoid cells (clonality)	Multiple myeloma, plasmacytoid lymphoma
Lysozyme	Granulocytes, monocytes, macrophages	Granulocytic and monocytic leukemias
α_1-Antitrypsin, α_1-antichymotrypsin	Monocytes, macrophages, granulocytes	Malignant histiocytosis, true histiocytic lymphoma
S100	Neural tissue, Langerhans cells, melanocytes	Histiocytosis X, melanoma
Leu M_1	Myelocytes	Reed-Sternberg cells, adenocarcinoma
Leu 7 (HNK$_1$)	Natural killer cells, neuroendocrine cells	FCC lymphomas, melanoma, oat cell carcinoma
Antihemoglobin A	Erythroid cells	Erythroleukemia

[a] LN-2 may react with epithelial cells, melanocytes, and other nonlymphoid cells.

fin sections of lymphoma, however, is assuming greater importance because of the newer markers appearing on the market at a fast pace. Surface immunoglobulins are not detected, but cytoplasmic immunoglobulins are recognized without difficulty in paraffin sections. Initially, this limited the use of paraffin-embedded cell blocks only to the detection of immunoglobulins and light chains in large cell lymphomas and plasma cell lesions. Currently, however, there are many lymphohistiocytic markers that do not require frozen sections for their utilization. The most useful of these is the leukocyte common antigen (LCA), namely, T200, recognizable by the T29/33 antibody,[279] which gives excellent results in smears as well as in B5-fixed paraffin sections of cell blocks (Fig. 14-25, Plate 14-29). The use of trypsinization has been attempted in an effort to uncover antigenic sites on the surface of cells and increase the sensitivity of LCA.[280] In our hands, however, trypsinization not only failed to accomplish this, but it led to fragmentation and floating of the sections and too uneven a splotching of the immunostain. A large cell lymphoma usually expresses only one of the immunoglobulins and either κ- or λ-light chains in a monoclonal pattern. This is also true for plasmacytomas, which may be diagnosed in cytologic specimens by the use of immunocytochemistry (Fig. 14-26, Plate 14-30).

Some newer antibodies can be reliably used in the separation between various types of lymphomas in paraffin sections. A few of these, such as LN-1, LN-2,[281] and MB2 are indicative of B-cell lineage, while UCHL-1,[282] MT1, and L60[283] favor a T-cell origin. L-26[284] is also a good indicator of B-cell derivation,

436 PRACTICAL CYTOPATHOLOGY

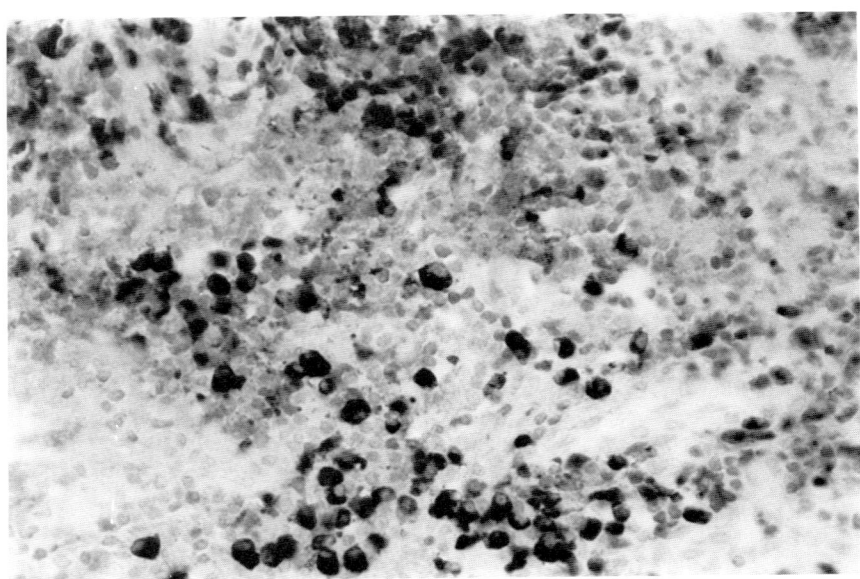

Fig. 14-25 Large cell lymphoma stained for LCA. Note bright red diffuse positivity accomplished with the use of AEC as the chromogen. (See Plate 14-29.)

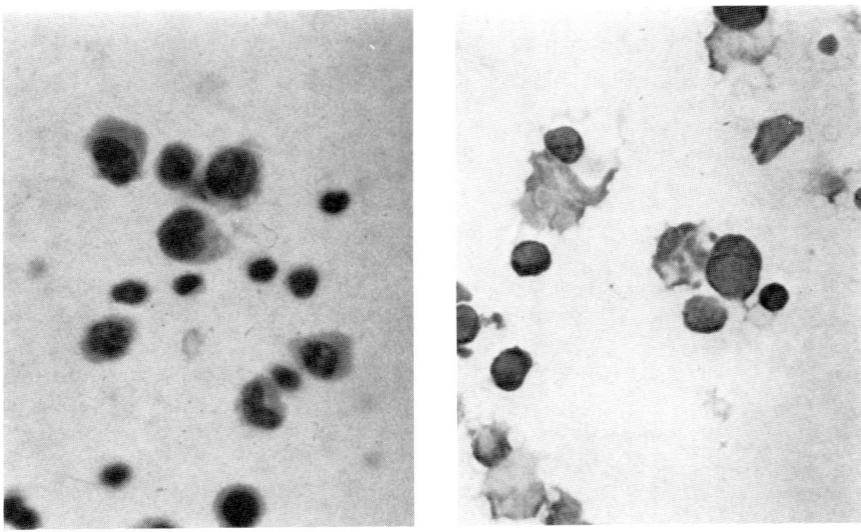

Fig. 14-26 Plasmacytoma in pleural effusion. (Left) Malignant cells with eccentric nuclei are delineated with Papanicolaou stain. (Right) Immunopositivity for κ chain only confirms the monoclonal nature of the proliferation. (See Plate 14-30.)

so that a combination of these various markers can be used in an attempt to establish the T- or B-cell origin of the lymphoma. Lymphohistiocytic markers are especially useful in the following circumstances: (1) differentiating lymphomas from other small cell neoplasms in the pediatric and adult age groups[285]; (2) distinguishing undifferentiated carcinoma from lymphoma, particularly in the head and neck area and in the retroperitoneum[50,286]; (3) assisting in the differential diagnosis between thymoma and lymphoma in the mediastinum, particularly when used in association with cytokeratin[287] (Fig. 14-27, Plate 14-31); and (4) separating reactive from possibly lymphomatous processes in newly discovered lymphadenopathies by demonstrating polyclonality in benign processes. For more definitive distinction and for the classification of lymphoma, we still recommend a combination of cytology and excisional biopsies, bearing in mind, however, that neither of these two approaches is useful if only routine Papanicolaou and H&E stains are used. Accordingly, both cytologic and biopsy samples can benefit tremendously from the use of ancillary techniques.

Immunocytochemistry markers are very useful in lymphomas, but they are not a substitute for expert interpretation of cytopathologic and surgically removed specimens. Furthermore, an extremely careful clinicopathologic correlation is needed in any lesion suspected of lymphoma. The degree of caution should be increased with regards to lymphomas in extranodal sites, particularly when the differential diagnosis is with granulomas and other inflammatory processes. Very often, histiocytes are involved in these processes and they may be difficult to evaluate by cytology alone. Certain markers identify cells derived from the bone marrow which are part of the monocyte/macrophage series. These include lysozyme, A_1AT, and A_1ACT, which are applicable to cytologic material.[288] In combination with epithelial markers, they are particularly useful in separating large pale cells into a histiocytic process or a metastatic clear cell carcinoma.[289] S100 protein identifies the reticulodendritic cells in lymph nodes but strong positivity for S100 excludes lymphoma from diagnostic considerations.[290] Also excluded are germ cell neoplasms, which may mimic a lymphoma or a histiocytic lesion. However, it should be noted that S100 positivity does not exclude carcinoma since poorly differentiated epithelial tumors may be positive for S100.[291] The marker is positive in a number of other

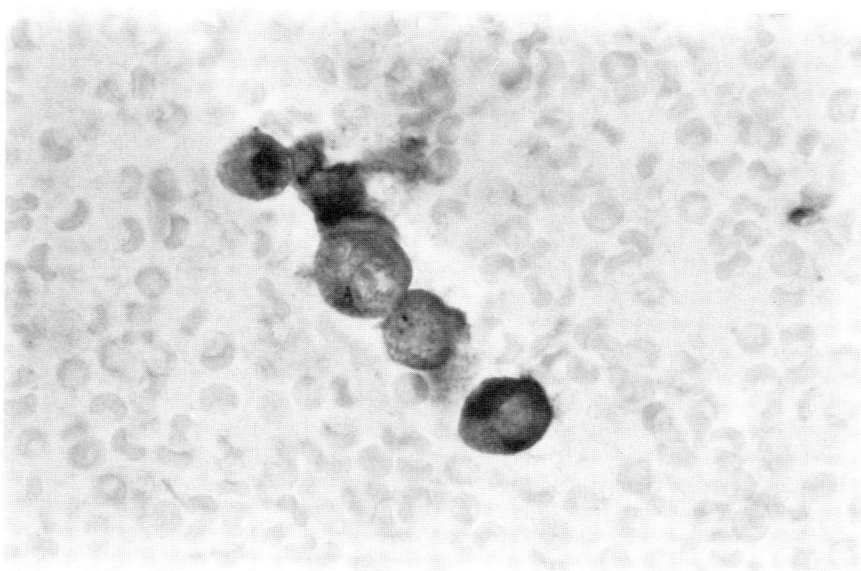

Fig. 14-27 Thymoma stained for cytokeratin. Notice positivity of the larger epithelioid cells while small lymphocytes in the background are virtually all negative. (See Plate 14-31.)

cells which are important to the cytopathologist. These include (1) melanocytes in fine needle aspirates or effusions suspicious of melanoma[292]; (2) chondrocytes in bone and cartilage tumors suspicious of chondrosarcoma[293]; and (3) physilliferous cells in neoplasms containing large pleomorphic cells, raising the possibility of chordoma.[294,295] Another diagnostic difficulty pertains to the differentiation of transformed histiocyte-like lymphocytes and Reed-Sternberg cells. Leu M_1 identifies Reed-Sternberg cells in nodal sites, but in extranodal location positivity has to be interpreted with caution because, as noted previously, Leu M_1 also stains malignant epithelial cells. A similar caution pertains to Leu 7, which identifies NK T cells in frozen sections of lymphoma, but is also positive for melanoma and neuroendocrine carcinoma in paraffin sections of solid tumors.

The differential diagnosis between lymphoma and carcinoma is accomplished by a combination of epithelial markers such as keratin, CEA and EMA and a panel of lymphohistiocytic markers such as LCA, L26, and $UCHL_1$. The use of three antibodies in the epithelial panel permits further characterization in case, for example, the CEA is strongly positive and keratin is not, an indication that the tumor may be an adenocarcinoma. If none of these markers is positive, vimentin, S100 and A_1AT/A_1ACT should be used next, to rule out the possibilities of a sarcoma, a melanoma, or a histiocytic process being responsible for the neoplasm. Likewise, the triple lymphohistiocytic combination permits distinction between T-cell and B-cell lineage in the event that LCA plus only L26 or $UCHL_1$ are positive.

MESENCHYMAL NEOPLASMS

In comparison with epithelial antibodies, mesenchymal markers are less numerous and much less thoroughly investigated.[296] In general, intermediate filament typing is of little assistance in soft tissue neoplasms because they are found indiscriminately in many subtypes of sarcoma and are difficult to demonstrate in paraffin-embedded sections.[297] Vimentin is of little help in recognizing these neoplasms, since it may be positive in epithelial tumors and fails to discriminate between the grades of sarcoma.[298] As with carcinomas, certain sarcomas coexpress vimentin and keratin, notably epithelioid sarcoma,[299] synovial sarcoma,[300] and leiomyosarcoma.[31] Likewise, actin and myosin are ubiquitous in neoplasms of both mesenchymal and epithelial origin.[301,302] Since neither actin nor myosin discriminates among the various nonepithelial tumors, a number of other antibodies have been tried in the workup of sarcomas (Table 14-14). Factor VIII-related antigen was initially heralded as an endothelial cell marker,[303] but we have detected positivity in other mesenchymal neoplasms.

Table 14-14 Antibodies Useful in the Study of Nonepithelial Neoplasms

Antibody	Applicable Neoplasm
Vimentin	Mesenchymal tumors (general)
Keratin	Synovial sarcoma, epithelioid sarcoma
Desmin	Myogenous tumors (smooth muscle, striated muscle)
Myoglobin	Rhabdomyoma, rhabdomyosarcoma
Factor VIII-related antigen, *Ulex europaeus* agglutinin	Vasoformative tumors (excluding Kaposi's sarcoma)
α_1-Antitrypsin, lysozyme, α_1-Antichymotrypsin	Malignant fibrous histiocytoma
S100 protein	Granular cell tumor, neurofibroma, schwannoma, clear cell sarcoma, malignant schwannoma, chondrosarcoma

Ulex europaeus lectin (UEL) has shown promise in the study of vascular neoplasms and may offer advantages over factor VIII-related antigen.[304] Angiotensin converting enzyme (ACE) is another endothelial cell marker, but its application in cytopathology has not been tested as yet.[305]

Myogenic differentiation can be detected by the presence of desmin, a broad indicator of cytoplasmic contractility noted in smooth muscle, striated muscle, and myoepithelial cells.[41] Desmin is most consistently and strongly positive in cells of leiomyosarcoma, but striated muscle cells display weak positivity.[306] However, it should be remembered that desmin is difficult to demonstrate in formalin- and B5-fixed specimen and works best in alcohol-fixed material (Fig. 14-28, Plate 14-32). This marker is an excellent discriminator between myogenous neoplasms and malignant fibrous histiocytoma.[307] Not infrequently this is the differential diagnosis in FNA's of soft tissue tumors.[308,309] MFH is generally negative for desmin but positive for vimentin, A_1AT, A_1ACT, and occasionally lysozyme[310] (Fig. 14-29, Plates 14-33 and 14-34). However, a few examples of MFH have been reported as positive for desmin.[8] A more precise identification of MFH may be accomplished with Factor XIIIa, a marker that was positive in all fifteen examples of the tumors studied.[311]

Myoglobin is the best indicator of rhabdomyosarcomatous differentiation,[312] which can also be demonstrated by antiskeletal muscle[313] and anti-Z-protein antibodies.[314] Both skeletal muscle actin and skeletal muscle myosin have been used in the immunocytologic diagnosis of rhabdomyosarcoma by FNA.[315] Unfortunately, no antibodies exist that discriminate between benign and malignant myoskeletal lesions.[316,317] The finding of Z bands by electron microscopy is typical of well-differentiated rhabdomyosarcoma, while poorly differentiated leiomyosarcoma reveal focal densities. In tissue sections, Masson's trichrome stain is very useful in distinguishing collagenous from myogenous extracellular matrix. A number of soft tissue tumors have been well studied by FNA, including liposarcoma,[318] Ewing's sarcoma,[319] neural-type neoplasms,[320,321] alveolar soft part sarcoma,[322,323] and others.[324] Some of these studies included the use of immunoperoxidase for detecting S100 protein,[325] but in general sarcomas have not been as thoroughly studied by immunocytopathology as have epithelial neoplasms.

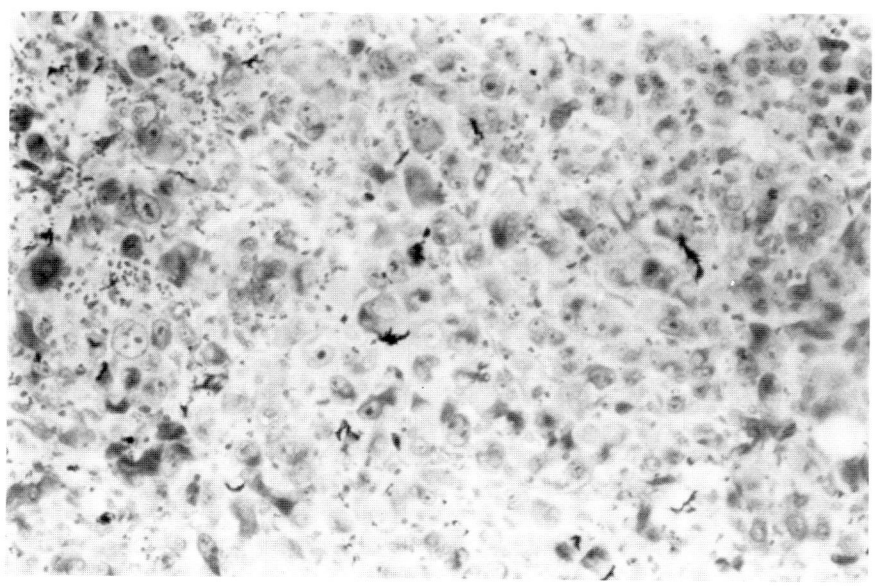

Fig. 14-28 Leiomyosarcoma in B5 fixed material stained for desmin. Note the faint, salmon-colored positivity of the large tumor cells. (See Plate 14-32.)

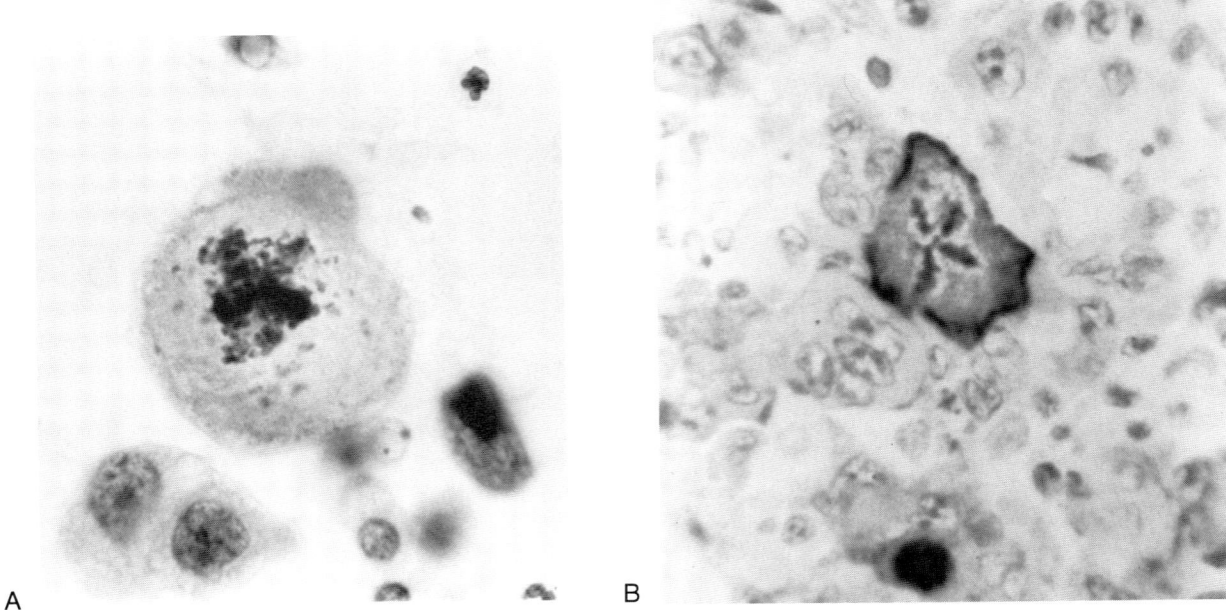

Fig. 14-29 Malignant cells with abnormal mitoses. **(A)** With Papanicolaou stain the giant cell is bizarre and undifferentiated. (See Plate 14-33.) **(B)** The strong A_1ACT positivity is typical of MFH. (Courtesy of B. Atkinson, M.D.) (See Plate 14-34.)

POORLY DIFFERENTIATED NEOPLASMS

Despite considerable experience in the field, cytopathologists now and then encounter neoplasms that defy classification or that fail to demonstrate an obvious epithelial, lymphohistiocytic, or mesenchymal origin. Keratin and vimentin are commonly coexpressed in these poorly differentiated tumors; even stalwarts of the older mesenchymal category such as Ewing's sarcoma have been known to demonstrate epithelial-like markers.[326] Within any of the main lineages, the presence of a marker acquires a different significance, depending on the cytomorphology of the neoplasm under study. It is helpful then to recognize basic distinctions among morphologic categories, such as those of small cell, large cell, pleomorphic, and spindle cell neoplasms. The large cell category, however, constitutes a very broad group within which many subtypes may share a common marker. A reliable LCA that does not cross-react with epithelial cells should be part of a panel used in order to exclude lymphoma. Positivity for keratin antibodies is not necessarily indicative of squamous differentiation in a large cell epithelial neoplasm.[327] If the antibody is polyclonal, both immature nonkeratinized cells as well as keratinized elements will demonstrate positivity. Monoclonal LMWK will be positive in poorly differentiated squamous cell carcinomas as well as in poorly differentiated adenocarcinomas in the areas of greatest cellular density. By contrast, HMWK is positive only in well-keratinized neoplasms and in mesothelioma. In our experience, LMWK but not HMWK stains an occasional intermediate-type small cell carcinoma of the lung, while NF is consistently negative in these neoplasms. An anti-EMA antibody of broad specificity should also be represented along with AFP, S100, and A_1CT. Together with cytomorphology, this panel will discriminate among the germ cell, melanocytic, and histiocytic lineages of large cell neoplasms, as shown in Table 14-15. Once the main lineage has been defined, subclassification may proceed based on the utilization of more specific antibodies combined with other methods. An overlooked tool is the examination of touch imprints or postexcisional aspirates from neo-

Table 14-15 Differential Diagnosis of Large Cell Neoplasms

	Poorly Differentiated Carcinoma	Germ Cell Tumor	Histiocytic Neoplasm	B-Cell Lymphoma	Melanoma	Sarcoma
CEA	+	+/−	−	−	−	−
EMA	+	−	−	−	−	−
Keratin	+	−	−	−	−	+/−
Vimentin	+/−	−	+/−	+/−	+	+
LCA	−	−	+/−	+	−	−
AFP	+/−	+	−	−	−	−
S100	+/−	−	−	−	+	+/−
A_1AT/A_1ACT	+/−	+	+	−	−	+/−

AFP, alpha-fetoprotein; CEA, carcinoembryonic antigen; EMA, epithelial membrane antigen; LCA, leukocyte common antigen.

plasms of difficult classification. Not only do they provide the appreciation of excellent cytologic detail, but they can be done quickly at the time of intraoperative consultation. They are particularly valuable for comparison with pre-existing cytologic material in the same patient or a library of rare cases. Needless to say, interpretation of morphologic features should go hand in hand with ICC and often actually supplant the value of the various markers in experienced hands.

A common problem in oncologic pathology is the differential between various pleomorphic neoplasms. These tumors may represent one of the germ cell neoplasms, malignant melanomas, anaplastic carcinoma, or a lymphohistiocytic malignancy. Another possibility, particularly in soft tissues, is a sarcoma with pleomorphic features, such as pleomorphic rhabdomyosarcoma and MFH. Vimentin is of no help, since it will stain all these neoplasms, except the germ cell tumors. The myogenic markers are consistently negative in melanoma and histiocytic neoplasms. So, if either desmin or myoglobin is positive, they point in the direction of a rhabdomyosarcoma. S100, may also be of help, since it will be negative in histiocytes as well as lymphocytes but positive in melanomas. The latter diagnosis can be confirmed by positivity for HMB-45, which appears to be rather specific for melanocytic lesions including melanoma. Rare sarcomas, such as malignant granular cell tumors, may be diagnosable by their S100 positivity, which should trigger a confirmatory ultrastructural examination. If S100 is negative and A_1AT and A_1ACT are positive, the possibility of MFH should be ruled out. The same epithelial markers discussed under large cell neoplasm can be applied to anaplastic carcinomas (Table 14-15). Poorly differentiated tumors may be composed of predominantly spindle cells, in which case a sarcomatoid carcinoma must be excluded by the use of keratin antibodies. If keratin is negative the various spindle cell sarcomas can be sorted out by the use of vimentin, S100, GFAP, NF, desmin, and myoglobin. The neural origin of spindle cell tumors can also be further discerned by the use of myelin basic protein, a useful marker that, if positive, excludes a glial origin for the neoplasm.[328]

METASTATIC WORKUP

The greatest application of immunocytochemistry is in identifying a possible primary site for a neoplasm. The mere recognition of a cell type may narrow the differential diagnosis considerably. Consequently, separation of tumors into the pleomorphic, spindle, round cell, large cell, and small cell categories just discussed plays an important supportive role in this process. ICC assists cytomorphology in determining the direction of differentiation of a given lineage as for example the classification of epithelial cells into squamous, glandular, and neuroendocrine subtypes. Frequently, however, the site of origin may still be undeciphered because certain pathways of differentiation are shared by many tumors. In these cases, correlation with clinical data and familiarity with the cytomorphologic appearance of various tumors will facilitate the task at hand. Because of its noninvasive nature, cytopathology plays a particularly important role in elucidating the primary site of widely metastatic tumors. This can be accomplished not only in malignant effusions but also in FNA specimens by the use of immunocytochemistry in conjunction with electron microscopy.

Fine Needle Aspirates

At my institution, we are frequently called to evaluate tumors that spread to the liver, the retroperitoneum or lymph nodes of the head and neck.[329] The same applies to lymph nodes of the supraclavicular and mediastinal areas and subcutaneous metastases presenting as lumps and bumps easily accessible to FNA. The combination of cytomorphology, ultrastructure, and immunocytochemistry pays handsome dividends in these cases. The differential diagnosis of metastatic tumors is given in Table 14-16, along with the most useful markers for the various types of neoplasms. In the liver, the finding of cells with squamous differentiation invariably represent metastatic lung carcinoma in male or female smokers. Second in frequency is cervical carcinoma in the female or esophageal carcinoma in the male. Metastatic adenocarcinoma must be differentiated from hepatocellular carcinomas. This can be accomplished by electron microscopy, with the demonstration of bizarre mitochondria and bile canaliculi in primary liver cell tumors, which are often positive for AFP. Adenocarcinomas from lung and the GI tract are usually CEA positive, whereas lactalbumin positivity favors breast carcinoma. CEA is only infrequently positive in tumors of prostatic origin, but is frequently positive in other adenocarcinomas (Fig. 14-30, Plate 14-35). However, results with CEA cannot be interpreted in absolute terms. By contrast, TGb and prostatic specific antigen are virtually pathognomonic for their respective sites or origin. Other very specific cell markers include GFAP, positive in tumors of glial origin, and surfactant apoprotein, positive in type II

Table 14-16 Metastatic Workup Applicable to FNA and Other Cytologic Specimens

Primary Neoplasm	Immunodiagnostic Markers	Ultrastructural Features
Lymphoma	LCA, LN1, LN2, L26, UCHL-1, MT-1, MB2, L-60	No cell junctions, no surface specializations
Prostate	PSA, PAP	Short microvilli, abundant organelles
Thyroid	Thyroglobulin, calcitonin, CEA	Complex nuclear contours, electron-dense granules
Breast	Lactoalbumin, estrogen receptors	Intracytoplasmic lumina
Lung	CEA, surfactant apoprotein	Fluffy granules, lamellar bodies
Kidney	Secretory piece, URO series	Glycogen granules, lipid droplets
Liver	AFP, HbsAg, A_1AT, CEA	Bile canaliculi, bizarre mitochondria
Pancreas	Du-Pan 2	Small secretory granules, short microvilli
Ovary	OC-125	Peripheralized secretory granules, abundant microvilli

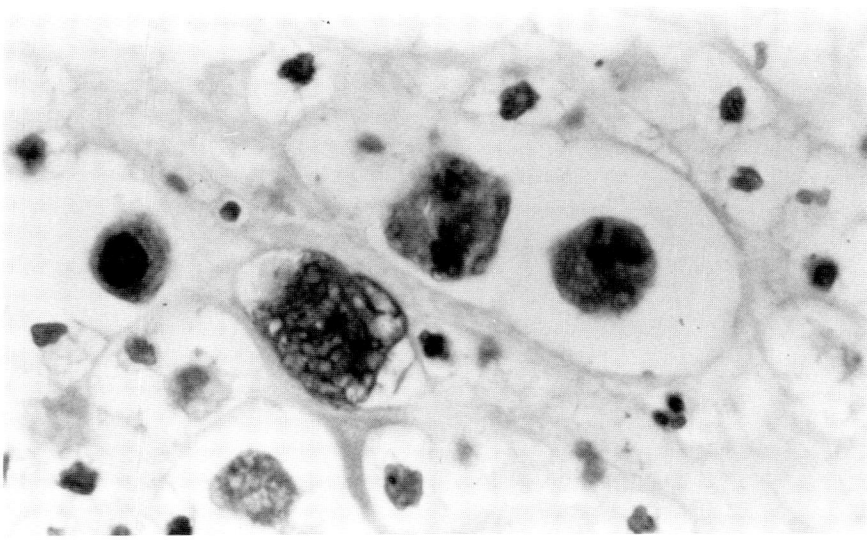

Fig. 14-30 Metastatic carcinoma stained for CEA. Strong positivity made a prostatic primary unlikely. A clinical search uncovered a primary in the lung. (See Plate 14-35.)

cell neoplasms of the lung. A number of monoclonal antibodies may also be of assistance as discussed under the organ-specific panels.

Body Fluids

One of the greatest challenges to the cytopathologist is the differentiation between mesothelioma and adenocarcinoma. This difficulty extends to surgical pathology, where both papillary and tubuloacinar neoplasms can be encountered. In cytologic material, very large individual cells with clear demarcation between endoplasm and ectoplasm favors mesothelioma. However, in cell clusters, adenocarcinoma and mesothelioma may form tridimensional structures, which are very difficult to distinguish from one another. The presence of intracytoplasmic lumina is not an absolute criterion for mesothelioma since adenocarcinomas, particularly of breast and lung origin, may also demonstrate this feature. By electron microscopy, however, such lumina as well as the entire perimeter of mesothelial cells are rich in long, slender, and bushy microvilli, not commonly seen in adenocarcinomas (Table 14-17). In the latter, short and stubby microvilli fail to intertwine and are distributed mainly at the apical pole of the cells.[330] Material for electron microscopy requires special handling and collection in glutaraldehyde, a fixative that is not routinely used in cytopathology. By contrast, ICC can be applied retrospectively to smears and cell blocks showing evidence of malignancy.

In practice, a panel composed of CEA, EMA, keratin, and HMWK provides useful information concerning malignant cells in effusions.[97,331] Recently, we added Leu M_1 to the battery with only a minor gain in sensitivity. Even allowing for differences in technique and in the antibodies utilized, strong positivity for CEA favors an epithelial malignancy.[332–334] Strong positivity for keratin is typical of mesothelial cells regardless of benignity or malignancy.[334] Mesotheliomas are invariably negative for CEA, frequently negative for EMA and show a two-tone positivity for LMWK and HMWK. Most investigators believe that diffuse strong positivity for EMA is not a characteristic of mesothelial cells but rather favors epithelial derivation[335] (Table 14-18). Adenocarcinomas are consistently and strongly positive for both CEA and EMA, diffusely but weakly positive for LMWK, and usually negative for HMWK. However, results with various markers will vary with the antibody, the mode of fixation and the technique of immunostain utilized. When immunocytochemistry is not available, mucin stain may also play a significant role in the recognition of adenocarcinoma.

Table 14-17 Ultrastructural Distinction Between Mesothelioma and Adenocarcinoma

Location	Mesothelioma	Adenocarcinoma
Cell surface	Microvilli evenly distributed around entire cell Slender bushy microvilli No glycocalyceal bodies	Microvilli concentrated at poles Short stubby microvilli Glycocalyceal bodies noted
Cell junctions	Apical tight junctions Well-developed desmosomes	Terminal bars near lumen Poorly developed junctions
Cytoplasm	Tonofilaments surrounding the nucleus Abundant glycogen No secretory granules	Irregularly distributed intermediate filaments Variable amount of glycogen Numerous secretory granules

Verification of the malignant status is difficult for individual groups of cells in effusions because: (1) even if these cells derive from patients with cancer, it does not follow that they are malignant, since mesothelial hyperplasia occurs in patients with effusions; (2) a negative biopsy of the nearest serosa is not a definitive proof of benignity since there may be a skip pattern of involvement and malignant cells may gain access to the cavity via the lymphatic circulation without seeding of the serous membrane; and (3) a

Table 14-18 Staining Characteristics of Mesothelioma and Adenocarcinoma

Type of Stain	Mesothelioma	Adenocarcinoma
Routine stains	Two-tone appearance with Papanicolaou stain Peripheral blebs with Romanowski's stain	Homogeneously distributed stain No peripheral blebs noted
Special stains	Cytoplasm contains PAS (+) digestible material Extracellular space contains Alcian blue (+) material removable by hyaluronidase	Glycogen content small No hyaluronic acid present in extracellular space
Immunostains	CEA consistently negative EMA variably positive with frequently "thick" membrane pattern Both low and high molecular weights keratin positive	CEA consistently positive EMA frequently positive in cytoplasm and cell periphery Positive only with low-molecular-weight keratin

CEA, carcinoembryonic antigen; EMA, epithelial membrane antigen; PAS, periodic acid-Schiff.

ploidy abnormality, as detected by flow cytometry, is not definitive either, since it depends on the proportion between benign mesothelial cells and malignant cells present in the effusion.[336] The sensitivity of flow cytometry also varies from study to study, so that cytomorphologic evaluation emerges as the gold standard in the interpretation of immunocytochemical results.[337]

Leu M_1 positivity in an effusion favors an adenocarcinoma and the pattern of positivity is very similar to that of EMA. B72.3 gives a strong diffuse positivity in carcinomas of the breast, lung and stomach.[338] A_1AT and A_1ACT may be positive in carcinomas, particularly those arising in breast, lung, and pancreas, in contrast to stomach and ovary.[121] The keratin positivity in mesothelial cells is stronger in alcohol-fixed smears and tissues than in cell blocks fixed in formalin. Squamous cell carcinoma exfoliates proportionately less tumor cells in effusions than do both mesothelioma and adenocarcinoma. The cells occur mainly as single elements and, if cell groupings are noted, they contain mostly spindle cells. CEA is frequently negative in squamous cell tumors but may be positive in transitional cell carcinomas. HMWK and LMWK are positive in squamous cell tumors, but lack the two-tone quality exhibited by mesothelioma. EMA is weakly positive in squamous cell carcinoma but without the linearity noted in adenocarcinoma. As noted previously, EMA is frequently negative but may be positive in a small proportion of mesotheliomas. However, in these cases, a very thick linear pattern of positivity has been noted due to the richness in microvilli of the mesothelial cells.[339] The exact significance of this finding awaits further investigation.

NUCLEUS AND MARKERS OF MALIGNANT TRANSFORMATION

Just as the cytoplasm reveals differentiation, the nucleus holds the secret of malignancy. Cytologists have been aware of this dogma for years, but sometimes in individual cases one cannot be conclusive as to the final diagnosis. An altered DNA content of the nucleus seems to be the most reliable parameter for ascertaining malignancy. The DNA amount can be measured reliably on slides by the Feulgen reaction or in cell suspensions by flow cytometry. Cytogenetic studies too, may reveal malignancy-associated changes, but this method is more tedious than ICC and electron microscopy.

Flow cytometry can be easily applied to body fluid or FNA specimens and has emerged as the technique of choice in assessing borderline lesions of difficult interpretation.[336] Aneuploidy, encompassing both a lesser and a greater amount of DNA in comparison with non-neoplastic cells, has been consistently detected in flow cytometric analysis of malignant tumors.[340] By analyzing the DNA histogram, the DNA index and the percentage of cells in the proliferative S-phase of the cell cycle can be calculated. A DNA index of 1.0 corresponds to diploid (euploid), non-neoplastic cells, while values different from 1.0 (aneuploid) occur in malignant neoplasms. A greater proportion of cells in the proliferative S phase of the cycle correlates well with a more aggressive behavior, particularly in breast cancer.[341] An estimate of kinetic activity can be obtained by immunostaining with the Ki-67 antibody. This marker binds to a nuclear antigen expressed by proliferating but not by resting cells.[342] Other markers, such as nucleolar antigen, have been linked to malignant transformation but results await confirmation in clinical cytologic material.[343] One must be skeptical of prominent nucleoli detected by morphologic means, since the largest size of nucleoli occurs in reparative, rather than neoplastic, conditions. It is not safe to generalize, but the nuclear size in relationship to the cytoplasm (N/C ratio) and the irregular deposition of chromatin beneath the nuclear envelope have been the most reliable criteria of malignancy in our hands. Neither necessitates ICC for appreciation. Both can be nicely demonstrated by electron microscopy, but one should not try to establish a malignant diagnosis in such a minute sample.

ACKNOWLEDGMENTS

I am grateful to former trainees Rosa Davila, Maria Mason and Clyniece Breland for their assistance during the preparation of this manuscript. Special thanks to Alan Silverberg, M.D., Colleen Fahey, and Denise Sandusky for the excellence of the cellular samples they obtained.

REFERENCES

1. Akhtar M, Ali MA, Owen EW: Application of electron microscopy in the interpretation of fine needle aspiration biopsies. Cancer 48:2458, 1981
2. Yazdi HM, Dardick I: What is the value of electron microscopy in fine-needle aspiration biopsy? Diagn Cytopathol 4:177, 1988
3. Farr A, Nakane, P: Immunohistochemistry with enzyme labeled antibodies: A brief review. Immunol Methods 47:129, 1981
4. Falini B, Taylor C: New developments in immunoperoxidase techniques and their application. Arch Pathol Lab Med 107:105, 1983
5. Angel E, Nagle RB: Magic markers: Practical problems in the use of immunoperoxidase histochemistry. Pathologist 39:13, 1985
6. Nadji M: The potential value of immunoperoxidase techniques in diagnostic cytology. Acta Cytol 24:443, 1980
7. Gupta PK, Myers JD, Baylin SB, et al: Improved antigen detection in ethanol-fixed cytologic specimens. Diagn Cytopathology 1:133, 1985
8. Chess Q, Hajdu S: The role of immunoperoxidase staining in diagnostic cytology. Acta Cytol 30:1, 1986
9. J-Jimenez D, Gangi MD: Application of diatex compound in cytology: Use in preparing multiple slides from a single routine smear. Acta Cytol 30:446, 1986
10. Hsu SM, Raine L, Fanger H: Use of avidin-biotin peroxidase-complex (ABC) in immunoperoxidase techniques: A comparison between ABC and unlabeled antibody (PAP) procedures. J Histochem Cytochem 29:577, 1981
11. Wood GS, Warnke R: Suppression of endogenous avidin-binding activity in tissues and its relevance to avidin-biotin detecting system. J Histochem Cytochem 29:1196, 1981
12. Bedrossian U, De Arce E, Bedrossian C: Immunoperoxidase to detect herpes simplex virus in cytologic specimens. Lab Med 15:673, 1984
13. Matutes E, Catovsky D: The fine structures of round lymphocyte subpopulations—A study with monoclonal antibodies and the immunogold technique. Clin Exp Immunol 50:416, 1982
14. De Arce E, Bedrossian C, Bedrossian U, et al: Detection of herpesvirus cervicovaginitis by a sequential Papanicolaou-immunoperoxidase technique. Diagn Cytopathol 1:23, 1985
15. Gupta M, Sharma B, Singh V, Luthra U: Immunocytological demonstration of HSV-II antigen on exfoliated cells from precancerous and cancerous lesions of the uterine cervix. Diagn Cytopathol 4:48, 1988
16. Masih A, Rennard SI, Bin Kley LI, et al: Detection of CMV in BAL specimens by cytology, tissue culture, fluorescent monoclonal antibodies and in-situ hybridization. Acta Cytol 31:648, 1987
17. Robey S, Gage W, Kuhajda F: Comparison of immunoperoxidase and DNA in-situ hybridization techniques in the diagnosis of cytomegalovirus colitis. Am J Clin Pathol 89:666, 1988
18. Bedrossian CWM, De Arce E, Bedrossian U, Kelly L: Herpetic tracheobronchitis detected at bronchoscopy: Cytologic diagnosis by the immunoperoxidase method. Diagn Cytopathol 1:292, 1985
19. O'Hara C, Gardner W, Bennett B: Immunoperoxidase staining of trichomonas vaginalis in cytologic material. Acta Cytol 24:448, 1980
20. Dorman S, Danos L, Caron B, et al: Detection of chlamydia trachomatis in Papanicolaou-stained cervical smears by indirect immunoperoxidase method. Acta Cytol 29:665, 1985
21. Kobayashi T, Ueda M, Araki H, et al: Immunocytochemical detection of Chlamydia infection in the urogenital tracts. Diagn Cytopathol 3:303, 1987
22. Gupta PK, Shurbaji MS, Mintor LF, et al: Cytopathologic detection of chlamydia trachomatis in vaginopancervical (fast) smears. Diagn Cytopathol 4:224, 1988
23. Kadish A, Burk R, Kress Y, et al: Human papillomaviruses of different types in precancerous lesions of the uterine cervix: Histologic, immunocytochemical and ultrastructural studies. Hum Pathol 17:384, 1986
24. Deligeorgi-Politi H, Mui K, Trotta K, et al: Immunocytochemical localization of human papilloma virus and cytomorphologic correlation in smears and biopies of cervical flat condylomata. Diagn Cytopathol 2:320, 1986
25. Bedrossian CWM, Bedrossian UK, Symington J, et al: HPV detection with antibodies against HPV-related synthetic nucleotides. (In preparation.)
26. Domagala W, Weber K, Osborn M: Diagnostic significance of coexpression of intermediate filaments in fine needle aspirates of human tumors. Acta Cytol 32:49, 1988
27. Lehto V, Miettinen M, Virtanen I: Varying expression of cytokeratin and neurofilaments in neuroendocrine tumors of human gastrointestinal tract. Lab Invest 52:429, 1985
28. Miettinen M, Lehto V, Dahl D, Virtanen I: Varying expression of cytokeratin and neurofilaments in neuroendocrine tumors of human gastrointestinal tract. Lab Invest 52:429, 1985
29. Ramaekers F, Haag D, Jap P, Vooijs P: Immunocytochemical demonstration of keratin and vimentin in cytologic aspirates. Acta Cytol 28:385, 1984

30. Herpers MJHM, Ramaeker FCS, Alderveireld J, et al: Coexpression of GFAP and vimentin-type intermediate filaments in human astrocytomas. Acta Neuropathol (Berl) 70:33, 1983
31. Brown DC, Theaker JM, Banks PM, et al: Cytokeratin expression in smooth muscle tumors. Histopathology 11:477, 1987
32. Churg A: Immunocytochemical staining for vimentin and keratin in malignant mesothelioma. Am J Surg Pathol 9:360, 1985
33. Caselitz T, Osborn M, Seifer G, et al: Coexpression of keratin and vimentin filaments in adenoid cystic carcinomas of the salivary gland. Virchows Arch [A] 403:337, 1984
34. Gould VE: The coexpression of distinct classes in intermediate filaments in human neoplasm. Arch Pathol Lab Med 109:984, 1985
35. Krepler R, Denk H, Artlieb U, Moll R: Immunocytochemistry of intermediate filament proteins present in pleomorphic adenomas of the human parotid gland: Characterization of different cell types in the same tumor. Differentiation 21:191, 1982
36. Gatter KC, Dunnill MS, Van Menjen GNP, Mason DY: Human lung tumors may coexpress different classes of intermediate filaments. J Clin Pathol 39:950, 1986
37. Altmannsberger M, Osborn M, Schafer H, et al: Distinction of nephroblastoma from other childhood tumors using antibodies to intermediate filaments. Virchows Arch [A] 45:112, 1984
38. Herman CJ, Moesker O, Kant A, et al: Is renal cell (Grawitz) tumor a carcinosarcoma? Evidence from analysis of intermediate filament types. Virchows Arch [B] 44:73, 1983
39. Henzen, Logmans SC, Mullin KH, et al: Expression of cytokeratin and vimentin in epithelial cells of normal and pathologic thyroid tissue. Virchows Arch [A] 410:347, 1987
40. Davila R, Bedrossian CWM, Silverberg A: Immunocytochemistry of the thyroid gland in surgical and cytologic specimens. Arch Pathol Lab Med 112:51, 1988
41. Molenaar WM, Oosterhuis JW, Oosterhuis AM, Ramaekers FCS: Mesenchymal and muscle-specific intermediate filaments (vimentin and desmin) in relation to differentiation in childhood rhabdomyosarcomas. Hum Pathol 16:838, 1985
42. Gould VE: The coexpression of distinct classes of intermediate filaments in human neoplasms. Arch Pathol Lab Med 109:984, 1985
43. Kasper M, Goertchen R, Stosiek P, et al: Coexistence of cytokeratin, vimentin and neurofilament protein in human choroid plexus: An immunohistochemical study of intermediate fluids in neuroepithelial tissues. Virchows Arch [A] 410:173, 1986
44. Lazarides E: Intermediate Filaments: A chemically heterogeneous, developmentally regulated class of proteins. Annu Rev Biochem 51:219, 1982
45. Moll R, Franke W, Schiller D: The catalog of human cytokeratins: Patterns of expression in normal epithelia, tumors and cultured cells. Cell 31:11, 1982
46. Gown A, Vogel A: Monoclonal antibodies to human intermediate filament proteins: Analysis of tumors. Am J Clin Pathol 84:413, 1985
47. Altmannsberger M, Osborn M, Schauer A, Weber K: Antibodies to different intermediate filament proteins: Cell type-specific markers on paraffin-embedded human tissues. Lab Invest 45:427, 1981
48. Domagala W, Lubinski J, Woyke S, et al: Decisive role of intermediate filament typing of tumor cells in the differential diagnosis of difficult fine needle aspirates. Acta Cytol 31:253, 1987
49. Denk H, Krepler R, Artlieb U, et al: Proteins of intermediate filaments. An immunohistochemical and biochemical approach to the classification of soft tissue tumors. Am J Pathol 110:193, 1983
50. Droese M, Altmannsberger M, Kehl A, et al: Ultrasound-guided percutaneous fine needle aspiration biopsy of abdominal retroperitoneal masses. Acta Cytol 28:368, 1984
51. Puts JJG, Vooijs GP, Huijsmans A, et al: Cytoskeletal proteins as tissue specific markers in cytopathology. Exp Cell Biol 54:73, 1986
52. Kahn H, Hanna W, Yeger H, Baumal R: Immunohistochemical localization of prekeratin filaments in benign and malignant cells in effusions. Am J Pathol 109:206, 1982
53. Osborn M, Weber K: Tumor diagnosis by intermediate filament typing: A novel tool for surgical pathology. Lab Invest 48:372, 1983
54. Miettinen M, Lehto VP, Virtanen I: Antibodies to intermediate filament proteins in the diagnosis and classification of human tumors. Ultrastruct Pathol 7:83, 1984
55. Cooper D, Schermer A, Sun T: Classification of human epithelia and their neoplasms using monoclonal antibodies to keratins: Strategies, applications, and limitations. Lab Invest 52:243, 1985
56. Battifora H: Recent progress in immunocytochemistry of solid tumors. Semin Diagn Pathol 1:251, 1984
57. Ramaekers FCS, Huysmans A, Moeker O, et al: Monoclonal antibodies to keratin filaments for glandular epithelia and their tumors. Lab Invest 49:353, 1983

58. Debus E, Weber K, Osborn M: Monoclonal cytokeratin antibodies that distinguish simple from stratified squamous epithelia characterization on human tissue. EMBO J 1:1641, 1984
59. Walts AE, Said JW, Shintaku IP, et al: Keratins of different molecular weights in exfoliated mesothelial and adenocarcinoma cells—An aid to cell identification. Am J Clin Pathol 81:442, 1984
60. Walts AE, Said JW, Banks-Schlegel SB: Keratin and CEA in exfoliated mesothelial and malignant cells: An immunoperoxidase study. Am J Clin Pathol 80:671, 1983
61. Bolen JW, Thorning D: Mesotheliomas: A light- and electron-microscopical study concerning histogenetic relationships between the epithelial and the mesenchymal variants. Am J Surg Pathol 4:451, 1980
62. Hammar S, Bockus D, Remington F, Cooper L: The unusual spectrum of neuroendocrine lung neoplasms. Ultrastruct Path (In press)
63. Ramaekers FCS, Haug D, Kant A, et al: Coexpression of keratin and vimentin-type intermediate filaments in human metastatic carcinoma cells. Proc Natl Acad Sci USA 80:2618, 1983
64. Azar HA: Attributes of neoplasms. p. 1. In Azar HA (ed): Pathology of Human Neoplasms. Raven Press, New York, 1988
65. Lee VM-Y, Wu H-L, Schlaepfer WW: Monoclonal antibodies recognize individual neurofilament triplet proteins. Proc Natl Acad Sci USA 79:6089, 1982
66. Leff EL, Brooks JSJ, Trojanowski JQ: Expression of neurofilament and neuron specific enolase in small cell tumors of the skin using immunocytochemistry. Cancer 56:625, 1985
67. Coakham HB, Brownell B, Harper EL, et al: Use of monoclonal antibody panel to identify malignant cells in cerebrospinal fluid. Lancet 1:1095, 1984
68. Kasper M, Goertchen R, Stosiek P, et al: Coexistence of cytokeratin, vimentin and neurofilament proteins in human choroid plexus: An immunohistochemical study of intermediate filaments in neuroepithelial tissues. Virchows Arch [A] 410:173, 1986
69. Kahn HJ, Yeger H, Baumal R, et al: Categorization of pediatric neoplasms by immunostaining with antiprekeratin and anti-vimentin antisera. Cancer 51:645, 1983
70. Christen B, Trojanowski JQ, Pietra GG: Immunohistochemical demonstration of phosphorylated and nonphosphorylated forms of NF subunits in human pulmonary carcinoids. Hum Pathol 18:997, 1987
71. Moll R, Osborn M, Hartschurch W, et al: Variability of expression and arrangement of cytokeratin and neurofilament in cutaneous neuroendocrine carcinomas (Merkel cell tumors). Ultrastruct Pathol 10:473, 1986
72. Roessmann U, Valasco ME, Garuketti P, et al: Neuronal and astrocytic differentiation in human neuroepithelial neoplasms: An immunohistochemical study. J Neuropathol Exp Neurol 42:113, 1983
73. Ducataman BS, Scheithauer BW: Malignant peripheral nerve sheath tumors with divergent differentiation. Cancer 54:1049, 1984
74. Blobel G, Gould VE, Moll R, et al: Coexpression of neuroendocrine markers and epithelial cytoskeletal proteins in bronchopulmonary neuroendocrine neoplasms. Lab Invest 52:39, 1985
75. Clark RK, Miethinen M, Leij L, Darynov V: Terminally differentiated derivatives of pulmonary small cell carcinomas may contain neurofilaments. Lab Invest 53:243, 1985
76. Ramaekers F, Broers J, Klein Rot M, et al: Detection of epithelial and neural type of intermediate filament proteins in human lung tumors. Acta Histochem (Jena) 34(suppl):45, 1987
77. McDowell EM, Wilson TS, Trump BF: Atypical endocrine tumors of the lung. Arch Pathol Lab Med 105:20, 1981
78. Schnipper LE: Clinical implications of tumor cell heterogeneity. N Engl J Med 314:1423, 1986
79. Garson JA, Coakham HB, Kemshead JT, et al: The role of monoclonal antibodies in brain tumor diagnosis and cerebrospinal fluid (CSF) cytology. J Neurooncol 3:165, 1985
80. Velasco M, Dahl D, Roessmann U, Gambetti P: Immunohistochemical localization of glial fibrillary acidic protein in human glial neoplasms. Cancer 45:484, 1980
81. Koskull H: Rapid identification of glial cells in human amniotic fluid with indirect immunofluorescence. Acta Cytol 28:393, 1984
82. Bigner SH, McLendon RE, Mensi DE, et al: Expression of glial fibrillary acidic protein in cytologic specimens from the central nervous system as demonstrated by monoclonal antibodies. Acta Cytol 29:919, 1985
83. Trojanowski J, Atkinson B, Lee V: An immunocytochemical study of normal and abnormal human cerebrospinal fluid with monoclonal antibodies to glial fibrillary acidic protein. Acta Cytol 30:235, 1986
84. Budka I: Non-glial specificities of immunocytochemistry for the glial fibrillary acidic protein (GFAP). Triple expression of GFAP, vimentin and cytokeratins in papillary meningioma and metastasizing renal carcinoma. Acta Neuropathol (Berl) 72:43, 1986

85. Ostrzega N, Cheng L, Layfield L: Glial fibrillary acid protein: Immunoreactivity in FNA of salivary gland lesions. Diagn Cytopathol 5:145, 1989
86. Collins V: Monoclonal antibodies to glial fibrillary acidic protein in the cytologic diagnosis of brain tumors: Acta Cytol 28:401, 1984
87. Ludwin SK, Kosec JC, Eng LF: The topographical distribution of S100 an GFAP in the adult rat brain. J Comp Neurol 165:197, 1976
88. Iwa N, Yutoni C, Ishibashi-Ueda H, Katayama Y: Immunocytochemical demonstration of GFAP in imprint smears of human brain tumors. Diagn Cytopathol 4:74, 1988
89. Dekmezian RH, Sneige N, Ordonez NG: Ovarian and omental ependymoma in peritoneal washings. Diagn Cytopathol 2:62, 1986
90. Osborn M, Weber K: Tubulin-specific antibody and the expression of microtubules in 3T3 cells after attachment to a substractum: Further evidence for the polar growth of cytoplasmic microtubules in vivo. Exp Cell Res 103:331, 1976
91. Ben-Ze'ev A: The cytoskeleton in cancer cells. Biochim Biophys Acta 780:197, 1985
92. Bedrossian CWM, Masood S, Prey MU: Immunocytochemical detection of myoepithelial cells in breast carcinoma: A comparative study between S100, HHF and smooth muscle actin in paraffin embedded tissue. Mod Pathol (In press)
93. Chen JC, Gnepp D, Bedrossian CWM: Adenoid cystic carcinoma of the salivary glands: An immunocytochemical analysis. Oral Surg 65:316, 1988
94. Bedrossian CWM, Maksem J, Desai K, Tannenbaum M: Immunocytochemistry of the prostate in cytologic and surgical specimens. Diagn Cytopathol (In press)
95. Gould VE: Histogenesis and differentiation: Evaluation of these two concepts as criteria for the classification of neoplasms. Hum Pathol 17:212, 1986
96. Dahlin DC, Beabout JW: Dedifferention of low grade chondrosarcomas. Cancer 28:461, 1971
97. Mason M, Bedrossian CWM, Fahey CA: Value of immunocytochemistry in the study of malignant effusions. Diagn Cytopathol 3:215, 1987
98. Boon M, Lindeman J, Meeuwissen A, Otto A: Carcinoembryonic antigen in sputum cytology. Acta Cytol 26:389, 1982
99. Kobayashi T, Yamaki T, Yoshino E, et al: Immunocytochemical demonstration of carcinoembryonic antigen in cerebrospinal fluid with carcinomatous meningitis from rectal cancer. Acta Cytol 28:430, 1984
100. Walts A, Said J: Specific tumor markers in diagnostic cytology: Immunoperoxidase studies of carcinoembryonic antigen, lysozyme and other tissue antigens in effusions, washes and aspirates. Acta Cytol 27:408, 1983
101. Holmberg V, Wahren B, Esposti PL: Carcinoembryonic antigen in cytological specimens of urothelial carcinoma. Cytometry 5:437, 1984
102. Gray A, Downing R, Hill R, et al: Demonstration of carcinoembryonic antigen in bone marrow from patients with carcinoma. J Clin Pathol 37:1090, 1984
103. Krykou K, Iatridis S, Athanassiadou P, et al: Detection of benign or malignant origin of ascites with combined indirect immunoperoxidase assays of carcinoembryonic antigen and lysozyme. Acta Cytol 29:57, 1985
104. Masuzawa M, Lee P-K, Kamada T, et al: Carcinoembryonic antigen, alpha-fetoprotein and carcinoplacental alkaline phosphatase in gastric carcinoma metastatic to the liver. Cancer 39:1175, 1977
105. Schwartz M, Randolph R, Panko W: Carcinoembryonic antigen and steroid receptors in the cytosol of carcinoma of the breast. Cancer 55:2464, 1985
106. Heald J, Buckley CH, Fox M: An immunohistochemical study of the distribution of carcinoembryonic antigen in epithelial tumors of the ovary. J Clin Pathol 32:918, 1979
107. Holden J, Churg A: Immunohistochemical staining for keratin and carcinoembryonic antigen in the diagnosis of malignant mesothelioma. Am J Surg Pathol 8:277, 1984
108. Yamamoto Y, Yasumura K, Murakoshi M, et al: Application of immuno-electron microscopy to the cytologic study of benign and malignant mammary lesions. Acta Cytol 29:257, 1985
109. Osamura R, Watanabe K, Akatsuka Y: Peroxidase-labeled antibody staining for carcinoembryonic antigen of cytologic specimens for light and electron microscopy. Acta Cytol 29:254, 1985
110. Jacobsen GK, Jacobsen M, Clausen PP: Distribution of tumor associated antigens in the various histologic components of germ cell tumors of the testis. Am J Surg Pathol 5:257, 1981
111. Morinaga S, Ojima M, Sasano N: Human chorionic gonadotrophin and alpha-fetoprotein in testicular germ cell tumors: An immunohistochemical study in comparison with tissue concentrations. Cancer 52:1281, 1983
112. Szymendera JJ, Zborzil J, Sikorowa L, et al: Value of five tumor markers (AFP, CEA, hCG, hPL and SP1) in diagnosis and staging of testicular germ cell tumors. Oncology 38:222, 1981
113. Wagener C, Menzel B, Breuer H, et al: Immunohistochemical localization of Alpha-Fetoprotein (AFP) in germ cell tumors: Evidence for AFP production by

tissues different from endodermal sinus tumor. Oncology 38:236, 1981
114. Hustin J, Reuter AM, Franchimount P: Immunohistochemical localization of HCG and its subunits in testicular germ cell tumors. Virchows Arch [A] 406:333, 1985
115. Inaba N, Renk T, Wurster K, et al: Ectopic synthesis of pregnancy specific beta-1 glycoprotein (SP_1) and placental specific tissue proteins in non-trophoblastic malignant tumors: Possible markers in oncology. Klin Wochensch 58:789, 1980
116. Wepsic HT, Onstad JW, Sell S: $Alpha_1$-Fetoprotein in a patient with a poorly differentiated carcinoma of the anterior mediastinum. Cancer 34:841, 1976
117. Wachner R, Wittekind C, Von Kleist S: Localization of CEA beta-HCG, Sp1 and Keratin in the tissue of lung carcinomas: An immunohistochemical study. Virchows Arch [A] 402:415, 1983
118. Eckert H. Immunohistochemical findings in intrathoracic tumors. II. Demonstration of A_1AT in tumor tissue. Z Erke Atmungsorg 161:319, 1983
119. Kojiro M, Kawano Y, Isomura T, Nakashima T: Distribution albumin and/or alpha-fetoprotein positive cells in hepatocellular carcinoma. Lab Invest 44:221, 1981
120. Reintoft I, Hagerstrand I: Demonstration of a_1-Antitrypsin in hepatomas. Arch Pathol Lab Med 103:495, 1979
121. Permanetter W, Wiesinger H: Immunohistochemical study of lysozyme, $alpha_1$ antichymotrypsin, tissue polypeptide antigen, keratin and carcinoembryonic antigen in effusion sediments. Acta Cytol 31:104, 1987
122. Pinkus G, Kurtin P: Epithelial membrane antigen—A diagnostic discriminant in surgical pathology. Hum Pathol 16:929, 1985
123. Sloane J, Ormerod M: Distribution of epithelial membrane antigen in normal and neoplastic tissues and its value in diagnostic tumor pathology. Cancer 47:1786, 1981
124. Battifora H, Kopinski: Distinction of mesothelioma from adenocarcinoma: An immunohistochemical approach. Cancer 55:1697, 1985
125. Ghosh AK, Spriggs AI, Taylor-Papadimitriou J, Mason DY: Immunocytochemical staining of cells in pleural and peritoneal effusions with a panel of monoclonal antibodies. J Clin Pathol 36:1154, 1983
126. To A, Dearnaley D, Ormerod M, et al: Epithelial membrane antigen: Its use in the cytodiagnosis of malignancy in serous effusions. Am J Clin Pathol 78:214, 1982
127. Thomas P, Battifora H: Keratins versus epithelial membrane antigen in tumor diagnosis. Hum Pathol 18:728, 1987
128. Walts A, Said J, Shintaku I: Epithelial membrane antigen (EMA) in the cytodiagnosis of effusions and aspirates: Immunocytochemical and ultrastructural localization in benign and malignant cells. Diagn Cytopathol 3:41, 1987
129. Burchell J, Durbin H, Taylor-Papadimitrious J: Complexity of expression of antigenic determinants, recognized by monoclonal antibodies HMFG-1 and HMFG-2, in normal and malignant human mammary epithelial cells. J Immunol 131:508, 1983
130. Hilkens J, Buijs F, Hilgers J, et al: Monoclonal antibodies against human milk fat globule membranes detecting differentiation antigens of the mammary gland and its tumors. Int J Cancer 34:197, 1984
131. Hilborne L, Cheng L, Nieberg R, Lewin K: Evaluation of an antibody to human milk fat globule antigen in the detection of metastatic carcinoma in pleural, pericardial, and peritoneal fluids. Acta Cytol 30:245, 1986
132. Szpak C, Johnston W, Lottich S, et al: Patterns of reactivity of four novel monoclonal antibodies (B72.3, DF3, B1.1 and B6.2) with cells in human malignant and benign effusions. Acta Cytol 28:356, 1984
133. Johnston W: Applications of monoclonal antibodies in clinical cytology as exemplified by studies with monoclonal antibody B72.3. Acta Cytol 31:537, 1987
134. Lyubsky S, Madariaga J, Lozowski M, et al: A tumor-associated antigen in carcinoma of the pancreas defined by monoclonal antibody B72.3. Am J Clin Pathol 89:160, 1988
135. Thor A, Ohuchi N, Szpak C, et al: Distribution of oncofetal antigen tumor-associated glycoprotein-72 defined by monoclonal antibody B72.3. Cancer Res 46:3118, 1986
136. Johnston W, Szpak C, Lottich S, et al: Use of a monoclonal antibody (B72.3) as an immunocytochemical adjunct to diagnosis of adenocarcinoma in human effusions. Cancer Res 45:1894, 1985
137. Martin S, Moshiri S, Thor A, et al: Identification of adenocarcinoma in cytospin preparations of effusions using monoclonal antibody B72.3. Am J Clin Pathol 86:10, 1986
138. Johnston W, Szpak C, Lottich S, et al: Use of a monoclonal antibody (B72.2) as a novel immunohistochemical adjunct of the diagnosis of carcinoma in fine needle aspiration biopsy specimens. Hum Pathol 17:501, 1986
139. Lundy J, Kline TS, Lozowski M, Chao S: Immunoperoxidase studies with Mab B72.3 applied to breast aspirates: Diagnostic considerations. Diagn Cytopathol 4:95, 1988
140. Prey M, Bedrossian CWM, Masood S: The value of monoclonal antibody B72-3 for the diagnosis of

breast carcinoma: Experience with the first available commercial source. Hum Pathol (In press)
141. Miettinen M, Lehto VP, Virtanen I: Immunofluorescence microscopic evaluation of the intermediate filament expression of the adrenal cortex and medulla and their tumors. Am J Pathol 118:360, 1985
142. DeLellis RA, Tischler AS, Lee AK, et al: Leu-enkephalin-like immunoreactivity in proliferative lesions of the human adrenal medulla and extraadrenal paraganglia. Am J Surg Pathol 7:29, 1983
143. Lloyd RV, Blaivas M, Wilson BS: Distribution of chromogranin and S100 protein in normal and abnormal adrenal medullary tissues. Arch Pathol Lab Med 109:633, 1985
144. Tanaka T, Yoshimi N, Iwata H, et al: FNA cytology of pheochromocytoma-ganglioneuroma of the organ of Zuckerkandle. Diagn Cytopathol 5:64, 1989
145. Lloyd RV, Shapiro B, Sisson JC, et al: An immunohistochemical study of pheochromocytoma: Arch Pathol Lab Med 108:541, 1984
146. DeLellis RA, Wolfe HJ: The pathobiology of the C-cell Pathol Annu 16:25, 1981
147. Holm R, Sobrinho-Simoes M, Nestland JM, et al: Medullary carcinoma of the thyroid gland: An immunohistochemical study. Ultrastruct Pathol 8:25, 1985
148. Sikri KL, Varndell IM, Hamid GA, et al: Medullary carcinoma of the thyroid. An immunocytochemical and histochemical study of 25 cases using 8 separate markers. Cancer 56:2481, 1985
149. De Stephano DB, Lloyd RV, Pike AM, Wilson BS: Pituitary adenomas: An immunohistochemical study of hormone production and chromogranin localization. Am J Pathol 116:464, 1984
150. Kovaks K, Horvath E, Ezrinc, et al: Adenomas of the human pituitary producing growth hormone and thyrotropin. A histologic, immunocytologic and fine structural study. Virchows Arch [A] 395:59, 1982
151. Fisher EC, Morris JH, Kettyle WM: Intrasellar gangliocytoma and syndrome of pituitary hypersecretion: Case report. J Neurosurg 59:1071, 1983
152. Ehya H, Lang WR: Cytology of granulosa cell tumor of the ovary. Am J Clin Pathol 85:402, 1985
153. Kurmann RJ, Andrade D, Goebelsmann U, et al: An immunohistological study of the steroid localization in Sertoli-Leydig cell tumors of the ovary and testis. Cancer 42:1772, 1978
154. Kurmann RJ, Goebelsmann U, Taylor CR: Steroid localization in granulosa-theca cell tumors of the ovary. Cancer 43:2377, 1979
155. Davey DD, Glant MD, Berger EK: Parathyroid cytopathology. Diagn Cytopathol 2:76, 1986
156. Ordonez NG, Ibanez ML, Samaan NA, Hickey RC: Immunoperoxidase study of uncommon parathyroid tumors. Am J Surg Pathol 7:535, 1983
157. Heitz PU, Kasper M, Polak JM, et al: Pancreatic endocrine tumors: Immunocytochemical analysis of 125 tumors. Hum Pathol 13:263, 1982
158. Tomita T, Friesen SR, Himmel JR, et al: Pancreatic polypeptide secreting endocrine tumors in a study of three cases. Am J Pathol 113:134, 1983
159. Bedrossian CWM, Weilbaecher D, Bentinck, Greenberg SD: Ultrastructure of human bronchioloalveolar cell carcinoma. Cancer 36:1399, 1975
160. Bedrossian CWM, Glick AD, Graham S, Mitchell L: Cytopathology and electron microscopy in the diagnosis of lung cancer by FNA biopsy. Patologia 22:367, 1984
161. Balis JV, Patterson JF, Paciga JE, et al: Distribution and subcellular localization of surfactant associated glycoproteins in human lung. Lab Invest 52:657, 1985
162. Harris JP, South MA: Secretory component: A glandular epithelial cell marker. Am J Pathol 105:47, 1981
163. Brooks JJ, Ernst CS: Immunoreactive secretory component of IgA in human tissues and tumors. Am J Clin Pathol 82:660, 1984
164. Pinkus GS, Thomas P, Said JS: Leu-M1—A marker for Reed-Sternberg cells in Hodgkin's disease. Am J Pathol 119:224, 1985
165. Wieczorek R, Suhrland M, Ramsay D, et al: Leu-M1 antigen expression in advanced (tumor) stage mycosis fungoides. Am J Clin Pathol 86:25, 1986
166. Pinkus GS, Said JW: Leu-M1 immunoreactivity in nonhematopoietic neoplasms and myeloproliferative disorders. Am J Clin Pathol 85:278, 1986
167. Sheibani K, Battifora H, Burke J, Rappaport H: Leu-M1 antigen in human neoplasm: An immunohistologic study of 400 cases. Am J Surg Pathol 10:227, 1986
168. Sheibani K, Battifora H, Burke JS: Antigenic phenotype of malignant mesotheliomas and pulmonary adenocarcinomas. Am J Pathol 123:212, 1986
169. Nadji M, Tabei SZ, Castro A, Chu TM, Morales A: Prostatic origin of tumors: An immunohistochemical study. Am J Clin Pathol 73:735, 1980
170. Keshgegian AA, Kline TS: Immunoperoxidase demonstration of prostatic acid phosphatase in aspiration biopsy cytology (ABC). Am J Clin Pathol 82:586, 1984
171. Katz RL, Raval P, Brooks TE, Ordonez NG: Role of immunocytochemistry in diagnosis of prostatic neoplasia by fine needle aspiration biopsy. Diagn Cytopathol 1:28, 1985
172. Nadji M, Morales AR: Immunohistochemical markers for prostatic cancer. Ann NY Acad Sci 420:134, 1983
173. Brawer MK, Peehl DM, Stamey TA, Bostiwick DG:

Keratin immunoreactivity in the benign and neoplastic human prostate. Cancer Res 45:3663, 1985
174. Ostrzega N, Cheng L, Layfield LF: Keratin immunoreactivity in FNA of the prostate: An aid in the differentiation of benign epithelium from well differentiated carcinoma. Diagn Cytopathol 4:38, 1988
175. Albores-Saavedra J, Nadji M, Civantos F, Morales AR: Thyroglobulin in carcinoma of the thyroid: An immunohistochemical study. Hum Pathol 14:62, 1983
176. Deftos LJ, Bone HG, Parthemore JG, Burton DW: Immunohistochemical studies of medullary thyroid carcinoma and C-cell hyperplasia. J Clin Endocrinol Metab 51:857, 1980
177. Davila R, Bedrossian CWM, Silverberg AB: Immunocytochemistry of the thyroid in surgical and cytologic specimens. Arch Pathol Lab Med 112:51, 1988
178. Gal R, Aronof A, Gertzmann H, Kessler E: The potential value of the demonstration of thyroglobulin by immunoperoxidase techniques in fine needle aspiration cytology. Acta Cytol (Praha) 31:713, 1987
179. Tuccari CT, Barresi G: Immunohistochemical demonstration of lactoferrin in follicular adenomas and thyroid carcinomas. Virchows Arch [A] 406:67, 1985
180. Bedrossian CWM, Davila RM: Lactoferrin demonstration in thyroid follicular and papillary carcinomas. Arch Pathol Lab Med 112:1176, 1988
181. Koelma IA, Nap M, VanSteenis GJ, Fleuren GJ: Tumor markers for ovarian cancer: A comparative immunocytochemical study of two commercial monoclonal antibodies. Am J Clin Pathol 90:391, 1988
182. Shishin J, Ghazizadeh M, Oguro T, et al: Immunohistochemical localization of CA-125 antigen in formalin-fixed paraffin sections of ovarian tumors with the use of pronase. Am J Clin Pathol 85:595, 1986
183. Kobayashi T, Teraoka S, Tsujioka T, Yoshida Y: Ciliated ovarian adenocarcinoma cells in ascitic fluid cytology: Report of a case with immunocytochemical features. Diagn Cytopathol 4:234, 1988
184. Charpin C, Bhan AK, Zurawski VR, et al: Carcinoembryonic antigen and carbohydrate determinant (CA 19-9) localization in 121 primary and metastatic ovarian carcinomas. Int J Gynecol Pathol 1:231, 1982
185. Mariani-Constantini R, Agresti R, Andreola S, et al: Characterization of the specificity by immunohistology of a Mab to a novel antigen of ovarian carcinomas. Pathol Res Pract 180:169, 1985
186. Bhattacharya M, Chatterjee SK, Barlow JJ, Fuji H: Monoclonal antibodies recognizing tumor-associated antigen of human ovarian mucinous cystadenocarcinomas. Cancer Res 42:1650, 1982
187. Walker RA: The demonstration of alpha-lactalbumin in human breast carcinomas. J Pathol 129:37, 1978
188. Rosiello R, Carriero J, Giordano GG: Distribution of ferritin, transferrin and lactoferrin in breast carcinoma tissue. J Clin Pathol 37:51, 1984
189. Fortt RW, Gibbs AR, Williams D: The identification of casein in human breast cancer. Histopathology 3:395, 1979
190. Bahn R, Mangkormkonok-Mark M, Albertson D, et al: Detection of alpha-lactalbumin in breast lesions and relationship to estrogen receptor and serum prolactin. Cancer 46:1775, 1980
191. Flower JL, Cox EB, Geisinger KR, et al: Use of monoclonal antiestrogen receptor content in fine needle aspiration breast biopsies. Ann Surg 203:250, 1986
192. Haagensen DE Jr, Mazoujian G: Utilization of the GCDFP-15 protein as a marker of breast carcinoma with apocrine features: Clinical and pathologic findings. Protides Biol Fluids Proc Colloq 31:567, 1983
193. Marianni-Constantini R, Menard S, Clemente C, et al: Immunocytochemical identification of breast carcinoma cells in effusions using a monoclonal antibody. J Clin Pathol 35:1037, 1982
194. Thor A, Simpson J, Ohuchi N, et al: Monoclonal antibodies and human carcinomas: Diagnostic and experimental applications. p. 165. In DeLellis RA (ed): Advances in Immunohistochemistry. Raven Press, New York, 1988
195. Espinosa CG, Balis JU, Saba SR, et al: Ultrastructural and immunocytochemical studies of bronchiolo-alveolar carcinoma. Cancer 54:2182, 1984
196. Tao LC: Aspiration biopsy cytology of mesothelioma. Diagn Cytopathol (In press)
197. Banner BF, Gould VE, Radosevich JA, et al: Application of monoclonal antibody 44-3A6 in the cytodiagnosis and classification of pulmonary carcinomas. Diagn Cytopathol 1:300, 1985
198. Tao LC, Ho CS, McLoughlin MJ, et al: Cytologic diagnosis of hepatocellular carcinoma by fine-needle aspiration biopsy. Cancer 53:547, 1984
199. Suen KC: Diagnosis of primary hepatic neoplasms by fine needle aspiration cytology. Diagn Cytopathol 2:99, 1986
200. Bedrossian CWM, Davila RM, Merenda G: Immunocytochemistry of the liver in cytologic and surgical specimens. Arch Pathol Lab Med (In press)
201. Ordonez NG, Manning JT: Comparison of alpha-1-antitrypsin and alpha-1-antichymotrypsin in hepatocellular carcinoma: An immunoperoxidase study. Am J Gastroenterol 79:959, 1979
202. Goodman ZD, Ishak KG, Langloss JM, et al: Combined hepatocellular cholangiocarcinoma: A histologic and immunohistochemical study. Cancer 55:124, 1985

203. Van Eyken P, Sciot R, Paterson A, et al: Cytokeratin expression in hepatocellular carcinoma: An immunohistochemical study. Hum Pathol 19:562, 1988
204. Klavins JV: Tumor markers of pancreatic carcinomas. Cancer 47:1597, 1981
205. Metzgar RS, Rodriguez N, Funn OJ, et al: Detection of pancreatic cancer associated antigen (DU-PAN2 antigen) in serum and ascites of patients with adenocarcinoma. Proc Natl Acad Sci USA 81:5242, 1984
206. Combs SG, Hidvegi DF, Ma Y, et al: Pleomorphic carcinoma of the pancreas with osteoclast-like giant cells expressing an epithelial associated antigen detected by monoclonal antibody 44-3-A6. Diagn Cytopathol 4:316, 1988
207. Haglund C, Roberts PF, Nordling S, et al: Expression of laminin in pancreatic neoplasms and in chronic pancreatitis. Am J Surg Pathol 8:669, 1984
208. Muraro R, Wunderlich D, Thor A, et al: Definition by monoclonal antibodies of a repertoire of epitopes on CEA differentially expressed in human colon carcinomas versus normal adult tissues. Cancer Res 45:5769, 1986
209. Holthofer H, Miettinen A, Passivuo R, et al: Cellular origin and differentiation of renal carcinomas. A fluorescence microscopic study with kidney specific antibodies, anti-intermediate filament antibodies and lectins. Lab Invest 49:317, 1983
210. Koprowska I, Zipsel S, Himes T, Herlijn M: The search for monoclonal antibodies to identify uterine epithelial neoplastic cells. Acta Cytol 29:920, 1985
211. Jothy S, Brazinsky SA, Chin-A-Lay M, et al: Characterization of monoclonal antibodies to CEA with increased tumor specificity. Lab Invest 54:108, 1986
212. Kline TS, Kannan V: Aspiration biopsy cytology and melanoma. Am J Clin Pathol 77:597, 1982
213. Walts AE: Malignant melanoma in effusions: A source of false negative cytodiagnosis. Diagn Cytopathol 2:150, 1986
214. Ordonez NG, Sneige N, Hickey RC, Brooks TE: Use of monoclonal antibody HMB-45 in the cytologic diagnosis of melanoma. Acta Cytol 32:684, 1988
215. Johnston WW, Borowitz MJ, Stuhlmiller GM, Seigler MD: Expression of a melanoma tumor-associated antigen as demonstrated by a monoclonal antibody (D6.1) in cytopathologic preparations of human tumor cells from effusions and needle aspirates. Anal Quant Cytol Histol 7:73, 1985
216. Angeli S, Koelma IA, Feuren GJ, Vanstechis GJ: Malignant melanoma in fine needle aspirates and effusions: An immunocytochemical study using monoclonal antibodies. Acta Cytol 32:707, 1988
217. Hammar S, Gould VE: Neuroendocrine neoplasms. p. 333. In Azar HA (ed): Pathology of Human Neoplasms. Raven Press, New York, 1988
218. Phalman S, Esscher T, Nilsson K: Expression of gamma-subunit of enolase, (neuron specific enolase) in human non-neuroendocrine tumors and derived cell lines. Lab Invest 54:554, 1986
219. Said JW, Vimadalal S, Nash G, et al: Immunoreactive neuron-specific enolase, bombesin and chromogranin as markers for neuroendocrine lung tumors. Hum Pathol 16:236, 1985
220. Nolan JA, Trojanowski JQ, Angeretti RH: Neurons and neuroendocrine cells contain chromogranins. J Histochem Cytochem 33:791, 1985
221. O'Connor DT: Chromogranin widespread immunoreactivity in polypeptide hormone producing tissues and in the serum. Regul Pept 6:263, 1983
222. Rode J, Dhillon AP, Doran JF, et al: PGP 9.5, a new marker for human neuroendocrine tumours. Histopathology 9:147, 1985
223. Gould VE, Wiedenmann B, Lee L, et al: Synaptophysin expression in neuroendocrine neoplasms as determined by immunocytochemistry. Am J Pathol 125:243, 1987
224. Swerdlow SH, Murray LF: Natural killer (Leu$_7^+$) cells in reactive lymphoid tissues and malignant lymphoma. Am J Clin Pathol 81:459, 1984
225. Lipinski M, Braham K, Caillaud JM, et al: HNK-1 antibody detects an antigen expressed on neuroectodermal cells. J Exp Med 158:1775, 1983
226. Szyfelbein WM, Ross JS: Carcinoids, atypical carcinoids and small cell carcinomas of the lung: Differential diagnosis of FNA biopsy specimens. Diagn Cytopathol 4:1, 1988
227. Horan DJ, Bonfiglio TA, Patten SF: Fine needle aspiration cytopathology of bronchial carcinoid tumors: An analytical study of the cells. Anal Quant Cytol 4:105, 1982
228. Caya JG, Wollenberg NG, Clowry LJ, Tieu TM: The diagnosis of pulmonary small cell anaplastic carcinoma by cytologic means: A 13 year experience. Diagn Cytopathol 4:202, 1988
229. Gould VE, Linnoila RI, Memoli VA, Warren WA: Neuroendocrine components of the bronchopulmonary tract: Hyperplasias, dysplasias and neoplasms. Lab Invest 49:519, 1983
230. Akhtar M, Ali MA, Sabbah R, et al: Aspiration cytology of neuroblastoma: Light and EM correlations. Cancer 57:797, 1986
231. Artlieb U, Krepler R, Wiche G: Expression of microtubule associated proteins (Map 1 and Map 2) in human neuroblastomas and differential diagnosis of immature neuroblasts. Lab Invest 53:684, 1985

232. Berthold F: Current concepts on the biology of neuroblastomas. Blut 30:65, 1985
233. Kay D, DeLellis RA, Dayal Y, et al: Ductal adenocarcinomas of the pancreas with neuroendocrine cells: An immunohistochemical study. Lab Invest 52:33, 1985
234. Chejfec G, Falkner S, Grimelius L, et al: Synaptophysin: A new marker for pancreatic endocrine cells and their neoplasms. Am J Surg Pathol 11:241, 1987
235. Nesland JM, Holm R, Johannessen JV, et al: Neuron specific enolase immunostaining in the diagnosis of breast carcinomas with neuroendocrine differentiation: Its usefulness and limitations. J Pathol 148:35, 1986
236. Briggs JC, Ibrahim NBN: Oat cell carcinoma of the oesophagus: A clinico-pathological study of 23 cases. Histopathology 7:261, 1983
237. Gnepp DR, Corio R, Brannon R: Small cell carcinoma of the major salivary glands. Cancer 58:705, 1986
238. Zak FG, Jindrak K, Capozzi F: Carcinoidal tumor of the kidney. Ultrastruct Pathol 4:51, 1983
239. Turbat-Herrera EA, Herrera GA, Gore I, et al: Neuroendocrine differentiation in prostatic carcinomas. Arch Pathol Lab Med 112:1100, 1988
240. Jaffee R, Santamaria M, Yunis EJ, et al: The neuroectodermal tumor of bone. Am J Surg Pathol 8:885, 1984
241. Dehner LP: Peripheral and central primitive neuroectodermal tumors: A nosologic concept seeking a consensus. Arch Pathol Lab Med 110:997, 1986
242. Sweeney EC, Barry-Walsh C, Robinson A: Sertoli-Leydig cell-tumor of the ovary with heterologous elements and carcinoid: an immunohistochemical and ultrastructural study. Ultrastruct Pathol 5:185, 1983
243. Wick MR, Schwithauer BW, Kovacs K: Neuron-specific enolase in neuroendocrine tumors of the thymus, bronchus and skin. Am J Clin Pathol 79:703, 1983
244. Inove M, Veda G, Yamasaki M, Tamaka Y, et al: Immunocytochemical demonstration of peptide hormones in endometrial carcinomas. Cancer 54:2127, 1984
245. Silva EG, Kott MM, Ordonez NG: Endocrine carcinoma, intermediate cell type of the uterine cervix. Cancer 54:1705, 1984
246. Miles PA, Herrera GA, Mena H, Trujillo I: Cytologic findings in primary malignant carcinoid of the cervix. Acta Cytol 29:1003, 1985
247. Tan TH, Young BW: Pheochromocytoma of the bladder: A case report. J Urol 87:63, 1962
248. Colby TV: Carcinoid tumor of the bladder: A case report. Arch Pathol Lab Med 104:199, 1980
249. Cefis F, Cattaneo M, Carnevale-Ricci PM, et al: Primary polypeptide hormone and mucin producing malignant carcinoid of the larynx. Ultrastruct Pathol 5:459, 1983
250. Foon KA, Todd RF: Immunologic classification of leukemia and lymphoma. Blood 68:1, 1986
251. Magidson JG, Cheng L, Hannah JB, Lewin KJ: Immunoperoxidase study of lymphomas-comparison of a one-step frozen section technique with indirect methods on paraffin sections. Am J Clin Pathol 84:166, 1985
252. Harris NL, Poppema S, Data RE: Demonstration of immunoglobulin in malignant lymphomas: Use of immunoperoxidase techniques in frozen sections. Am J Clin Pathol 78:14, 1982
253. Domagala W, Emeson EE, Koss LG: T and B lymphocytes enumeration in the diagnosis of lymphocyte-rich pleural fluid. Acta Cytol 25:108, 1981
254. Ghosh AK, Spriggs AL, Mason: Immunocytochemical staining of T and B lymphocytes in serous effusions. J Clin Pathol 38:608, 1985
255. Robey SS, Cafferty LL, Beschorner WE, Gupta PK: Value of lymphocyte marker studies in diagnostic cytopathology. Acta Cytol (Praha) 31:453, 1987
256. Yam LT, Lin DG, Janckila AJ, Li CY: Immunocytochemical diagnosis of lymphoma in serous effusions. Acta Cytol (Praha) 29:833, 1985
257. Martin SE, Zhang HZ, Magyarosy E, et al: Immunologic methods in cytology: Definitive diagnosis of non-Hodgkin's lymphomas using immunologic markers for T and B cells. Am J Clin Pathol 82:666, 1984
258. Harris NL, Khan AK: B-cell neoplasms of the lymphocytic, lympoplasmacytoid and plasma cell types. Hum Pathol 16:829, 1985
259. Taylor CB, Russell R, Chandor S: An immunohistologic study of multiple myeloma and related conditions, using an immunoperoxidase method. Am J Clin Pathol 70:612, 1978
260. Garcia CF, Weiss LM, Warnke RA: Small noncleaved cell lymphoma: An immunophenotypic study of 18 cases and comparison with large cell lymphoma. Hum Pathol 17:454, 1986
261. Hsu SM, Zhang HZ, Jaffee ES: Utility of monoclonal antibodies directed against B and T lymphocytes and monocytes in paraffin-embedded sections. Am J Clin Pathol 80:415, 1983
262. Marder RJ, Variakojis D, Silver J, Epstein AL: Immunohistochemical analysis of human lymphomas with monoclonal antibodies to B cell and Ia antigens reactive in paraffin sections. Lab Invest 52:497, 1985
263. Weiss JW, Winter MW, Phyliky RL, Banks PM: Peripheral T-cell lymphomas: Histologic, immunohis-

tologic and clinical characterization. Mayo Clin Proc 61:411, 1986
264. O'Hara MF, Cousar JB, Glick AD, Collins RD: Multiparameter approach to the diagnosis of hematopoietic-lymphoid neoplasms in body fluids. Diagn Cytopathol 1:33, 1985
265. Ramzy I, Rone R, Schultenover SJ, Buhaug J: Lymph node aspiration biopsy: diagnostic reliability and limitations—An analysis of 350 cases. Diagn Cytopathol 1:39, 1985
266. Young JA, Crocker J: Pleural fluid cytology in lymphoplasmacytoid lymphoma with numerous intracytoplasmic immunoglobulin inclusions. Acta Cytol 28:419, 1984
267. Collins RD: T-neoplasms: Their significance in relation to the classification system of lymphoid neoplasms. Am J Surg Pathol 6:755, 1983
268. Nathwani BN, Kim H: Rappaport: Malignant lymphoma, lymphoblastic. Cancer 38:964, 1976
269. Neiman RS: Immunoblastic sarcoma. Am J Surg Pathol 6:755, 1983
270. Lutsner M, Edleson R, Schein P, Green I, et al: Cutaneous T cell lymphomas: The Sézary syndrome, mycosis fungoides and related disorders. Ann Intern Med 83:534, 1975
271. Friedman M, Kim U, Shimaoka K, et al: Appraisal of aspiration cytology in management of Hodgkin's disease. Cancer 45:1653, 1980
272. Qizilbash A, Elavathil LJ, Chen V, et al: Aspiration biopsy cytology of lymph nodes in malignant lymphoma. Diagn Cytopathol 1:18, 1985
273. O'Dowd GJ, Frable WJ, Behm FG: Fine needle aspiration cytology of benign lymph node hyperplasias-diagnostic significance of lymphohistiocytic aggregates. Acta Cytol 29:554, 1985
274. Silverman JF: Fine needle aspiration cytology of cat scratch disease. Acta Cytol 29:542, 1985
275. Katz RL, Raval P, Manning JT, et al: A morphologic, immunologic, and cytometric approach to the classification of non-Hodgkin's lymphoma in effusions. Diagn Cytopathol 3:91, 1987
276. Feinberg MR, Bhaskar AC, Bourne P: Differential diagnosis of malignant lymphomas by imprint cytology. Acta Cytol 24:16, 1980
277. Wilkerson JA: Intraoperative cytology of lymph nodes and lymphoid lesions. Diagn Cytopathol 1:46, 1985
278. Levitt S, Cheng L, DuPuis MH, Layfield LF: Fine needle aspiration diagnosis of malignant lymphoma with confirmation by immunoperoxidase staining. Acta Cytol 29:895, 1985
279. Battifora H, Trowbridge IS: A monoclonal antibody useful for the differential diagnosis between malignant lymphoma and non-hematopoietic neoplasms. Cancer 51:816, 1983
280. Kurtin P, Pinkus GS: Leucocyte common antigen: A diagnostic discriminant between hematopoietic and non-hematopoietic neoplasms in paraffin sections using monoclonal antibodies. Hum Pathol 16:353, 1985
281. Linder J, Ye Y, Armitage JO, Weisenburger DD: Monoclonal antibodies marking B cell non-Hodgkin's lymphoma in paraffin-embedded tissue. Mod Pathol 1:29, 1988
282. Norton AJ, Ramsay AD, Smith SH, et al: Monoclonal antibody ($UCHL_1$) that recognizes normal and neoplastic T cells in routinely fixed tissues. J Clin Pathol 39:399, 1986
283. Wieczorek R, Buck D, Bindl J, Knowles DM: Monoclonal antibody Leu 22 (L60) permits the demonstration of some neoplastic T-cells in routinely fixed and paraffin-embedded tissue sections. Hum Pathol 19:1434, 1988
284. Cartun RW, Coles BF, Pastuszak WT: Utilization of monoclonal antibody L26 in the identification and confirmation of B cell lymphomas. Am J Pathol 129:415, 1987
285. Andres TL, Kadin ME: Immunologic markers in the differential diagnosis of small round cell tumors from lymphocytic lymphoma and leukemia. Am J Clin Pathol 79:546, 1983
286. Spagnolo DV, Michie SA, Crabtree GS, et al: Monoclonal anti-keratin (AE1) reactivity in routinely processed tissue from 166 human neoplasms. Am J Clin Pathol 84:697, 1985
287. Finley JL, Silverman J, Strausbauch PH, et al: Malignant thymic neoplasms: Diagnosis by fine-needle aspiration biopsy with histologic, immunocytochemical, and ultrastructural confirmation. Diagn Cytopathol 2:118, 1986
288. Walts AE, Said JW: Specific tumor markers in diagnostic cytology: Immunoperoxidase studies of CEA, lysozyme and other tissue antigens in effusions washes and aspirates. Acta Cytol 4:408, 1983
289. Strauchem JA, Dimitrious-Bona A: Malignant fibrous histiocytoma: Expression of monocyte/macrophage differentiation antigens detected with monoclonal antibodies. Am J Pathol 124:303, 1986
290. Kahn H, Hanna W, Yeger H, Barmal: Role of antibody to S100 protein in diagnostic pathology. Am J Clin Pathol 79:341, 1983
291. Drier JK, Swanson PE, Cherwitz DL, Wick MR: S100 protein immunoreactivity in poorly differentiated carcinomas. Arch Pathol Lab Med 111:447, 1987
292. Pinto MM: An immunoperoxidase study of S100 protein in neoplastic cells in serous effusions: Use as a marker for melanoma. Acta Cytol 30:240, 1986

293. Nakamura Y, Becker LE, Marks A: S100 protein in tumors of cartilage and bone: An immunohistochemical study. Cancer 52:1820, 1983
294. Kontozoglou T, Qizilbash AH, Sianos J, Stead R: Chordoma: Cytologic and immunocytochemical study of four cases. Diagn Cytopathol 2:55, 1986
295. Finley JL, Silverman JF, Dobbs DJ, et al: Chordoma: Diagnosis by FNA biopsy with histologic immunocytochemical and ultrastructural confirmation. Diagn Cytopathol 2:330, 1986
296. Brooks JJ: Immunohistochemistry of soft tissue tumors. Progress and prospects. Hum Pathol 13:969, 1982
297. Miettinen M, Lehto VP, Bedley RA, et al: Expression of intermediate filaments in soft tissue sarcomas. Int J Cancer 30:541, 1982
298. Ramaekers F, Haag D, Jap P, Vooijs P: Immunochemical demonstration of keratin and vimentin in cytologic aspirates. Acta Cytol 28:385, 1984
299. Chase DR, Enzinger FM, Weiss SW, Langloss JM: Keratin in epithelioid sarcoma: An immunohistochemical study. Am J Surg Pathol 8:435, 1984
300. Fisher C: Synovial sarcoma: Ultrastructural and immunocytochemical features of epithelial differentiation in monophasic and biphasic tumors. Hum Pathol 17:996, 1986
301. Bussolati G, Guliotta P, Fulcheri E: Immunohistochemistry of actin in normal and neoplastic tissues. p. 325. In DeLellis RA (ed): Advances in Immunohistochemistry. Masson, New York, 1984
302. Macartney JC, Trevithick MA, Kricka L, Cuvian RC: Identification of myosin in human epithelial cancers with immunofluorescence. Lab Invest 41:437, 1979
303. Mukai K, Rosai J, Burgdorf WHC: Localization of factor VIII related antigen in vascular cells using an immunoperoxidase method. Am J Surg Pathol 4:273, 1980
304. Ordonez NG, Batsakis JG: Comparison of *Ulex europaeus* lectin with Factor VIII related antigen in vascular lesions. Arch Pathol Lab Med 108:129, 1984
305. Auerbach R, Alby L, Grieves, et al: Monoclonal antibody against ACE: Its use as a marker for murine, bovine and human endothelial cells. Proc Natl Acad Sci USA 79:7891, 1982
306. Altmannsberger M, Weber K, Droste R, et al: Desmin is a specific marker for rhabdomyosarcoma of human and rat origin. Am J Pathol 118:85, 1983
307. Kindblom LG, Jacobsen GK, Jacobsen M: Immunohistochemical investigation of tumors of supposed fibroblastic-histiocytic origin. Hum Pathol 13:834, 1982
308. Golough R, Us-Krasovec. Differential diagnosis of the pleomorphic aspiration biopsy sample of non-epithelial lesions. Diagn Cytopathol 1:308, 1985
309. Walaas L, Agervall L, Hagmar B, et al: A correlative cytologic and histologic study of MFH: An analysis of 40 cases examined by FNA cytology. Diagn Cytopathol 2:46, 1986
310. du Boulay CEA: Demonstration of alpha-1 antitrypsin and alpha-1 antichymotrypsin in fibrous histiocytomas using the immunoperoxidase technique. Am J Surg Pathol 6:559, 1982
311. Nemes Z, Thomazy V: Factor XIIIa and the classic histiocytic markers in malignant fibrous histiocytoma: a comparative immunocytochemical study Human Pathol 19:822, 1988
312. Brooks JJ: Immunocytochemistry of soft tissue tumors: Myoglobin as a marker for rhabdomyosarcoma. Cancer 50:1757, 1982
313. Om A, Ghose T: Use of antiskeletal muscle antibody from myasthenic patients in the diagnosis of childhood rhabdomyosarcomas. Am J Surg Pathol 11:272, 1987
314. Mukai K, Iri H, Torikata C, et al: Immunoperoxidase demonstration of a new muscle protein (Z protein) in myogenic tumors as a diagnostic aid. Am J Pathol 114:164, 1984
315. deJong ASH, van Kessel-van Vark M, van Heerde P: Fine needle aspiration biopsy diagnosis of rhabdomyosarcoma. Acta Cytol 31:573, 1987
316. Popok SM, Naib ZM: Fine needle aspiration cytology of myositis ossificans. Diagn Cytopathol 1:236, 1985
317. Dahl I, Kerman M: Nodular fasciitis: A correlative cytologic and histologic study of 13 cases. Acta Cytol 25:215, 1980
318. Akerman M, Rydholm A: Aspiration cytology of lipomatous tumors: A 10 year experience at an orthopedic oncology center. Diagn Cytopathol 3:295, 1987
319. Akhtar M, Ali M, Sabbah R: Aspiration cytology of Ewing's sarcoma: Light and electron microscopic correlations. Cancer 56:2051, 1987
320. Dahl I, Hapmar B, Idvall I: Benign solitary neurilemmoma: A correlative cytologic and histological study of 28 cases. Acta Pathol Microbiol Immunol Scand [A] 92:91, 1981
321. Hood IC, Qizilbash AH, Young JM, Archibald SD: Needle aspiration cytology of a benign and a malignant schwannoma. Acta Cytol 28:158, 1984
322. Kapila K, Chopra P, Verma K: Fine needle aspiration cytology of alveolar soft part sarcoma: A case report. Acta Cytol 29:559, 1985

323. Nieberg RK: Fine needle aspiration cytology of alveolar soft part sarcoma: A case report. Acta Cytol 28:198, 1984
324. Rhydholm A, Akerman M, Idvall I, et al: Aspiration cytology of soft tissue tumors: A prospective study of its influence on choice of surgical procedure. Int Orthop 6:209, 1982
325. Van Stapel MJ, Gatter K, deWolf, et al: New sites of human S100 immunoreactivity detected with monoclonal antibodies. Am J Clin Pathol 85:160, 1986
326. Moll R, Lee I, Gould VE, et al: Immunocytochemical analysis of Ewing's tumors: Patterns of expression of intermediate filaments and desmosomal proteins indicate cell type heterogeneity and pluripotential differentiation. Am J Pathol 127:288, 1987
327. Ramaekers F, Puts J, Kaut J, et al: Differential diagnosis of human carcinomas, sarcomas and their metastases using antibodies to intermediate-sized filaments. Eur J Cancer Clin Oncol 18:1251, 1982
328. Mogollon R, Penneys NS, Albores-Saavedra J, et al: Malignant Schwannoma presenting as a skin mass: Confirmation by the demonstration of myelin basic protein within tumor cells. Cancer 53:1193, 1984
329. Bedrossian CWM, Martinez F, Silverberg A: Fine needle aspiration. p. 25. In Gnepp D (ed): Pathology of the Head and Neck. Churchill Livingstone, New York, 1988
330. Lobzik L, Antman KH, Warhol MJ: The distinction of mesothelioma from adenocarcinoma in malignant effusion by electron microscopy. Acta Cytol 29:219, 1985
331. Silverman JF, Nance K, Phillips B, Norris HT: The use of immunoperoxidase panels for the cytologic diagnosis of malignancy in serous effusions. Diagn Cytopathol 3:134, 1987
332. Sehested M, Ralfkjaer E, Rasmussen J: Immunoperoxidase demonstration of carcinoembryonic antigen in pleural and peritoneal effusions. Acta Cytol 27:125, 1983
333. Orell SR, Dowling KD: Oncofetal antigens as tumor markers in the cytologic diagnosis of effusions. Acta Cytol 27:625, 1983
334. Cibas ES, Corson JM, Pinkus GS: The distinction of adenocarcinoma from malignant mesothelioma in cell blocks of effusions: The role of routine mucin histochemistry and immunohistochemical assessment of carcinoembryonic antigen, keratin proteins, epithelial membrane antigen, and milk fat globule-derived antigen. Hum Pathol 18:67, 1987
335. To A, Dearnaley DP, Orerod MG, et al: Epithelial membrane antigen: Its use in the cytodiagnosis of malignancy in serous effusions. Am J Clin Pathol 78:214, 1982
336. Unger K, Raber M, Bedrossian CWM, et al: Analysis of pleural effusion using automated flow cytometry. Cancer 52:873, 1983
337. Stonesifer KJ, Xiang J, Wilkinson EJ, et al: Flow cytometric analysis and cytopathology of body cavity fluids. Acta Cytol 31:125, 1987
338. Martin SE, Moshiri S, Thor A, et al: Identification of adenocarcinoma in cytospin preparation of effusions using monoclonal antibody B72.3. Am J Clin Pathol 86:10, 1986
339. Leong A S-Y, Parkinson R, Milios J: "Thick" cell membrane revealed by immunocytochemical staining: A clue to the diagnosis of mesothelioma. Diagn Cytopathol (In press)
340. Barlogie B: Abnormal cellular DNA content as a marker of neoplasia. Eur J Cancer Clin Oncol 20:1123, 1984
341. Bedrossian CWM, Raber M, Barlogie B: Flow cytometry and cytomorphology in primary resectable breast cancer. Anal Quant Cytol 3:112, 1981
342. Henry MJ, Stanley MW, Swenson B, et al: Cytologic assessment of tumor cells kinetics: Applications of monoclonal antibody Ki-67 to fine needle aspiration smears. Diagn Cytopathol (In press)
343. Busch A, Gyorkey F, Busch RK, et al: A nucleolar antigen found in a broad range of human malignant tumor specimens. Cancer Res 39:3024, 1979

Index

Page numbers followed by f refer to figures; those followed by t refer to tables.

Abscess
  pancreatic, 288
  subareolar, 173
Acantholysis, in pemphigus vulgaris, 263
Acid-secreting glands, stomach, 266
Acinar cell, 424
  adenocarcinoma, grading of, 324t
  carcinoma
    pancreatic, 280–281, 286, 286f
    salivary gland, 255, 257f, 258
  salivary gland, 252
Acinar component, atrophy of, 283
Acinar formations, in islet cell neoplasms, 287
Acinar units, lobular, 252
Acquired immune deficiency syndrome (AIDS), patients at risk for, lymph node fine needle aspiration in, 398
Actin, 412
  skeletal muscle, 439
  smooth muscle, 414
Actinomyces
  infection, female genital tract, 31, 32f–33f
  israelii, 31
  sp., IUD and, 92
Actinomycosis, respiratory tract, 196
Acute lymphocytic leukemia, 387
Adenoacanthoma, endometrial, 107, 109f, 109, 110f–111f
Adenocarcinoma
  of colon, 275–276f
  cytologic features, 217t
  cytoplasmic characteristics in, 11, 14f–15f, 16
  differentiated from
    mesothelioma, 443
    squamous carcinoma, 209t
  ductal, 280
  endocervical, 82–86, 114
  endometrial, 101
  clear cell cancer, 107, 108f
  cytologic findings, 101–103, 103f–106f
  diagnostic considerations, 101
  serous papillary, 103, 107f
  esophageal, 266, 267f
  gastric, 266, 269–271
  keratin expression in, 410, 411
  liver, 299–300
  lung, 127, 128f, 211, 212–219
    diagnostic pitfalls, 216–219
    metastatic, 216, 218f, 219, 225
    tumor markers in, 426–427
  metastasis to brain, 364t, 372, 374f, 375f, 376
  metastatic, in effusions, 344, 345, 346
  metastatic workup, 442
  pancreatic, 288
  periampullary, 273, 274, 274f
  prostatic, 326, 329f–332
    acinar, grading of, 342t
    histologic grading of, 323–324, 324t
    response to hormonal therapy, 333t, 333
  renal, metastasis to liver, 300
  salivary gland, 259
  scar, 184
  secretory markers in, 421, 421f, 422f, 422–424
  thyroid
    follicular, 238
    papillary, 238–241
  urothelial, 319–320
  uterine, 129
  vaginal, 49
Adenohypophysis, neoplasms, 419
Adenoid cystic carcinoma
  cells from, 9–10, 10f
  of salivary gland, 258–259
Adenoma
  colon, 275
  liver cell, 295, 297
  monomorphic, of salivary glands, 254, 255
  pituitary, 419
  pleomorphic, See Pleomorphic adenoma
  thyroid
    colloid, 236–237
    microfollicular and trabecular, 237–238
Adenomatous hyperplasia, endometrial, 99
Adenosis, vaginal, 47, 48f
Adenovirus, pneumonia from, 203
Adrenal gland, tumors, hormones produced by, 419
Adriamycin, cytopathology of, 159
Aerosol-type fixative, 16
AIDS, See Acquired immune deficiency syndrome
Air-drying, 164
  artifacts in, 1, 3f, 16, 18
Alcian blue, 18, 405, 421
Alcohol-based fixatives, 404
Alkaline phosphatase-antialkaline phosphatase (ALP) technique, 404, 404t, 405
Alpha-fetoprotein (AFP), 358
  in adenocarcinoma, hepatic, 299, 300
  in effusions, 354
  levels, in hepatocellular carcinoma, 297
  as tumor marker, 415, 416
α-1 antichymotrypsin, in hepatocellular carcinoma, 14–25
Alveolar spaces, in herpes virus infection, 200
Amelanotic melanoma, 300
American Burkitt's lymphoma, 389
Amphophilia, cytoplasmic, 146, 146f
Anaplastic carcinoma, of thyroid gland, 242, 244
Aneuploidy, 445
Antibodies, *See also* specific antibody
  directed at infectious agents, 406, 406t

459

Antibody methods
    direct labeled, 404
    unlabeled, comparison of, 404, 404t
Antibody panels, multiple, 404
α_1 Antichymotrypsin (A_1ACT), 414, 438
    in carcinomas, 445
        hepatocellular, 427
    in mesenchymal tumor, 439
Antigen(s), multiple, 404
Antigen antibody staining, in human papillomavirus infection, 40, 43f, 44f
Antigenicity, preservation of, 403
Antiskeletal muscle, 429
α_1 Antitrypsin (A_1ACT), 414, 416, 438
    in carcinoma, 445
        hepatocellular, 427
    in mesenchymal tumor, 439
Anti-Z-protein antibodies, 439
Apocrine cells, breast, 166, 167f
Apocrine carcinoma, of breast, 178
APUD, tumors of, 385
Arias-Stella phenomenon, 94, 96f
Artifact
    air-drying, 1, 3f, 16, 18
    of cytocentrifugation, 17
    in Papanicolaou-stained slides, 18
Asbestos bodies, 187, 187f
Ascaris lumbricoides, 47
Ascites, 337
    in extrauterine cancers, 133
    in liver cirrhosis, 341
Aspergillosis pneumonia, 194, 194t, 195f–196
Aspirates
    fine needle, in metastatic workup, 442–443
    postexcisional, 440, 441
Aspiration, *See also* Fine needle aspiration
    endometrial, 87, 133
Astrocytoma, brain, 365, 366f–368f
Atypical cells, in breast cancer, 178–179
Autolysis, cytoplasmic, 146
Avidin-biotin complex (ABC) technique, 404, 404t, 405

B-cell immunoblastic sarcoma, 393, 394f
B-cell lymphoma
    classification of, 382t, 382
    gastric, 271
    markers for, 433, 434
B5, 405
B72.3, 417
Bacterial infections
    of female genital tract, 28t, 28–31, 32f–33f
    of lung, 204

Balloon catheter, esophageal screening with, 261–262
Barrett's epithelium, 266
Barrett's esophagus, 263, 264, 265f
Basal cells
    prostate, 424
    respiratory tract, 185, 186f
Basophilic inclusion, in cytomegalovirus pneumonia, 202, 202f
"BB shots," 40, 45f
BCG, 318
Benign cells
    breast, 174
    radiation effects on, 149, 150
Bile duct, granular cell tumors of, 274
Bilirubin, 292
Binucleation
    in macrophages, 339
    post-irradiation, 145f–146f, 147, 148f
Bischlorethylnotrosourea (BCNU), cytopathology of, 159
Bladder
    carcinoma, metastatic, from cervical carcinoma, diagnosis, radiation effects on, 158
    cyclophosphamide effects on, 159
    lesions, 303–304
        metastatic, 320
    mapping, 315
    papillary tumors, of, grading of, 307, 307t
Bland cells, in acinar cell carcinoma, of salivary gland, 258
Blast crisis, 387
Blast-like cells, in granulocytic sarcoma, 398, 400f
Blastomyces
    dermatitidis, 193
    differentiated from Cryptococcis, 193, 194
    lung inflammation from, 189t
Blastomycosis, North American, lung, 193–194
Bleomycin, cytopathology of, 159
"Blue blobs," 244
    extracellular, 2, 3f
    in thyroiditis, 244, 246f
Blue round cell tumors, small, differential diagnosis of, 413, 413t
Body cavities
    anatomy and histology of, 337
    fluids, *See* effusions
Bombesin, 430
Bone marrow, cells from, in lymphoma, 437
Bowen's disease, *See* Carcinoma in situ, of vulva
Brain tumors
    metastatic, 372, 373f–376

primary, 363
    gliomas, 365, 366f–371f
    meningioma, 372, 374f
    midline tumors, 365t, 371, 372, 373f
    neural crest tumors, 365t, 369f, 371, 372f, 373f
Breast
    adenocarcinoma of
        cell relationships in, 11, 14f–15f, 16
        metastasis from brain, 364f
        metastasis to lung, 216, 218f, 219
    carcinoma
        metastatic, in effusions, 346, 348f, 349
        of Paget's disease of nipple versus benign papilloma, 169–170
        tumor markers in, 425, 426
    fine needle aspiration cytology, 163–164
        in cancer, 173–179
        of cysts, 166
        of fat necrosis, 172, 172f
        of fibroadenoma, 166, 167–169
        of fibrocystic change, 164, 165–166, 167f
        of gynecomastia, 172
        of inflammation, 173
        of nipple secretions, 173
        of normal breast tissue, 161, 164f, 165f
        of papillary lesions, 170, 170f
        in pregnancy and lactation, 170, 171–172
        of radiation changes, 172, 173
        of subareolar abscess, 173
Bronchi, methotrexate effects on, 160
Bronchial aspirates and sputum, cell preservation in, 17
Bronchioloalveolar carcinoma, 184, 211, 212, 214, 215f–216
    subclassification of, 421
Bronchoalveolar lavage, in lymphoma of lung, 225
Bronchogenic adenocarcinoma, 212–214
Bronchogenic squamous carcinoma, 216, 216f
Brush(es), endocervical, 24
Brush cytology
    in colon specimen collection, 274, 275
    in duodenal specimen collection, 272
    esophageal, 261, 262, 263f
Burkitt's lymphoma, 387
    classic, 389
    differentiation of, 434
    gastric, 271
Busulfan (Myleran)
    cytopathology of, 159

in squamous cell carcinoma, 210t, 210, 211
urothelial atypia from, 318, 319

CA-1, 422
Ca-19.9, 425
CA-125, 425, 426
Calcific concretions, 187
Calcitonin, 419
Calcium oxylate crystals, 196
Calyces, 304
Campylobacter pylori, 269
Cancer cells, characteristics, in breast cancer, 174, 175, 175f
Candida, 182
  albicans
    esophagitis, 262
    female genital tract infection, 40, 44f–45f
    gastric infection, 269
    yeast forms of, 40f, 44f–45f
Candidiasis
  respiratory tract, 196
  uterine cervix, 54–55
"Cannonballs," 40, 45f
Carbowax fixative, 17
Carcinoembryonic antigen (CEA), 358, 405, 419, 438
  in effusions, 354
  in metastatic workup, 442, 443
  nonsecretory, 411
  as tumor marker, 415, 421
Carcinoid cells, atypical, 224
Carcinoid tumors
  immunocytochemistry of, 405
  lung, 224–225
  metastasis to liver, 300
  pancreatic, 287, 288
Carcinoma, *See also* specific type, specific body area
  differentiation of mesothelioma from, 417
  metastatic, *See* Metastatic carcinoma
  recurrent, post-irradiation, 157
  vimentin expression in, 411
Carcinoma in situ
  breast, 178, 179
  of cervix, *See* Cervix, uterine, dysplasia and carcinoma in situ
  urinary tract, radioresistant, 158
  urothelial, 311, 315, 316f
  of vulva, 51f–52f, 53
Carcinomatosis, meningeal, 359
Carcinomatous cells, post-irradiation, 157
Cardia, 266
Carnoy's fixative, 16

Catheterization
  in carcinoma in situ, urothelial, 315
  in urothelial cytology, 323
Cavities, of body, *See* Body cavities
Cell(s)
  arrangements of, in dysplasia and carcinoma in situ of cervix, 64, 65f
  characteristics, in breast cancer, 174–175
  clusters, from breast cancer, 174, 175f
  desquamation of, factors influencing, 133
  normal cytology of, 5–9
  relationships, in malignancy, 11
  size and shape
    cytoskeletal determinants of, 408, 408t
    estimating of, 5
    radiation effects on, 147, 148, 148f, 150f
Cell balls, 11, 16f
  from clear cell adenocarcinoma, 107, 108f
Cell block, 17
  in adenocarcinoma, renal, 300
  advantages of, 17–18
  in effusions, 353
  in hepatocellular carcinoma, 297
  in immunocytochemistry, 404, 405
Cell membrane, disintegration, post-irradiation, 144f, 147
Cellular pleomorphic adenoma, 252
Cellular specimens, 403
Cellularity, in breast cancer, 174
Central nervous system, cytology of, 357 *See also* Cerebrospinal fluid
  cellular patterns, 359–360, 360f
  clinical history, 357–358
  metastatic tumors, 376f, 376–377
  special studies, 358
  specimen collection, 358
  specimen preparation, 358
  tumors of, 359t, 363, 364f, 365t, 366t
    brain, *See* Brain, tumors
Centrifugation, 17
Cerebrospinal fluid (CSF)
  lymphoid cells in, cytomorphology of, 366t
  physiology of, 358
  source of, 357
  specimens, 17
    collection, 358
  tumor in, cytomorphologic characteristics of, 365t
  tumor cells in, 359
Cervical intraepithelial neoplasia (CIN), 18, 61
Cervical scrape, 87

Cervical-vaginal smears, 28
  cancer cells in, post-irradiation, 156, 157
Cervical-vaginal-endocervical (CVE) smear, 1, 17, 24, 28
  during menstruation, 88, 88f
  endometrial cells in, 87
  in ovarian neoplasms, 16, 117f, 118f, 119f
Cervicitis, follicular, 36f, 37
Cervix, uterine
  atrophy, 58, 59f
  cancer
    bladder metastasis, 158
    development of, 24
    microinvasive, cytologic features of, 72, 73, 74f–75
    vaginal smear cytology, postirradiation, 151
  carcinoma
    bladder metastasis, 158
    microinvasive, cytologic features of, 72, 73, 74f–75
  chemotherapy effects on, 159
  dysplasia and carcinoma in situ, 60
    biology of cervical neoplasia, 61, 64–65
    cytologic features of, 65–70
    keratinizing dysplasia, 70, 72f, 72
    morphologic features and subclasses of, 60–61, 62f–63f, 64t
    nonkeratinizing dysplasia, 70, 71f, 72f
    severity, cytologic evaluation of, 66, 67f–70
  endocervical adenocarcinoma, 82–86
  folic acid deficiency effects, 58
  hyperkeratosis of, 57
  infectious diseases of, 53–57, 57f
  irradiation of, 58
  parakeratosis of, 57
  reparative changes, 58, 60
  small cell carcinoma of, 80f, 81
  squamous cell carcinoma of,
    cytologic manifestations of, 75–81
    differential diagnosis of, 81–82
    recurrent, post-irradiation, 155f
  squamous metaplasia of, 57, 58f, 58
Charcot-Leyden crystals, 187
Chemotherapy, *See also* specific agent
  cytopathology of, 141, 142f, 158–160
  in squamous cell carcinoma, 210t, 210, 211
Chlamydia, 407, 407f
  infection, of uterine cervix, 54
  trachomatis infection, female genital tract, 31, 34f–37
"Chinese character configuration," 197
Chlorambucil, cytopathology of, 159

Chloroma, *See* Granulocytic sarcoma
Cholangiocarcinoma
  of liver, 299
  markers for, 427
Cholecystitis, chronic, 272, 273
Cholelithiasis, 272, 273
Chondroblasts, in Müllerian tumors, endometrial, 113
Choriocarcinoma
  endometrial, 113, 114f
  oncofetal markers in, 415, 415t, 417f
Choroid plexus
  cells
    in neonatal head trauma, 363f
    neurofilament expression in, 412
  papillomas, 365
Chromatin, 10
  in breast cancer cells, 174
  in cervical dysplasia and carcinoma in situ, 66, 66f
  in cytomegalovirus, 37
  in herpes simplex virus, 37, 38f
  in lymphoma, 386
  in pancreatic duct carcinoma, 283
  in squamous cell carcinoma, cervical, 74f, 75f, 77
  in ovarian carcinoma, 116
  in thyroid cell, 234, 235
Chromatolysis, 147
Chromogranin, in neuroendocrine markers, 430
Chronic lymphocytic leukemia, 388, 388f
Chronic myelogenous leukemia (CML), 387
Chylothorax, 337
Cilia, 6f
Ciliated columnar cells, respiratory tract, 183, 184, 185f
Cirrhosis, liver, 293
  ascites in, 341
  cytologic changes in, 297
  diagnosis, 293, 294f
CK1-CK4 antibodies, 410
Clara cells
  in bronchioalveolar carcinoma, 214
  neoplasms derived from, 421
  respiratory tract, 184
Clear cell(s), 49
Clear cell carcinoma
  endometrial, 107, 108
  metastatic, in effusions, 349
  of vagina, 49, 50f
Clonorchis sinensis infection, 299
Clue cells, in *Gardnerella (hemophilus) vaginalis,* 28, 31, 54
Coccidioides
  immitis, 190

lung inflammation from, 189, 190t
Coccidioidomycosis, lung, 190, 191, 191f–192f
"Cockleburrs," 94, 97f
Cohesive cells, malignant, 385
Colitis, ulcerative, *See* Inflammatory bowel disease, idiopathic
Collagen, in smear background, 405
Colloid carcinoma, breast, fine needle aspiration, 176–177
Colon
  adenocarcinoma, metastatic
    to brain, 364f
    in effusions, 349
    to liver, 299
    to lung, 216, 218f
  carcinoma, 118, 124f–127
  cytology of, 274
    of pathologic conditions, 275, 276f
    specimen collection, 274, 275
Colonoscopy, 261
Columnar cells
  in adenocarcinoma, esophageal, 266
  atypical, shedding of, in pregnancy, 94
  in Barrett's esophagus, 263, 264f
  in carcinoma, colonic, 118, 127f, 127
  endocervical, 5, 6f
  gastric, 7
  metaplastic, in *Chlamydia trachomatis,* 31, 34f–35f
  respiratory tract, 183, 184f, 184, 185f
Computerized tomography (CT), in central nervous system studies, 357, 358
Concretions, 187
Condyloma, 55, 64
  acuminatum, of vulva, 53
  atypical, 55, 56f, 58f
  uterine cervix, 59f
Congestive heart failure, pleural effusion from, 342
Core needle biopsy
  hepatic, 291, 293
  pancreatic, 279
Corpora amylacea, 187
Cotton swab specimens, 24
Cowdry type A inclusions, 201f, 201
Creola bodies, 184, 216
Crohn's disease, *See* Inflammatory bowel disease, idiopathic
Cryptococcosis, lung, 191, 192f, 193
Cryptococcus
  differentiated from *Blastomyces,* 193, 194
  differentiated from *Histoplasma,* 193
  lung inflammation from, 189, 190t

  neoformans, 191
Curschmann's spirals, 186, 186f, 187
CVE smears, *See* Cervical-vaginal-endocervical smears
Cyclophosphamide (Cytoxan)
  cytopathology of, 142f, 159–160
  urothelial atypia from, 318
Cyst
  breast, 173
    fine needle aspiration of, 166
  mucoepidermoid carcinoma and, 259
  pancreatic, 281
  salivary gland, 253
  thyroglossal duct, 247–249
  thyroid, 237
Cystadenocarcinoma
  ovarian, 132
  pancreatic, 281, 288–289
    mucinous, 281
Crystadenoma, pancreatic,
    mucinous, 281
    serous (microcystic or glycogen-rich), 289
Cystic endometrial hyperplasia, 99
Cystic masses, pancreatic, 288–289
Cystic papillary carcinoma, thyroid, 236
Cystitis
  cystica, 304
  hemorrhagic, 157
Cytocentrifugation, 17, 358
  artifacts of, 17
Cytochemistry, in effusion, 354
Cytohormonal evaluation, of female genital tract, 25–27
  abnormal hormonal patterns, 27–28
  maturation index, 27, 27t
Cytohormonal pattern, in extrauterine cancer, 133
Cytokeratin, 409, 410
Cytologic methods and techniques, 16–18
Cytomegalovirus (CMV), infection, 5f
  female genital tract, 37, 39f
Cytomegalovirus esophagitis, 262
Cytomegalovirus pneumonia, 202–203
Cytopathology, defined, 1
Cytoplasm
  adenocarcinoma
    endocervical, 84, 85f
    endometrial, 103, 104f, 105f
  autolysis, 146
  in carcinoma, pancreatic duct, 283
  features, in malignancy, 11, 14f–15f
  in breast cells, in pregnancy and lactation, 171
  in cervical dysplasia and carcinoma in situ, 65, 66, 67f, 70, 71f

in medullary carcinoma, of thyroid gland, 242, 244f
of mesothelial cells, 339
organelles, cell type differentiation by, 414
in papillary carcinoma, of thyroid, 239, 240f, 241f
radiation effects on, 142, 143–146, 147
in thyroid hyperfunction, 235
Cytoplasmic amphophilia, 146, 146f
Cytoplasmic deposits, 147
Cytoplasmic extensions, 365
Cytoplasmic inclusions, in cytomegalovirus pneumonia, 201, 202f
Cytoplasmic membrane system, of neoplastic cells, 416, 417–419
Cytoxan, See Cyclophosphamide

Debris, necrotic, 389
Decidual cells, shedding of, in pregnancy, 94, 95f
Decoy cells, 307
Desmin, 412
  in mesenchymal neoplasms, 438t, 439
  tumors coexpressing, 409t
Desquamation, of cells, factors influencing, 133
Diarrhea, 275
Diathesis, tumor, 221
  oat cell carcinoma, 219, 221
  squamous cell carcinoma, 206, 209f
Diethylstilbestrol (DES), vaginal tumors and, 47, 49
Differentiation, indicators of, 414–415
  epithelial membrane antigens, 416, 417–419
  hormones, 419–420
  oncofetal markers, 415–416
  secretory markers, 421–424
DNA
  in human papillomavirus, 40
  in malignant nuclei, 10
  nuclear content, 445
  staining of, 18
  in urothelial tumors, 307
Döderlein bacilli, 54
Donovan bodies, 30f, 31, 49
Drugs, See also specific agent
  urothelial neoplasms induced by, 317–319
Duodenum, cytology of, 261
  normal, 272, 273f
  of pathologic conditions, 272, 273–274
"Dust cells," 1, 9
Dysgerminoma, oncofetal markers of, 415, 415t
Dyskeratocytes, 55

Dysplasia, post-irradiation, 152f, 153f, 153–157
Dysplastic cells, 92

Echinococcus, 2
Ectocervical smear, 28
Ectopic pregnancy, 94
EDTA, 430
Effusions
  benign conditions in, cytology of, 339–342, 354
  causes of, 339
  classification of, 337, 339
  malignant tumors in, cytology of, 342
    leukemia, 349
    lymphoma, 349, 350f
    mesothelioma, 345, 345f
    metastatic tumors, 345, 346–349, 351, 352f
    myeloma, 349, 350f, 351
  practical considerations
    clinical correlations, 353–354
    cytohistologic correlations, 353
    differential diagnosis, 352
    special procedures, 354–355
  terminology, 337
  types, 338–339
Electron microscopy
  in effusions, 353f, 354
  of mesothelioma, 345, 345f
  of metastatic carcinoma, in effusions, 349
  of pneumocytes, 186
Endocervical brushes, 24
Endocervical cells
  columnar, 5, 6f, See also Columnar cells
  differentiated from endometrial cells, 91f, 92
  during menstruation, 91f
Endocervical smear, 28
Endocervix
  adenocarcinoma, 114
  radiation effects on, 150
Endocrine neoplasms, hormone and markers in, 418t, 419
Endometrial cells
  abnormal shedding of, 92–99
  differentiated from endocervical cells, 91f, 92
  during menstruation, 89f
Endometrial hyperplasia, cell changes in, 94, 98f–100f
Endometrium, cytology of
  aspiration techniques, 133
  of benign disorders, 87–101
    abnormal shedding of endometrial cells, 92–99

  diagnostic considerations, 87–92
  polyps, 94, 98f
  of malignant diseases, 113
    adenoacanthoma and adenosquamous carcinoma, 107, 109f, 109, 110f–111f
    adenocarcinoma, 101–103, 104f–107f
    carcinoma, 49, 84t, 128
    clear cell carcinoma, 107, 108f
    differential diagnosis, 115, 115t
    metastatic, 113, 114f
    Müllerian tumors, 109, 111f, 113
    radiation effects, 150
    sampling techniques, 24, 87
    serous papillary carcinoma, 103, 103f, 104f
Endometrium "wreath," during menstruation, 89f
Endometrioid carcinoma, prostatic, 332, 333
Endoplasmic reticulum, rough, 414
Endoscopic retrograde cholangio-pancreatography (ERCP), 272, 281, 282
Endospores, coccidioidomycosis, 191
Endothelial cell, hepatic, 292, 292f
  in hepatocellular carcinoma, 297, 297f
Enolase, neuron specific, 358, 413
Entamoeba histolytica, 275
  infection, female genital tract, 47
Enterobius vermicularis, 47
Enzyme-secreting glands, stomach, 266
Eosin, See Hematoxylin and eosin stain
Ependymoma, 363, 365, 368f, 369f
Epidermoid carcinoma, of lung, 206–211
Epithelial atypia, gastric, 268f, 268
Epithelial cells
  biliary, in adenocarcinoma, hepatic, 299
  columnar, See also Columnar cells
    bronchial, 5, 6f
  differentiation of, 415
  during menstruation, 90f
  in extrauterine cancer, 117f–118f, 120f–123f, 129f, 129
  in fine needle aspiration specimens, 381
  intermediate filaments in, 408t
  malignant, detection of, 417
  in mammary dysplasia, 165, 165f
  in monomorphic adenoma of salivary gland, 254
  pancreatic duct, 282
  in pancreatitis, 283f, 283
  in pleomorphic adenoma, of salivary glands, 254, 255f

Epithelial cells (*Continued*)
  in prostatic hyperplasia, 324, 326f, 327f
  in reflux esophagitis, 262
Epithelial dysplasia, gastric, 269
Epithelial hyperplasia, atypical, respiratory tract, 184, 185t
Epithelial membrane antigen, 348
  differentiation by, 416, 417–419
Epithelial repair
  in squamous cell carcinoma, cervical, 81, 81f
  thyroid gland, 247
Epithelioid cells
  histiocytes, 385
  in leiomyosarcoma, gastric, 271
  in thyroiditis, 246
Epithelium
  adenomatous, of colon, 275
  gastric, 266, 267f
  human, Moll's keratin subfamilies in, 409, 410f
  from normal breast tissue, 164, 165f
  in prostatitis, 326, 328f
Esophagitis
  Candida albicans, 262
  herpetic, 200
  reflux, 262, 263f
  viral, 262
Esophagus
  cyclophosphamide effects on, 159
  cytology of
    of neoplastic lesions, 263, 264–266, 267f
    of non-neoplastic lesions, 262–263, 264f
    normal, 261
    specimen collection, 261–262
  radiation effects on, 157–158
  squamous carcinoma of, 211
Estrogen, squamous cell response to, 25
Ethanol, for smear fixation, 16, 17, 404
Ewing's sarcoma, 387
  markers for, 440
Exocrine carcinoma, markers for, 428
Extrauterine cancer, *See* Genital tract, female, extrauterine cancer
Exudates, 339

Factor VIII-related antigen, 438, 438t
Fallopian tube, tumors, 28
False-negative smears, in adenocarcinoma of endometrium, 101
Fast smear, 24
  vaginal component of, 28
Fat
  necrosis, breast, 172, 172f

  vacuoles, in hepatocellular carcinoma, 296
Fat cells, breast, fine aspiration of, 164, 164f
Fecal material, in prostatic cytology, 332
Female, genital tract, *See* Genital tract, female
Ferruginous bodies, 187, 187f
Fetal calf serum, 379
Fibroadenoma, of breast, 179
  fine needle aspiration of, 166, 167–169
Fibroblasts, 414
Fibrocystic change, of breast, 164–166
Fibrolamellar carcinoma, diagnosis, 297
Filament typing, 354
Filling defects, urothelial, 303
Filter preparations, 17
Filtration methods, in central nervous system studies, 358
Fine needle aspirates, in metastatic workup, 442–443
Fine needle aspiration, 1, 18–19
  of breast, *See* Breast, fine needle aspiration of
  of liver, *See* Liver, fine needle aspiration of
  of lymph nodes, *See* Lymph nodes, fine needle aspiration of
  of pancreas, *See* Pancreas, fine needle aspiration of
  of prostate gland, *See* Prostate gland, fine needle aspiration of
  of salivary glands, *See also* Salivary glands
  of thyroid gland, *See* Thyroid gland, fine needle aspiration of
Fixation
  in immunocytochemistry, 403, 404
  rapid, 16, 17
  of female genital tract cells, 24
Fixative
  aerosol-type, 16
  Carbowax, 17
"Flame cells," 235
Flow cytometry, 445
  for lymphoma classification, 433
Fluids
  body
    collection, 17
    in metastatic workup, 443–445
    processing of, 17
    specimens, preservation of, 16–17
  body cavity, *See* Effusions
FNA, *See* Fine needle aspiration
Focal nodular hyperplasia, 195
Folic acid, deficiency, 58, 141
Follicular adenoma, thyroid, 246
Follicular carcinoma
  thyroid, 233, 238

  vimentin expression in, 411, 412f
Follicular cells, thyroid, 234, 234f
  in thyroiditis, 246
Follicular center cells (FCC), 383
Follicular structures, in thyroid
  multinodular, 236f, 236
  uninodular, 236–238
Fontana-Masson panel, 428, 430
Formaldehyde solutions, 404
Formalin, 404
Franzen needle and guide, 323
Fungal infections, female genital tract, 28t, 40, 44f–45f
Fungal pneumonias, invasive, 194–196
Fungi, 182
  causing granulomatous inflammation in lung, 188, 189–194
  variably producing disease, 196–199

Gardnerella (hemophilus) vaginalis, 28, 29f, 31, 54
Gastric columnar cells, normal, 7f
Gastrin, islet cell tumors stained for, 431f
Gastritis, 269
Gastrointestinal tract, cytology of
  colon, 274, 275, 276f
  duodenum, 272–274, 274f
  esophagus, 261–266, 267f
  salivary glands, 251–261
  stomach, 266, 267–272f
Genital tract, female, cytology of, 23–24
  bacterial infections, 28t, 28–31, 32f–33f
  cervix, *See* Cervix, uterine
  Chlamydia trachomatis infection, 31, 34f–37
  cytohormonal evaluation, 25–28
  cytopathologic reporting, 24–25
  of endometrium, *See* Endometrium
  extrauterine cancer, 115, 127, 128f
    associated findings, 128–133
    colonic neoplasms, 118, 124f–127
    factors influencing desquamation of cells, 133
    incidence, 115–116
    mammary neoplasms, 118, 120f–123f
    ovarian neoplasms, 116, 117f–118f, 119f
  fungal infections, 40, 44f–45f
  parasitic infestations, 28t, 40, 44f–47
  radiation therapy cytopathology, *See* Radiation therapy
  sampling techniques, 24
  vaginal, 47–49

viral infections, 37–40, 41f–44f
vulva, 49, 51f–57, 57f
Germ cell tumors, 437
  oncofetal markers of, 415, 415t
Germinoma, of pineal area, 371, 373f
Giant cells
  in adenocarcinoma, periampullary, 274
  in effusions, 341
  in herpes pneumonia, 201
  in measles virus pneumonia, 202, 203f
  syncytiotrophoblast, 94, 97f
Giardia lamblia infection, duodenal, 272, 273f
Glandular cells, atypical, 184, 185f
  in urothelial lesions, 304
Glandular structures, in hepatocellular carcinoma, 297
Glial cells, intermediate filaments in, 408t
Glial fibril(s), 365
Glial fibrillary acidic protein (GFAP), 354, 358
  in immunocytochemistry, 413, 414
  tumors coexpressing, 409t
Glioblastoma multiforme, 365
Glioma, 363, 365, 366f–371f
  distinguished from pituitary adenoma, 419
Glycogen-rich cystadenoma, pancreatic, 289
Glycoproteins, in pancreatic cancer, 428
Goblet cells
  hyperplasia, 184
  nonciliated, respiratory tract, 184, 185f
Gonads, neoplasms, hormone-producing, 420
Gonorrheal vulvitis, 49
Granular cell tumors, bile duct, 274
Granulation, in medullary carcinoma, of thyroid gland, 242, 244f
Granulocytic sarcoma, cytology of, 398, 399f
Granuloma
  in cryptococcosis, 191, 193
  inguinale, 30f, 31, 49
  lung, sarcoidosis, 188
Granulomatous conditions, 188
  in lung, fungi causing, 188, 189–194
  in lymph node, fine needle aspiration of, 385, 385f
Granulomatous prostatitis, 326, 329f
Granulosa-theca cell tumors, 420
Granulocytic sarcoma, 387
Grave's disease, 235, 237
Ground-glass nuclei, in herpes simplex virus, 55, 56f
Gupta bodies, 31

Gupta lesions, 31
Gynecomastia, fine needle aspiration of, 172

H&E, *See* Hematoxylin and eosin stain
Hamman-Rich syndrome, 184
Hazardous chemicals, handling of, 20
Head
  squamous carcinoma, 211
  trauma, neonatal, choroid plexus cells in, 363f
Hemangioendothelioma, epithelioid sclerosing, of liver, 301
Hematoxylin, 405
Hematoxylin and eosin (H&E) stain, 163, 164
  in effusions, 358
  in pancreatic disease, 281
Hemosiderin pigment, 292, 294
Hepatitis, acute, diagnosis, 293
Hepatocellular carcinoma, diagnosis, 293, 294f, 294, 296–299
  markers for, 427, 428f
  sclerosing, 297
Hepatocytes
  in cirrhosis, 293, 294f
  in hepatocellular carcinoma, 296, 296f
  smear of, 292, 292f
Herpes genitalis, 49
Herpes simplex virus infection, of female genital tract, 37, 38f
  uterine cervix, 55, 56f
Herpes virus infection
  immunocytochemistry application to, 406, 406t, 406f, 407
  Type I, respiratory, 200–201
HHF-35, 414
High molecular weight (HMWK) keratin antibodies, 410, 411, 440
Histiocytes
  benign, 8f, 9
    distinguished from tumor cells, 214, 216
  during menstruation, 88, 91f, 92
  epithelioid, 385
  in lymphoma, 388, 389, 437
  post-irradiation, 150, 151
Histiocytic lymphoma, classification of, 382t, 382
Histiocytosis, cerebral, 362f
Histogram, DNA, 445
Histoplasma
  capsulatum, 189
  differentiated from cryptococcus, 193
  lung inflammation from, 188, 189t
Histoplasmosis, lung, 189, 190, 190f
History
  in fine needle aspiration, 295

in central nervous system cytology, 357–358
  in fine needle aspiration, 295
  incomplete, 1
HMB-45, 430, 441
Hobnail cells, 49
Hodgkin's disease, 386
  classification of, 434
  cytology of, 393, 396–398
  lymphocyte depleted, 396
  lymphocyte-predominant, 396
  mixed cellularity, 396
  nodular sclerosing, 396, 397f
Honeycomb exudate, 197, 198f
Hormonal patterns, abnormal, 27–28
Hormonal therapy, prostatic cancer response to, 333t, 333
Hormonal values, maturation index, 27t
Hormones
  in islet cell neoplasms, 287, 411, 420
Host response, radiation changes in, 149, 150
β-Human chorionic gonadotropin (BhCG), 415, 416
Human milk fat globule (HMFG), 417
Human papillomavirus (HPV) infection, 307
  of female genital tract, 37, 40, 41f–44f
  of uterine cervix, 61, 64–65
  immunocytochemistry application, 407–409
Hürthle cell, 236
  nodules, 247
  in thyroiditis, 244, 245f, 246f, 247
  tumors, 246–247, 247f
Hypercalcemia, 296
Hyperchromasia, 61
Hyperkeratosis, 72
  of uterine cervix, 57
Hypocellular specimens, 403

ID3, 425
ID5, 425
Immigration, neutrophilic, 144f, 145f, 146
Immunoblast(s), in lymphoma, 387
Immunoblastic lymphoma, gastric, 271
Immunoblastic reactions, in lymphoma, 392, 392f, 393
Immunoblastic sarcoma
  B-cell, 393, 394f
  T-cell, 393, 395f, 396f
Immunocompromised patient
  pneumocystis in, 197
  viral infections in, 199
Immunocytochemical panel, 427
Immunocytochemistry
  application to cytologic specimen, 18, 403–405

Immunocytochemistry (*Continued*)
  in cervical dysplasia and carcinoma in situ, 64
  cytoskeletal determinants of cell shape, 408, 408t
  in effusions, 354
  indicators of histogenesis and differentiation, 414–424
  infections, 406–408
  intermediate filaments, *See* Intermediate filaments
  lymphohistiocytic markers, 433–438
  mesenchymal neoplasms, 438–439, 440f
  metastatic workup, 441–445
  neuroendocrine markers, 430–433
  nucleus and markers of malignant transformation, 445
  organ-specific markers, 424–430, 431f, 432f, 433f
  poorly differentiated neoplasms, 440–445
  technical aspects, 403–405
Immunoelectron microscopy, of epithelial membrane antigen, 417
Immunoenzymatic method, 404
Immunogold technique, 405
Immunohistochemical evaluation, in hepatocellular carcinoma, 298
Immunoperoxidase studies, in pancreatic duct carcinoma, 285
Indian-file arrangements, in carcinoma, mammary, 118
Infarction, pulmonary, 342
Infection
  esophageal, 262
  gastric, 269
  immunocytochemistry application to, 406–408
Infectious agents, 2
Infectious diseases
  respiratory tract, *See* Respiratory diseases
  of uterine cervix, 53–57, 57f
Infectious specimens, handling of, 20
Inflammation
  breast, 173
  in squamous cell carcinoma, cervical, 81, 81f
Inflammatory bowel disease, idiopathic, 275
Inflammatory conditions
  in cerebrospinal fluid, 359t
  in effusions, 349
Inflammatory mass lesions, of liver, 301, 301f
Inflammatory process, in effusions, 341
Influenza virus, pneumonia from, 204

Intercellular spaces, 9
Intermediate cells
  multinucleated, from radiation, 143f, 144f
  in small cell carcinoma, 219
Intermediate filaments, 408–409
  cytoskeletal components, 414
  glial fibrillary acidic protein, 413, 414
  neurofilament, 412–413
  tumors coexpressing, 409t
  vimentin, 411–412
Intestines
  metaplastic cells, 268, 269
  methotrexate effects on, 160
  radiation effects on, 158
Intranuclear inclusions, in adenovirus pneumonia, 203
Intraparotid lymphoid hyperplasia, 253
Intrauterine devices (IUD)
  Actinomyces infection from, 31
  endometrial cell shedding and, 92, 93f
Invasive procedures, for central nervous system studies, 357
Iodine-233 (^{233}I), 234
Irrigation smears
  female genital tract, 24
  in urothelial cytology, 323
Islet cell, 282
  hormones, production in, 287, 420
  tumors, 281, 286, 287–288, 420
    metastasis to liver, 300
    stained for gastrin, 431f

Karyopyknosis, 147
Karyopyknotic vaginal smears, 49
Keratin, 285, 412
  cells positive for, 424
  in hepatocellular carcinoma, 298
  in immunocytochemistry, 409–411
  in mesenchymal neoplasms, 438, 438t
  in poorly differentiated neoplasms, 440
  stain specific for, 164
  tumors coexpressing, 409t
Keratinaceous material, in adenocarcinoma, endometrial, 109, 110f
Keratinization, excessive, 53
Keratinizing squamous cell carcinoma, of cervix, 75, 76f
Keratinizing dysplasia
  cervical, 65, 70, 72f, 72
  in small cell carcinoma, cervical, 81
  of uterine cervix, 61, 63f
Keratinizing squamous cell carcinoma, of uterine cervix, cytologic manifestations of, 77, 78f
Ki-67 antibody, 445
Kidney, 304
  tumors, 304, 319–320

adenocarcinoma, metastasis to liver, 300
Kiel classification, of lymphoma, 382t
Koilocytes, 55, 307
  in human papillomavirus, 407f, 408
Koilocytosis, 61, 64
Kulchitsky cell, 219
Kuppfer cell, nuclei, 292

L-26, 435, 438
Laboratory, organization of, 19–20
Lactalbumin, 426
  in breast carcinoma, 426
  in metastatic workup, 442
Lactation, breast in, 170, 171–172
Laminin, 428
Large cell carcinoma
  anaplastic, of thyroid gland, 242
  undifferentiated, of lung, 221, 223f
Large cell malignant lymphoma, 391, 392–393, 394f
Large cell tumors, immunocytochemistry for, 440
Large cleaved follicular center cell lymphoma, 391, 391f
Large noncleaved follicular center cell lymphoma, 391, 392–393, 394f
Lateral vaginal wall, smear, 25
Lavage technique
  saline, 275
  stomach specimen collection by, 267
Leiomyosarcoma
  endometrial, 113, 113f
  gastric, 271, 272f
  metastasis to liver, 301
Lennert's lymphoma, 387
Leptothrix bacteria, 40, 45f–46f, 47
  in trichomonal infection, 55, 55f
Leu 7, 431
Leu M_1, 421, 438
  in adenocarcinoma differentiation, 443, 445
Leukemia
  acute lymphocytic, 387
  cells of, in effusions, 349
  central nervous system involvement in, 373f, 376–377, 387
  chronic lymphocytic, 388, 388f
  chronic myelogenous, 387
  lung involvement in, 225, 226f
Leukocyte(s)
  in effusions, 354
Leukocyte common antigen (LCA), 358, 412
Leukocytic invasion, post-irradiation, 144f, 145f, 146, 147
Leukoplakia 53, *See also* Hyperkeratosis

Leukorrhea, infections, of vagina, 47
Leydig cell, 420
Lillie-Mayer hematoxylin, 405
Lipase, levels, in acinar cell carcinoma, pancreatic, 280
Lipofuscin granules, 332
Lipofuscin pigment, 234
Lipoma, salivary gland, 252
Lithiasis, 317
Liver
    fine needle aspiration of, 291–292,
        diffuse liver disease, diagnosis, 293–294
        inflammatory mass lesions, 301, 301f
        mass lesion diagnosis, 294–296, 299–300
        metastatic neoplasms, 300–301
        normal cytology of, 292, 292f
        overview of pathology, 292, 293
        problems in, 295–296
    tumor markers in, 427, 428f
Liver cell, pigments, 292
LN-1, in lymphoma, 435
LN-2, in lymphoma, 435
Lobular acinar units, 252
Lobular carcinoma, of breast, fine needle aspiration of, 177
Low molecular weight keratin (LMWK) antibody, 410, 411
    monoclonal, 440
Lower respiratory tract, radiation effects on, 157
Lukes-Collins, classification of lymphoma, 382, 382t
Lung
    cellular components of, 181
    granulomatous inflammation in, fungi causing, 188, 189–194
    neoplasms, 204–205, 225
        adenocarcinoma, 127, 128f, 211, 212–219
        bronchioalveolar carcinoma, tumor markers in, 416, 426–427
        classification of, 205–206
        carcinoid tumors, 224–225
        diagnostic tests for, 205, 205t
        large cell undifferentiated carcinoma, 221, 223f
        lymphomas and leukemia, 225, 226f
        metastatic carcinoma, 225
        miscellaneous and rare, 225, 226f
        precursors of, 413
        small cell carcinoma, 219–221
        squamous (epidermoid) carcinoma, 206–211
    tumor markers in, 415, 426–427
    viral infections, 199–204
Lupus serositis, 341
Lymph nodes, fine needle aspiration of, 379–380
    differential diagnosis in, 383–386
    indications for, 379, 379t
    lymphoma classification, 381–383
    in patients at risk for AIDS, 398
Lymphocyte(s)
    abnormal populations of, 386
    in effusion, 353, 354
    lymphomas containing, 387–389
    salivary gland lesions containing, 253
    in Warthin's tumor of salivary gland, 255
Lymphocyte-depleted Hodgkin's disease, 396
Lymphocyte-like cells, in small cell carcinoma, 219
Lymphocyte-predominant Hodgkin's disease, 396
Lymphoglandular bodies, 2, 3f, 175, 382, 384f, 385
Lymphogranuloma venereum, 49
Lymphohistiocytic markers, 422, 433–438
Lymphoid cells
    in cerebrospinal fluid, cytomorphology of, 366t
    in thyroiditis, 244
Lymphoid hyperplasia
    intraparotid, 253
    reactive, fine needle aspiration in, 386f, 386
Lymphoid stroma, in thyroiditis, 244
Lymphoma
    breast, 174, 175
    central nervous system involvement in, 376f, 376–377
    classification, 381–383
    cytology, 380–381
        of granulocytic sarcoma, 398, 399f
        of Hodgkin's disease, 393, 396–398
        of large cell lymphoma, 391, 392–393, 394f
        of large cleaved follicular center cell lymphoma, 391, 391f
        of lymphoma of small lymphocytic cells, 387–389
        of malignant lymphoma-lymphoblastic, 398, 399f
        of small cleaved follicular center cell lymphoma, 389, 389f
        of small noncleaved follicular center cell lymphoma, 389,
    diagnosis of, 387
    in effusions, 349, 350f
    gastric, 271, 271f
    of lung, 224, 226f
    lymphohistiocytic markers in, 433–438
    metastasis to liver, 301
    secretory markers in, 422
Macronucleoli, in squamous cell carcinoma, cervical, 77
Macrophages, 389
    in cerebrospinal fluid, 359t
    in effusions, 339–341, 342
    in fibrocystic change, 166
    in lymphoma, 392
Magnetic resonance imaging (MRI), in central nervous system studies, 357, 358
Magnification, for slide screening, 2
Malignancy
    cytologic criteria of, 9–16
    nuclear criteria of, 10–12
Malignant cells
    exfoliation of, 101
    radiation effect on, 149, 150
Malignant transformation, nucleus and markers of, 445
Mammary carcinoma, 118, 120f–123f
Mammary dysplasia, fine needle aspiration of. See fibrocystic change, of breast
Masson's trichrome stain, 439
Mast cells, in Warthin's tumor of salivary gland, 255, 256f
Mastitis, 173
Maturation index, 27, 27t
May-Grünwald-Giemsa (MGG) stain
    in lymph node studies, 379
    in pancreatic disease, 281
    for prostatic cytopathology, 333
    in thyroid hyperfunction, 333
Measles virus pneumonia, 202, 203f
Medullary carcinoma
    of breast, fine needle aspiration of, 177, 177f
    of thyroid gland, 233, 241, 242, 243f, 244f
Medulloblastoma, 363, 369f, 371, 372f
Melanoma
    breast, 174
    of lung, 225, 227f
    metastasis
        to brain, 372, 375f, 376
        in effusions, 352f
        to liver, 300
    organ markers in, 428–430
    of vulva, 53
Melphalan, cytopathology of, 159
Meningioma
    brain, 372, 374f
    in cerebrospinal fluid, 359

Meningitis, 359, 361f
  in neonate, 363
Menstruation
  endometrial cells during, 87–88
  endometrial changes during, 88–91f, 92
Merkel cell tumor, 411, 413
Mesenchymal cells
  differentiation of, 414
  intermediate filaments in, 408t
Mesenchymal neoplasms, immunocytochemistry in, 438–439, 440f
Mesothelial cells
  benign, 9
  body cavity, 337, 338t
  in body fluid, 338f, 339, 341
  in effusions, diagnosis, 352
  normal, 5, 8f, 9
  shedding of, 346
Mesothelioma
  differentiated from
    adenocarcinoma, 443
    carcinoma, 417
  in effusions, 342–345, 345f
    versus, metastatic carcinoma, 354
  epithelial, 342
  fibrous, 342, 343
  keratin expression in, 411
Metaplastic cells, intestinal, 268–269
Metaplastic dysplasia, uterine cervix, 61, 62f
Metaplastic-type cells, in human papillomavirus, 40, 43f
Metastatic tumors
  in effusions, 345, 346–349
    mesothelioma versus, 354
  endometrial, 113, 114f
  in effusions, 351, 352f
  liver, 294
Metastatic workup, in immunocytochemistry, 441–445
Methotrexate, cytopathology of, 142f, 160
Methyl green pyronin (MGP), 18
Microcysts, pancreatic, 289
Microfilaments, 414
  antibody to, 405
Microfilariae, 47
Microtubules, 414
Microvilli, in effusions, 345, 345f
Milk fat globule, 358
  human, 417
Mitomycin, mitomycin C, 318
  cytopathology, 160
Mitosis
  abnormal, 61
  cells in, 405, 405f
Mitotic figures, abnormal, 61
Molluscum contagiosum, in female
    genital tract, 40, 44f, 49
Monoclonal antibodies
  in *Chlamydia trachomatis* infection, 35f, 37
  in Hodgkin's disease, 398
  against intermediate filaments, 408, 409
  against keratin, 410
  in lymphoma, 434, 435
Monocyte, central nervous system, 361f
Monomorphic adenoma, of salivary gland, 254, 255
Mouth, squamous cells from, benign, 182
Mucicarmine stain, 18, 405
  in adenocarcinoma, 421, 423f
Mucin
  in adenocarcinoma, 344
  extracellular accumulation of, in colon carcinoma, 118, 125f
  intracytoplasmic, 269, 270f
  in mesothelioma, 344
  production, 18
Mucinous cystic neoplasms, pancreatic, 281, 288–289
Mucocele, of breast, fine needle aspiration of, 176, 177
Mucoepidermoid carcinoma, of salivary gland, 258, 259, 260f
Mucormycosis (phycomycosis) pneumonia, 196
Mucus, in colloid cancer of breast, 176
Müllerian tumors, malignant, endometrial, 109, 111f, 113
Multinucleation
  in cytomegalovirus, 37
  in herpes simplex virus, 37, 55
  post-irradiation, 145f–146f, 147, 148f
Muscle tumors, in effusions, 354
Muscular cells, intermediate filaments in, 408t
Mycelia, in aspergillosis, 195
Mycetoma, 196
  in squamous cell carcinoma, 210t, 210
Myeloma, effusion associated with, 349, 350f, 351
Myleran, *See* Busulfan
Myogenous cells, contractile proteins in, 414
Myoglobin, in mesenchymal tumors, 439
Myosin, skeletal muscle, 439

National Cancer Institute, grading of lymphomas, 380, 381t
Neck, squamous carcinoma, 211
Neisseria gonorrhoeae, 28

Neonate
  head trauma, choroid plexus cells in, 363f
  meningitis, in, 363
Neural crest, tumors, 365t, 369f, 371, 372f, 373f
Neuroblastoma, 386
  neuroendocrine markers for, 433
Neuroendocrine differentiation, markers for, 430–433
  in islet cell neoplasms, 287
Neuroendocrine tumors
  site of origin of, 433t
  carcinoma, small cell, undifferentiated, esophageal, 266
  site of origin of, 433t
Neurofilament (NF), 412–413, 430t, 431
  tumors coexpressing, 409t
Neuron-specific enolase (NSE), 413
Neuronal cells, intermediate filaments in, 408t
Neutrophils, fecal, 275
Nipple
  Paget's disease of, versus benign papilloma, 169–170
  secretions, 173
Nocardiosis, respiratory tract, 196–197
Nodular sclerosing Hodgkin's disease, 396, 397f
Non-Hodgkin's lymphoma
  classification of, 382, 382t
  diagnostic criteria for, 385t, 385, 386
  grading of, 380, 381t
  salivary gland, 253
Normal cells, cytology of, 5–9
NSE, 430t, 431, 432f
Nuclear criteria, of malignancy, 10–12
Nuclear envelopes, in cervical dysplasia and carcinoma in situ, 70, 71f
Nuclear folds and clefts, in lymphoma, 389, 389f
Nuclear membrane, wrinkling of, 147
Nuclear molding, in herpes simplex virus, 55, 56f
Nucleoli
  in adenocarcinoma, endometrial, 103
  in carcinoma
    mammary, 118, 119f
    ovarian, 116
    small cell, cervical, 80f, 81
    squamous, 74f, 75, 206, 207
Nucleus, nuclei
  adenocarcinoma, endocervical, 82, 83f, 85
  in carcinoma, mammary, 118
  in cervical dysplasia and carcinoma in situ, 65, 66, 70, 71f

changes, from radiation, 143f, 145f–146f, 147, 148f
  in malignant transformation, 445
  naked, breast, 166f, 166
    in fibroadenoma of breast, 168, 168f, 169
  pyknotic, in squamous cell carcinoma, 77, 78f
  size, estimating of, 5

Oat cell carcinoma, 376
  markers for, 431, 433
  neurofilaments in, 413
OC-125, 425
OCP-125, 422
Oligodendroglioma, brain, 365, 370f, 371, 371f, 312
Oncocytes, in Warthin's tumor of salivary gland, 255
Oncocytoma, of salivary gland, 255, 257f, 258
Oncofetal markers, 415–416
Oral cavity, radiation effects on, 157
Organ-specific markers, 424–430, 431f, 432f, 433f
Ovarian carcinoma cells, 49
Ovary
  serosal inclusion cyst, psammoma bodies in, 129, 130f
  tumor, 116, 117f–118f, 119f
    cystadenocarcinoma, 132
    tumor markers in, 425, 426f
Oxyphilic cell, 236

Paget's disease, of nipple, versus benign papilloma, 169–170
Palpable masses, fine needle aspiration of, 18
Pancervical specimen, 24
Pancreas
  fine needle aspiration of, 279–280
    acinar cell carcinoma, 286, 286f
    classification of neoplasms, 280, 280t
    cystic masses, 288–289
    ductal carcinoma, 283–385f
    islet cell neoplasms, 286, 287–288
    of normal pancreas, 282, 282f
    pancreatitis, chronic, 282, 283
    overview of pathology, 280–281
    types of cytologic samples, 281–282
  radiation effects on, 158
  tumor markers in, 428
Pancreatic duct
  adenocarcinoma, 280

  aspirates, 282
  carcinoma, 283–285f
Pancreatic juice, aspirate of, 281
Pancreatic specific antigen (CA-1), 422
Pancreatitis, 272, 273
  chronic, 281, 282, 283
Papanicolaou stain, 18, 19t, 163, 164
  for prostatic cytology, 333
Papillary cancer
  breast, 177, 178
  of lung, 214, 214f
  of thyroid gland, 233, 238–241, 241f, 242, 242f, 243f, 246
Papillary formations, in effusions, 346–349
Papillary tumors, of bladder, grading of, 307, 307t
Papilloma
  of breast
    fine needle aspiration of, 170, 170f
    of nipple, Paget's disease versus, 169–170
  of choroid plexus, 365
Papillomavirus, human, See Human papillomavirus
Parabasal cells, 58
Paracentesis, 337
Paracoccidioides brasiliensis, 204
Paragonimus westermanii, 204
Parakeratosis, 72
  pleomorphic, 77, 78f
  of uterine cervix, 57
Parakeratitic changes, in human papillomavirus infection, 40, 42f
Paranuclear vacuole, from radiation, 144
Parasitic agents, in female genital tract, 28t, 40, 44f–47
Parasitosis, vaginal, 47
Parathyroid hormone, 420
Parathyroid tumors, hormone secretion in, 420
Paraurethral glands, lesions, 304
Parenchyma, involvement in herpes virus infection, 200
Parietal cells, gastric, 266
Peau d'orange, 173
Pelvis, 304
Pemphigus vulgaris, 263
Periampullary adenocarcinoma, 273, 274, 274f
Pericardial cavity, 337
Pericardiocentesis, 337
Perinuclear halo, 40, 42f
Peritoneal cavity, 337
  fluid in, 337
Peroxidase-antiperoxidase (PAP) technique, 404, 404t, 405
Phagocytes, in multinodular thyroid, 235, 236f, 236

Phagocytosis, post-irradiation, 146, 149
Pheochromocytoma, 419
Phycomycosis, See Mucormycosis
Phylloides sarcoma, of breast, 178
Pineal area, germinoma of, 371, 373f
Pinealoma, 371, 373f
Pinocytic vesicles, 414
Pituitary gland
  adenoma, 419
  tumors, hormones produced by, 419, 420
Plant cells, 183
Plasma, 404
Plasmacytic differentiation, 414
Plasmacytoid lymphocytic lymphoma (immunocytoma), 389
Plasmacytosis, immunocytochemistry for, 435, 436f
Pleocytosis, reactive, 362f
Pleomorphic dysplasia, uterine cervix, 61
Pleomorphic neoplasms
  adenoma, of salivary gland, 252, 253–254, 254f, 255f
  differentiation of, 441
Pleomorphism
  in adenocarcinoma, endometrial, 103
  in islet cell neoplasms, 287
  in squamous cell carcinoma, esophageal, 265f, 265
Pleomorphic spindle cells, endometrial, 109, 112f, 113
Pleural cavity, 337
Pleural effusion, causes, 342
Pneumocystis
  carinii, 2, 197
  respiratory tract, 197–199
Pneumocytes
  respiratory tract, 185, 186
  Type I, 185
  Type II, 186
Pneumonia
  fungal, invasive, 194–196
  necrotizing acute, 197
  progression of, 193
  viral, 199–204
Pneumonic process, 188
  in adenocarcinoma of lung, 216, 216f
Pneumothorax, 337
"Poly ball," 151f
Polykaryocytes, in measles virus pneumonia, 202
Polymorphonuclear leukocytes
  squamous cell and post-irradiation, 144f, 145f, 146, 147
  in Trichomonas vaginalis, 40, 45f
Polymorphous cell population, in lymphoma, 434
Polyoma virus, 307

Polyps, endometrial, benign, 94, 98f
Pregnancy
    breast in, 170, 171–172
    endometrial cell shedding during, 92, 94, 95f–97f
Prostate gland
    adenocarcinoma, metastasis to bladder, 320f–321f
    carcinoma, metastatic, in effusions, 349
    fine needle aspiration of, 323, 324
        of adenocarcinoma, 326, 328f–332
        of atypical hyperplasia, 326
        of benign prostatic hyperplasia, 324–326, 327f
        of carcinoma, unusual types of, 332, 333, 333t
        complications, 334
        diagnostic accuracy, 334, 334t
        diagnostic pitfalls, 332, 332t
        of granulomatous prostatitis, 326, 329f
        histologic grading, 323–324, 324t
        of neoplasms, microscopic features of, 325t
        of prostatitis, 326, 328
        radiotherapy response, 333, 334
        response to hormonal therapy, 333t, 333
        stains, 333
        technical aspects, 323
    tumor markers in, 424
Prostate-specific antigen (PSA), 424
Prostatic-specific acid phosphatase (PSAP), 424
Prostatitis, 326, 328
    granulomatous, 326, 329f
Psammoma bodies, 4f
    in adenocarcinoma, endocervical, 84, 86f
    in extrauterine cancer, 129–133
    in papillary carcinoma, of thyroid, 240, 241f
    in respiratory tract, 187
Pseudocyst, pancreatic, 288–289
Pseudoeosinphilia, 146
Pseudolymphoma, 271
Pulmonary infarction, effusions in, 342
"Pus balls," 149, 151f
Pyelogram, intravenous (IVP), 303
Pyknosis, nuclear, 58
    in squamous cell carcinoma, 77, 78f
Pyloric antrum, 266

Radiation
    acute reaction, 142–150f
    breast changes from, 172, 173
    esophageal changes from, 263

urothelial cellular atypia from, 319
"Radiation-persistent cancer," 157
Radiation reaction
    intermediate, 149, 151f
    in squamous cell carcinoma, 210t, 210
Radiation therapy
    cytopathology of, 141
        cell membrane changes, 144f, 147
        cell size and shape changes, 147, 148, 148f, 150f
        of cervicovaginal mucosa, 142, 143–146
        chronic (late, persistent) changes, 149
        dysplasia, 152f, 153f, 153–157
        endometrium and endocervix changes, 150
        extragenital tissue effects, 157–158
        host response, 149, 150
        intermediate radiation reaction, 149, 151f
        nuclear changes, 145, 146f, 147–150f
        smear appearance, 150, 151, 153
        smear background effects, 149, 150f, 151f
    prostatic cancer response to, 333, 334
    to uterine cervix, 58
Reactive atypia, distinguished from periampullary adenocarcinoma, 273, 274
Reactive conditions, in cerebrospinal fluid, 359t
Reactive process, in adenocarcinoma of lung, 216, 216f
Rectal mucosa, 332, 332t
Red blood cells (RBC), 5
    hemolyzation of, 16
Reed-Sternberg cell, in lymphoma
    in Hodgkin's disease, 393, 396, 397f, 398
    identification of, 438
Reflux esophagitis, 262, 263f
REG-53 antibodies, 410
Renal cell carcinoma, diagnosis, 319–320
Renal pelvis, urothelial lesions of, 303, See also Urothelial lesions
"Repair" cells, respiratory tract, 182–183
Reserve cells
    hyperplasia, 186f
    respiratory tract, 185, 186f
Respiratory diseases, cytologic diagnosis of, 181, See also Lung, Pneumonia
    cell changes currently not associated with neoplasia, 181–186
    infectious diseases, 187, 188

    sarcoidosis, 188, 189f
    tuberculosis, 188
Respiratory syncytial virus, 203–204
Rhabdomyoblasts, in Müllerian tumor, endometrial, 113
Rhabdomyosarcoma, differentiation, 439
RNA, staining of, 18
Romanowsky-stained smear, in fibroadenoma of breast, 167
Rosettes, 158, 365
Round cell tumors, blue small
    differential diagnosis, 413, 413t
    neuroendocrine differentiation, 430

S100, 412
Saline lavage, 275
Salivary glands, cytology of, 251–252
    benign lesions, 252–253, 253f, 254f
    masses, 252
    normal appearance on FNA biopsy, 252, 253f
    tumors
        adenoid cystic carcinoma, 258–259
        adenocarcinoma, 259
        acinic cell carcinoma, 255, 257f, 258
        monomorphic adenoma, 254, 255
        mucoepidermoid cancer, 259, 260f
        oncocytoma, 255, 257f
        pleomorphic adenoma, 253–254, 254f, 255f
        Warthin's tumor, 255, 256f
Sarcoidosis, salivary gland, 253
Sarcoma, 438
    Ewing's, 387, 440
    granulocytic, 387, 398, 399f
    immunoblastic
        B-cell, 393, 394f
        T-cell, 393, 395f, 396f
    lung, 225, 227f
    metastasis to liver, 300–301
    phylloides, of breast, 178
    stromal, endometrial, 109, 112f, 113
    vimentin expression in, 411
Scar adenocarcinoma, 184
Scintigraphy, in thyroid carcinoma, 234
Secretory markers, differentiation by, 421–424
Secretory piece, 421
Seminal vesicle cells, 332, 332t
Seminoma, 225
Sensitization response (SR), 145
Serotonin, 420
Serous cavities, radiation effects on, 158
Serous papillary carcinoma, endometrial, 103, 103f, 104f
Sertoli-Leydig cell, 420
Sialadenitis, 252, 253
Sialosis, 252

Signet ring configuration, in adenocarcinoma, 11, 15f
Sjögren's syndrome, 253
Slide, screening of, 2
Small blue round cell tumors, neuroendocrine differentiation, 430
Small cell neoplasms, central nervous system, 360f
Small cell carcinoma
  anaplastic (undifferentiated), of lung, 219–221, 222t
  anaplastic, of thyroid gland, 244
  of lung, 219–221, 222t
  metastatic, in effusions, 346
  neurofilaments in, 413
  undifferentiated (neuroendocrine)
    esophageal, 266
    metastasis to liver, 300
  of uterine cervix, cytologic manifestations of, 80f, 81
Small cleaved follicular center cell lymphoma, 389, 389f
Small noncleaved follicular center cell lymphoma, 389, 390f, 391
Smear
  appearance, post-irradiation, 150, 151, 153
  aspirate, preparation of, 18
  background of, 2
    in extrauterine cancer, 117f–118f, 120f–124f, 128f, 129f, 129, 130
  direct, 17
  female genital tract, unsatisfactory, 24
  radiation effects on, 149, 150f, 151f
  rapid fixation of, 16, 17
Smooth muscle actin (SMA), 414
"Smudge cells," 203
Southern blot, 40
Specimens
  limitations in, 1, 2
  origins of, 1, 2t
  problems in, 405
Spherules, coccidioidomycosis, 191
Spiderlike cells, post-irradiation, 149
Spindle cells(s), 9
  in adenocarcinoma, periampullary, 274
  malignant, 14
  pleomorphic, 109, 112f, 113
Spindle cell sarcoma, differentiation, 441
Splendore-Hoeppli phenomenon type tissue reaction, 31
Sputum, specimens, 17
Squamous cell(s)
  in adenocarcinoma, endometrial, 109, 110f
  benign, in respiratory tract, 182–183
  in candidiasis, 54f, 55

female genital tract, cytohormonal evaluation of, 25, 25f, 26f, 27
  in human papillomavirus infection, 40, 41f
  intermediate cells, 25
  post-irradiation, 155, 156f
    polymorphonuclear leukocyte and, 144f, 145f, 146, 147
  superficial, 25, 25f
    post-irradiation, 150
  in *Trichomonas vaginalis*, 40, 45f–46f, 55, 55f
Squamous cell carcinoma, 2
  in cerebrospinal fluid, 359
  cervical atrophic changes mimicking, 58
  classification of, cytoplasmic features for, 11, 14f
  diagnostic pitfalls associated with, 210t, 210–211
  distinguished from adenocarcinoma, 209t
  esophageal, 211, 263, 264–266
  of head and neck, 211
  keratin expression in, 410
  lung, 191f, 216, 216f, 260–261
    metastatic, 225
  metastasis to liver, 300
  metastatic, in effusions, 346
  metastatic workup, 445
  urothelial, 319–320
  uterine, 129
  of uterine cervix, 54
    cytologic manifestations of, 75–81
    differential diagnosis of, 81–82
    microinvasive, 72, 73, 74f–75
    recurrence, post-irradiation, 155f, 156f
  of vagina, 49
  of vulva, 53
Squamous epithelium
  development, disordered, 61
  in urothelial lesions, 304
Squamous metaplasia
  post-irradiation, 157
  respiratory tract, 183, 183f
  of uterine cervix, 57, 58f
    atypical, 57, 58
Staining characteristics, radiation effects on, 146
"Starry sky" background, 389
Steroids
  liver neoplasms and, 297
  mucormycosis from, 196
  squamous cell response to, 25
  use, history of, 295
Stomach
  cytology of
    of neoplastic lesions, 266, 269–272f

of non-neoplastic lesions, 267, 268f–269
normal, 266, 267f
specimen collection, 17, 266, 267
radiation effects on, 158
Stroma
  in adenoid cystic carcinoma of salivary gland, 258
  in fibroadenoma of breast, 168f, 168
  lymphoid, 244
  in pleomorphic adenoma, of salivary gland, 254, 254f
Stromal balls, in adenoid cystic carcinoma of salivary gland, 258
Stromal cells
  during menstruation, 88, 90f, 92
  shedding of, in pregnancy, 94
Stromal fragments, in fibrocystic change, 166
Stromal sarcoma, endometrial, 109, 112f, 113
Strongyloides stercoralis, 204
Subareolar abscess, fine needle aspiration of, 173
Sulfur granules, in *Actinomyces* infection, 31
Superimposition of neutrophils, 146
Surgery, radical, pancreatic, 279
Syncytiotrophoblastic giant cells, in pregnancy, 94, 97f

T-cell immunoblastic sarcoma, 393, 395f, 396f
T-cell lymphoma, 385, 387, 399f
  classification of, 382t, 382
  markers for, 433, 434
  morphology of, 391
"Tadpole" cells, 11
  in squamous carcinoma of lung, 206, 207f
TAG 72.3, 417
Technetium-99m (^{99m}Tc) pertechnetate, 234
Terminal bars, 65
Thiotepa (triethylemthiophosphoramide), 318
  cytopathology of, 160
Thoracentesis, 337
Thrombin, 404
Thymoma, lymphohistiocytic markers in, 437, 437f
Thyroglobulin (TGb), 419, 422, 424, 425
Thyroglossal duct, cysts, 247–249
Thyroid gland
  carcinoma, hormones produced by, 419, 419f

Thyroid gland (*Continued*)
  fine needle aspiration of, 233
    anaplastic carcinoma, 242, 244
    clinical uninodular thyroid, 236–238
    diagnostic tests for carcinoma, 234
    epidemiology of thyroid carcinoma, 233–234
    epithelial repair, 247
    flow chart, 248t
    follicular carcinoma, 238
    Hürthle cell tumors, 246–247, 247f
    hyperfunctional thyroid, 235
    medullary carcinoma, 241, 242, 243f, 244f
    multinodular thyroid, 235–236
    normal thyroid, 234–235
    papillary carcinoma, 238–241, 241f, 242f, 243f
    thyroglossal duct cysts, 247–249
    thyroiditis, 244–246
  tumor markers in, 424, 425
Thyroiditis
  chronic, 244–246, 247
  subacute, 246
Thyroxin (T_4), 248t
Tigroid-lace-like background, 2, 4f
Toluidine blue, 405
Touch imprints, 440, 441
Toxoplasmosis, 385
Trabecular formations, in islet cell neoplasms, 287
Tracheobronchitis, herpetic, 200
Transitional cell(s)
  atypia, urothelial, 306f
  exfoliation of, 5, 7f
Transitional cell carcinoma
  metastatic, in effusions, 346
  prostatic, 333, 333t
  urothelial, grading of, 307, 307t, 307f, 310f, 312f, 313f, 314f, 316f, 317f
Transitional epithelium, in urothelial lesions, 304–305
Transudates, 338, 339
Trichomonads, 55, 55f
Trichomonas, 407
  vaginalis, 40, 45–47
Trichophyton, female genital tract, 40
Triethylenethiophosphoramide, *See* Thiotepa
Triple smear method, *See* Cervical-vaginal-endocervical smear
Trophoblasts, in pregnancy, 94
Trophozoites, giardia, 272, 2733f
Tuberculous effusions, 341
Tubular carcinoma, breast, fine needle aspiration of, 177, 178f
Tumor cell
  differentiation, *See* Differentiation
  smears, suspended, 17

Tumor debris
  in squamous carcinoma, 206, 209f
Tumor diathesis, *See* Diathesis, tumor
Tumor markers
  CK1-CK4 antibodies, 410
  in malignant transformation, 445
  neuroendocrine, 430–433
  oncofetal, 415–416
  organ specific, 424–430, 431f, 432f, 433f
  RGE-53 antibodies, 410
  secretory, 421–424

UCHL, 438
UCHL-1, 435
Ulcer, gastric, 269
Ultrasonography, for thyroid carcinoma, 234
Umbrella cells, 305
Upper urinary tract, urothelial lesions in, *See* Urothelial lesions
Ureter, 304
  metastatic lesions to, 320
  urothelial lesions of, 303, *See also* Urothelial lesions
Urethra, lesions, 304
Urinary cytology, diagnostic yield of, 322
Urinary tract
  radiation effects on, 158
  regions of, 304
Urine
  collection, 17
  specimens from, 17
Urologic cytology
  prostate gland, *See* Prostate gland
  urothelial lesions, *See* Urothelial lesions
Urothelial atypia, 310f
Urothelial hyperplasia, 308f
  atypical, 308f, 309f, 311
Urothelial lesions, cytologic detection of, 303–304
  anatomic considerations, 304–305
  benign atypias, 305–307
  carcinoma in situ, 311, 315, 316f
  correlation with histology, 320, 333
  cytologic atypia, drug-induced, 317–319
  diagnostic yield of urinary cytology, 322
  grading of, 307, 307t
  high-grade lesions, 311, 312f
  ileal loop, 315, 317f, 317
  lithiasis, 317
  of low-grade tumors, 307, 308f–311
  radiation-induced cellular atypia, 319
  specimen collection and processing, 322–323

  unusual lesions, 319–320
Uterus
  adenocarcinoma, 129
  cervix, *See* Cervix, uterine
  squamous cell carcinoma, 129

Vacuoles
  in *Chlamydia trachomatis,* 35f
  from IUD, 92
  in liver cells, 292
  in lobular carcinoma of breast, 177
  in macrophages, 339
  post-irradiation, 154
Vacuolization, post-irradiation, 142, 143f–146, 147, 150
Vagina, cytology of, 47
  of benign tumors, 47–49
  malignant tumors, 49
Vaginal pool smears, 24, 25, 87
Vaginal smear, cytology, postradiotherapy, 151
Vaginal wall, scrapings, 28
Vaginopancervical (Fast) smear, 24
Varicella zoster virus pneumonia, 202
Vasopressin, 419, Oxytocin, 419
Vesicular nucleus, in trichomonas vaginalis, 46f, 47
Vimentin, 354, 438, 441
  in immunocytochemistry, 411–412
  in mesenchymal neoplasms, 438, 438t, 439
  in poorly differentiated tumors, 440
  tumors coexpressing, 409t
Viral antigen, 64
Viral esophagitis, 262
Viral infections
  female genital tract, 28t, 37–40, 41f–45f
  lung, 199–204
Virchow-Robin spaces, tumor cells in, 359
Vitamin B12, 269
Vulva, cytology of
  benign tumors, 53
  malignant tumors, 49, 51f–52f, 53
Vulvitis, gonorrheal, 49

Waldenström's macroglobulinemia, 389
Warthin's tumor, salivary gland, 255, 256f, 258
Warts
  genital, 61, 64
  human papillomavirus, 37
"Windows," mesothelial, 9
Wright's stain, 225

Yeast forms, of *Candida* organisms, 40f, 44f–45f